THE COMPLETE BOOK OF NATURAL
PREGNANCY
AND CHILDCARE

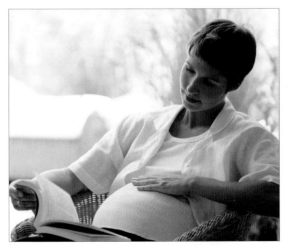

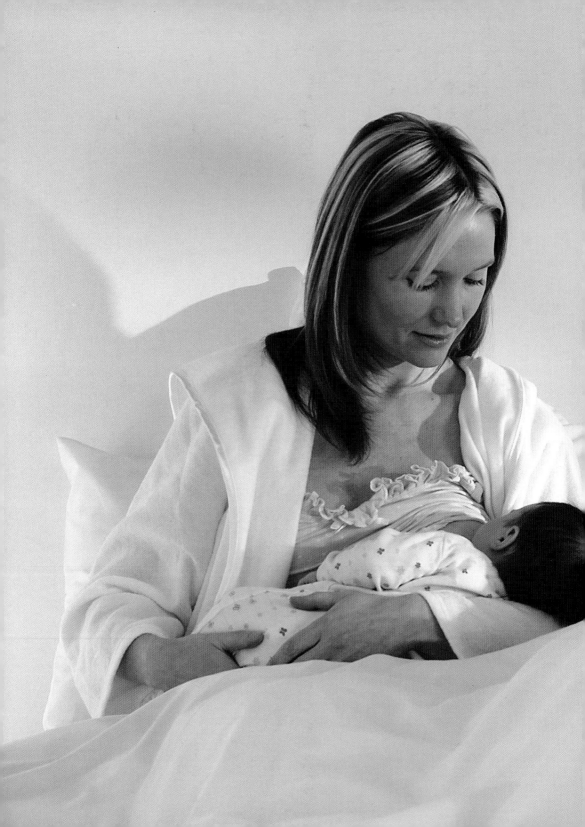

THE COMPLETE BOOK OF NATURAL
PREGNANCY
AND CHILDCARE

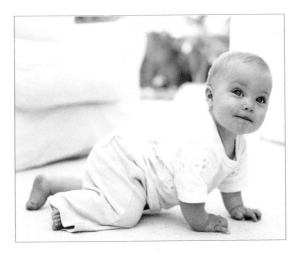

Conceiving, giving birth, and raising your
child the way nature intended, from birth
right through to age 5; an essential
companion for every parent and carer

Anne Charlish and Kim Davies

southwater

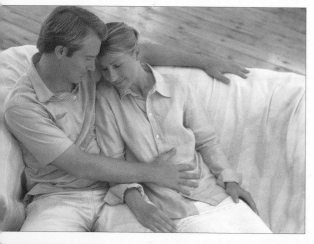

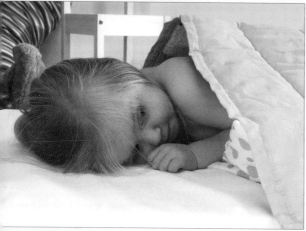

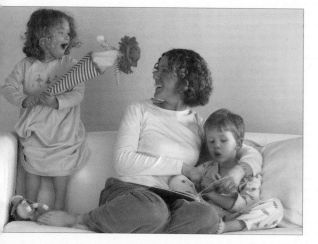

This edition is published by Southwater

Southwater is an imprint of Anness Publishing Ltd
108 Great Russell Street, London WC1B 3NA
www.annesspublishing.com; info@anness.com
twitter @Anness_Books

If you like the images in this book and would like to investigate using
them for publishing, promotions or advertising, please visit our website
www.practicalpictures.com for more information.

Publisher: Joanna Lorenz
Editorial Director: Helen Sudell
Executive Editor: Joanne Rippin
Designer: Nigel Partridge
Cover Design: Adelle Morris

PUBLISHER'S NOTE
The author and publishers have made every effort to ensure that all
instructions contained within this book are accurate and safe, and
cannot accept liability for any resulting injury, damage or loss to
persons or property, however it may arise. If you or your child do have
any special needs or problems, consult your doctor or another health
professional. This book cannot replace medical consultation and should
be used in conjunction with professional advice. Check the advisability
of any complementary therapies or remedies with your doctor before
using them.

contents

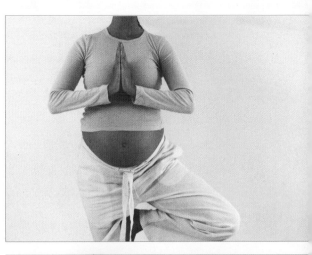
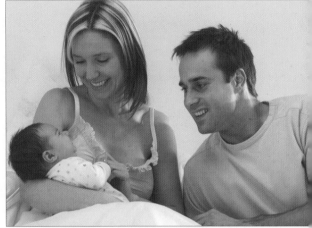
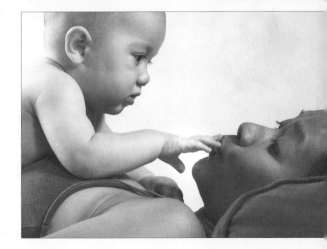

Introduction

There is nothing more natural than pregnancy and giving birth, and many parents would tell you that there is no life experience more rewarding. The sense of achievement that many women feel when they look back on childbirth is unlike any other – even if the birth turned out very differently than they expected – and many years after the event, most fathers can recall every detail of the moment they saw their child being born.

The gestation and birth of your child, however, is just the beginning of the journey of being a parent. Raising a son or daughter is a lifelong project, one that involves, over the course of the years, thousands of separate judgements and decisions that will affect the way your child grows up, and the kind of person he or she becomes. Those decisions, when repeated each year across the population, also have far-reaching effects on the world at large.

This book follows the progress of conception, birth, and caring for your baby from the first day up to pre-school age. The first section looks at how you can prepare for pregnancy through improving diet and well-being. It then takes you through each and every stage of this extraordinary life event, from the moment of conception, explaining what is happening to your body at every stage, and on to giving birth.

Advice and information is given on all the basic ways you will care for your new baby, and then as he or she grows, how to enjoy and manage each exciting new developmental stage. Throughout there are lots of ideas on healthy eating, play and stimulation, behaviour and cognitive development, at every age. A practical reference section at the end of the book gives advice on natural, ways to make your child's home environment a healthy, place, and a wealth of healthy eating ideas and recipes from first weaning solids to delicious, nutritious meals for the whole family to enjoy together.

The contents of this book are intended to help parents to make choices that are natural, responsibly ecological and soundly sensible. Childcare, like any other social activity, is subject to fashion – but this book is not a trendy guide to green parenthood, and has no ideological axe of its own to grind. The aim of the book is primarily to give parents the means to bring up their children in a way that does as little harm to the environment and the community as possible, but more importantly in a way that is also good for the child.

In practice, natural childcare is an amalgam of old practices (such as cooking real meals rather than using jars of processed babyfood) and of the best new thinking in paediatrics (such as the revelation that cold, fresh air is the best treatment for croup). There is nothing regressive about using time-honoured methods, nor is it a denial of

The nine months of pregnancy is the start of your life as a parent; in keeping yourself properly rested and eating healthily you are also beginning to care for your baby, giving him or her the best start in life.

Natural remedies can help you treat some of the common problems that pregnancy brings.

Your closeness, touch and communication are the most precious gifts you give your newborn.

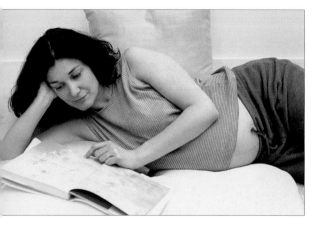

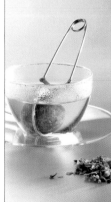

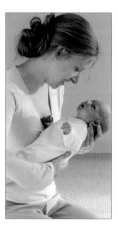

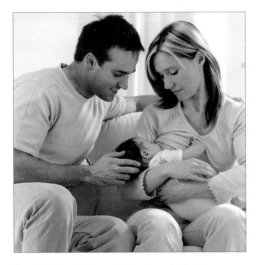

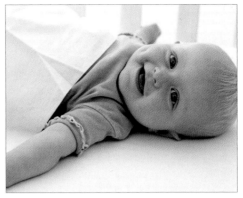

Parents have to make thousands of decisions when they bring up their children. But ultimately the most important thing is that the child feels loved and special.

Breastfeeding is the most natural way to feed your new baby, and there is plenty of support out there to help you get the hang of it, and continue.

modern technology. The much-stated claim, for example, that breastmilk is the best food for your baby is undeniable; but formula milk and other options are there if you cannot manage it at any point and for any reason. The business of using 'real' nappies is much easier in today's society than it was a generation ago: there are commercial laundry services, there are shaped washable nappies with poppers that are almost as easy to put on as disposables. All these nappy choices are better for the world and are also better for your baby's skin than the

bleached, indestructible, chemical-rich disposables that were once seen as a mother's best friend, and only option.

Any mother or father who aims to take a natural approach to childcare will find much guidance in these pages – but this is not a manual, and the advice contained in the book should not be seen as a blueprint. From the moment of birth, every child is an individual with a unique personality and set of circumstances, and every parent has an instinctive way of caring for their child. The most natural thing a mother or father can do is to rely on their growing knowledge of their own child's way of being, to learn from experience as much as possible, and above all to trust to instinct. Follow these principles, and you won't often go far wrong.

Protect your child from chemicals by using natural cleansers instead.

Every child has a unique personality that needs to be appreciated.

One of the best parts of looking after a toddler is seeing how their sense of fun develops, especially when they learn that they are amusing and entertaining you.

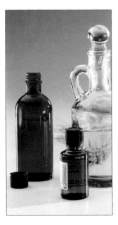

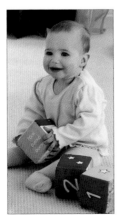

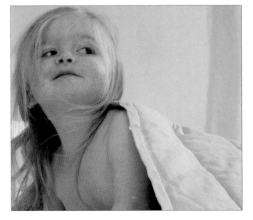

section one

fertility and conception

The desire to conceive is one of the most basic and powerful of human instincts, shared with all the living things on our planet. Once you have decided to embark upon this incredible journey, then a whole new world opens up to you. When you are trying to conceive, or boosting your fertility, gather as much information as you can, and maintain optimum physical well-being and a healthy mental outlook.

Preparing for pregnancy

❝ Enjoy all the new things that you will be discovering about yourself. **❞**

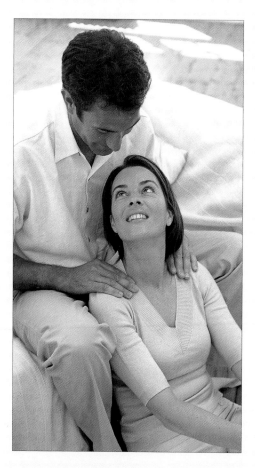

Having a child is a wonderful event, but of course it is also a life-changing one. The decision to try for a baby is one that no one else can take for you – only you know whether this is a course that you truly wish to embark on.

As you explore this exciting potential change in your life, consider both the emotional and practical issues. Think about the strength of the relationship with your partner, and discuss possible parenthood thoroughly with them. Weigh up your age, your current income and work prospects, your living arrangements and whether there is sufficient space for a baby. Discuss how you will adapt to the changes you will have to make, as an individual and also as a couple. Ask yourself whether or not you feel ready to become responsible for a new life. After all, a child will be with you for many years to come.

Find out as much as you can about pregnancy, labour, and being a parent. Talk to other parents, and spend time with people who have young children so that you get a real taste of just what it may be like.

If you have a partner, your relationship will need to be strong as you start along the road to parenthood. Many decisions lie ahead, which should be made together.

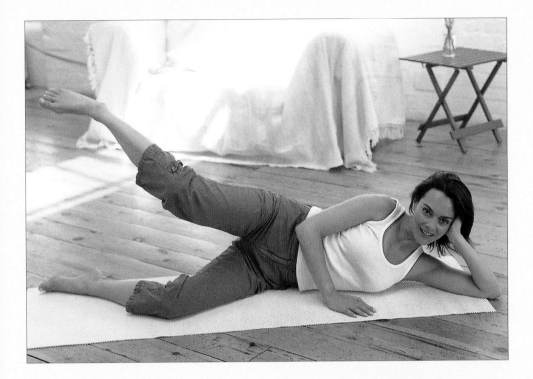

The decision to have a child involves both instinct and reason. Don't worry if you have doubts, as no one can be totally certain of any choice that they make. We can only decide what feels right for us and then pursue our chosen goal in a positive spirit.

If you decide to go ahead, you will want to prepare as well as possible. You may need to do something radical, such as give up smoking or radically reduce your alcohol consumption, or improve your general health or fitness or lose or gain weight before trying to conceive. Look into ways of eating healthy, natural foods and find out about the wide choice of complementary therapies that will help to keep you in top mental and physical shape. Above all, enjoy all the new things that you will be discovering about yourself and the journey ahead of you.

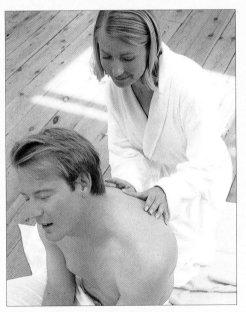

Top: Keep yourself in good physical shape, but avoid suddenly starting a tough routine that you have never tried before, and seek advice from your doctor first.

Help to strengthen your relationship, and keep stress at bay, by making time to enjoy relaxing and sensual pleasures such as a soothing massage.

Deciding to have a baby

Choosing to have a baby is without question the most momentous decision of your life. No other will have such far-reaching, and yet such potentially rewarding, implications over the years to come.

Some people feel an absolute certainty that they are ready to have a baby. Others feel more ambivalent about the effect that a child may have on their lifestyle or relationship. In addition, partners often feel differently about exactly when or if they want to become parents.

Discussing all the issues is essential. It is important that you ask yourself some searching questions before going ahead, and that you and your partner are honest about any hopes and fears that you have.

WHY YOU WANT TO HAVE A BABY

Talking about your reasons for wanting a baby can help you to pinpoint any assumptions that you have about the role a child will play in your life. For example, do you see a baby as something that will enhance an already happy life – or as a way of filling an emotional void? Are you hoping he or she will strengthen a loving partnership – or cement over the cracks in a rocky one?

It would not be wise to conceive a child in order to repair problems in your relationship or simply because you want to have someone to love. If there are tensions between you and your partner, having a baby will almost certainly exacerbate them – lack of sleep and having more to do at home soon cause tempers to fray.

Caring for a baby can be an isolating experience, especially if you do not have a loving partner to lean on. Many people bring up their children as lone parents – and do a wonderful job. Ideally, though, you will be in a committed, loving relationship that is strong enough to withstand the challenges of bringing up a child.

PROGRESSING TO PARENTHOOD

One of the most important things for you and your partner to consider is whether or not you feel ready to welcome another person into your relationship. Are you sufficiently certain of each other's feelings for one another to be able to care for a helpless and dependent baby?

Think, too, about whether your partner is the person you want to parent your child. Do you consider him or her to be sufficiently mature, kind, compassionate, intelligent, and sensitive to be your co-parent? As a hypothetical question, would you have liked your partner as a parent yourself? Try to imagine it just for a moment.

YOUR LIFESTYLE

Before trying to conceive, discuss how you see your lives adapting to a new child. Consider some of the practical issues. Is your home a suitable place for a child, for example, or will you have to move? Is one of you planning to stay home with the baby for the first years? If so, is the other prepared to become sole breadwinner for a time?

If your career is important to you, think about whether you can take some time off without damaging your future prospects. Consider, too, how you will cope with both the costs of having a child and the likely reduction in your income as a result of working less or paying for childcare.

Take some time to think about how you see your lives in five or ten years' time. Is what you want in terms of

FERTILITY ISSUES TO CONSIDER

When considering whether or not this is the right time to try for a baby, you may need to consider biological factors. Most important of these is the age of the woman.

A woman's fertility decreases as she gets older, particularly after the age of 35. Fertility starts to decrease about ten years before a woman's periods stop, and most women start the menopause around 45–55 (though it can be much earlier). There is no way of knowing exactly when the menopause will start, so it is wise not to put off conceiving for too long, particularly if you are already in your thirties.

From a biological point of view, a woman is most likely to conceive between 20 and 25 years of age. If you delay having a child until later, be aware that you are more likely to experience delays in conception than younger women. However, age usually brings with it greater stability and maturity, which are vital factors where parenthood is concerned.

Many different factors may be involved in the timing of your pregnancy. If both you and your partner feel that you are ready to have a child together, then this is probably the right time for you to go ahead, irrespective of work, finances or any other concerns.

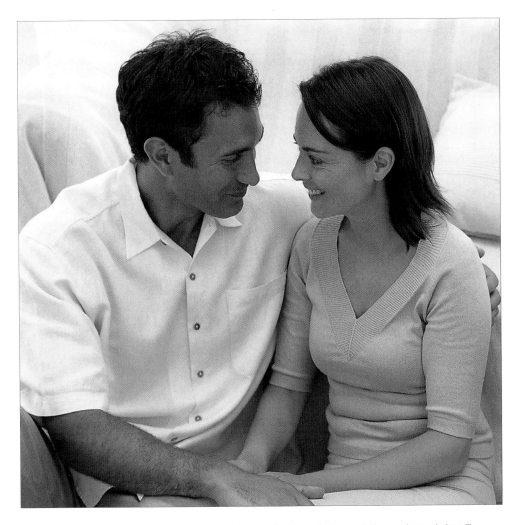

home and career compatible with what your partner wants? Are you agreed on how you see your future lives?

None of these issues is likely to be the deciding factor in whether or not you try to start a family. However, discussing them can help to build up a picture of how you and your partner feel about starting a family, and whether or not you need to make changes to your lifestyle first.

YOUR SUPPORT NETWORK

Family and close friends can be a vital support when you have a baby – particularly in the first few months when you are adjusting to your new lifestyle. It is a good idea to discuss with your partner the role that each of your families may play in helping you. Do you have supportive friends or relatives near to where you live at the moment? If not, would you consider moving?

Deciding whether, and when, to have a baby will probably be the biggest and most important event of your lives together – and the most exciting.

MAKING A DECISION

Ultimately, only you and your partner can know if this is the right time for you to try for a baby. Give yourselves plenty of time to make the decision, and listen carefully to what your inner voice tells you.

Listen just as carefully to what your partner says – and make sure that you hear what he or she actually says, rather than what you wish to hear. It is easy to imagine that your partner's aims are the same as yours, but this isn't always the case. Having a baby is a long-term commitment and both partners need to be sure that this is what they really want.

How pregnancy happens

For pregnancy to occur, both the man's and the woman's reproductive system must be in good working order, the couple must make love at the right time of the woman's menstrual cycle, and her body must produce a complex chain of hormones in order to keep the pregnancy going.

When a man ejaculates during sexual intercourse, millions of sperm are released into the woman's vagina. They move up the vagina and through the cervix into the uterus, propelled both by the force of ejaculation and by moving their tails like tiny fish. From there, the sperm make their way to the Fallopian tubes. This process is like a frantic race, as only one sperm among the millions can fertilize the egg. The rest fall away before they reach the goal, or else arrive too late.

If sexual intercourse has taken place without contraception, some sperm may reach the Fallopian tube and a single one may fertilize the waiting egg. The fertilized egg then makes its way towards the woman's uterus (womb), where it attaches itself to the lining. Here, it develops first into a tiny embryo, then a fetus and, eventually, into a baby.

THE WOMAN'S REPRODUCTIVE SYSTEM

A woman's reproductive system lies within her pelvis, and consists of the ovaries, the Fallopian tubes, the uterus, the cervix, the vagina and the vulva.

Baby girls are born with all their eggs in place in the ovaries – about 2–3 million of them. The ovaries are dormant during childhood and start to function only as puberty and menstruation begins. From then, women of childbearing age produce an egg every four weeks or so. This monthly timetable is called the ovulatory or menstrual cycle. About 400–500 eggs are produced during a woman's childbearing years – before ovulation ceases at menopause, usually in the woman's forties or fifties.

At the beginning of the ovulatory cycle, a number of eggs begin to grow in the ovaries. After about 14 days, one egg is mature enough to be released into the Fallopian tube. The ovulated egg enters the Fallopian tube and travels towards the uterus. It is during this journey that the egg may be fertilized. If not, some 14 days after ovulation the lining of the uterus is shed into the vagina – that is, the woman has her period. Then the entire cycle begins again.

CONCEPTION AND HORMONES

Hormones are chemicals that the body produces to regulate all kinds of natural processes. They act as messengers, telling the ovaries, for example, when to release an egg.

Two hormones play a crucial role in ovulation and pregnancy. Each month, follicle-stimulating hormone (FSH) stimulates an egg to mature, then luteinizing hormone (LH) causes the egg to be released into the Fallopian tubes, where it is ready to be fertilized. The hormones FSH and LH are produced in the brain, in an organ called the pituitary gland. The cells around the egg produce two other hormones – oestrogen and progesterone. These hormones cause the lining of the uterus to thicken – to create an environment in which an implanted, fertilized egg can thrive and grow. It is the monthly drop in the level of progesterone which, in the absence of a fertilized egg, brings on a woman's period.

The regular ebb and flow of different hormones throughout the menstrual cycle means that there are only a few days in each month when a woman is likely to conceive. This 'window of opportunity' is known as the fertile period.

FEMALE REPRODUCTIVE SYSTEM

The woman's egg is released from the ovary. It travels down the Fallopian tube to the uterus.

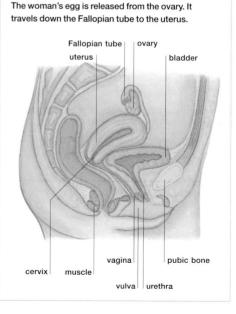

Fallopian tube | ovary
uterus | bladder
cervix | muscle | vagina | pubic bone
vulva | urethra

If the woman is menstruating but is not producing eggs for some reason, conception cannot occur. However, women can conceive even if they are not having periods – although conception is less likely.

THE MAN'S REPRODUCTIVE SYSTEM

A man's reproductive system consists of the penis, the testicles, and the various tubes that connect the two and carry sperm. Sperm is produced in the two testicles, which are contained within the scrotum. Men do not start making sperm until they reach puberty.

Thousands of microscopic tubes within the testicles connect to the two tubes – which are known as the efferent ducts. These lead into one single tube, the epididymis. The epididymis is part of the route through which sperm leaves the man's body. It is about 12 metres (40 feet) in length, and it is narrower than a fine piece of thread.

THE SPERM'S JOURNEY

Men, unlike women, are physiologically primed to reproduce at any time, and so sperm are in constant production. A series of muscular contractions in the wall of the epididymis serves to transport them along its length. During this time, the sperm are modified so that they become capable of fertilization. They also acquire their ability to move (which is known medically as motility) while they are in the epididymis. The sperm now pass

> **" Seven days after fertilization, the egg becomes implanted in the lining of the uterus. This is the moment when conception is said to take place. "**

through a tube called the vas deferens, which moves them quickly into the urethra, which passes through the penis. The urethra is the tube through which urine is passed outside the body. During sexual arousal and ejaculation, the opening between the urethra and the bladder shuts, and sperm-containing semen is rapidly transported along it.

THE RACE TO THE EGG

It takes only one sperm to fertilize an egg. When a man ejaculates during sexual intercourse, between 100 million and 300 million sperm are discharged into the woman's vagina – at about 45km (28 miles) per hour.

Each sperm is genetically unique, meaning that no two contain exactly the same set of genes. The millions of individual sperm are now in competition with each other as they race to fertilize the egg.

The route to the egg is hazardous. This is why sperm are produced in such large numbers. To stand a chance of fertilizing the egg, the sperm have to be able to withstand the environment of the woman's vagina and cervix. The acidity of this environment protects against bacteria and potentially dangerous infections, but it is also inhospitable to sperm. Weak or damaged ones will not make it.

In addition, the force of gravity means that millions of sperm simply leak out of the woman's vagina – as few as 5 per cent of them reach the cervix. Of these, only 200 or so make it as far as the woman's Fallopian tubes. Any sperm that make it this far have covered a huge distance that is, in terms of its own length, equivalent to several hundred miles.

The last few superfit sperm now proceed to the outside of the egg. Of these sperm, just one will break through the surface, leaving its tail behind. This is the moment of fertilization. In the instant that it occurs, the egg's surface becomes impenetrable to other sperm.

Fertilization of the egg may take up to 24 hours. It then undergoes a series of complex changes until eventually, seven days after fertilization, it becomes implanted in the lining of the uterus. This is the moment when conception is said to take place.

Sperm can survive for quite a long time inside the woman's body – perhaps up to 48 hours – so fertilization can still take place even if the egg is not ready when they first reach the Fallopian tube.

MALE REPRODUCTIVE SYSTEM

Sperm travels from the testicles through the epididymis, vas deferens and urethra to the penis.

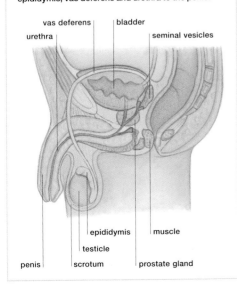

vas deferens | bladder
urethra | seminal vesicles
epididymis | muscle
testicle
penis | scrotum | prostate gland

Aiding conception

A baby can be conceived only around the time of ovulation, during the woman's fertile period. The egg is usually fertilized by the man's sperm within 48 hours of being released by the ovary. There are various ways in which a woman can judge when she is ovulating. By identifying this fertile period a couple can make a point of having intercourse and maximize the chance of conceiving.

WHEN DO I OVULATE?

Women ovulate about 14 days before the start of their next period. This is not the same as saying that ovulation takes place 14 days after the last period because the length of the menstrual cycle varies. Women may have a cycle as short as 21 days or as long as 38 days rather than the standard 28-day cycle.

There are various methods that you can use to calculate when ovulation is likely to occur. However, bear in mind that these serve as a rough guide only. Many experts and researchers in the field of infertility are sceptical about the effectiveness of the methods used. Even if you are certain that you know when you are ovulating, you should continue to make love at other times if you want to get pregnant.

Your menstrual cycle

If you have a regular monthly cycle, you will know when the next period is likely to start. Count back 14 days from that date – this is the day on which you are likely to ovulate.

> **YOUR CHANCES OF CONCEIVING**
> Conception is more likely to take place if:
> - The woman is between the ages of 20 and 34; the ideal age is 20–25.
> - The man produces healthy sperm.
> - Intercourse takes place at the right time in the woman's menstrual cycle.
> - Both partners are fit and well, and are following a healthy lifestyle.
> - Both partners are a healthy weight, with a good waist-to-hip ratio (see page 51).
> - Both partners avoid smoking, alcohol and caffeine.

Working out your probable fertile time means keeping a record of your periods for some months, in some cases up to a year, to establish the normal length of your cycle.

Cervical mucus

If your periods are irregular, you may be able to establish when you ovulate by studying your cervical mucus (produced by glands in the cervix's lining). Just before ovulation, it is transparent, thinner and more profuse, and takes on an jelly-like consistency, so that a drop will stretch between your fingers without breaking. After ovulation less, more milky coloured, mucus is produced.

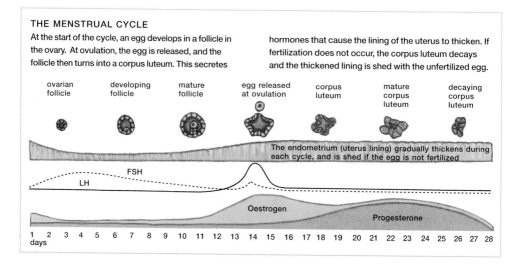

THE MENSTRUAL CYCLE
At the start of the cycle, an egg develops in a follicle in the ovary. At ovulation, the egg is released, and the follicle then turns into a corpus luteum. This secretes hormones that cause the lining of the uterus to thicken. If fertilization does not occur, the corpus luteum decays and the thickened lining is shed with the unfertilized egg.

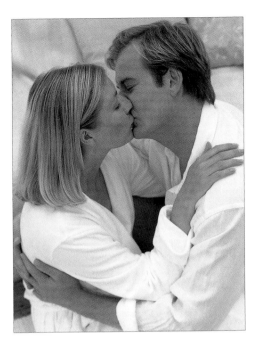

Making love around the time of ovulation will maximize your chances of becoming pregnant. All methods for establishing ovulation are approximate, so you should continue to make love at other times.

Body temperature

You can measure changes in your basal body temperature to determine when you are at your most fertile. Basal body temperature (BBT) is your temperature immediately on waking in the morning, before you have got up or eaten or drunk anything. BBT drops just before ovulation and then rises again some 12–24 hours later, once ovulation has occurred. If you record the changes in your BBT each day for several months on a special chart, a pattern is likely to emerge. You can use this to help you predict the time of ovulation.

Remember that your temperature can rise and fall for other reasons. For example, if you are ill or if you take your temperature later in the day, your reading is likely to be inaccurate. Doing both the temperature and cervical-mucus methods at the same time tends to give more accurate results than either method done alone.

Ovulation kits

You can also establish the day of ovulation by using an over-the-counter ovulation prediction device. These kits work by measuring the amount of the LH hormone being produced, which helps to establish when ovulation is about to occur. All you need to do is a urine test. If plenty of LH hormone is being produced, a chemical will change colour. This means you are likely to be ovulating. However, like all the methods, ovulation kits are not foolproof. They can produce a false positive result. They are also expensive.

Remember that the consistency of cervical mucus may change for other reasons – for example, if you have an infection. For greater accuracy, it is best to combine this method with the body temperature method.

To test your mucus, insert your finger into your vagina, then gently withdraw it. If the mucus is clear, moist and stretchy, you are probably close to ovulation. Making love within the next 24–36 hours could give a good chance of conception.

BODY TEMPERATURE CHART

In the temperature method, a basal thermometer is used to detect minute changes in a woman's body temperature during the ovulatory cycle; regular thermometers are not sensitive enough.

Most basal thermometers are supplied with a chart like this one. Make several copies so that you can keep a record of temperature changes over a few months. You may need help from an expert in order to interpret the results and pinpoint your fertile period.

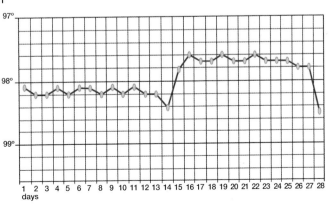

Preconceptual care

Ideally, both you and your partner should start to prepare for conception a few months before you try for a baby. Nobody can guarantee you a healthy baby but if you and your partner are fit and healthy at the point of conception, you are giving your pregnancy the best start possible.

Your diet, weight and fitness can all impact on your fertility and on the pregnancy. Maintaining a regular fitness programme, eating a healthy diet and reducing stress can all aid your chances of conception, and will also help the woman's body to cope better with pregnancy. The months before conception are also a good time to give up smoking, reduce or give up alcohol, and attend to any other health issues.

The majority of women do not need any supplements other than folic acid either before conception or during their pregnancy. However, it is important that you start taking folic acid, which substantially reduces the risk of spina bifida, as soon as you start trying for a baby – the current recommended dose is 400 micrograms every day.

DENTAL CHECK

Before conceiving, have a full dental check-up. Try to get any treatment done straight away so that you can avoid having X-rays or anaesthetics during pregnancy. Pregnant women are also advised not to have any amalgam (silver) fillings put in or removed during pregnancy since they may leak tiny doses of mercury, which is toxic.

MEDICAL CHECK-UP

Tell your doctor that you want to conceive. Ask about any supplements or medication you are taking – both over-the-counter and prescribed drugs could affect the health of your baby. Your doctor will also be able to provide advice on your diet, health and lifestyle, and advise you on losing or gaining weight, if necessary.

If you have diabetes, epilepsy or any other chronic condition that requires you to take long-term medication, your doctor may recommend changing the drugs or reducing the dosage before conception. He or she may also suggest genetic counselling if you or your partner have a family history of genetic disorders.

SEXUAL HEALTH CHECKS

Some sexually transmitted infections can affect your fertility as well as your general health. As they do not necessarily cause symptoms, you may be unaware that you have been infected. For this reason, all women wanting to conceive are advised to have a 'well-woman'

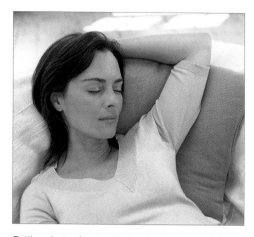

Getting plenty of rest and relaxation is an essential element of preconceptual health care. You should also make sure that you have all the vital health checks.

screening test. This checks for signs of:
- Bacterial infections such as chlamydia, gonorrhoea and syphilis, which can be cured with antibiotic treatment.
- Viral infections such as warts, herpes, hepatitis, and HIV, which can usually be treated to improve symptoms.

Untreated chlamydia, in particular, is a major cause of female infertility and ectopic pregnancies. It may cause pain on intercourse but is often present without other symptoms, so many women only visit their doctor when they have problems conceiving. Up to a third of people are thought to be infected with chlamydia at some point in their lives.

SEXUALLY TRANSMITTED INFECTIONS
Symptoms may include any of these:
- Pain in the lower abdomen.
- Pain during or after sex.
- Bleeding after sex.
- Spotting or bleeding between periods.
- The sudden onset of much heavier periods after starting a new sexual relationship.
- Pain when passing urine.
- Increased or foul-smelling vaginal discharge.
- Rash, spots, lumps, itching or ulcers around the genital area.

RUBELLA

Before you try to get pregnant, you should have a test to ensure that you are immune to rubella (German measles). Rubella is a viral disease that can cause severe abnormalities in babies if their mothers catch it during pregnancy. Have the test even if you are sure that you had rubella as a child – rubella is frequently misdiagnosed, and it is not clear how long immunity achieved in this way lasts. If you are not immune, you can be vaccinated and then retested to make sure that the vaccine has worked. You should not attempt to conceive for at least one month after the vaccination.

ALCOHOL AND FERTILITY

If you want to get pregnant, then consider cutting out alcohol completely. There is research to suggest that even light drinking may reduce your chances of conception, though many doctors believe that having an occasional drink will do no harm. All experts agree that regular, heavy drinking or binge drinking can have adverse effects on fertility – and one study found that having two drinks a day could reduce a woman's fertility by almost 60 per cent. Regular or heavy drinking carries high risks for the baby, and alcohol is also linked to an increased risk of miscarriage in the first trimester.

Men trying to conceive should drink no more than three to four units a day (that's two pints of lager or roughly two 175ml/6fl oz glasses of wine if you opt for lower-strength drinks). Heavy drinkers may produce weak, inferior sperm, which are unable to negotiate the journey to meet the woman's egg. They may also produce babies with serious defects.

Alcohol crosses the placenta, so a baby is exposed to alcohol when the mother drinks. Babies born to mothers who are heavy drinkers may be affected by fetal alcohol

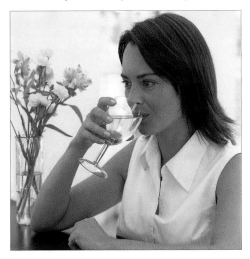

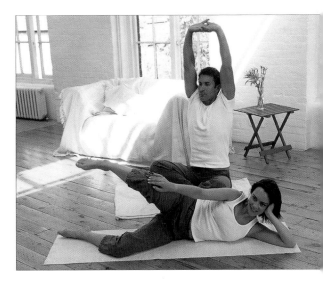

Yoga increases your stamina, strength and suppleness as well as helping you achieve deep relaxation.

syndrome. This can cause severe defects such as growth deficiency, facial abnormalities, problems with co-ordination and movement, and mental impairment. In addition, the babies may be born addicted to alcohol – and may suffer withdrawal symptoms and fail to thrive.

Researchers are not sure whether it is safe to drink any alcohol in pregnancy because the effects vary depending on the individual woman's health, the speed at which her body absorbs alcohol, her diet and so on. To be on the safe side, women are advised not to drink at all. If you do drink while pregnant, then you should still avoid all alcohol in the first three months and thereafter your maximum limit should be no more than one or two units of alcohol once or twice a week; two units is roughly equivalent to one 175ml/6fl oz glass of wine or to a pint of beer, assuming you choose drinks with a lower alcohol content.

GIVE UP SMOKING

If you smoke, you should give up before trying to conceive. As well as affecting your general health, smoking reduces your fertility. If you smoke while pregnant, you have a higher risk of miscarriage and stillbirth; you also face an increased risk of having a premature or low-birthweight baby. Your partner should also give up to avoid the risk of passive smoking to both mother and baby. See your doctor if you want help with giving up smoking.

For optimum fertility and a healthy baby, it is best to give up alcohol entirely.

Time with your partner

Before you welcome a new baby into your life, it is important to devote special time and energy to your relationship with your partner. The time before conception – as well as the months of pregnancy itself – can be a marvellous opportunity to strengthen the bonds between you, and to work through unresolved emotional issues.

It can be very easy for partners to become focused on the baby that they want, and to forget that they are life partners as well as potential parents. Couples who enjoy each other's company, and respect each other's strengths and aims, tend to make happy and committed parents.

A loving relationship and good communication can help you to face possible delays in conception as well as the challenges that pregnancy can bring. In the weeks and months to come, you may have to undergo a number of tests and checks. Some may raise difficult questions – for example, how you would react if there was something wrong with the baby. The time that you invested in each other before conception will help you cope together, as loving partners.

WORKING TOGETHER

The months before conception may be a good time to complete projects that you wish to carry out in the house or garden. Working together for the future can deepen the relationship and can also help you to prepare both practically and mentally for the likely changes to your lifestyle when you have a family.

Practical projects are also better done before the pregnancy is advanced, and certainly before you have a new baby to care for. Any unresolved long-term problems – such as clearing up financial affairs – would also best be dealt with now rather than later, when you will have less time and energy to devote to them.

ENJOY ONE ANOTHER

How you celebrate and enjoy your relationship with your partner will depend on what you both like doing. You may like to cook delicious food together, go for long walks in the fresh air, swim or exercise, have friends in for dinners and barbecues, or enjoy other shared interests.

Making love is, of course, a wonderful way to express your affection. For many couples, this is the first time that they are able to enjoy sex without having to worry about contraception, which can heighten the pleasure as well as the sense of connection between you.

SHARING MASSAGE

Gentle massage is a great way of deepening the closeness between you and your partner. It is also highly beneficial for pregnant women or those wishing to conceive. Anyone can give a pleasurable massage, and the basic techniques are not difficult to learn. You may like to enrol in a short course to learn from an expert. As well as being extremely relaxing, massage is helpful during pregnancy since it can alleviate common complaints such as backache, insomnia and even morning sickness.

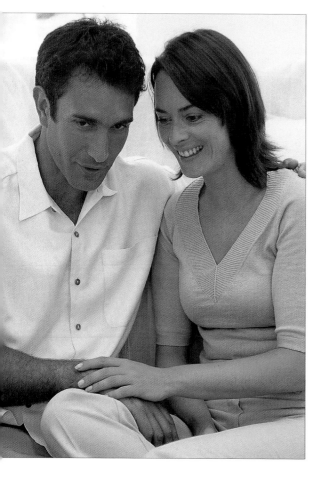

Pregnancy can be an emotional time, with many ups and downs. A close and loving relationship will help you to face any difficulties together.

Giving a relaxing massage

The key to good massage is focus and feedback. Concentrate on what your hands are doing and enjoy the pleasure that you can give. Use the following basic techniques, alternating them in whichever way feels right to you. Ask your partner whether or not the touch feels good – or if they would prefer a lighter or firmer pressure. Then let your intuition guide you. Do not massage over a joint or the spine. Avoid using fast, rhythmic movements on a woman who is pregnant or trying to conceive.

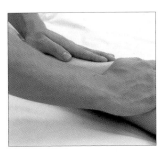

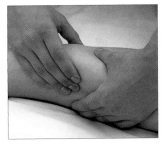

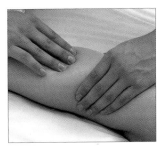

1 Start with slow, rhythmic, stroking movements, using the whole hand. Try applying light pressure with your fingertips, or use your thumbs or knuckles for deeper pressure. If you want to use oil, stroke it evenly over the area that you are massaging.

2 Gently grasp handfuls of flesh or muscle, particularly where you can feel that a muscle is hard or contracted. Use your thumbs and fingers to knead and roll the area, rather like dough. Keep checking that the touch feels good for your partner, and alternate with strokes.

3 Work specific areas by making a series of small circular movements with one or several fingers, the pads of the thumbs, or the heel of the hands. This helps to stimulate the circulation. Alternate with stroking movements, and remember to ask for feedback.

Aromatic massage

Adding a few drops of aromatherapy oil to your massage oil can heighten the pleasure and well-being that receiving a massage can bring. The main, immediate effect of aromatherapy is relaxation, which is very beneficial in conception and pregnancy – neroli or rosewood are excellent soothing oils. You can also use oils in a vaporizer, to create either an uplifting or soothing atmosphere in a room.

Aromatherapy oils can have a powerful effect and not all of them are suitable for women intending to conceive. See pages 212–213 for advice on using aromatherapy oils safely, and a list of oils to avoid in pregnancy.

When not to massage

There are some circumstances in which you should not have a massage. For example:

- If you have an infection.
- If you have a high temperature.
- If you have severe back pain, especially if the pain shoots down the arms or legs.
- If you have a skin infection.

Massage is one of the easiest ways to de-stress and release the tensions of the day. It's also a great way to pamper your partner and enjoy time together.

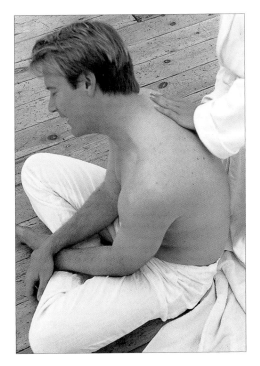

Avoiding hazards

We know that some environmental substances, in particular toxins and radiation, may hinder conception and endanger pregnancy. The research currently available is not clear-cut, and it is by no means the case that all women exposed to a potential hazard will necessarily develop a problem. However, it seems sensible to reduce your exposure to hazards wherever you can, as a safeguard for yourself and your child. If you are trying to conceive or are pregnant, here are some of the things you should avoid.

X-RAYS

Having an X-ray exposes you to a tiny dose of radiation. The dose given is too small to cause problems to you, but it can sometimes have an adverse effect on the developing fetus. Always tell your doctor and your dentist if you are trying to conceive or know that you are pregnant. Wherever possible have any medical or dental investigations carried out before you attempt to conceive to avoid exposing the fetus to any risk.

If you had an X-ray before realizing that you were pregnant, talk to your doctor about the potential effects. In most cases, there is unlikely to be a problem.

OTHER SOURCES OF RADIATION

Computers, VDUs and televisions are sometimes cited as a hazard because they give out small amounts of radiation. However, the general advice is that the radiation you are exposed to in this way is not in sufficient quantity or strength to have an effect on fertility or pregnancy.

The research concerning the effect of mobile phones on the brain and the nervous system is not yet clear, but it would be wise to reduce your use to a minimum. Avoid chatting for long periods and use a hands-free model whenever possible. Do not chat with the mobile held next to your head while in an enclosed area such as a car.

CATS AND KITTENS

The faeces of kittens and young cats may carry the parasite toxoplasmosis. If this is passed to a pregnant woman, it can harm a developing fetus and cause a variety of abnormalities. The faeces is infectious only when kittens or young cats first acquire toxoplasmosis – which is usually while hunting during the first year of life. They then develop antibodies to the infection and excrete the parasite, in which case they are no longer infectious. To protect yourself, avoid contact with kittens and young cats wherever possible. Always wear gloves if you have to

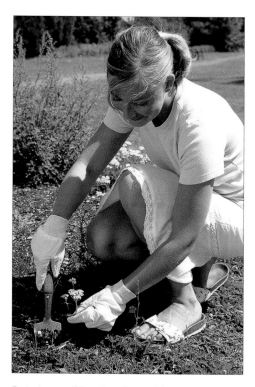

Protect yourself from toxoplasmosis by wearing gloves while gardening, and washing your hands afterwards. Check that your tetanus immunization is up to date.

TOXOPLASMOSIS

This is a form of infection that causes few symptoms – those affected may think they have a mild case of flu. So if you know that you been exposed to kitten faeces, see your doctor for an immunity test straight away. This can detect antibodies to toxoplasmosis in the blood, and will help to establish whether or not you are immune. Unfortunately, the test can sometimes provide borderline results.

If toxoplasmosis is caught during pregnancy, it can cause a miscarriage. It may also cause damage to the unborn baby, including to the brain. If you have already been infected and are immune, toxoplasmosis will not affect future pregnancies.

> ❝ Complete any renovations before you try for a baby. Chemicals in some decorating products are harmful. ❞

empty a cat-litter tray, and disinfect it with boiling water for five minutes every day. There may also be toxoplasmosis in the soil so wear gloves for gardening. Wash your hands thoroughly after contact with soil.

APPLIANCES
It is worth getting appliances such as microwave ovens or gas heaters checked to make sure that they are working properly and are not leaking radiation or carbon monoxide into your home.

CHEMICAL PRODUCTS
Certain room deodorizers, furniture polish, oven cleaners, weedkillers and other products may contain poisonous substances. Always read labels carefully, and seek out household cleaning and garden products that are non-toxic and environment-friendly.

Take special care if you are exposed to chemicals at work – for example, if you are a hairdresser or a gardener. Talk to your doctor or midwife about whether or not any substances you come into contact with could be harmful to your pregnancy.

LIVESTOCK
Do not touch pregnant livestock if you are trying to conceive or may already be pregnant. They may carry bacteria that can cause miscarriage.

LONG-HAUL FLIGHTS
Sitting in one position for a long period – as you do when flying – increases your risk of deep vein thrombosis (DVT). In DVT a blood clot forms in the leg or pelvis. This clot can then become detached and travel to the lungs, a condition that can be life-threatening. It is now known that women are at greater risk of developing DVT when they are pregnant.

To help prevent DVT, get up from your seat every hour or so and move around. At regular intervals in between, flex your wrists and ankles and stretch your neck to left, to right and downwards in order to keep freshly oxygenated blood flowing around the body. Drink plenty of water before, during and after the flight – dehydration has been shown to increase the risk of DVT – and make sure that you do not drink any alcohol.

Home renovations are best done before you start trying for a baby. Choose products that are environment-friendly, to reduce your exposure to toxic substances.

IS YOUR HOME SAFE?
Take time before trying to conceive to make sure your home is a safe place to be. This is a good time to get done any jobs that could expose you to risk in pregnancy – for example, stripping old, lead-based paint from walls. Try to complete any renovations before you try for a baby – chemicals in some home-decorating products, such as paint thinners, strippers and glues are potentially harmful. Wherever possible, choose paints and other products that are child- and environment-friendly.

Many women find it difficult to bend down even early on in their pregnancies, so it is a good idea to complete any jobs that will require you to do so before conceiving. You should also fix any obvious hazards such as loose carpeting on the stairs.

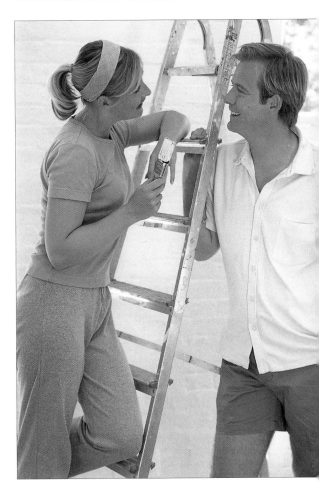

Common Qs and As

Q: How will having a baby change our lives?

A: Almost every aspect of your lifestyle will change to a greater or lesser extent when you have a child to look after. You will have to consider the child as well as yourself in every decision that you make, whether short or long term. For example, whenever you go out of the house, you will have to take a bag with extra clothing, spare nappies and other equipment with you. You may need to wait until the baby has fed, slept or been changed. You will be unable to go to some places, such as the cinema and theatre, with the baby – for those you will need to hire a babysitter or arrange for a friend or relative to look after the baby for you. In general, spontaneous outings will be much more difficult to achieve.

Although you will have less disposable cash and less free time, you will probably find that you will enjoy spending money on the baby and relish the time that you have with him or her. Parenthood often brings with it a very profound change in attitudes and priorities. You may find that your feelings about your career change and that you want to prioritize family life over your work. It may be that you start to feel that you have less in common with certain friends and that you actively seek out other parents to spend time with, or become closer to your family. Whatever the changes in store, many parents say that the joy of having a baby and bringing up a child profoundly outweighs the sacrifices they make.

Q: Once I have a baby, will I ever have time for myself again?

A: You will, but it will take more organization than before, and you will need the help of others to make sure you get it. It is a good idea to persuade your partner or a member of your family or a close friend to look after the baby for a few hours each week to make sure that you get your valuable 'me' time.

Q: My partner is very keen to have a baby and believes that it is a part of any normal human relationship to have children together. I am not so sure... and I don't know what to do.

A: You could say that it is part of most human partnerships to have a baby, but not all. There is nothing abnormal in not having children of your own. If you have doubts about having a child, give yourself and your partner more time to think things over. You may come to realize that your doubts simply reflect a certain anxiety on your part about how you will adapt to parenthood. You may also realize that there are other things you want to do with your life before you have children. Over time, you may discover that you are prepared to welcome this new challenge.

Q: My sister-in-law tells me that having children is nothing but drudgery. She says that if she had known what it is like, she would have thought twice about having her children at all. What do you think?

A: It may be that you caught your sister-in-law at a bad time. Perhaps she was feeling tired after work and knew she was behind with all the washing and housework. It may be that she thought back to her single life, before children, and wished for the luxury of time to herself. If you talked to her again, you might discover that she is happy and proud of her children and would not be without them. On the other hand, it may be that she really does yearn for the apparent freedom and luxury of a child-free life. It is important to remember that whatever someone else feels is no indication of how you would feel in a similar situation.

Q : My mother and my mother-in-law keep telling us that it is best to have children as young as possible. We would like to wait for a few years. Is this safe?

A : The ideal time to conceive is in your twenties. However, many women are having babies in their early thirties without problems. After the age of 32 a woman's fertility does start to decrease, but it is only from the age of 35 that this decline speeds up. Should any problem present itself, it could take time to be resolved and, at over 35, time starts to be against you. That said, many women have healthy babies in their late thirties and even their forties.

You should remember that mothers and mothers-in-law are often eager for grandchildren, and this may colour their judgement as to what's best for their daughters and daughters-in-law. You must be your own judge; only when you and your partner feel the time is right should you go ahead.

Q : I am concerned that my partner is talking about giving up her job after she has our baby. I don't think this will be helpful for her sanity or for our finances. What can I say to her?

A : It may be that a compromise solution in which she works part-time is the best option for you both. You may find it helpful to sit down together and work out three different budgets: one based on her returning to work, one on her working part-time and the other on her staying at home.

Your partner will need to work out how much money she will need from you if she is to stay at home full-time. This will help her to appreciate the impact this has on your joint finances. Be sure to include everything in your budget, and allow for extras such as holidays. When you have completed the budget, add at least 10 per cent as a contingency figure.

Q : I have recently got married to a man who has been married before and has two children by his first wife. I do not have any children and would love to start a family. My husband is reluctant to have a baby on the grounds that it could upset his children. I feel that this goes against my nature and is unfair. How can I persuade him?

A : This is an extremely complex issue, made more tricky because it affects a number of people who are bound up together in a potentially sensitive situation. First, it must be said that if you really want to have a child but do not act on that desire, you could regret it for the rest of your life. So it is important that you make it absolutely clear to your husband how important having a child is to you.

Fathers who no longer live with their children, through divorce, often suffer considerable guilt and anxiety as a result. Once they become calm and settled within their new marriage, they are often much more likely to consider positively the idea of having another child. It will help if you tell him that you understand these issues and also that you are in no way trying to cancel out his former marriage by creating another family. Take positive steps to show him that there will always be time and space in your lives for his first two children.

Ask your husband if he would like to encourage some kind of open dialogue with his children, if they are old enough to appreciate the issues. You may also find it beneficial to have one or two counselling sessions, attended by both you and your husband.

Healthy eating

❝ What you eat will affect the growth and development of every part of your baby. **❞**

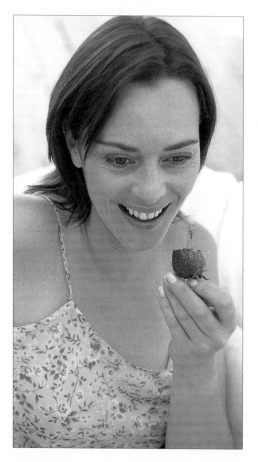

From the very first moment of conception, your baby will benefit from your healthy eating habits, as well as those of your partner. What you eat will affect the growth and development of every part of your baby: his or her bones, muscles, joints, teeth, senses and brain. Many people also believe that certain foods can even boost fertility.

Eating healthily and well is not nearly as complicated as some magazines and books lead us to believe. As you will see in the following chapter, good nutrition depends on a very simple formula indeed: eating a wide range of healthy foods and avoiding junk food.

Certain foods and toxins should be completely avoided before (if possible) and during pregnancy and these are described in detail in the following pages. As far as food supplements are concerned, there are very few – other than folic acid – that the woman who is pregnant or hoping to conceive needs to take, so long as she maintains a varied and healthy diet.

If you get hungry between meals, try to snack on fruit rather than the many tempting – but usually unhealthy – alternatives that are all too readily available.

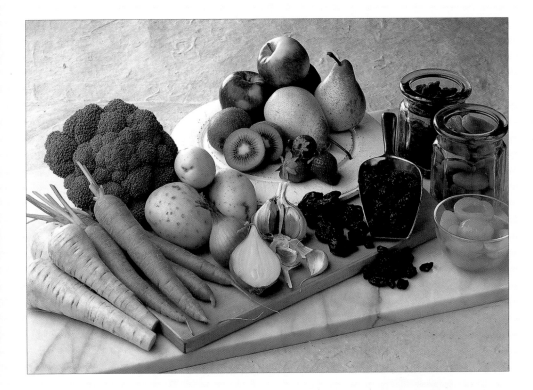

Food hygiene and how you prepare food is an important concept for pregnant women and is, in any case, something that all of us need to be fully aware of. Some food bugs may adversely affect the baby's healthy development and in some cases prove fatal to the unborn baby.

We have so much information available to us these days about the effects of food on our bodies that all of us can work out what we need for optimum health, growth and development. We are also now much better informed about the foods that pregnant women should avoid. Use this chapter as your guide to what and how much to eat and drink, what your weight should be, and how you can treat yourself to a cleansing detox day.

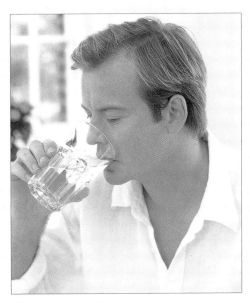

Top: A healthy diet is a well-balanced one, with a good proportion of fruit and vegetables. Make sure that you eat five portions of fruit and vegetables each day.

Drinking plenty of water cannot be over-emphasized. Even those of us who think we drink a great deal are probably not consuming enough.

Sensible eating

Healthy eating is a major cornerstone of preconceptual care. If you are trying for a baby, both partners should eat a healthy diet that provides a good supply of all the vital nutrients. This helps to boost your immune system, aids cell-repair and renewal, and keeps the reproductive organs in good working order.

Do not restrict your food intake in order to lose weight before conception or during pregnancy. Dieting can adversely affect fertility because you may not be taking in enough nutrients to keep the body functioning properly and producing the necessary hormones. If you do want to lose weight, it is generally better to increase your physical activity rather than restricting the amount that you eat. At the same time, do not overeat. Being overweight and eating a poor diet have both been shown to have an adverse effect on fertility.

You should also ensure that you keep to healthy eating habits, which you can then go on to share with your children. Make time for meals, do not rush your food, and

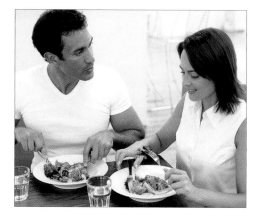

Make time to prepare and enjoy healthy meals made from fresh ingredients. Sitting at the dining table to eat will get you in the habit of taking good, regular meals.

stop eating when you have had enough. Make sure that you do not miss meals. Eat little and often – having four or five small meals a day is much easier on the digestion than eating a couple of larger ones.

EATING IN PREGNANCY

To a degree, your baby's health depends on what you eat and drink just before and during pregnancy. Because of this, mothers-to-be were traditionally advised to 'eat for two'. Experts no longer regard this as sensible advice, but that is not to say that the opposite is true. Some women eat too little during pregnancy to keep their weight down. Undereating can lead to problems such as a more difficult labour and underweight babies and an insufficient supply of nutrients and energy to support the pregnancy, and an increased risk of osteoporosis later.

Pregnancy can have a huge effect on your eating habits. Some women go off foods they once loved, while others keep eating the same dish or develop highly eccentric tastes. All of this is normal, so long as you have a balanced diet, and eat enough to maintain your energy levels.

In general, women who gain a reasonable amount of weight tend to have easier pregnancies and labours, and a lower risk of miscarriage and neonatal death (death around the time of delivery). Heavier babies are often healthier

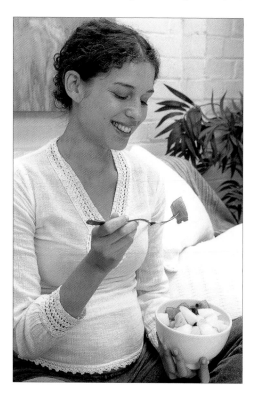

Remember to eat at least five helpings of fresh fruit and vegetables every day.

ARE YOU A HEALTHY WEIGHT?

Here we provide two ways for you to check whether you are a healthy weight. One quick method is by using the chart on the right. Simply find the point where your height and weight meet and then check the key below. The other method (using the body mass index) is explained below.

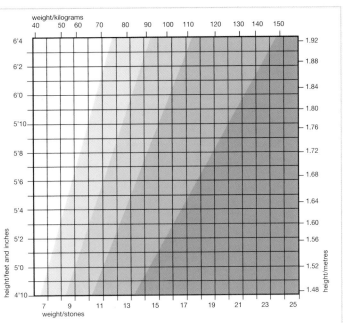

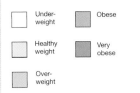

- ☐ Under-weight
- ☐ Healthy weight
- ☐ Over-weight
- ☐ Obese
- ☐ Very obese

Body Mass Index (BMI)

Healthcare professionals often use a calculation called the body mass index to work out whether a person is a healthy weight for his or her height. You can do this just as easily for yourself.

BMI = your weight in kilograms divided by (your height in metres) squared. (To convert weight from pounds to kilograms multiply by 0.4536; to convert height from feet to metres multiply by 0.3048.)

For example, Sue weighs 65 kg and is 1.64 metres tall, so her BMI is: $65 \div (1.64)^2 = 24.17$

A BMI of over 40 will adversely affect your fertility and is also a serious health risk. The ideal is a BMI of 20–25. Over 30 and you need to lose weight. If your BMI is under 20, concentrate on gaining weight through eating protein and carbohydrate, and having a full cooked breakfast and a generous lunch and dinner.

---

than those with a low birthweight, and are usually better able to resist common childhood illnesses. However, pregnant women who gain an excessive amount are at greater risk of developing diabetes, as are their babies.

WHY WOMEN GAIN WEIGHT IN PREGNANCY

Women lay down fat early in pregnancy as preparation for milk production and breastfeeding. This fat remains after the baby is born, but should gradually disappear, providing that you are following a healthy diet and exercising regularly. Other weight gain comes from the placenta, the fluids surrounding the baby and the baby itself, which accounts for more than half of the total weight gain. During pregnancy, women produce more blood, and this also increases their overall weight. The extra blood is needed to support a healthy pregnancy.

Everyone is different and so there are no strict rules about how much weight pregnant women should put on. Most women tend to gain around 9–13.5kg (20–30lb)

during pregnancy. However, someone who is already overweight may not need to put on as much weight during her pregnancy as a woman who is underweight. That said, the overweight woman should not try to diet once she knows that she is pregnant. Your weight will be monitored through your pregnancy as part of your antenatal checks and advice will be given on whether your weight gain is healthy.

RATE OF WEIGHT GAIN

The following is a rough guide to the rate of weight gain through a normal pregnancy:

0–12 weeks	10 per cent
13–20 weeks	25 per cent
21–28 weeks	45 per cent
29–36 weeks	20 per cent
37–40 weeks	0 per cent

A balanced diet

Eating healthily is a vital part of preconceptual care for men and women, helps women cope better with the demands of pregnancy, and gives a growing baby a healthier diet, too. General guidelines for healthy eating are:

- Eat a balanced diet, including food from each of the main food groups every day.
- Eat five helpings of fruit and vegetables every day.
- Minimize your intake of animal fats and sugars.
- Drink six to eight glasses of water every day.
- Have regular meals.
- Choose natural unprocessed foods wherever possible.
- The only supplement that all women need to take is folic acid.

GROUP 1: BREADS AND OTHER CEREALS

These foods are excellent sources of carbohydrate, which gives us energy, and fibre, which helps to keep the digestive tract healthy. They also provide us with B vitamins, some calcium and iron. Eat whole grains wherever possible – for example, wholewheat breakfast cereals without added sugar, wholemeal bread and wholewheat pasta. Choose brown or wild rice, which have undergone less processing than white varieties.

GROUP 2: FRUIT AND VEGETABLES

Eat five helpings of fruit and vegetables each day. A helping can be a glass of juice, a piece of fruit such as an apple or banana, a small salad or a portion of vegetables. Fruits and vegetables contain a wide range of vitamins and minerals, have almost no fat and are a good source of fibre. Eat them raw or lightly cooked to gain their full nutrient value.

GROUP 3: MEAT, FISH AND ALTERNATIVES

Beef, lamb, pork and bacon are good sources of protein, which the body needs for vital functions such as cell-repair. They also provide minerals such as iron and zinc, and B vitamins. Opt for lean cuts and trim off visible fat. Grill, roast or microwave meat, so that some of the fat drains off. Add more vegetables than meat to stews and casseroles to gives you a healthier dietary balance.

Fish and poultry also provide protein. Oily fish such as mackerel, salmon and sardines are rich in nutritious fish oils, so try to eat two portions a week. However, avoid eating more than one fresh tuna steak or two medium-sized cans of tuna a week, due to the mercury content (excess mercury can harm a fetus' nervous system). Grill, steam, microwave or bake fish rather than deep frying it.

Nuts, peas, lentils, soya and pulses also contain protein but, unlike meat or fish, they do not contain all the essential amino acids needed for growth. To maximize their nutritional value, serve them with plant foods and whole grains such as wholemeal bread. Some people class pulses as a distinct food group, but nutritionally speaking, they cannot be considered as good for you as meat or fish.

GROUP 4: MILK AND OTHER DAIRY PRODUCTS

Dairy produce such as eggs, cheese, milk and milk products provide calcium, which builds teeth and bones, and some protein. Pregnant women need lots of calcium to build their baby's skeleton. Low-fat dairy products are generally better for you. If you worry about weight gain, reduce your butter intake and avoid cream. Natural yogurt is a healthy option. Women who wish to conceive or who are pregnant should avoid raw or lightly cooked eggs and soft cheeses such as Brie and Camembert, because of the risk of food poisoning.

GROUP 5: FAT AND SUGAR

We need some fat in our diet. There are two main types of fat: saturated, which is solid at room temperature, and unsaturated, most of which remain liquid. Saturated fats, such as butter and lard, can increase blood cholesterol and

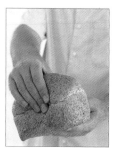

Try this test to check how healthy a brown loaf is: take the bread between your hands and squeeze gently. If it gives easily, it probably doesn't provide much fibre. As a general rule, the denser the bread, the more fibre it contains – so the healthier it is for you.

ORGANIC FOOD

Many people believe that organic produce tastes better and is more nutritious for you than conventionally grown food. Buying organic means that you are reducing your exposure to chemicals in the foods that you eat: organic fruit and vegetables are produced without the use of chemical fertilizers and pesticides, while animals used for organic meat are not given routine antibiotics or growth hormones.

THE MAIN FOOD GROUPS

This shows the proportions of the five main food groups that parents-to-be should aim to eat.

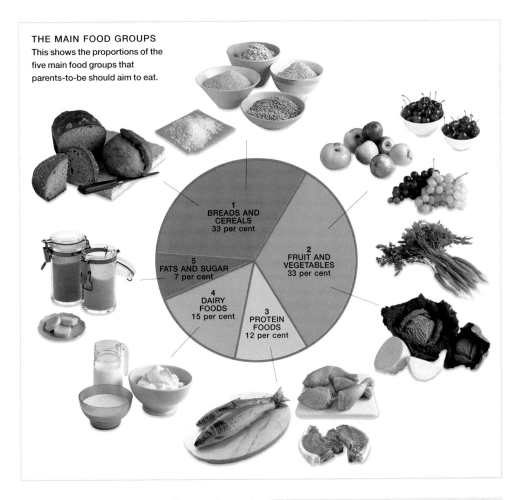

1 BREADS AND CEREALS
33 per cent

2 FRUIT AND VEGETABLES
33 per cent

3 PROTEIN FOODS
12 per cent

4 DAIRY FOODS
15 per cent

5 FATS AND SUGAR
7 per cent

with it the risk of heart disease. The two forms of unsaturated fat – monounsaturated and polyunsaturated – are better for you and may decrease cholesterol levels. Monounsaturated fats include olive oil and avocado, while polyunsaturated fats include most vegetable oils, fish oil and nuts. As a general rule, pick low-fat dairy products and use olive oil in place of butter.

Sugary foods provide a short-term energy boost, but little nutritional value. Eat sparingly, if at all.

WHY WE NEED FIBRE

Fibre is an indigestible substance that we get from nuts, cereals, fruit and vegetables. It is not broken down or digested in the body, but is vital for speeding up the passage of waste products through the bowel and removing toxins. Constipation is common during pregnancy, when bowel movements slow down, but plenty of fibre-rich food and water will help to prevent this.

DRINK WATER

Make sure that you are drinking enough water to maintain and repair all the body's systems, including the reproductive system. To avoid dehydration, which can lead to irritability, headache, tension, swollen ankles and a bloated stomach, you need to drink six to eight glasses of water every day – more if the weather is very hot. This may seem like a lot of water, but after just a few days your body will become accustomed to it.

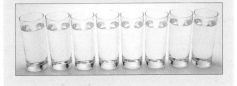

Can foods boost fertility?

Whether or not certain foods can boost fertility is a matter of great debate. Some natural health practitioners strongly believe that they can. However, many doctors and other health experts profoundly disagree. Leading fertility specialists maintain that no food in the world can actually make you more likely to conceive.

To a certain extent, this is a matter of interpretation. If your diet lacks certain important nutrients, this could lead to fertility problems. A deficiency of zinc, for example, has been linked to low sperm counts. In such cases, eating zinc-rich food – such as eggs and whole grains – may help to improve the man's fertility. In general, however, most health professionals agree that following a healthy balanced diet, drawing on all the main food groups every day, is the best route to optimum fertility for both partners. Remember, too, that this must be combined with regular, sustained exercise.

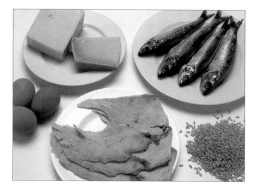

Foods that are rich in zinc, which is important for male fertility, include sardines, turkey, eggs, brown rice and cheeses such as Parmesan and Cheddar.

FERTILITY FOODS FOR MEN

Prospective fathers should eat a healthy, nutritionally balanced diet that includes foods rich in vitamins A, B, C and E, and essential fatty acids (which are found in oily fish and polyunsaturated fat). Men also need to eat foods that contain the minerals zinc and selenium.

Zinc and vitamin C play particularly important roles in the question of male fertility. Zinc is needed for the production of sperm and the male hormones: several prominent research studies have found that the male sex glands and sperm contain high concentrations of zinc.

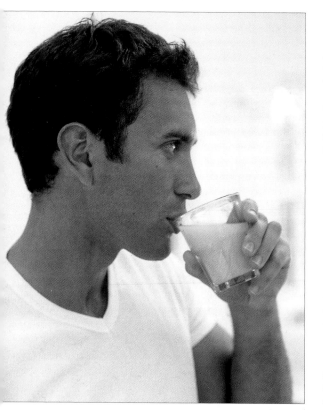

> **HERBAL TEAS FOR FERTILITY**
> Herbalists recommend the following teas, singly or in combination, three times daily:
> - cinnamon
> - cramp bark
> - ginger
> - ginseng
> - lemon balm
> - lady's mantle
> - motherwort
> - vervain
> - winter cherry

Men can play their part by sticking to five portions of fruit and vegetables a day. A glass of orange juice counts as one portion.

> **Drawing on all the main food groups every day is the best route to optimum fertility.**

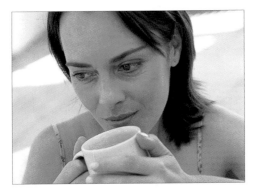

To enhance your preconceptual health, make sure you drink enough – but of the right kinds of drinks such as fruit juices, smoothies, herbal teas and lots of water.

Vitamin C is thought to reduce the tendency of sperm to clump together in the woman's body – a common cause of infertility. Modern diets are often low in zinc, and stress, smoking, pollution and alcohol deplete the body's levels further. Zinc-rich foods include oysters and shrimps, as well as other shellfish, sardines, turkey, duck and lean meats. Parmesan and Cheddar cheese are good sources of zinc, as are eggs, wholegrains, brown rice and nuts.

Citrus fruits, strawberries, kiwi fruit and peppers are excellent sources of vitamin C and should be included as part of your five servings of fruit and vegetables a day. Citrus fruits also provide selenium, another nutrient that is needed for fertility. One of the best sources of vitamin A is liver (not to be eaten by pregnant women or those trying to conceive), also found in egg yolks, dairy products, carrots, red peppers and leafy vegetables. You can get B vitamins from meat, green vegetables and wholegrains. Vitamin E is found in nuts and most vegetable oils.

FERTILITY FOODS FOR WOMEN

Any woman who is wanting to conceive should ensure that they follow a balanced, healthy diet. This diet should include foods rich in fatty acids, vitamin C, zinc, iron and folic acid – all easy to obtain from everyday foods. Iron-rich foods include meat, fish, eggs, dark green leafy

The best way to up your intake of vitamin C is to eat as much fruit as possible. Take melon, for example, for breakfast with muesli or as an after-dinner dessert.

vegetables and dried fruit. Good supplies of folic acid are found in green leafy vegetables, and also in nuts and pulses (see also pages 34–35).

If you have been taking the contraceptive pill, it may be helpful to increase your intake of foods containing the mineral manganese (good sources include oats, rye bread and peas) and also vitamin B6 (green vegetables and wholegrain cereals). These foods help to break down oestrogen, an excess of which may be associated with infertility. Eating zinc-rich foods might also be helpful (although shellfish should be avoided).

KEEP IT FRESH AND RAW

Another vital aspect of healthy eating is choosing fresh, unprocessed foods. There is still much research to be done on the effects of an over-refined, chemical-laden diet on fertility and pregnancy, but fresh produce, with fruits and vegetables raw or lightly cooked, is as beneficial to the prospective parent as it is to all of us.

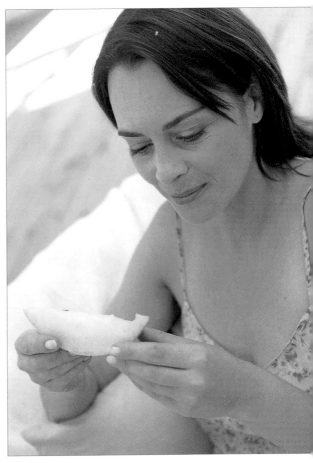

Do I need supplements?

You need more of certain nutrients before conception and during pregnancy. For example, your iron requirement almost doubles while your baby is growing. Many experts believe that pregnant women and those trying for a baby can obtain all the minerals and vitamins they need from a healthy, balanced diet. However, many women are still routinely prescribed supplements of iron.

All women need to take supplements of folic acid. This is needed before conception and during early pregnancy in an amount that is difficult to derive from our food.

Some women may be advised to start taking other supplements such as calcium as the pregnancy progresses. However, this is only if they cannot obtain sufficient supplies from their diet.

FOLIC ACID

An essential B vitamin, folic acid (folate) cannot be produced by the body, so it must be obtained through diet or supplements. Women hoping to conceive and in the early stages of pregnancy need 400 micrograms (mcg) of folic acid every day, to help the baby's spine and brain to develop properly. To ensure that you are getting enough, take a 400mcg supplement before conception and for the first 12 weeks of pregnancy. You should also eat plenty of folate-rich foods such as Brussels sprouts, wholemeal bread and orange juice. If you get your folic acid via a multivitamin, check that it has the recommended amount and that it does not contain vitamin A, which can be harmful. A higher dose of 500mcg is recommended if you have diabetes or there is a family history of neural tube defects and possibly if you take anti-epilepsy medication – see your doctor for advice.

FOODS HIGH IN FOLIC ACID

- spinach and other leafy vegetables
- broccoli
- green peas
- asparagus
- Brussels sprouts
- orange juice
- tomato juice
- oranges
- strawberries
- bananas
- grapefruit
- wholemeal bread

Folate levels decrease over time and with cooking, so do not store fruit or vegetables for long periods before eating. Cook vegetables lightly by steaming, microwaving or stir-frying.

FOLIC ACID AND THE NEURAL TUBE

Women hoping to conceive need 400mcg of folic acid a day, to ensure the healthy development of the baby's spine and spinal cord.

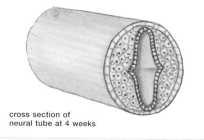

cross section of neural tube at 4 weeks

What folic acid does

Folic acid protects the neural tube – which will go on to form the spine and spinal cord – and helps it to close properly. This helps ensure normal brain and spinal cord development. Folic acid can help protect an unborn baby from developing spina bifida (an abnormal development of the spinal cord) and anencephaly (absence of most of the brain). Infants born with anencephaly die shortly after birth, and babies with spina bifida are born with partial or total paralysis.

The neural tube should close between the 25th and 30th day after conception, when women may not realize they are pregnant. This is why all sexually active women of childbearing age should take folic acid each day.

NUTRIENTS AND PREGNANCY

It is important that you obtain a sufficient amount of all vitamins and minerals before and during pregnancy. However, some minerals have particularly important roles to play in the health of both mother and baby, so you should pay particular attention to ensuring that you are getting enough. Eating foods that are rich sources of these minerals is the most natural way of upping your intake, but some women may need to take supplements.

Calcium

You should make sure that you are getting enough calcium before you conceive because once you are pregnant the baby will deplete the reserves of calcium in your bones and teeth. Calcium is essential for the healthy development of your baby's teeth and bones, which

Take a short walk every day so that you receive exposure to sunlight. This enables the body to manufacture vitamin D, which in turn aids the absorption of vitamin C.

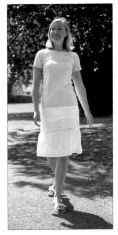

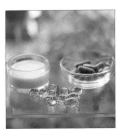

begin to form from around weeks four to six.

Your body absorbs calcium more efficiently during pregnancy, and your baby is unlikely to go short. The baby will take what calcium it needs, but this may not leave you enough for your own requirements.

Make sure that you eat and drink plenty of calcium-rich foods before conceiving and throughout your pregnancy. You will need the equivalent of 600ml (1 pint) milk a day. A small pot of yogurt or 25g (1oz) hard cheese contain as much calcium as about 200ml (⅓ pint) milk.

Vegans and women who never drink milk, either because they are allergic to it or because they simply don't like it, may need calcium supplements. If you are eating well, 600 milligrams (mg) should be enough, but 1200mg may be advised in some cases.

Vitamin D helps the body to absorb vitamin C properly. This vitamin is found in milk, butter and eggs. More importantly, however, the body can manufacture its own vitamin D if it is exposed to the sun. You should therefore take a short walk outdoors each day to expose your face, hands and arms to daylight. Women in the UK are recommended to take 10mcg vitamin D daily during pregnancy and while breastfeeding. In other countries, such as the USA and Canada, milk is fortified with vitamin D, so more can be obtained through diet.

Iron

During pregnancy, your body manufactures extra blood, and your requirement for iron increases at the same time. You will probably need almost twice as much iron as you did before you became pregnant.

Iron is needed for the formation of haemoglobin, the oxygen-carrying pigment in red blood cells. If you don't have enough haemoglobin in your blood, insufficient oxygen may be transported to your organs and your baby. This will also result in your becoming very tired.

Make sure that you are eating plenty of iron-rich foods

Supplements such as iron come in a number of different forms. Chelated supplements are said to be more rapidly absorbed by the body.

before conception, particularly red meat and dark poultry meat. Vitamin C helps the body to absorb iron from other, plant-based sources more efficiently, so it is a good idea to have a glass of orange juice or a tomato salad with meals. Another simple way of increasing iron intake is to use iron pans when cooking.

Pregnant women are routinely prescribed iron tablets in some countries. A supplement may not be necessary if you eat a good diet with sufficient iron-rich foods (although it may be still necessary if you are expecting two or more babies). If you are worried about iron intake, or feel tired for no apparent reason, see your doctor. A simple blood test will determine if you are deficient (anaemic). It can be hard to get enough iron if you do not eat red meat, so vegetarians and vegans are often advised to take iron and B12 supplements.

Zinc

You need zinc to help the baby develop – there is evidence to suggest that an inadequate intake is linked to low birthweight. Make sure you are eating enough zinc-rich foods before conceiving; the body's levels of zinc can fall by as much as 30 per cent during pregnancy.

Foods to avoid and food safety

During pregnancy and the months before you conceive (both men and women), avoid taking in toxic substances if possible. You cannot combat environmental health hazards such as emissions from industrial sites, but you can make sure that you do not spend time in smoky atmospheres and that you avoid foods that may be harmful, are highly processed or lack nutritional value.

WHAT TO AVOID

The following substances may cause harm to you or your baby and should ideally be avoided completely.

- **Soft rinded or blue-veined or unpasteurized cheese** such as Brie and goat's cheese, due to the risk of listeriosis.
- **Raw or lightly cooked eggs and poultry,** as hens may be infected by salmonella and other bacteria. Cook eggs and chicken well to prevent infection.
- **Raw beef** including steak tartare, rare beef and undercooked beefburgers, regardless of where the meat comes from, because of the risk of BSE.
- **Certain fish,** because they contain mercury, which can harm the developing nervous system in an unborn child. Avoid shark, swordfish and marlin and eat no more than one tuna steak or two medium cans of tuna each week.
- **Shellfish and raw fish,** which carry a higher-than-average risk of food poisoning.
- **Liver,** liver pâté and liver sausage. They are high in vitamin A, which can cause damage to the fetus.

OESTROGEN AND FERTILITY PROBLEMS

The female hormone oestrogen, used in some contraceptive pills, plays a vital role in reproduction. Research suggests that some women who take an oestrogen-containing pill for several years may suffer reduced fertility for a few weeks or months when they stop. Oestrogens are also found in non-organic dairy produce and meat, fish from polluted waters, pesticides, plastic containers and clearfilm.

Increased exposure to synthetic oestrogens may be one reason for the rise in fertility problems. In men, too much oestrogen can lower sperm count, while an excess in women is thought to be associated with conditions such as endometriosis and ovarian cysts, both of which adversely affect fertility.

- **Unpasteurized milk,** which may harbour highly harmful bacteria, including salmonella and listeria (see also section on preventing food poisoning).

Minimize your intake of the following foods and drinks:

- **Alcohol,** which may impede the uptake of B-vitamins, zinc and iron, lower hormone levels, inhibit ovulation and the ability of sperm to move, and harm a fetus.
- **Tea and coffee,** whose caffeine content may harm female fertility. A lot of tea can impede iron uptake.
- **Sugary foods** such as cookies, cakes and other sweet snacks and drinks, which contain few nutrients.

BANISHING CAFFEINE

If you want to conceive, it is a good idea to cut out or cut down on caffeine, tea and chocolate. Researchers have found that they can have an adverse effect on female fertility.

One study found that taking in more than 300mg of caffeine a day lowered a woman's chance of conceiving by as much as 27 per cent. Even modest consumption appears to hinder conception: women who drink only one to two cups daily lowered their chances of conceiving by about 10 per cent.

Another study found that an intake of more than 300mg of caffeine a day may be associated with miscarriage. In addition, pregnant women who drank eight or more cups of coffee a day were found to have double the risk of stillbirth as women who did not drink coffee.

It is helpful if you have some way of measuring 300mg of caffeine. This 300mg limit is roughly equivalent to the following items:

- Four cups or three mugs of instant coffee.
- Three cups of brewed coffee.
- Six cups of tea.
- Eight cans of regular cola drinks.
- Four cans of energy drinks.
- Two 200g (7oz) bars of chocolate.

There are all kinds of non-caffeine hot drinks available today that form good alternatives to tea and coffee, from herbal tea to barley-based drinks.

- **Fried foods and junk food**, which are high in unhealthy fats and should be avoided where possible.
- **Salt**, from adding salt to food or eating salty snacks such as crisps (US potato chips). Excess salt increases the risk of high blood pressure, which can be harmful.
- **Convenience foods and takeaway meals**, as these have poor nutrient value. Eat fresh, natural foods.

PREVENTING FOOD POISONING

Poor food hygiene is responsible for thousands of cases of food poisoning every year. Most people suffer a bout of diarrhoea or sickness and have no long-term effects. However, pregnant women need to take great care to avoid food poisoning, since there is a real threat to the unborn baby. Infants and children are also at risk.

Food poisoning is usually the result of eating food that has been contaminated by bacteria. These precautions will help prevent bacteria from spreading and multiplying:
- Wash your hands with hot water and an antibacterial soap before and after handling food, especially poultry, raw meat, fish, seafood, salads, vegetables and eggs.
- Wash your hands with hot water and antibacterial soap after handling cats, dogs and other domestic pets.
- Disinfect kitchen surfaces with an antibacterial solution, to kill potentially harmful bacteria.
- Use plastic, not wooden, chopping boards, and disinfect them after each use. Use separate boards for cooked and raw foods.
- Fridges should be kept at under 5°C (41°F). Use a fridge thermometer to be sure the temperature is right.
- Store raw foods separately from ready-to-eat and cooked foods (place raw meat and fish on the bottom shelf of the fridge). Always abide by use-by dates.
- Regularly clean taps, telephones and any gadgets in the kitchen, using an antibacterial solution.

Avoiding listeriosis

Listeriosis is caused by the bacterium *Listeria monocytogenes*. If caught during pregnancy, it can result in miscarriage, stillbirth or severe illness in the baby.

High levels of listeria have been found in some foods, so it is advisable to avoid these. They include:
- Unpasteurized milk.
- Pâté made from meat, fish or vegetables.
- Mould-ripened and blue-veined cheeses.
- Soft-whip ice cream from ice-cream machines.
- Pre-cooked poultry and cook-chill meals unless thoroughly reheated.
- Prepared salads, unless washed thoroughly.

Avoiding Campylobacter pylori

The bacterium *Campylobacter pylori* is the chief cause of food poisoning in both the UK and the USA – it accounts for more than 2.5 million cases of food poisoning in the USA every year. The bacterium is found in raw meat, poultry, wild birds and unpasteurized milk. This is one reason why pregnant women need to avoid raw and lightly cooked eggs and undercooked chicken.

Avoiding salmonella

Salmonella is a bacterium commonly found in hens. Be sure to cook poultry and eggs thoroughly when you are trying for a baby and during pregnancy. Do not eat foods containing raw egg, such as fresh mayonnaise.

Avoiding toxoplasmosis

Toxoplasmosis is an infection caused by a parasite that can cause miscarriage or damage to the unborn baby. It may be present in soil, so fresh fruit, vegetables and lettuce are all potential sources of infection. They should be thoroughly washed under running water.

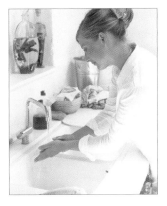

Be sure to wash your hands with antibacterial soap both before and after handling foods.

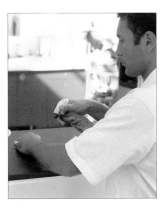

Always disinfect kitchen surfaces and chopping boards after preparing food on them.

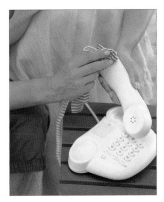

Use an antibacterial solution to wipe over taps, telephones and kitchen surfaces regularly.

A healthy day

You want to be as healthy and fit as possible before conceiving a baby. This cleansing programme offers a gentle way to eliminate toxins from the body without putting it under any stress. Undertaking a preconceptual cleanse with your partner can also be a pleasurable way to relax and spend some time together.

Some people associate cleansing with total fasting. However, it is very important that you do not take any extreme measures before conception and during pregnancy. Fasting is not good for the body, and should be avoided, in particular, by anyone wishing to conceive.

This programme emphasizes exercise, rest and relaxation together with healthy eating. Feel free to adapt it according to your individual needs. No special equipment is used, but you will need a soft-bristled brush for the skin, and essential oils of your choice.

A day of cleansing

Set aside a whole day – or even a weekend – for your cleanse. Choose a time when you know that you won't be interrupted, so you can focus totally on yourselves.

1 As soon as you wake up, drink a glass of hot water with a slice of lemon in it. Lemon possesses cleansing properties so will aid the cleansing process. (Drinking hot water with lemon when you wake up is a good habit to acquire.) Then eat a piece of fruit or a slice of wholemeal bread – don't add any butter or spread. This will get your digestive system moving.

2 Do some gentle stretching, yoga or warm-up exercises. Then, do 30 minutes of brisk exercise. This could take the form of running, fast walking or any other exercise that makes you slightly breathless (you should still be able to keep up a conversation). Brisk exercise speeds up your circulatory system, bringing oxygen and nutrients to all areas of the body and helping to eliminate toxins. Afterwards, drink a large of glass of water, and some juiced or liquidized fruit or vegetables.

3 Next, dry-brush your whole body in order to remove dead skin cells – either brush your own body or do this for your partner. Brush upwards, using long strokes on the arms and legs. Spend at least five minutes doing this, then take a warm shower. Use a body scrub to help slough off more dead skin cells in the water.

4 After the shower, deep-cleanse your face. Pour some boiling water in a large bowl, add a few drops of essential oil (chamomile, lavender or lemongrass are good oils to choose), then place a towel over your head. Let the steam soak into your skin for a few moments, then remove the towel and pat your face dry. Splash your face with cold water a few times to tighten up the pores again.

5 You and your partner may like to give one another a massage at this point. Massage helps to boost the circulation, which speeds up the elimination process. Enjoy a full body massage, or concentrate on the legs and feet, where toxins tend to collect. A foot massage is easy to do if you are on your own and improving the circulation here will have a knock-on effect for the whole system.

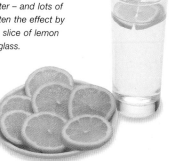

The most important aspect of cleansing is to drink water – and lots of it. Heighten the effect by adding a slice of lemon to each glass.

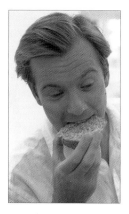

Wholemeal bread without butter is a wake-up call for the body's digestive system. Drink at least one glass of water, with lemon, beforehand.

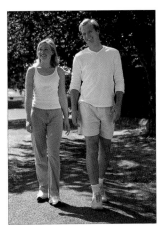

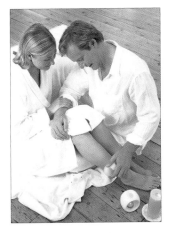

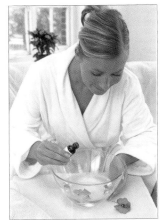

Exercise and fresh air are not only an essential part of detoxification, but are important elements of a healthy and enjoyable lifestyle.

Use a soft-bristled brush to energize your skin and remove dead cells. You and your partner can do this for each other if you like.

Give yourself a mini face treatment. Add a drop or two of essential oil to a bowl of boiling water, then allow the steam to cleanse your skin.

6 Spend some time relaxing after your massage; give yourself 30 minutes or an hour of total rest. Then do some gentle yoga or stretching to re-energize yourself. Stretching helps to mobilize the joints; it also increases the flow of blood, and brings nutrients and oxygen to different areas of the body.

7 Have a small lunch of fruit, vegetables and cereals. Stay sitting upright for at least 15 minutes after eating, to help your digestion. Then, go out for a short walk.

8 Do some meditation at this point, or simply sit quietly and focus on your breathing. Breathing deeply helps to get more oxygen to the muscles and organs. Wait two hours after eating, then do another session of exercise.

9 Have a salt rub. Waste products are excreted through the skin and massage, exfoliation and salt rubs all help keep the pores clean and healthy. You can use any type of salt mixed with a little olive oil. Rub into the skin with a circular motion, moving away from the heart. This aids the circulation and elimination systems.

10 Have a long aromatic bath, with your partner or by yourself. Dilute a couple of drops of aromatherapy oil in a carrier and add to the water. Afterwards, moisturize your skin. Combine this with another massage if you like.

11 Spend the rest of the evening quietly, perhaps incorporating some more yoga or stretching. Go to bed early to be sure that you get plenty of rest.

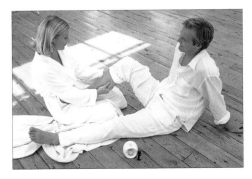

Take it in turns to give each other a relaxing massage. Try a leg and foot treatment, then a back massage.

ESSENTIAL ELEMENTS OF A HEALTHY DAY
Throughout the day:
- Drink only water. You should have at least 2 litres (3½ pints) and preferably more. Have a large bottle for each of you on hand so that you can keep topping up. This will also help you to monitor how much you have drunk.
- Eat lightly every two or three hours. Choose fibre-rich foods: fresh fruits, raw or lightly steamed vegetables, and whole-grain cereals.
- Remember that this is your time to relax – do not read, watch television or answer the telephone, and try not talk about anything contentious.

Common Qs and As

Q: I have found all sorts of weird foods and food remedies for boosting fertility on the Internet. Do they work?

A: Most fertility specialists and gynaecologists would recommend that you eat a wide variety of healthy foods every day with plenty of vegetables and plenty of water. There is no need to single out any one particular food. Refer to pages 32–35 to ensure that you are not missing out on any nutrients.

Q: I have heard that cleansing is a necessary part of preconceptual care. Why?

A: Many people feel healthier, more active and invigorated after cleansing for a short period, say a weekend. One of the great strengths of cleansing is the focus upon drinking plenty of water and exercising, both of which are very good for us. However, a healthy lifestyle that you can maintain every day is likely to be much more helpful than the occasional short cleanse.

Q: I was anorexic when I was younger. Could this make a difference to my chances of conceiving now?

A: Provided that your periods have returned to a normal pattern, your previous anorexia shouldn't affect your chances of conceiving. However, in view of your medical history, you may be wise to consider a combined multivitamin and multimineral supplement. Check this with your family doctor, and make sure that any supplement you do take is suitable for pregnant women.

If your periods have not returned to normal, you should consult your family doctor without delay. If necessary, ask your doctor for a referral to a consultant gynaecologist.

Q: I have a very fast-paced job and tend to eat on the wing. Could this adversely affect my chances of conceiving?

A: Eating in this way may not affect your chances of getting pregnant, but it will certainly not help either. Eating snacks hurriedly is not a good or healthy dietary habit, and it makes it hard for you to ensure that you are getting all the nutrients you need. If you have any other underlying medical problem, poor nutrition will tend to exacerbate the problem.

You may like to consider starting to pace yourself now for life with a baby, by eating regularly and well. Snacking as you go will become increasingly difficult and impractical once you have a child to consider.

Remember, too, that stress can affect your fertility and your ability to cope with pregnancy, so you might want to consider slowing down your lifestyle as part of your preconceptual care.

Q: I don't usually want to eat much in the morning, as early-morning eating makes me feel a bit queasy. Now I am trying for a second baby, I want to make sure that I get into eating habits that give me enough nutrients. How can I try to achieve this?

A: First and foremost, ask yourself if there are any foods that seldom make you feel queasy in the morning. You do not have to eat standard 'breakfast' fare. If you find the only thing you can eat is chicken tandoori, so be it. Secondly, make sure you have plenty of fluids, especially water, and try drinking juices or smoothies, for their extra nutritional value. Thirdly, make sure that your other meals include plenty of protein foods such as meat and fish, as well as wholegrain bread and pasta, and fruits and vegetables. These foods will help to keep you going.

Q: I have noticed that most of my friends manage to control their weight gain quite well with their first baby. Once it comes to the second baby, though, some of them have blown up by three stone (nearly 20kg) or more. How can I stop this happening to me?

A: The best thing you can do is to exercise regularly for the duration of the pregnancy and afterwards as well – swimming two or three times a week is ideal. Mothers who are at home with the first baby may find it difficult to take time out to exercise. If this is the case with you, try walking for a good 30 minutes a day with your first baby in a pushchair. Avoid high-calorie foods such as chocolate, biscuits, pastries, cakes, sugary foods, salty foods, fried foods, crisps, peanuts and alcohol.

Q: I shall be going abroad soon for a long vacation. I am worried about what we eat and how it is prepared since we are trying for a baby. Are there any precautions I should take?

A: You should always take care with what you eat and follow good hygiene practices when travelling in a developing country. In particular:

- Do not eat snacks from street stalls.
- Do not eat any salads or peeled fruit or fruit salad.
- Do not eat shellfish, pâté, raw steak, undercooked poultry, raw or lightly cooked eggs, or soft rinded or blue-veined or unpasteurized cheeses.
- Do not drink local water or have any ice in your drinks. All water should be bought bottled or thoroughly boiled before use.
- Clean your teeth with bottled water.

Check to see if there are any inoculations you need for your country of destination – and how far in advance you need to have them. Ask your doctor how these could impinge upon pregnancy first.

Q: There seems to be a new health scare almost every week about some food or other that pregnant women must not eat. I am becoming increasingly worried about my diet. How can I be sure that what I eat is safe?

A: This is a good question, but nobody can give you a cast-iron assurance that your diet is absolutely safe. The reason for this is that medical research, scientific research and research into nutrition is going on all the time. Scientists do make new discoveries, which they then publish. Newspapers can then seize upon this information and make the most of it – sometimes inflating it into scare stories. This can have the effect of making us think that none of the food we eat is really safe.

It is impossible to live without exposing yourself to any risk at all. The best you can do is to be pragmatic and to take precautions where you can. It has been well-established, for example, that some foods are unsafe or carry a higher risk in pregnancy, so it is sensible to avoid them. These include raw eggs, liver, some soft cheeses and some fish and meat. We also know that a diet including whole cereals, fresh fruit and vegetables, most fish, well-cooked chicken and other foods will give you a good range of nutrients, which helps your baby to develop. Making sure that you are following a balanced, healthy diet is therefore very important.

You should also take care to observe the rules of food hygiene. It can be a good idea to avoid eating out or getting takeaways unless you can be sure that good standards of hygiene are practised in the restaurant. Other than that, the best thing to do if you read any stories in the media that worry you is to have a talk with your midwife or doctor. They will help you to decide what, if any, changes to your diet you need to make.

Top fertility factors

❝ There is seldom any need to worry if pregnancy doesn't happen right away. ❞

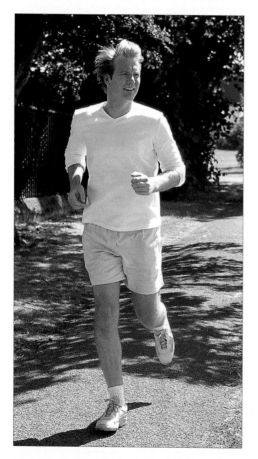

Some women become pregnant while barely thinking about it – it just happens. Others plan the pregnancy and find that they are pregnant within a few months. The remaining few may take more than a year to conceive and some of those may encounter a delay that is even longer than that.

There is seldom any need to worry if pregnancy does not happen straight away – this is very common, and many couples take the best part of a year to conceive. In fact, infertility is officially defined as over a year of regular, unprotected sexual intercourse without conception.

There are many ways in which you can boost your fertility level, as you will see throughout this chapter. De-stressing through complementary therapies and using positive thinking techniques are especially beneficial, not only before conception but also during pregnancy. In addition, you can prepare to eliminate the common causes of infertility before you even attempt to become pregnant. For example,

Keeping in good physical shape – and this includes your partner as well as yourself – is a key aspect of preparing the body properly for conception.

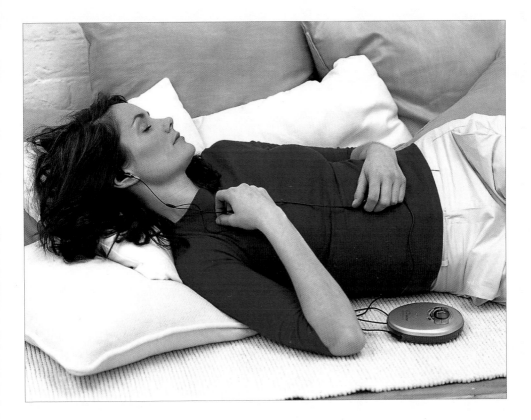

giving up smoking and cutting out alcohol are vital steps towards a healthy conception and pregnancy. Your weight is another important consideration: levels of extreme thinness and, conversely, carrying excessive weight, both adversely affect fertility levels in both women and men. As with everyone, attention to diet is the key issue here, combined with regular exercise, and sufficient levels of sleep.

There are much rarer causes of infertility, such as inherited diseases. In these cases, specialist genetic counselling may provide the way forward, and is readily available. There may also be a medical reason that hinders or delays conception, which will need to be referred to a fertility specialist.

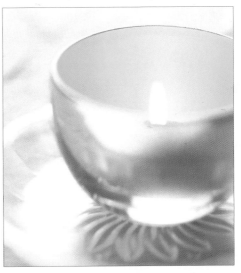

Top: Listening to soothing music is a really easy way to relax and unwind – it is thought that stress is a common cause of decreased fertility.

Simply using candles to create soft light and a calm atmosphere is another way to alleviate the build-up of stress that can creep up on all of us.

Getting pregnant

The best way of achieving a healthy pregnancy is to have sex as frequently as possible during the woman's fertile period, and for both partners to look at all the aspects of their lifestyle with a view to achieving optimum health and vitality.

HOW OFTEN SHOULD YOU HAVE SEX?

It used to be thought that a man would produce weaker sperm if he had sex very frequently. However, doctors now know that this is a myth, and so there is nothing to gain by you and your partner abstaining from sex with a view to producing more vigorous sperm. In fact, it is now well established that the more often you make love, the better the chance you have of getting pregnant.

Statistically, the chances of becoming pregnant in any one act of intercourse are low. However, you can increase your chances of conception by making love every day during the woman's fertile period. It is important to remember that many experts and researchers in the field of infertility are sceptical about the effectiveness of the various methods for calculating the fertile period. So, even if you think that you know when your fertile period is, you should still continue to have regular, unprotected sex at other times.

HOW LONG WILL IT TAKE TO CONCEIVE?

One important study into conception found that couples having sex once a month between the woman's periods took an average of 43 months in which to conceive. With couples having sex three times a month, the average time for conception was 15 months. If the couple made love ten times a month, the average delay was reduced

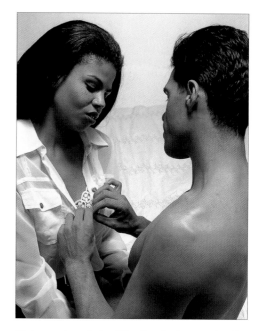

Give yourselves plenty of time to enjoy happy, relaxed lovemaking. The more often that you have sex, the more likely you are to conceive.

to five months. In couples who had sex 15 times or more each month, conception took an average of just three and a half months.

About one in six couples experience some delay or difficulty in becoming pregnant. You should not worry if it takes time for you to conceive, provided that the delay has not continued for more than a year. However, you should ensure that you are making love at least every other day during the woman's fertile period. Eighteen out of every twenty couples who are trying for a baby manage to achieve a pregnancy within a year. Another one in twenty conceive within two years. Others may succeed after trying for more than two years.

Nobody knows why conception can sometimes take a long time, or sometimes fail to happen at all. Many couples who have been trying for a year or two to become pregnant are perfectly healthy and have no obvious fertility problems. Ultimately, you may have to accept that conceiving a baby involves an element of chance – and it sometimes takes time.

THE PILL AND YOUR FERTILITY

Some women experience a delay in conception if they have been taking the Pill before they start trying for a baby. The majority of women find that their periods return to normal within three months of stopping the contraceptive pill, but a few may find it takes longer. If you are planning to conceive in the near future, some experts recommend that you stop the Pill and use alternative methods of contraception for three months before you try to get pregnant.

> **❝ There is nothing to gain by abstaining from sex with a view to producing more vigorous sperm. ❞**

EMOTIONAL FACTORS

It is often impossible to know why a woman does not conceive, but it is certain that emotional factors and stress as well as medical problems can play a part. Events such as moving house, starting a new job or suffering a bereavement in the family can all cause stress. This can reduce your desire to make love, and can also have a temporary effect on your fertility.

Sometimes the very fact that couples are trying for a baby can cause anxiety and so delay the wished-for conception. This is what lies behind the stories everyone has heard of couples who stop trying, and then quickly find that they conceive.

WHEN TO SEEK HELP

Medically, infertility is defined as the inability to conceive after more than a year of regular, unprotected sexual intercourse. You and your partner should see a doctor together if you have not conceived within a year of starting to try – or earlier if you think there may be a medical reason for the delayed conception.

It is a good idea to take a record of the start and finish dates of each period from the time that you started to attempt conception. This will help your GP and any specialist to understand your normal cycle.

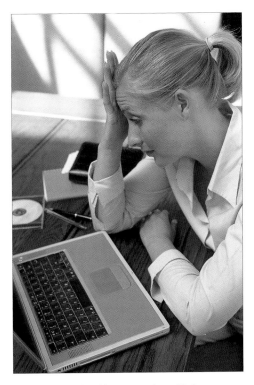

Feeling overwhelmed by your work can hinder your chances of conception – you may be too busy to make love at the right time, and stress can affect fertility.

Aside from medical problems, the causes for a delay in conception may include:

- Your age.
- Being overweight.
- Being underweight.
- Having a sexually transmitted disease.
- Drinking alcohol.
- Having a high caffeine intake.
- Smoking.
- Having intercourse at the wrong time – for example, being too busy to have sex during the fertile period.

Your doctor may give you individual advice on how to maximize your chance of conception, for example by helping to pinpoint the woman's fertile period or by advising you to, say, lose weight.

If appropriate, you may also be referred to a specialist for further investigations into the causes (see next chapter). Doctors do not usually refer couples for further treatment until after they have been trying to conceive for a year or more, unless there is a good medical reason to do so.

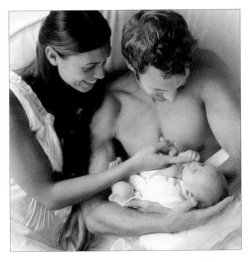

Don't be surprised if you do not conceive straight away. Many couples take more than a year to become pregnant, even when they are making love regularly.

Risk factors

Nobody knows why some women have difficulty conceiving, develop problems in pregnancy or give birth to babies with certain disorders or defects. But research has established a number of risk factors for pregnancy; these are listed opposite. Being affected by one or more of these risk factors does not mean that you cannot or should not become pregnant. However, it can mean that you may need closer monitoring and more detailed or frequent antenatal care than other women.

ASSESSING THE RISK
The many different risk factors may look daunting, so it is important to remember that over 97 per cent of pregnancies result in a healthy baby. If the medical staff involved in your care know of any risk factors, they can offer you appropriate tests and be fully prepared for any complications that may arise.

In some cases, women and their partners may benefit from genetic counselling before trying to conceive. Genetic counselling gives an individual assessment of your chances of having a baby affected by a congenital (developmental) disorder. This is usually offered to prospective parents who have a medical history that could affect a pregnancy. It may also be offered to women over 35 in order to evaluate the risk factor of age, and to women who have had three or more successive miscarriages.

HIGH BLOOD PRESSURE AND DIABETES
Established diabetes or high blood pressure can put the mother at a higher-than-average risk during pregnancy. These conditions can also develop during pregnancy, and this is one of the reasons that pregnant women need to attend regular antenatal checks before the birth.

High blood pressure
During pregnancy, high blood pressure is risky because it may lead to pre-eclampsia. This condition is one of the most common causes of miscarriage or stillbirth, so it needs to be carefully monitored by medical staff. Pre-eclampsia also poses a risk to the mother since it can lead to eclampsia, a serious condition that causes convulsions and can be fatal.

Symptoms include high blood pressure, swelling (in the face, ankles, wrists and sometimes all over the body) and the appearance of protein in the urine. This is one reason why urine is tested as part of a woman's antenatal care. Pre-eclampsia often develops at 30–34 weeks' pregnancy but it can start earlier or later.

Diabetes
There is no reason why women with diabetes should not bear a child, but they need careful supervision to ensure that their blood sugar and insulin levels are kept under control. Because of this, diabetic women are likely to attend antenatal clinics more frequently than usual. They usually have repeated blood and urine tests, so any problem can be promptly identified and treated.

Women with diabetes have a greater than average risk of such complications as stillbirth, pre-eclampsia, urinary infection and excessively large babies. For these reasons, pregnant women with diabetes are encouraged to attend hospital antenatal care and to have a hospital delivery so that specialist medical staff are on hand to assist.

Pregnancy diabetes is a form of the disease that occurs only in pregnancy and clears up soon after the birth. It carries the same risks as established diabetes.

RUBELLA AND RHESUS INCOMPATIBILITY
Both rubella and rhesus incompatibility can cause serious birth defects. These problems are more common than genetic and chromosomal disorders. However, you can be screened before conception so that both hazards can be avoided. Pregnant women are screened for rubella and rhesus incompatibility as part of their antenatal care.

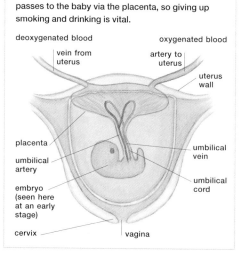

MOTHER AND BABY'S BLOOD SYSTEM
Whatever enters the woman's bloodstream passes to the baby via the placenta, so giving up smoking and drinking is vital.

deoxygenated blood   oxygenated blood

vein from uterus

artery to uterus

uterus wall

placenta

umbilical vein

umbilical artery

umbilical cord

embryo (seen here at an early stage)

cervix

vagina

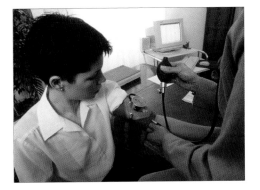

Your blood pressure will be taken regularly once you are pregnant, because high blood pressure can lead to problems in the pregnancy.

Rubella

Also known as German measles, rubella is a highly infectious viral disease. If a pregnant woman contracts rubella, the virus can attack the baby's nervous system and heart, causing deformities, miscarriage or stillbirth.

Rubella can exist in a very mild form and it is easy to mistake for a cold. Ideally, women should be checked for immunity to rubella before they attempt to become pregnant. If you are not immune, you can be vaccinated and then be checked again to make sure that the vaccine has worked. You should have the rubella immunity test, even if you think that you had rubella as a child. The disease is often misdiagnosed, and the duration of immunity acquired through illness is unknown.

Rhesus incompatibility

The rhesus factor is a substance found in blood: most people have it, and so are described as rhesus positive, but about one in six people do not have rhesus factor in their blood, and are rhesus negative.

Problems can arise when a rhesus-negative woman carries a rhesus-positive baby. In this case, some of the fetal blood cells can pass from the baby's body into yours. This provokes your body to make antibodies to fight the alien cells and destroy them. This reaction does not usually harm either you or the baby. The problem arises with a subsequent pregnancy if the baby is again rhesus positive. The woman's body now contains antibodies to fight and destroy rhesus-positive cells. These antibodies may pass into the circulation of the second baby and attack its blood cells, leading to severe anaemia, heart failure, jaundice or mental impairment. In an extreme case a baby would need a transfusion in the uterus, but women can be monitored for this situation and there are now injections available that help to prevent serious problems from arising.

FACTORS THAT MAY AFFECT YOUR PREGNANCY

The risk factors associated with conception and pregnancy include:

Age
- Being under 18.
- Being 36 or over.

Reproductive medical history
- Previous problem affecting the uterus, such as fibroids.
- Previous Caesarean or myomectomy (removal of fibroids from the uterus).
- Having an IUD in place at conception.
- Three or more miscarriages that occurred before existing pregnancy.
- Four or more previous deliveries.
- In a previous pregnancy, early labour, cervical stitch, late miscarriage, late termination, two or more terminations, stillbirth or neonatal death.
- Previous small or large baby.
- Congenital fetal abnormality in previous baby.
- Developing rhesus antibodies in previous pregnancy.
- Developing problems such as high blood pressure, proteinuria, pre-eclampsia in a previous pregnancy.
- Severe bleeding after giving birth to previous baby or manual removal of placenta.
- Very short labour (less than 2 hours) or long labour (over 12 hours) in previous pregnancy.
- Postnatal depression after birth of previous baby.

Other medical factors
- High blood pressure (140/90 or more, taken after you have been lying down for five minutes).
- Diabetes.
- Hepatitis B, HIV or AIDS.
- Family history of or congenital fetal abnormality.
- Having a heart murmur.
- Pelvic or abdominal abnormalities.
- Being underweight or overweight.
- Being less than 1.5m (5ft) tall.

Lifestyle factors
- Smoking.
- Drinking more than ten units of alcohol a week.
- Illegal drugs taken by either parent.
- Having had a high number of sexual partners or a partner who is bisexual.

Race
- If you are of Afro-Caribbean origin, a test for sickle-cell anaemia is suggested.
- If you or your family is of Mediterranean or Asian origin, a test for thalassaemia is suggested.

What is the best age?

The best time biologically for a woman to have a child is when she is aged between 20 and 25. However, biological fertility is not the only thing that women have to consider when deciding when to try for a baby. Many women do not meet the person they wish to have children with until much later in life, or they may feel unable to cope with the demands of a new baby when they are younger. Women may also wish to concentrate on other aspects of life, such as building a career or ensuring they are financially stable, before they have a family.

Women's fertility decreases with age, particularly after they reach 35. Statistically speaking, both mother and baby also face increased risks as the years go by. However, it is important to remember that statistics give an indication only of the likelihood of a problem occurring in particular circumstances; they cannot predict what will happen to individual women. In other words, women over the age of 35 will not necessarily experience difficulty in conceiving a healthy pregnancy, nor are women guaranteed a problem-free pregnancy if they have children in their twenties. Many women have experienced the successful delivery of a healthy baby when in their late thirties and early forties.

PROBLEMS WITH CONCEPTION

Older women may take longer to conceive for several reasons. Most important is the fact that age can affect the general fertility of both partners. In addition, older couples may make love less frequently, and conception depends on regular and frequent sexual intercourse. At the same time, the menstrual cycle is more likely to become irregular as the woman ages, which may make it more difficult to pinpoint the fertile period.

One problem for women over 35 is that any delay or difficulty with conception may take time to resolve. If, for example, a 36-year-old woman tries to conceive, it will probably be a year before she realizes that there is a problem. She will therefore be 37 by the time that she seeks help. Fertility tests, too, can take time, so she may be 38 by the time a problem is identified. During all this

> **Many women have experienced the safe and successful delivery of a healthy baby when in their late thirties and early forties.**

AGE AND THE LIKELIHOOD OF A DOWN'S BABY
The risk of a woman bearing a baby with Down's syndrome rises sharply as she ages.

Age	Risk factor
20	1 in 2000
25	1 in 1205
30	1 in 885
35	1 in 365
37	1 in 225
39	1 in 140
40	1 in 109
42	1 in 70
45	1 in 32
49	1 in 12

time, the woman's fertility will have continued to decrease. Women who decide to undergo artificial insemination or assisted conception also discover that these procedures are time-consuming. In an ideal world, any fertility treatments and assisted conception should be embarked upon earlier rather than later in the woman's childbearing years.

AGE-RELATED PROBLEMS IN PREGNANCY

One of the most common concerns felt by older mothers is that the baby will have Down's syndrome, a genetic error that causes both physical and mental impairment. The impairment can be such that the child can never lead an independent life. As people with Down's syndrome may live to over the age of 50, this can place an exceptional burden upon the parents.

The possibility of having a Down's syndrome baby is not the only consideration for older mothers. Other risk factors that are linked to age include the increased possibility of:

- High blood pressure, which can lead to pre-eclampsia.
- Diabetes developing in pregnancy.
- Miscarriage and genetic defects – the likelihood of miscarriage rises with age in the same way as the incidence of Down's syndrome, but it is not known why this is so.
- Babies of low birthweight.

Women over the age of 35 are also more likely to develop other general medical ailments that may have an impact on a developing baby. Some disorders may need treating with medication that may be inappropriate during

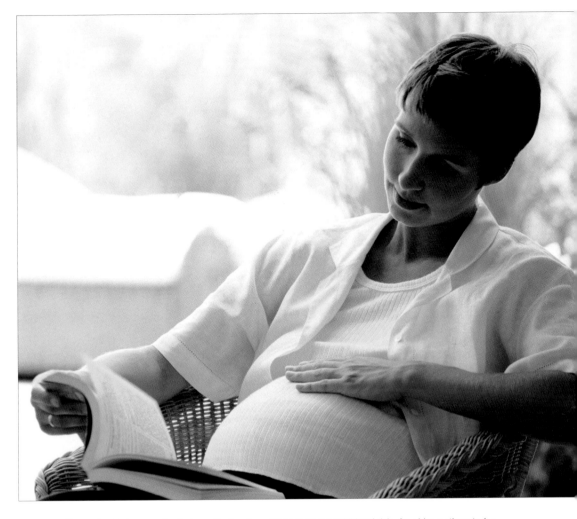

pregnancy. The mother-to-be may also feel very tired and suffer severe fatigue during labour. Pregnancy can also exacerbate any underlying medical condition, such as back pain or anaemia, because of the burden that it exerts upon the mother's body.

AN INDIVIDUAL PERSPECTIVE

All of this may seem highly alarming to the woman over 35 who is pregnant or who hopes to become so. However, you should be aware that all the risks discussed here are based on statistics – your individual risk may actually be much lower. After all, a large number of women over 35 do have extremely successful and trouble-free pregnancies. In general, it may be that the older mother takes a little longer to conceive and that there are more potential health risks both to her and the

While there are additional risks for older mothers-to-be, age brings with it an increased maturity and confidence that will be helpful during pregnancy and parenthood.

baby, but the important thing to remember is that with good antenatal care risks can be identified promptly, monitored and treated.

When it comes to younger mothers-to-be, women under 20 may be physically healthy, but this is not usually the best time to have a baby. The woman's body may not be fully developed, she may not have completed her education and she and the father may not be emotionally mature enough to cope with the demands of bringing up a child. Young mothers also tend to be less aware of the risks of smoking and drinking in pregnancy, and they may be less likely to attend antenatal care.

Your weight

Research shows that women who are underweight or overweight may have difficulty conceiving, and there is also some evidence to show that men's weight can affect their fertility.

THE EFFECT OF BEING UNDERWEIGHT

Being excessively thin may be the result of restricting food intake or of exercising too much. Both can upset the hormonal balance in the body with the result that your fertility is affected. Women need a certain amount of body fat in order to produce the hormones that control ovulation. This is why women who are very thin may stop ovulating and having periods altogether. Men who are very thin may suffer reduced sperm count or function.

The best way to achieve a healthy weight if you are too thin is to add plenty of complex carbohydrates such as wholewheat pasta and bread to a healthy, balanced diet. Do not increase your intake of high-fat foods.

THE EFFECT OF BEING OVERWEIGHT

Excess weight in men can affect their ability to produce sperm, while overweight women may experience difficulty conceiving. Pregnant women who are overweight are at greater risk of suffering birth complications. Also, if you are overweight, it will probably take you longer to recover from the labour and delivery and you will be prone to fatigue both during pregnancy and during the first few months of motherhood.

All of the health risks associated with being overweight can have an adverse impact on conception, on the course

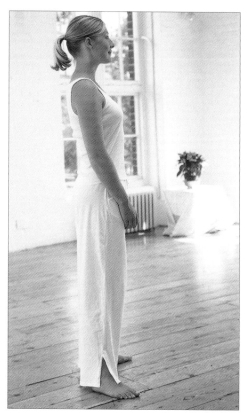

Being a healthy weight helps you to maintain good posture, which in turn reduces fatigue and aids the elimination of toxins from the body.

of the pregnancy and on the delivery itself – the most notable health risks in trying to become pregnant and maintaining a pregnancy are high blood pressure, diabetes and kidney disease.

LOOK TO THE FUTURE

Prospective parents may want to consider the long-term risks of being overweight, both for their own health and for the future well-being of their children. People who are overweight are more likely to die prematurely – and the risks rise with every extra stone that they carry.

If, for example, you weigh 85kg (about 13 stone) instead of the 65kg (10 stone) that would be ideal for your

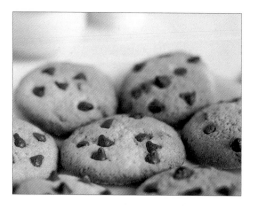

Being overweight reduces the chance of conceiving. If you weigh more than is ideal, cut out fatty, sugary foods.

height and build, your risk of dying within a given period increases by 60 per cent – statistically speaking, you are likely to die five years before your time.

All parents want to see their children through to a happy, independent adulthood. By looking after yourself, you will maximize the time you have with your children (and grandchildren) and the time they have with you.

CHECKING YOUR WEIGHT

The body mass index (BMI) provides a quick method of assessing whether you are a healthy weight for your height. Being under- or overweight may be harmful to your health and undermine your chances of conceiving. Check the box on page 29 to find out your BMI.

Your waist-to-hip ratio, which shows how much fat is stored in the abdomen, is another guide that you can use to assess your general health. To check your waist to hip ratio, divide your waist circumference by your hip circumference. The ratio should be less than 1 for men and less than 0.8 for women. For example, a man with a 80cm (32in) waist and 92cm (36in) hips would have a ratio of 0.88, which is fine. If his waist was 104cm (41in) and he had a hip measurement of 102cm (40in), the ratio would be 1.02, signifying he was overweight.

Both the BMI and the waist-to-hip ratio should be used as a rough guide only to your health and weight. If you are worried about your weight, it is a good idea to see your doctor for individual advice.

KEEP HEALTHY AND CONTROL YOUR WEIGHT

Diet and exercise should be the twin pillars of any weight-control programme that you may undertake. Natural therapies can help to strengthen and support your physical and emotional well-being, as well as aid weight control. If you want to lose weight, do so slowly and steadily – avoid any rapid weight-loss programmes, food supplements, diet pills or any diet that is based on a particular food group, such as all-protein meals. Ideally, you should reduce your weight to its optimum level and maintain it for several months before conception. You should not be dieting when you are trying to conceive or are pregnant.

- Eat healthily every day, and cut out sugar, salt, alcohol, cakes, biscuits, sweets, chocolate and peanuts. Your doctor may refer you to a dietician if you feel you need help with developing a healthy eating plan.

- Consider acupuncture to stimulate your energy levels, bolster your immune system and boost your lymphatic drainage system, which helps to eliminate toxins. A course of six or twelve sessions with a qualified acupuncturist may be the booster you need to set you on course for a controlled weight loss.

- Try the Alexander technique, a system of posture and balance that improves energy levels, strengthens all the muscles of your body, increases suppleness and helps you to move properly. All these factors may assist your weight control.

- Use essential oils (aromatherapy) to enhance your energy levels. Some oils help to eliminate toxins and some help you to relax and thus improve your posture and movement. Always check that the ones that appeal to you are safe to use during conception and pregnancy before buying.

- Visit a chiropractor or osteopath, who can help to correct poor postural habits and so strengthen muscles. Manipulation of the skeletal and muscular system can also help to remove energy blocks – thus assisting the efficient functioning of the body's processes.

- Take regular exercise at least every other day, but don't exhaust yourself. Walking and swimming are good ways to start exercising. Dance therapy is a fun method you may like to try.

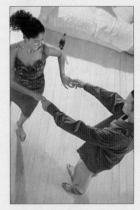

- Consult a herbalist for herbs that help to stimulate the lymphatic draining system and the elimination of toxins. Check that any you use are safe during conception and pregnancy.

- Try a massage or shiatsu. Both techniques can greatly improve the lymphatic drainage system. Toxins are eliminated and your vitality increases, which helps to speed up your metabolism and reduce hunger.

- Practise yoga for increased suppleness so that the muscles start to work at their optimum and your digestive system functions more efficiently.

- Consider homeopathy, focusing on those remedies that help cleanse the system and relieve fatigue. Check that your choices are safe to use in pregnancy.

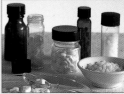

Fertility hazards

Smoking and drinking are two of the biggest risk factors for conception and pregnancy, but they are under your control. It is essential that you and your partner do not smoke at all if you are trying for a baby or if you are pregnant, and you should not drink more than a small amount before conception.

You should also try to avoid other harmful substances wherever possible. For example, avoid doing anything that brings you into contact with toxic substances and do not take any medication or supplements without discussing this with your doctor. In addition, you should be aware of any signs of poor health that you experience, and see your doctor promptly if you think that you are ill.

SMOKING AND INFERTILITY

It has been shown that smoking by either partner directly affects the chances of conceiving. Both partners should give up smoking some months (ideally at least four months) before attempting to conceive. This gives some time for your bodies to recover from the effects of smoking and also allows you to cope with any withdrawal symptoms that you may experience.

Smoking in the first few months of pregnancy is likely to have a more harmful effect on a baby's health than any other aspect of your lifestyle. Carbon monoxide and other poisonous chemicals will cross the placenta from your bloodstream directly into the baby's. This may affect development, and may make the baby more vulnerable to infection and disease.

Women who smoke during pregnancy are more likely to miscarry or to have a stillbirth. If they carry the baby to term, the baby is likely to be underweight (this is usually referred to as low birthweight) and he or she is more likely to suffer with infections of the respiratory tract, such as bronchitis and colds, in childhood. The child's ability to concentrate and learn may also be affected as may be his or her capacity for memory.

If you are already pregnant and still smoking, don't be tempted to think that it is too late to stop. It is not. You can minimize the damage to your baby by giving up now. Nicotine is a drug, which, like many others, is addictive, and it is undeniably difficult to stop smoking. Your doctor or midwife will offer you advice on good ways to quit. While you are doing so, it may be helpful to remember two things. First, if you give it up now, you will never have to go through the withdrawal symptoms again. Second, you are now doing your best to make sure that you give birth to a healthy child.

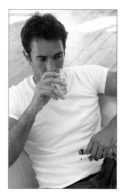

The occasional drink may do no harm, but both men and women should give up smoking before conception. Smokers and heavy drinkers may produce weak sperm that are unable to complete the journey to fertilize the woman's egg.

BREATHING IN TOXINS: WHAT SMOKING DOES

Tobacco smoke contains dozens of carcinogens. It also contains carbon monoxide, which is a poisonous gas that lowers the amount of oxygen carried around the body by the blood. Tobacco smoke also contains nicotine, which makes the heart beat faster and work harder than it should. Nicotine adversely affects blood-clotting factors, and so may play a part in heart attacks. In addition, tobacco smoke contains radioactive compounds, which are known to cause cancer. It contains hydrogen cyanide, which kills cilia, the tiny hairs that move together in waves to help keep the lungs clean and working efficiently. All of these toxins are entering your baby's bloodstream via the placenta each time you smoke.

DRINKING ALCOHOL

Fertility experts have different views on whether women trying to conceive should abstain completely from alcohol or merely cut down to a sensible level. Some experts believe that the occasional glass of wine or beer is unlikely to cause harm, but the official advice is for women to cut out alcohol.

It's important to avoid alcohol in the first three months because of the increased risk of miscarriage. if you do drink after that, then one small glass of wine or beer once or twice a week is probably a good limit to observe. The man should drink a maximum of two pints of lower strength beer or two glasses of wine a day, and preferably less than that.

Strive for a healthy lifestyle, good general fitness and relaxation. A happy, well-balanced relationship is vitally important if you are going to create a new life.

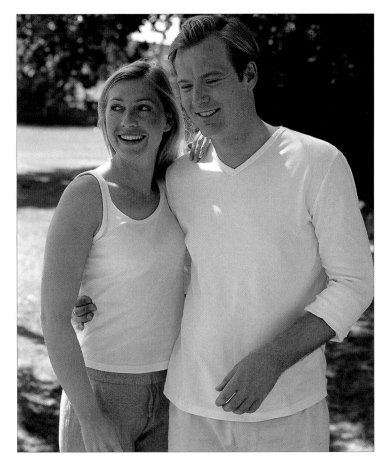

If you are experiencing any difficulty in conceiving – that is, if you have been having regular, unprotected intercourse for a year or more but have not achieved a pregnancy – then both partners should definitely consider abstaining from alcohol completely. Heavy drinking can affect both your chances of conception and the pregnancy itself. Men who are heavy drinkers may produce weak sperm and can also produce babies with serious defects. Women who drink excessively around the time of conception and during pregnancy can give birth to severely damaged babies. If you do drink heavily and wish to try for a baby, it is a good idea to see your doctor for advice beforehand. He or she may advise you to give up alcohol for several months before attempting to conceive.

YOUR GENERAL HEALTH

Ideally, both partners should be in good physical health before conceiving a child. This will give you the best chance of achieving a healthy pregnancy. A good level of health and fitness will also help the woman's body to cope with the demands of pregnancy and labour. It is worth seeing your doctor for a check-up, so you can sort out any health problems before conception. This will also help to reduce your risk of having to take medication during pregnancy. Look at the list of symptoms below, and let your doctor know if any apply to you:

- Aches, pains and inflammations.
- Allergy.
- Apathy, feeling overtired, having less zest for life.
- Asthma or shortness of breath.
- Bloating.
- Constipation or other bowel problems, such as diarrhoea.
- Cough, persistent.
- Dark circles under eyes.
- Dental abscess.
- Fluid retention (swollen ankles, legs or fingers).
- Regular indigestion.
- Swelling and pain in the joints.

The role of the genes

Everyone resembles their parents. You only have to look at a family photo album to see how obviously and how often human characteristics are passed on from one generation to the next.

The mechanism by which these resemblances pass down the generations is the gene. Every human being has around 70,000 genes, and each gene contains a piece of information about one detail of a person's inherited make-up. For an embryo in the uterus, the data contained in the genes function as instructions: they tell the growing organism how to organize the multiplying cells into a human baby (as opposed to a frog or a rose); and they make that baby an individual, with a unique set of identifying characteristics inherited from its parents.

These genes are responsible for all that we are at the moment of our birth. They determine physical details such as our build, hair colour and facial features. Genes also govern, for good and ill, our natural propensities. A bookish nature, a gift for football, playing the violin or painting – all these talents can be learned, but they tend to be inborn. That is, somewhere in those 70,000 genes there is one for intelligence, athleticism, musicality or artistry that comes to a child as a birthday gift from its father or mother.

WHERE GENES ARE

There is a complete set of genes within every cell of a human body. Each drop of blood, every hair – every tear, even – contains millions of copies of the total blueprint for each individual. This is why blood tests can tell doctors so much about a person's genetic make-up: all the information about who you are is there to be decoded.

Genes are stored in long strings of DNA, and DNA forms part of the 46 pairs of chromosomes in the core of every cell. Every person inherits 23 chromosomes from their father (via the specialized sex cells in sperm) and 23 from their mother (via the sex cells in ova). The mix is random, and unique from the very moment of conception. Each child in a family gets a different set of 46, and so a different collection of genes. This is why brothers and sisters are not clones of each other.

WHAT CAN GO WRONG

Copies of chromosomes are laid down within sex cells, ready to be passed on to the next generation. But sometimes the copying process can go wrong and a gene mutates. This can have no effect at all, or it may result in an abnormality that manifests itself as a disease in the next generation. If that disease is not fatal, and the person

THE SPIRAL OF LIFE
Genes are stored in the double helix of DNA. There is a complete set of genes in every human cell.

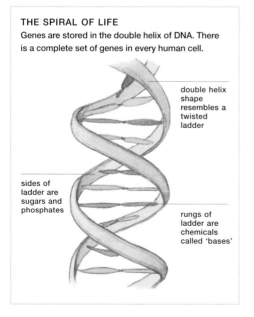

double helix shape resembles a twisted ladder

sides of ladder are sugars and phosphates

rungs of ladder are chemicals called 'bases'

INHERITED DISORDERS
Some of the most common inherited disorders include the following:
- Congenital heart defects.
- Diabetes, type 1.
- Cleft lip and palate.
- Colour blindness.
- Thalassaemia (blood disorder).
- Fragile-X syndrome (the leading cause of mental impairment).
- Sickle-cell anaemia.
- Cystic fibrosis.
- Muscular dystrophy.
- Haemophilia (blood-clotting disorder).
- Polycystic kidney disease.
- Haemochromatosis (iron storage disease).
- Achondroplasia (disorder of bone growth).
- Huntington's disease/Chorea (brain disorder).
- Albinism (lack of the pigment melanin).
- Marfan's syndrome (disorder affecting the heart, eyes and skeleton).
- Tay-Sachs disease (disorder affecting the brain).

affected grows up and has children, then the mutated gene can be passed on with all the others, perpetuating the illness in subsequent generations. So, a hereditary illness represents a tiny flaw in the genetic make-up of a person who may have lived generations ago. That person passed the flaw on by chance, in the natural way, and now it has become a fixture of the genetic make-up of some of his or her descendants.

However, there is another kind of disorder affecting the genetic process. Sometimes something goes wrong not with an individual gene, but with the entire chromosome. Some chromosomal disorders inevitably result in miscarriage, because some vital piece of genetic information has been lost. There are some chromosomal disorders which are not fatal or life-threatening, but do result in illness or some other medical disorder for the child. The best-known example is Down's syndrome, which results when an embryo inherits an extra chromosome from the parents, and so has 47 instead of the usual 46.

It is important to understand that chromosomal disorders are not hereditary. A hereditary disorder is one where all the genetic information has been passed on correctly to the embryo, but it just so happens that one of the characteristics that has been passed on is flawed or damaged from a health point of view. A chromosomal disorder, on the other hand, is one where the process has gone awry at the moment of conception. It is a genetic accident, not an inherited condition.

These disorders are rare: about one in every 100 births includes such a single gene disorder. Chromosomal abnormality occurs in about one in every 150 births.

WHAT IS GENETIC COUNSELLING?

Genetic counselling is a consultation with a doctor at which the possible effects of any genetic disorder, as well as your individual risk of passing a particular disorder on to your children, will be explained to you. You may also want to talk about the effect an inherited disorder may have on your child's quality of life; and how that disorder could be treated afterwards.

You may be offered genetic counselling if there is any condition within your own personal medical history, or the medical history of your partner or either of your families, that could suggest a risk. Genetic counselling may also be offered to older women, particularly those over 40, whose babies are statistically more prone to chromosomal disorders. Couples who are first cousins may be offered counselling, because they share a greater proportion of the same genes (inherited from their mutual grandparents) so there is more chance of any hereditary disorder being passed on.

Sometimes, entire communities are at greater risk of specific disorders. These are groups that, historically,

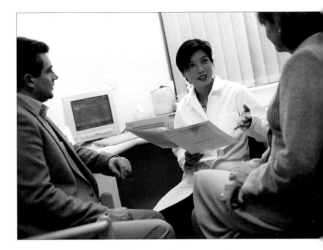

A genetic counsellor will help you and your partner to interpret scans and test results, in the context of your two families' histories. You will be given probabilities rather than forecasts; genetics cannot predict the future.

tend to intermarry for strong cultural or religious reasons, with the result that all the families in the group are genetically related to each other.

The genetic consequence of this is that the gene pool is smaller, and this has the effect of increasing the chance that any disorder that may exist will become more widely distributed than usual within the community. This increased risk will persist even after the cultural circumstances that created it have changed. So, for example, Ashkenazi Jews are more at risk than other people of Tay-Sachs disease. People of Mediterranean or Asian origin are statistically more likely to inherit thalassaemia.

GENETICS AND PROBABILITY

On its own, the fact that there is an inherited disorder in your family does not mean that you are a carrier of the disease, nor that you will inevitably pass it on to the next generation. Remember, only half your genes come from each parent, so there is only a 50:50 chance of any single gene being passed from a parent to you, or from you to your child. Moreover, the mere presence of a gene in your genetic make-up does not of itself mean that you will display that characteristic: not all genes are active in every person or every generation.

In the case of some hereditary diseases, you can be tested to determine whether or not you or your partner is a carrier. This is done by means of a blood test. You cannot be given a simple yes or no answer to the question 'Will my child develop a hereditary disease?'. All that can be determined is a statistical probability, and this can be used to advise you.

Relaxation and fertility

Stress and anxiety can delay conception, so it is important that you incorporate plenty of rest and relaxation into your life when you are trying to conceive. Exercise, too, is an essential part of your preconceptual and pregnancy care. Moderate physical activity not only contributes to general good health, but it also relieves stress and tension, thus helping to keep your hormones and menstrual cycle functioning normally.

EXERCISE

Incorporate three or four exercise sessions of about 30 minutes into every week. Walking in the fresh air and swimming are good options for women who are pregnant or hoping to become so, because they can be done for long periods without causing excessive tiredness. Whichever activity you choose, avoid exhausting yourself. Make sure that you combine your fitness programme with a healthy diet and drinking plenty of water.

SLEEP

How much sleep we need varies depending on our age, health and particular constitution. Most adults need about eight to ten hours a night in order to feel fully rested. Good-quality regular sleep is an absolute must for good health. As we sleep, our blood pressure decreases. The

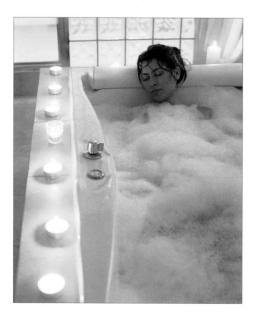

> ❝ Exercise can relieve stress and tension, thus helping to keep your hormones and menstrual cycle functioning normally. ❞

body's repair systems work more quickly and efficiently, so sleep is the time when damage is repaired. In addition, the body's natural elimination systems (the liver, the kidneys and the circulation) can carry out their work without having to process more toxins from the air we breathe or food we eat.

To help ensure a good night's rest, try the following:
- Establish a good sleep routine. Go to bed and get up at roughly the same time each day, even if you have had a bad night.
- Eat your last meal of the day at least three hours before bedtime. You can have a small snack before bed if necessary.
- Avoid stimulants in the evening, such as tea, coffee, alcohol and nicotine. Having a milky drink before bed can help you to get to sleep.
- Make sure the bedroom is well ventilated – open the window a little at night.
- Clear any daytime clutter, such as a computer, TV, newspapers or work papers, from the bedroom. If you can't clear them away, cover them up with a throw.
- Make sure that your bed gives you good support without being too hard.
- Avoid having stimulating discussions or arguments before bedtime – put them off until the next day.
- If you can't sleep, get up and go into another room. Try again in a few minutes or when you feel sleepy.

ACHIEVING PEACE OF MIND

Relaxation and peace of mind are important elements of your preconceptual care. Some psychologists say that there are three basic elements of happiness: having a good relationship, having something to do and having something to look forward to. Those are three important goals to work towards, but, whatever your circumstances, you can develop a relaxed attitude.

One step to peace of mind is to look at your present problems, worries, and dilemmas. If you feel anxious

Relaxation is an important aspect of improving your fertility. An aromatherapy bath, with candles, can be a wonderful way to release the strains of the day.

about any area of your life, sit down and write a list of the issues that worry you. Put them into categories: practical, financial, emotional, family and so on.

Now consider how you may be able to deal with those worries. Nagging long-term problems can be both destructive and extremely fatiguing: it is much better to deal with them if you are able to, or at least try and adopt a more relaxed attitude towards them. If you feel overwhelmed by a particular problem, it may be worth getting some additional help from either a complementary therapist or a counsellor.

Assess your priorities and take steps to deal with them in order of importance. List problems, too, so that you can seek help if necessary to resolve them.

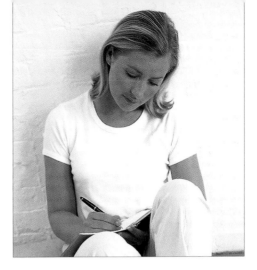

MONITOR YOUR STRESS RATING

Everybody has some stress in their life. However, it is possible to put a figure on your stress levels, as shown in this test devised by Holmes and Rahe in 1967.

Tick those events you have experienced in the last year, then add up your total. This will give an indication of the source and degree of stress in your life.

EVENT	SCORE
Death of spouse	100
Divorce	73
Marital separation	65
Prison term	63
Death of a close family member	63
Personal injury or illness	53
Marriage	50
Loss of job	47
Marital reconciliation	45
Retirement	45
Change in family member's health	44
Pregnancy	40
Sex difficulties	39
Addition to family	39
Business readjustment	39
Change in financial state	38
Death of a close friend	37
Change to different type of work	36
More or fewer marital arguments	35
Taking out a large mortgage or loan	31
Foreclosure on mortgage or loan	30
Change in work responsibilities	29
Son or daughter leaving home	29
Trouble with in-laws	29
Outstanding personal achievement	28
Spouse begins or stops work	26
Starting or finishing school	26
Change in living conditions	25
Change of personal habits	24
Trouble with boss	23
Change in work hours or conditions	20

EVENT	SCORE
Change in residence	20
Change in school	20
Change in recreational habits	19
Change in church activities	19
Change in social activities	18
Taking out a small mortgage/loan	17
Change in sleeping habits	16
More or fewer family gatherings	15
Change in eating habits	15
Holiday	13
Christmas	12
Minor violation of the law	11

TOTAL SCORE

Assess your stress rating by adding up the figures for each life event that you have experienced. If your total comes to less than 150, your rating is normal. If your rating comes to 150–299, you are experiencing more stressful events than the average person. A high level of stress can undermine your chances of getting pregnant, and you may be at risk of developing a stress-related condition. A score of 300 or more is very high, and your risk of becoming ill is much greater than normal.

If you have a high stress rating – or if you are feeling anxious, stressed or overwhelmed – make sure that you dedicate time each day to de-stressing and relaxing. There are many ways to do this – what is important is to find one that works for you. For example, you may need to do more exercise, take up yoga or meditation, or simply incorporate some 'me-time' into your day.

Preconception yoga stretches

Many doctors recommend yoga exercises such as these as an effective way to relax, which may help those trying to conceive. These exercises also increase blood flow (and so the supply of oxygen and nutrients and removal of accumulated waste products, which may cause imbalances), flexibility and strength in areas vital to conception, pregnancy and birth – the pelvic region, hips, abdomen and spine. Many yoga instructors believe that this approach encourages energy to flow freely around the body in a way that makes it more open to conception.

Pelvic movements with focused awareness

These relaxing movements encourage increased awareness, blood flow and flexibility in the pelvic area.

Feel that you are opening up to new healing energy and letting go of any tension there.

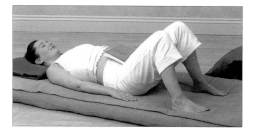

1 Lie down, with a large book and three cushions beside you. Place one cushion under your head and tuck in your chin to lengthen the neck. Bend your knees and plant the feet hip-width apart on the floor. Place the book on your lower abdomen, so it is evenly balanced on the hip and pubic bones. Place your arms alongside your body, with palms facing down to support you. As you breathe in, press on your hands and arch your lower back so that the navel and hip bones rise and your pelvis (and the book) tips towards your feet.

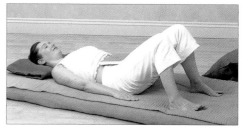

2 As you breathe out, gently pull in the navel towards the spine and press on your hands to lift the sitting bone (coccyx) just off the floor. With this movement, the pelvis (and the book) is now tipped backwards, towards your head. Keep your waist against the floor and move the lower spine only. Repeat these two movements several times. As you do so, bring real awareness of thought to your body. This will help you to do the movements in a focused way. Breathe naturally as you work; do not hold your breath.

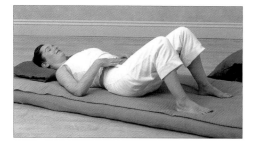

3 Now place your hands, in a relaxed pose, on top of the book. Breathe deeply, bringing your awareness to the pelvic region. Feel the movements of the book over the pelvic area as you breathe in and out slowly for several minutes.

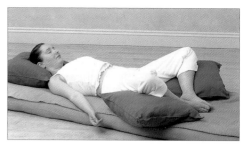

4 Remove the book and bring the soles of your feet together so that your knees fall outward. Support them with the remaining two cushions. Place your hands, palms up, beside you in a gesture of openness and complete surrender. Relax for several minutes.

Improving flexibility and muscle tone in the lower body

These three simple exercises improve flexibility in the spine and hips and strengthen the abdominal muscles. Work gently at first; your strength and flexibility will improve with practice. Relax afterwards and feel the effect of the exercises on your muscles and breath. Keep your coccyx on the floor throughout.

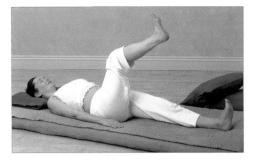

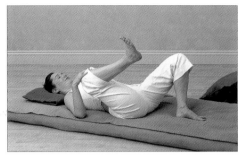

1 Lie on your back with a cushion under your head and your arms, palms down, alongside the body. Bend your right leg, keeping the left leg stretched with the ankle flexed. Make large cycling circles with your right leg until you feel tired. Then rest for a few moments with both legs stretched out – be aware of the muscles in the right side of the lower abdomen. Repeat the same number of circles with your left leg, and then rest again.

2 With your left knee bent and your left foot planted firmly on the floor, take hold of your right knee and move the right leg in circles from the hip. This releases any tightness in the groin and hip joint. Keep breathing naturally and work very gently, especially if the area feels stiff. It doesn't matter if the movements are very small, since your flexibility will gradually improve. Rest, then repeat the movements on the other side.

3 Now work with both knees and the breath. Breathe in as you take the knees out to the sides. Breathe out as you pull your knees close to your chest to stretch your lower back. Again, work very gently and build up your ability slowly – in yoga the point is always to work with the body, not to force it into uncomfortable positions. Repeat several times, then rest.

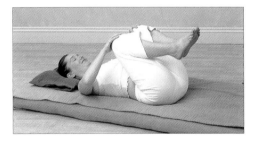

Lying twist

This powerful but simple twisting exercise opens up and relaxes both the shoulders and the hips. This in turn helps to make the entire spine more flexible, creating space between the vertebrae.

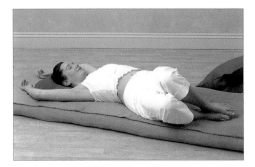

Lie down, raise your arms, bend them at the elbows, and place them on the floor above or beside your head. This position opens and lifts the chest. Bend your knees and place your feet together on the floor. Breathe in. As you breathe out, lower both knees to the right, ensuring that you keep them together. The aim is to place your right knee on the floor without letting your left elbow leave the floor, but only take it as far as feels comfortable. As you breathe in, raise your knees to the centre, still keeping them pressed together. As you breathe out, lower them to the left and raise them again as you breathe in. Repeat several times, then relax for several minutes.

Common Qs and As

Q: I had a pregnancy terminated when I was 17 – I am now 29 and married and wish to have my first baby. But I am worried that I may not be able to conceive because of the termination.

A: There is probably no reason for you to worry: many women have had a termination – even several terminations – and then gone on to have a healthy baby later on. The best advice is to go ahead and start trying, although you may wish to visit your family doctor to discuss your particular medical history.

Q: I have had thrush and a number of other infections in the past and wonder if this will affect my chances of becoming pregnant.

A: Many women suffer from regular thrush, and there is no reason why this should stop you from conceiving. However, a sexual health check is recommended for all women before attempting to conceive. Explain your circumstances to your family doctor and make sure that you have the full range of checks – especially the one for chlamydia, which often has no symptoms but frequently causes infertility.

Q: I have had two miscarriages early on in my pregnancies. I am now trying to conceive for the third time. Is it likely to happen again?

A: Miscarriage is very distressing, and it is not surprising that you are anxious about conceiving again. However, you may find it reassuring to know that having two successive miscarriages is quite common – you have only a slightly higher than normal risk of having another one. Doctors do not consider that you have a problem until you have had three successive miscarriages.

Get plenty of support before and after conception. If using natural therapies, choose a practitioner who is experienced in treating pregnant women.

Q: How do you know if you have one of the risk factors for pregnancy?

A: Most risk factors cause unusual symptoms. If you notice anything worrying, you should see your family doctor so that any problem can be identified and treated.

Some conditions, however, cause few or no distinctive symptoms. These include fibroids and ovarian cancer. If you are aware of any conditions that have affected members of your family, you should tell your doctor. He or she may recommend a specialist check-up before you try to become pregnant.

Q: We are always so busy, we are often too tired to make love, but I desperately want to have a baby.

A: So, something has to give. Take a look at your daily routine and your weekly schedule – both your own and your partner's – and decide what you can edge out in order to make more time for you and your partner. Beware leaving it too late: if you should encounter problems in conceiving, you may need additional months (or more) for these to be resolved.

You might find it helpful to make a list of all the things you have to do. Put them in order of priority to you. Now see whether you can leave any undone – if so, delete them. Think whether any can be delegated to other people – and do so. Then set yourself a reasonable timescale in which to achieve the rest.

Talk together with your partner and make a pact that certain times of the week are dedicated to being together. Stick to the arrangement and don't let other commitments or activities take priority over it.

Perhaps you also need to talk about how much you want to have a baby. Is there a subconscious reason that is stopping you giving conception a real chance?

Q: We want to start a family but I am terrified when I read about all the things that can go wrong.

A: Remind yourself that 97 per cent of all pregnancies result in the safe and successful delivery of a normal and healthy baby. With today's antenatal care (which represents preventative health care at its best), problems can be detected and resolved. You really have no reason to be terrified. Starting a family is one of life's great adventures.

Q: We want to start a family but I am scared of the pain of birth.

A: There are now a wide range of pain relief options for labour and delivery. You will be able to tell those responsible for your care that you want maximum pain relief and make sure that that statement is entered on your hospital birth plan. You may also want to consider a water birth, which is thought to reduce the pain. At this stage, it is a good idea for you to confide in your partner and perhaps an additional friend or relative as well.

You may wish to discuss with them who you would like to be with you for the labour and delivery. You could, for example, have your partner as well as your mother or sister or good friend. You may wish to have an acupuncturist or hypnotist with you as well as – or instead of – your partner or relative. It would also be a good idea for your partner to accompany you to antenatal checks and, of course, to the antenatal (parent craft) classes as well.

On the issue of fearing the pain and discomfort of childbirth, there is another reason for you to act now and not delay conceiving. This is because, the younger you are when you give birth, the easier it is likely to be for you. As you get older, your energy levels will be lower and your muscles and joints will be weaker and less flexible.

Q: I have read that Pilates and yoga are particularly helpful in conception and pregnancy. Why is this?

A: Pilates is a system of conditioning exercise that focuses on low impact and relaxing routines. In essence it consists of a series of controlled movements performed within the frame of your body so that no movement will pull you from the centre of your body. Yoga also teaches you to focus, balance and 'centre' both your mind and body. Relaxing Pilates and yoga routines are especially helpful because relief from stress is of vital importance during pregnancy, and when trying to conceive.

If you want to practise Pilates or yoga when you are pregnant, it is important that you start before you conceive, and build up your strength, flexibility and body awareness. Experts say that you should not start Pilates, yoga or any other new form of exercise in the first three months of pregnancy. However, if you already have an established routine, you can usually continue provided that you modify certain positions – a trained yoga or Pilates teacher must advise you on how to do this.

Pilates and yoga also increase the circulation to your growing baby rather than diverting blood from it like other exercises. They develop your overall muscle strength and also increase your flexibility. This helps to prevent lower back pain during pregnancy and also improves your balance. Because Pilates and yoga help you to relax and teach you to breathe deeply and evenly, delivery may prove easier. These forms of exercise can also strengthen the abdominal muscles, making it easier for you to recover from childbirth and regain your pre-pregnancy fitness.

Women who are overweight may find Pilates and yoga particularly useful means of starting to exercise. Having improved their muscle strength and flexibility, they can then progress more easily to regular walking and swimming regimes.

Delayed conception

> **"** Professional help often resolves the problem, leading to a successful pregnancy. **"**

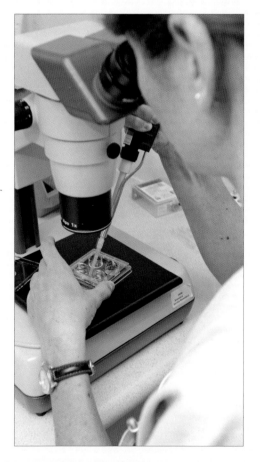

If you and your partner experience a delay in conceiving, remember first and foremost that this is not at all unusual, and you may just need a more rigorous tracking of your fertile time of the month. For especially long delays help can often resolve the problem, leading to a successful pregnancy.

Many people immediately think of IVF (in-vitro fertilization) as the solution to infertility, but this is very much a last-resort solution with a fairly low success rate. Infertility can be caused by all kinds of different problems, outlined in the following pages, and some of these can be resolved relatively simply.

The first step is for both partners to consult the family doctor and ask for a referral to a specialist. In the meantime, the chances of becoming pregnant will be enhanced by both partners doing everything they can to improve their general health and fitness. This means of course giving up smoking, cutting out alcohol, eating healthily, and exercising regularly. Relaxation is also a prime consideration. It can be difficult to maintain a happy, balanced attitude to life

All kinds of tests and investigations can be undertaken to understand infertility, so do not worry needlessly without seeking medical advice.

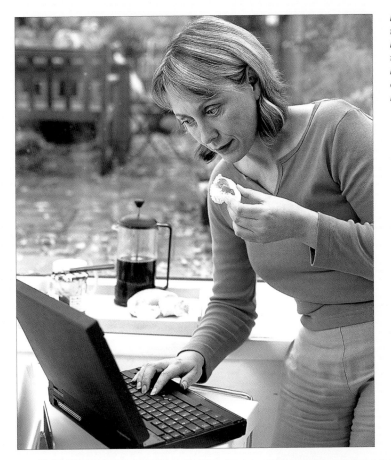

Many people believe that a stressful modern lifestyle, trying to juggle too many tasks and not taking time out for ourselves, contributes to infertility problems.

Meditation is the perfect way to relax and cope with the anxieties that may accompany infertility problems. The simplest form of meditation is simply to focus on gazing at an object such as a flower or crystal.

while trying to deal with your feelings about delayed conception. However, do whatever you can to relax and have fun with your partner by focusing on those things that you normally enjoy together. Choose activities that you enjoy out of the home to try and take the focus off lovemaking.

About one-third of infertility problems are caused by the woman's reproductive system, one-third by the man's and one-third may be unexplained. Once the problem is found, a relatively simple surgical procedure may be the answer. Even unexplained infertility often gives way to unexplained fertility after a period of time. There are lots of very good reasons to feel hopeful.

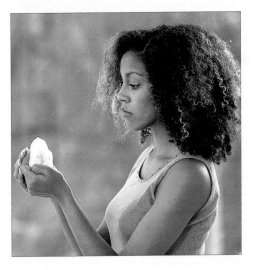

Problems with conceiving

Many couples naturally start to worry if conception does not happen within the first two or three months of trying for a baby. However, delayed conception is extremely common and there is very often no need for a couple to feel anxious.

The months of trying to get pregnant can be an extremely stressful time for both partners. It is all too easy to allow your thoughts to be dominated completely by your desire to have a baby, and to become increasingly worried when conception does not occur. Unfortunately, anxiety can become part of the problem and delay conception still further.

SEEKING MEDICAL HELP

You should see your family doctor if you have been having regular, unprotected sex for a year or longer but have not conceived. Your doctor may check that you are making love at the correct time, and will also ask about your general health and lifestyle – in particular whether you smoke or drink. He or she may also carry out some preliminary tests to rule out some of the obvious causes of infertility.

If these tests do not provide answers, ask to be referred to a consultant gynaecologist. It is very important that both partners attend all these consultations – because the problem may be with either partner or, sometimes, with both of you. In one-third of cases, failure or delay in conceiving arises from the woman's reproductive system; in another third there is a problem with the man's reproductive system; in the remaining third the problem lies with both partners or its cause simply cannot be identified. A gynaecologist will take a detailed medical history and will also check lifestyle factors that could be the reason for

> **66** Delayed conception is extremely common and there is very often no need for a couple to feel anxious. **99**

delayed conception. Various checks may be done on your blood and on the man's blood and semen. The reproductive organs of both partners are likely to be checked for damage, blockages and other problems.

These investigations may be invasive and time-consuming. However, they and any subsequent treatment can be very fruitful: up to 40 per cent of couples who seek specialist help achieve a pregnancy within two years. The major causes of infertility, together with their treatments, are discussed on the pages that follow.

MISCARRIAGE

In some cases, the woman may actually have conceived, but she may have had a miscarriage without realizing it. A high proportion of miscarriages occur within the first two months of pregnancy, often before the woman knows that she is pregnant. The loss of a baby through early miscarriage is much more common than many people believe, and may account for many cases of what is thought to be delayed conception. It could be that as many as over a half of all early pregnancies end in miscarriage.

The warning signs for an impending miscarriage include vaginal bleeding, abdominal cramps and backache similar to those of a period. Excessive vomiting can also be a symptom. Once a miscarriage starts, there is little that can be done to halt it. However, it is important that you seek medical advice immediately because there is a risk of infection and complications.

INVESTIGATING MISCARRIAGE

Having a miscarriage can be a very traumatic experience. For some women it is just as distressing as a bereavement, even when it occurs in the early stages of pregnancy. It may be of some comfort to know that miscarriage, particularly in the early months, is very common. It does not mean that there is anything inherently wrong with you, or that you are likely to miscarry next time you become pregnant. The vast majority of women go on to have successful pregnancies after experiencing a miscarriage. For this reason, having one or even two early miscarriages is not usually seen as a reason for medical investigation.

WORKING TOGETHER

Trying for a baby can involve many moments of both expectation and disappointment. It is difficult to cope with a specific problem with conception, but also hard to bear a failure to conceive where the cause simply cannot be identified. It is extremely important that you both find ways to relax as much as you can and to enjoy your relationship fully, so that trying for a baby does not become a negative and unhappy experience.

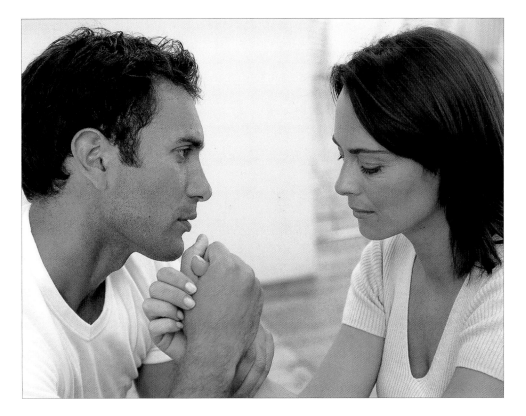

Tests are usually done if a woman experiences repeated miscarriages: this is defined as three or more successive miscarriages with no successful pregnancy occurring in between. After suffering three miscarriages, you should seek specialist help and advice. A late miscarriage – one that occurs after 14 weeks – should also be investigated.

Your family doctor will be able to refer you to a consultant gynaecologist if you have had recurrent miscarriages. In some cases, couples may then be referred to a genetic counsellor. Genetic counselling may help to determine the level or risk of future pregnancies, and to discuss the best way forwards.

WHY MISCARRIAGE HAPPENS

Doctors do not know why so many pregnancies end unsuccessfully, and determining the cause of a miscarriage can be very difficult or even impossible. Some of the known causes of early miscarriage include:

- A major abnormality in the baby. About three in every five early miscarriages are thought to be connected to fetal abnormality.
- The mother contracting rubella, listeriosis or chlamydia during the pregnancy.

It can be very distressing for both partners when pregnancy does not happen straight away, especially if you have delayed having a baby. It is essential to be totally supportive of each other.

- The failure of the fertilized egg to implant successfully in the lining of the uterus.
- The mother having a low level of progesterone, which is needed to sustain the pregnancy.

Later miscarriage (after 14 weeks) can be the result of:
- An abnormality in the uterus, such as a large fibroid.
- A weak (incompetent) cervix. This is a condition in which the cervix dilates instead of remaining tightly closed during pregnancy.
- Certain antenatal tests; amniocentesis, for example, carries a 1 in 200 risk of miscarriage.
- The mother having diabetes, epilepsy, asthma, kidney disease or high blood pressure.

Miscarriages are more common in very young women or women over 35. Many people think that minor injuries or distress can cause a miscarriage, but there is no medical evidence to support this.

WOMEN'S REPRODUCTIVE PROBLEMS

The conditions listed below include the most common reasons for female infertility. However, that is not to say that all women affected by them necessarily become infertile – some women with small fibroids, say, may have successful pregnancies without treatment. Treatment is an option in the case of most disorders.

Polycystic ovaries

This is a common condition in which many small cysts form in the ovaries. Polycystic ovary syndrome affects about one in ten women. Some of these women will encounter a variety of hormone-related problems, including infertility.

Women with polycystic ovaries may have no symptoms – with the result that they only know that they have the condition when fertility tests are done. However, symptoms can include:

- Obesity.
- Excessive hair growth on the face or body.
- Acne.
- Infrequent or no menstrual periods.
- Male-pattern baldness (the form of hair loss that is most commonly found in males – namely, losing hair first from the temples and then from the crown, with the bald area on the crown gradually widening).

Drug treatment is sometimes used to induce ovulation in women with polycystic ovaries. Otherwise, the cysts may be treated by being cauterized with a needle. This procedure is done by laparoscopy, in which a fibre-optic tube is inserted into the pelvic area through a small incision made just below the navel. This enables doctors to examine the woman's reproductive organs, take samples and carry out some minor surgery. A general anaesthetic is given.

Endometriosis

One in ten of all women referred for fertility testing turns out to be affected by endometriosis, making it a major cause of infertility. In this condition, cells similar to those of the lining of the uterus (the endometrium) become established outside it. They can grow anywhere in the pelvic area – for example, on the ovaries, in the Fallopian tubes, bladder, uterus, bowel, peritoneum or on the pelvic wall.

These stray endometrial cells respond to natural changes in hormone levels in the same way as those inside the uterus. That is, they increase during part of the month and break down when the lining is being shed (the period). However, because these cells are trapped inside the pelvic area, they cannot leave the body. Instead, they become inflamed and cause adhesions, which can cause one internal organ to become stuck to another. They may also form swellings which fill with dark blood – chocolate cysts.

ENDOMETRIOSIS

If you suffer with severe back ache, abdominal pain or strong cramps during menstruation, ask your doctor to refer you for a specialist check for endometriosis. In this condition, cells like those of the uterus lining grow elsewhere in the pelvis, in the areas shown below.

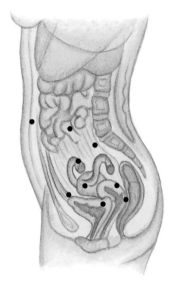

Possible endometriosis sites include: abdominal wall, intestines, Fallopian tubes, ovaries, appendix, uterus, peritoneum (lining of abdomen), cervix, rectum, bladder and vulva.

Many women who are affected by endometriosis think that they merely have painful periods, with the result that the condition often goes undetected for a long time – until fertility testing starts, in fact. The symptoms of endometriosis can include severe backache, abdominal pain and cramps during periods, and pain at ovulation, during bowel movements and during sex. The woman may sometimes also experience nausea and dizziness. Endometriosis is diagnosed by close examination of the pelvis, using a laparoscope.

The condition is usually treated by hormone therapy or by surgery. The procedure known as thermal coagulator treatment uses helium gas ionized by an electric current to dry out the endometrial cells. This procedure has had good results, and its other advantage is that it can be performed quickly.

Pelvic inflammatory disease (PID)

Infection can often cause inflammation in the uterus, Fallopian tubes and ovaries – a condition known as pelvic inflammatory disease. This is a common cause of infertility and other pregnancy-related complications. It is estimated that women who have suffered with PID have a seven-fold risk of ectopic pregnancy.

The bacteria that cause gonorrhoea and chlamydia are thought to be the main causes of PID, although bacteria that normally exist harmlessly in the bowel or gut may also be the culprit. The bacteria enter the body through the vagina and then work up through the cervix into the pelvic cavity. The infection may occur as a consequence of sexually transmitted chlamydia, childbirth, miscarriage, termination or the fitting of an IUD.

In some cases, PID causes no symptoms other than the woman's inability to become pregnant. It is therefore often not detected until fertility testing starts. The condition is also sometimes misdiagnosed as either endometriosis or appendicitis because it can cause similar symptoms. Where symptoms occur, they can include abdominal pain, exhaustion, high temperatures and very heavy, painful periods. The pain has been described as a dull ache across the lower abdomen. In some cases, it may be so intense that the woman is unable to move. The scar tissue caused by PID can increase the risk of recurrent infection and it can cause pain during sex.

PID is diagnosed by means of an internal examination and a laparoscopy. It is usually treated with antibiotics. In severe cases, the woman may need to be admitted to hospital so that antibiotics can be given to her intravenously (directly into the veins).

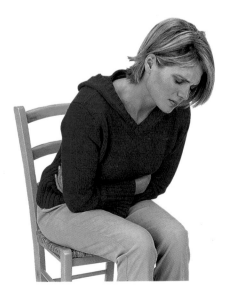

ECTOPIC PREGNANCY

Sometimes a pregnancy can start to develop in the Fallopian tubes rather than in the uterus. An ectopic pregnancy is normally accompanied by severe abdominal pain, and the woman will need emergency treatment to remove the pregnancy.

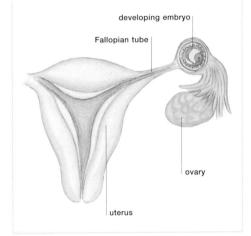

developing embryo

Fallopian tube

ovary

uterus

Ectopic pregnancy

An ectopic pregnancy is one that starts to develop in one of the Fallopian tubes or, more rarely, in another site in the abdominal cavity rather than in the uterus. It can cause permanent damage to the tube, leading to infertility. Doctors do not know why an ectopic pregnancy occurs. However, it is more common if the Fallopian tube has already been damaged by infection, surgery or by a previous ectopic pregnancy.

An ectopic pregnancy can be extremely serious, even life-threatening, and so the woman must get immediate medical treatment. The symptoms can include intense pain in the abdominal area and vaginal bleeding. Ectopic pregnancies are sometimes initially diagnosed as appendicitis or miscarriage.

An ectopic pregnancy cannot develop normally. Once an ectopic pregnancy is confirmed, surgery is needed to remove it. Sometimes, part of the Fallopian tube and part of the ovary may have to be removed as well, although doctors will avoid this whenever possible. Women who have suffered one ectopic pregnancy are at a higher risk of experiencing another one. However, many women who have had an ectopic pregnancy go on to have a perfectly healthy pregnancy.

Many women suffer menstrual cramps. However, severe abdominal pain should always be investigated. It may be a sign of one of several serious conditions.

Polyps and fibroids

Different forms of benign (non-cancerous) tumours or growths, polyps and fibroids can cause infertility in women. Doctors do not know why these grow.

Polyps have a stalk by which they attach themselves to the membrane lining the cervix or uterus. They may cause no symptoms, or the woman may experience a watery discharge streaked with blood between her periods and after intercourse.

Fibroids are bundles of muscle fibres that develop in the muscular wall of the uterus. They can vary in size from a small marble to a large ball. Fibroids are very common – one in five women over the age of 30 develops them. Like polyps, they may cause no symptoms. Where symptoms do occur, they may include long-lasting periods and heavy menstrual bleeding, including flooding and passing clots. The woman may also develop anaemia because of the excessive blood loss, which can then lead to feelings of exhaustion, breathlessness and depression. Other symptoms include severe cramps, incontinence, constipation and cystitis.

Polyps and fibroids are diagnosed by internal examination, ultrasound scan or laparoscopy. The woman may also be given a hysteroscopy, in which a viewing instrument is passed up the vagina into the uterus, or she may be offered a hysterosalpingogram, in which a dye is injected through the cervix so that X-rays of the reproductive organs can be taken. Polyps and fibroids are usually removed surgically. Drug treatment may be recommended to shrink large fibroids before surgery.

Early menopause

The menopause usually starts in the woman's late forties but some women may stop having periods in their thirties or even in their twenties. Women affected may at first think that they are pregnant. However, as well as the periods stopping, other symptoms can include hot flushes, night sweats, insomnia, vaginal drying, painful intercourse, loss of libido, genito-urinary infections, thinning of the skin, splitting of the nails, aches and pains, and incontinence. Women may also experience mood changes, anxiety, irritability, poor memory and poor concentration as well as subsequent loss of confidence.

If a doctor suspects premature menopause, the woman will be referred for a laparoscopy. In this procedure, the ovaries are examined by a laparoscope (a fibre-optic tube); this allows the doctor to see if the woman's ovaries contain follicles with eggs. Women who experience premature menopause may still achieve a pregnancy, but only through assisted conception.

Incompatibility

Failure to conceive may be due to an incompatibility between a man's sperm and a woman's cervical mucus. In these cases, the mucus contains antibodies that destroy the man's sperm before it can reach the egg. A post-coital test may be needed in which a sample of fluid is taken from the woman's cervix six to thirty-six hours after intercourse. This may be treated with drugs or the man's semen may be injected into the woman's uterus to avoid contact with the cervix. Assisted conception may also be an option.

INFERTILITY IN MEN

The reason for male infertility is usually defective sperm or a problem with delivering the sperm to the woman's vagina. It is rare for there to be no sperm at all. Usually the problem is that not enough sperm are being produced or that they are not strong enough to make the journey.

Abnormal sperm production

Sperm may be defective in:
- Quantity – if there are fewer than 20 million sperm per millilitre of ejaculate, the sperm count is said to be low.
- Motility – at least 40 per cent of the sperm should be moving in a healthy sample.
- Normality – the sperm should not be deformed.

If you are having difficulty conceiving, the man's semen will be analysed under a microscope for numbers of

---

FIBROIDS

These are bundles of muscle that have grown in the muscular wall of the uterus. They can delay or prevent conception, so early treatment is essential for women wishing to have a family.

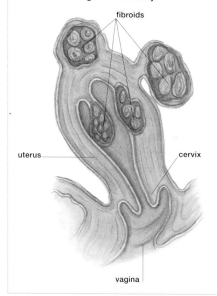

fibroids

uterus

cervix

vagina

sperm, motility, normality, infection and antibodies. The temperature of the testicles may be assessed by thermography. Some experts maintain that temperature is a defining factor in fertility, while many others disagree.

The man will also be screened for a number of diseases such as diabetes and kidney disease, for example, which can affect sperm production. Other male fertility tests include testicular biopsy and testicular X-ray in case of a genetic problem or childhood disease such as mumps, which may have led to problems with the sperm. Often the cause of low sperm count cannot be identified, and so cannot be treated. In some cases, therefore, assisted conception may be recommended.

Sperm delivery problems

There can be problems that stop the sperm from reaching the vagina. The major one is impotence, but another cause may be damage to the man's reproductive tubes, which may be due to a sexually transmitted disease or to some other cause.

Some cases of impotence and erectile problems may be treated by medication such as Viagra. Counselling may be offered if the impotence is thought to have a psychological cause. More often, however, male impotence is associated with a physical problem. Some of these conditions can be quite serious – they include heart disease, narrowing of the arteries, diabetes and high blood pressure – so it is important that men suffering from impotence should see their doctor. If the cause of the impotence is not treatable, artificial insemination may be an option.

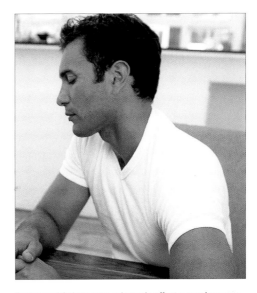

Stress and fatigue may adversely affect a man's sperm count and the quality of the sperm he produces, as well as diminishing his desire to make love.

Damage to the tubes that transport sperm – the epididymis or vas deferens – may be remedied by microsurgery. If the man has had a vasectomy, this can be reversed. However, the chances of this reversal procedure being successful are relatively low.

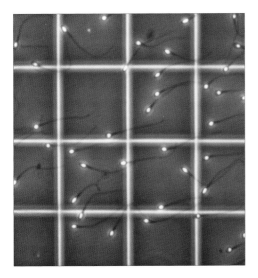

This shows human sperm occurring in a normal quantity – at least 30 million sperm per millilitre ejaculate. The lines on the screen assist counting.

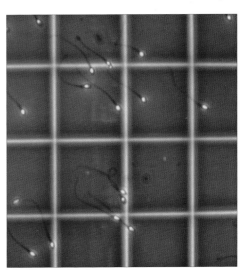

By comparison, this sample shows a low sperm count of under 20 million sperm. A temporary low count may be caused by excess alcohol, smoking, stress or illness.

Fertility treatment

Many couples who have sought professional help with conception go on to have a child naturally. Others may learn that the cause of the infertility cannot be treated or that it cannot be explained. In these cases, assisted conception may be an option. It should be remembered that infertility investigations and treatments can take a great deal of time, and they can also be very intrusive. It is important that both partners take steps to care for themselves and to support each other during what can be a difficult time.

SEEING A SPECIALIST

Various tests need to be done before a decision is made to start fertility treatment. Your family doctor may carry out some preliminary investigations. These tests may uncover a simple problem that the doctor can treat. If not, you should be referred to a specialist for further investigation.

A specialist will want to ensure that the woman is ovulating, the man is producing healthy sperm in sufficient quantities and that the sperm and egg are able to meet. The specialist will investigate the woman's menstrual cycle and ovulatory cycle, the health of her reproductive system and her general health. If the specialist suspects that she is not ovulating, he or she may take blood tests to check her hormone levels at frequent intervals during her menstrual cycle; her ovaries may also be scanned using ultrasound to check when and if ovulation takes place.

The man will be asked to provide two or more samples of semen. These will be analysed under a microscope to check that there is a sufficient quantity of sperm and that they are healthy. If the sperm count is low, the man's testosterone levels may be checked – a lack of this hormone can affect sperm production.

If the woman is ovulating and there is not a problem with the man's sperm, the doctor will carry out further tests to see why sperm and egg are not meeting. A sample of cervical mucus may be collected after the couple have sex and tested to see if there is any obvious incompatibility. The woman's reproductive system may be examined by laparoscopy to detect any blockages or damage, and the man's reproductive organs will also be checked.

Before starting fertility treatment, a specialist will discuss your general health and lifestyle to ensure that these are not factors in any delay in conception. Sometimes you may be given general health advice to carry out before or during treatment, which may include the following guidelines.

Common health advice for men

A specialist may advise:
- Losing weight if overweight.
- Stopping smoking – if you continue to smoke while receiving fertility treatment, it may be less effective.
- Reducing alcohol intake.
- Avoiding caffeine.
- Abstaining from any drugs – cannabis and cocaine, for example, affect sperm quality and quantity.
- Avoiding excessive exercise.
- Having a healthy diet.
- Monitoring the temperature of the testicles – overheating may affect sperm production.
- Reducing stress and getting enough rest.
- Stopping any non-essential medication that may interfere with sperm production.

In general, the man should comply with this advice for about 70 days before the semen analysis takes place. This is the length of time that it takes to produce sperm.

Common health advice for women

A specialist may advise:
- Losing excess weight if overweight.
- Stopping smoking.
- Giving up alcohol for the time being.
- Avoiding caffeine.
- Abstaining from drugs.
- Having a healthy diet.
- Taking regular, moderate exercise.
- Getting enough regular sleep and relaxation.

ROUTINE FERTILITY TREATMENTS

In many cases, the problem is straightforward and treatable. Fertility treatments may include the following:
- Fertility medication to stimulate ovulation.
- Hormone treatment to encourage sperm production.
- Drug treatment with corticosteroids to suppress production of antibodies to the man's sperm.
- Microsurgery – for example, to repair damage to the Fallopian tubes or male reproductive tubes.
- Other surgery – for example, to remove fibroids.

ASSISTED FERTILITY

If the specialist thinks that a couple are unlikely to achieve a pregnancy naturally, he or she may recommend that they start assisted fertility treatment. This treatment may take the form of artificial insemination or one of the other

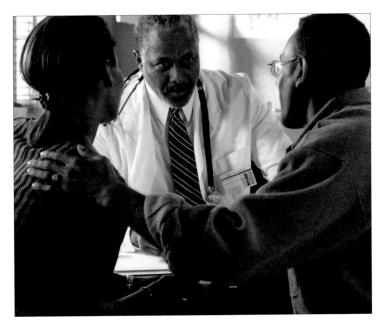

When a couple first consults a fertility specialist, he or she will check their general health and lifestyle before starting investigations.

methods listed, depending on the cause of the problem. It is extremely important that a couple understand exactly what is involved in any assisted fertility treatment. They need to appreciate its chances of success, and the financial cost that they will need to bear. They will be offered counselling, which is intended to help them to explore their feelings and to be honest with each other about their anxieties and fears.

ARTIFICIAL INSEMINATION

AI, or artificial insemination, involves introducing the partner's sperm into the woman's cervical channel or directly into the uterus when she is ovulating. This is done in hospital, using a syringe. No anaesthetic is necessary for this procedure. Sometimes the semen may be treated in order to remove defective or poor-quality sperm before they are inserted into the woman's body.

Artificial insemination is a useful method for couples in which the woman's body makes antibodies to her partner's sperm, and also for couples who experience sexual difficulties such as impotence or premature ejaculation, low sperm count or blockages in the male reproductive organs. It is sometimes used for cases of unexplained infertility.

DONOR INSEMINATION

Sometimes a donor's sperm may be used instead of that of a male partner. This is known as donor insemination (DI). The method can be used in cases of impotence or defective sperm, as well as by single and lesbian women who wish to have a child.

❝ In many cases, the cause of infertility is straightforward and treatable, but it may take time to identify it. ❞

IN-VITRO FERTILIZATION (IVF)

So-called test-tube babies are a result of this procedure, which involves mixing the woman's eggs with sperm outside her body.

Before IVF is carried out, the woman will take fertility drugs to stimulate her ovaries into producing more than one egg. The eggs are then collected. One method of doing this involves inserting a laparoscope through a small cut in the abdomen to draw off the egg-producing follicles. This is done under general anaesthetic. Alternatively, a needle is inserted through the abdomen and is then guided with ultrasound to draw off the follicles. This method requires only a local anaesthetic.

The eggs are mixed with sperm in a laboratory and left to incubate for two days at normal body temperature. Provided that both the eggs and the sperm are healthy, 60 per cent of the eggs may be fertilized. One or more of the resulting embryos will then be inserted into the uterus via a syringe. No anaesthetic is needed for this procedure. If there are additional eggs that have been fertilized, they may be frozen for future attempts.

The embryo or embryos then need to attach themselves to the lining of the uterus – implantation – for a pregnancy to take place.

When IVF is used

In-vitro fertilization may be used if the man is producing poor quality sperm, if the woman's body is making antibodies to the sperm, or if she has blocked or scarred Fallopian tubes or irregular ovulation. It is also sometimes recommended for cases of unexplained infertility. IVF can be done using the male partner's or a donor's sperm. Donor eggs can also be used if the woman is not producing her own. In some cases, donor embryos – that is, embryos made from both donor sperm and eggs – may be used.

IVF was successfully used for the first time in 1978, in the UK. It resulted in the birth of the world's first test-tube baby – Louise Brown. Like all assisted conception methods, the success rate of IVF is not high. When two embryos are transferred, there is a one in four (25 per cent) chance of a pregnancy occurring. However, just as pregnancies achieved naturally can end in miscarriage, so too can those that occur as a result of IVF. The percentage of IVF treatments that end in the delivery of a baby is just over 30% for women under 35. As the woman gets older her chances of a successful pregnancy reduces. Women over 44 years have a 5% success rate. Most couples who opt for IVF have to go through several treatment cycles.

GAMETE INTRA-FALLOPIAN TRANSFER (GIFT)

GIFT is a variation of IVF that is used when no reason can be found for female infertility, or if the man has a low sperm count. In this procedure, the eggs and sperm are collected as in IVF. Doctors examine the eggs to ensure they are healthy and select up to three for insertion. The eggs are mixed with the sperm, and are then placed immediately in one of the Fallopian tubes, where they are left to fertilize naturally. This procedure is done by laparoscopy, under a general anaesthetic. It has a success rate of about 25 per cent, but it is an invasive treatment and is now no longer practised in many fertility units.

ZYGOTE INTRA-FALLOPIAN TRANSFER (ZIFT)

This method is very similar to GIFT; the woman's eggs are collected and the eggs mixed with sperm in the same way. However, in this method doctors check that fertilization has taken place before injecting the fused eggs and sperm into the Fallopian tubes.

ZIFT is used when GIFT either hasn't worked or is considered unlikely to work. Again, the woman's Fallopian tubes must be healthy and functioning. The success rate is about 25 per cent. Both GIFT and ZIFT can be done with donor eggs or sperm.

In GIFT, the gynaecologist places selected eggs and sperm in the woman's Fallopian tube, with the aim of fertilization followed by implantation in the uterus.

INTRA-CYTOPLASM SPERM INJECTION (ICSI)

This technique is especially suitable when the man has a low sperm count or produces sperm either of poor quality or low motility. In ICSI, the eggs and sperm are collected in the same way as for IVF. A single sperm is then injected into an egg to ensure that fertilization takes place. The resulting embryo is then placed in the uterus so that implantation can take place. The success rate for each ICSI treatment is similar to IVF rates and is dependent upon the age of the patient.

DONOR SPERM, EGGS AND EMBRYOS

Sometimes, donated sperm is needed to facilitate a pregnancy. This may be because the male partner may pass on a genetic disease or has a very low sperm count. Donor sperm is also used by lesbian and single women who wish to conceive a child. The donor may be known to the couple. However, more often, the sperm comes from an anonymous donor via a sperm bank.

Another woman's eggs may be used in fertility treatment. The eggs may be fertilized by the male partner's sperm or that of a donor. A few of the resulting embryos are placed in the woman's uterus and she is given hormonal drugs to help maintain the pregnancy.

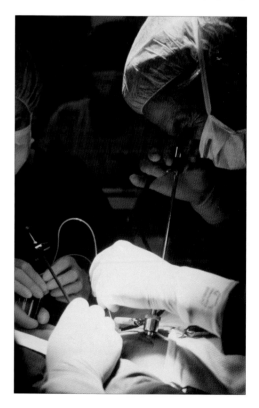

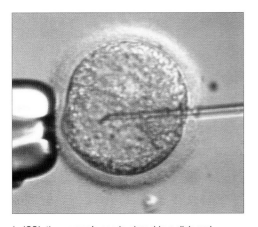

In ICSI, the woman's egg is placed in a dish and injected with a sperm before being transferred into the uterus in the hope of successful implantation.

Egg donation is the only assisted conception technique available for women who are not producing eggs at all, although surrogacy and adoption may be considered. Egg donation may also be used by women who may pass on a genetic disorder to their children.

Egg donation is a complex procedure, requiring the same drug treatment and monitoring as IVF or GIFT. Egg donors are usually women under the age of 35 who have already had their own children. The donor may be a relative or close friend of the couple, or may be anonymous. The use of the technique is limited because of a shortage of donors.

Donor embryos are also used in fertility treatment. They may come from couples who are themselves undergoing fertility treatment and have produced several viable embryos during IVF or other methods. They may also be produced by fertilizing donated eggs with donated sperm. They are used when neither the woman's eggs nor the man's sperm can be used to achieve a healthy pregnancy.

OTHER OPTIONS

Surrogacy and adoption are two options when assisted conception fails. In surrogacy, another woman is used to carry the fertilized egg and give birth to the baby. In some cases, the surrogate conceives using her own egg and the male partner's sperm, and then hands over the baby at birth. Surrogacy can be fraught with legal difficulties, and it works only if all parties are in full agreement about the arrangement and stick to it. Payment is illegal in some countries, including the UK.

Another alternative is adoption. The legal situation surrounding adoption is much clearer than that of surrogacy. However, there are many more couples wanting to adopt a baby than there are babies available. Often, older couples are not eligible for adopting babies.

ACCEPTING THE SITUATION

Some couples may decide to go ahead with fertility treatments, but others may choose not to do so. Still more may call a halt to the treatment after undergoing several unsuccessful attempts. Counselling should always be offered to couples who considering undergoing fertility investigations and treatments. It may also be beneficial to seek support from a complementary therapist as well.

It is sometimes the case that a couple who accept their infertility suddenly conceive – much to their joy and surprise. Others come to terms with their infertility, finding other ways to have a fulfilling and happy life.

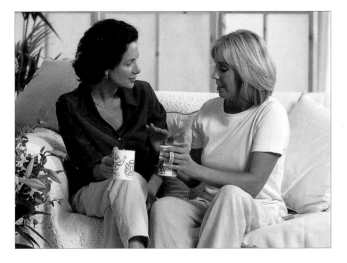

Infertility, which may continue for many years, almost always proves distressing and exhausting. A close friend can be a good source of support. However, be prepared to seek professional counselling via your family doctor if you feel the need to talk through the complex and deeply personal issues involved.

How natural therapies help

Some complementary practitioners believe that therapies may actively assist conception. Most infertility experts and gynaecologists would dispute this. However, there is no doubt that the natural therapies have their part to play in supporting people during the time that they are attempting to conceive.

First and foremost, many complementary therapies, including acupuncture and reflexology, encourage good general health and well-being. They may be useful to those trying to give up smoking and reduce their alcohol consumption, or they may simply help you to feel healthier and more alive, as with the detoxing effects produced by lymphatic massage. Many natural therapies, including massage, aromatherapy, reflexology and yoga, help with relaxation and de-stressing, which can play an important part in conception.

USING THERAPIES FOR EMOTIONAL SUPPORT

Natural therapies, and especially meditation, yoga and relaxation techniques, can be very helpful if you are having difficulty conceiving, allowing you space to express your feelings and come to terms with them. Some people are able to accept the difficulties in becoming pregnant with calm and equanimity, but others are deeply distressed by any delay and need extra support. There is plenty of research and anecdotal evidence to suggest that you are more likely to conceive if you are relaxed, at peace with yourself and able to deal with any negative feelings and anxieties. For example, it is not uncommon for women who have had problems conceiving to get pregnant once

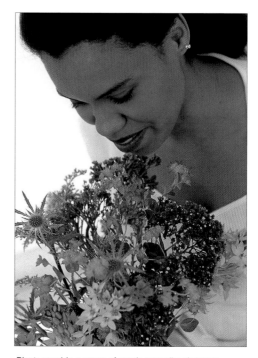

Plants provide a range of gentle remedies that may support conception. For example, certain Bach Flower Remedies aim to promote the kind of relaxed, open state of mind said to increase the chances of falling pregnant.

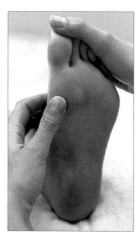

Reflexology can help to boost immunity and energy levels, creating a state of optimum health that is ideal for conception. Always seek medical advice before receiving reflexology during pregnancy (especially within the first three months) or possible pregnancy.

they are on a referral list for specialist advice – the pressure has been taken off them slightly. Negative feelings can all too easily take over. Women who have difficulty conceiving may rapidly find their lives dominated by thoughts of their ovulatory cycle. The start of each month may bring new hope, and the woman may feel determined to ensure that lovemaking coincides with her fertile period. As the time for menstruation approaches, she may become alternately anxious and hopeful, only to feel bitterly disappointed when she knows that she has not conceived. All this can be exhausting and stressful, and her self-esteem may drop.

Having children is seen as a natural process. Many women, in particular, feel very angry when it does not happen for them. It can be particularly hard to accept if they have spent years using contraception so as not to become pregnant at the wrong time or with the wrong partner. At the same time, a woman may start to feel guilty or inadequate. She may look for reasons in her past – wondering, for example, if the delay is somehow due to a previous termination or a past infection. Doctors can often be reassuring on these points.

At the same time, the man may be unhappy about the way his sex life with his partner is dominated by ovulation charts. He may feel taken for granted, wonder if his partner is more interested in having a child than in a happy relationship, and suppress his own feelings about a longed-for conception so that he is able to support the woman. From a conception standpoint, he too may benefit from supportive natural therapies, to improve his general well-being and keep him de-stressed.

Part of the holistic approach to health means that, as well as specific therapies, partners must learn to open up and speak to each other, in order to receive loving support and reassurance from each other. Friends or relatives can also be very helpful, although it is important to remember that not everyone has sufficient understanding and sensitivity in this situation. It can be an excellent idea to seek help from a professional counsellor, who will help you to explore any complex feelings and emotions you may have.

USING AFFIRMATION AND VISUALIZATION

Controlled breathing, meditation, visualization and affirmation work can all help both partners to get into the best mental and physical state to deal with the pre-conception period. Try the following exercise, adapting it to suit your personal situation:

- Choose a place where you will not be interrupted. Sit comfortably, with your back straight, perhaps sitting on a cushion cross-legged, or seated in a chair.
- Take a few deep breaths. Close your eyes. As you breathe, relax your shoulders and your face muscles. Concentrate on your breathing. You can focus on the air passing in and out of your nostrils or the rise and fall of your chest – whichever is easier for you.
- Bring your attention to the centre of your chest, the heart area. Notice how it feels as your breathe in and out – is there tension or pain here? Just notice the feeling, but don't try to change it. If you find focusing difficult, place your hands on your chest, and feel them rise and fall with your breath.
- As you continue to breathe, wish yourself well. There are several ways you can do this: some people like to imagine a pink light in the heart area that slowly expands and grows to encompass their entire body; others like to repeat affirmative phrases in their head. Try the following phrases: "May I be happy, May I be well, May I be safe, May I be at ease in the world". If you prefer, make up your own affirmation.
- Continue for a few minutes. Now visualize your partner in front of you. Imagine the pink light growing

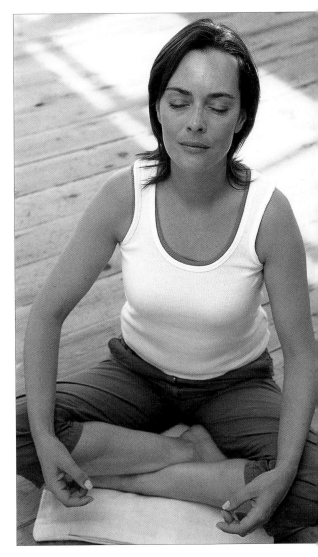

Feel completely free to include whatever elements you wish in pre-conception meditations or visualizations – only you know what feels calming and positive.

to encompass you both, and spend a few moments enjoying its warm loving embrace. If you are using the affirmation technique, turn your good wishes towards your partner: "May you be happy…" etc. After a few minutes, wish both yourself and your partner well: "May we be happy…" etc.

- Now, slowly let the pink light or the words fade away. Bring your attention back to your breathing. Continue sitting quietly for a minute or two, then get up slowly.

Common Qs and As

Q: After several months of trying to get pregnant, I am now starting to think about nothing else. I wait for my fertile period, both of us have cut out alcohol and my partner drinks very little, I make sure that neither of us is tired out before my fertile period... and then within two or three weeks, I get yet another period. I am starting to feel depressed about this and am beginning to believe that we will never have a family. What can we do?

A: First and foremost, try to relax, by any means that appeals to you. Make sure that you get enough exercise, and join a yoga or relaxation class. Make sure that both you and your partner are sleeping well: invest in a better bed if necessary.

Some couples do not become pregnant for two or more years, even though there is nothing wrong with either partner. Most gynaecologists know of hundreds of cases in which conception is delayed and, then, for no obvious reason, the problem resolves and the woman becomes pregnant.

The single most important thing for couples in this situation to remember is that they should never give up hope. What is known as unexplained infertility can just as easily, in time, give way to unexplained fertility. In the meantime, it is important to recognize the effect of repeated monthly disappointments on one's partner and the impact of delayed conception on you in respect of your other relationships and your family, as well as on how you manage at work.

Beware of damaging your relationship with your life partner for the sake of a need that may develop into an obsession with fertility and having children at some time in the future. If you are not pregnant after one year of trying, consult your family doctor with a view to a specialist referral.

Q: We have been trying for a baby now for four months and I am becoming increasingly worried and upset. Should we visit our family doctor, or is it too soon?

A: One in six couples experience delays and difficulties in conception. This is nothing unusual. It may take a year or more for you to become pregnant. See your doctor now if you prefer to do so, but you could probably afford to wait for a few months. It may well be that you find yourself pregnant before you see him or her.

Q: We have been trying for a baby for over one year now. I want to consult our family doctor but my partner is unwilling to do so. What can I do? Do you think this is a sign that he is less committed to the idea of starting a family than I am?

A: The fact that you are not yet pregnant may be worrying him. He may be feeling inadequate and disappointed. Talk to him and try to find out why he is so unwilling. He may fear that the issue lies with him, rather than you. Tell him that male fertility problems account for only one-third of cases – even a low sperm count, if that is what it turns out to be, does not make pregnancy impossible. Explain that there may be a relatively simple problem, such as a cyst or a blocked tube. Once he knows some of the facts, he may be more willing to seek help.

It might be helpful to drop the subject and concentrate on reassuring your partner and showing him that you love him for a month or so. However, you would be wise to see your doctor before too much more time passes. If your partner is still unwilling, make an appointment for yourself.

Q : I am getting very worried that there is a problem with me as my wife and I have been trying to get pregnant for nearly a year now, with no success. I'm concerned that I may be doing something wrong. I eat well and have given up smoking, but I have had a very pressured time at work over the last year and am probably drinking more than I should. I also had some kidney problems a year or so ago.

A : There are many reasons why conception does not happen straight away, but it may well be that your sperm count is low as a combined result of tiredness and alcohol. Alcohol has been shown to contribute to lower sperm counts, and fatigue can also do this, at least partly because it is probably making you less inclined to make love. However, kidney disease is another possible factor, as it can also lower sperm production, so do consult your family doctor about this.

Q : Both of my aunts had fibroids and this affected their ability to get pregnant. How do you know if you have them?

A : Fibroids are tumours that grow in the uterus (womb). They are benign, which means they are not cancerous, and are made up of muscle fibre. Fibroids can be as small as a pea and can grow as large as a melon. It is estimated that 20–50% of women have, or will have, fibroids at some time in their lives.

The problem with fibroids (non-cancerous growths) is that you don't always know they are there. There is no associated pain, and the only symptoms tend to be heavy menstrual bleeding, including flooding, or very long-lasting periods. You may also suffer from feelings of exhaustion or depression. If you notice any of these symptoms, you should see your family doctor without delay for diagnosis and treatment.

Q : My partner and I are discussing the possibility of assisted conception treatment. We are concerned that the success rates are so low, and are not sure whether it is worth going ahead or not.

A : Assisted conception treatments do have a low success rate, and most couples have to undergo several cycles of treatment before conceiving. There are obviously no guarantees of success here.

Some couples decide that assisted conception is not for them, and find other ways of coming to terms with their infertility. Only you can decide whether or not you want to go ahead. You should be offered counselling so that you can explore the issues fully – ask your specialist for a referral.

Q : I am not sure how keen my partner is to start a family, although he has agreed that we should and we have been trying for a while. Almost like clockwork, as soon as my fertile period is about to start, we have a row and do not make love for a few days. Then – once I am no longer fertile – we make it up. I have been thinking that it is simply coincidence, but now I am not sure. How can I stop this happening?

A : Consider whether your anxiety about conceiving is playing a part in this situation. It could be that you feel so tense when approaching your fertile period that a disagreement becomes inevitable. Alternatively, it could be that your partner does have real doubts about having a family.

The only way through this is to talk about the issue. Choose a time when you are both calm, and make sure that you listen to what he has to say. You may find it helpful to seek relationship counselling (via your family doctor or specialist organizations) to explore the issues further.

delayed conception

section two

your
natural
pregnancy

Understanding exactly what is taking place during each stage
of your pregnancy makes it even more thrilling and fascinating
than it already is. Knowledge of how your baby is growing,
what is happening to your body, and how diet, natural
therapies and other treatments can support your pregnancy is
all part of the journey of discovery on which you and your
partner are now embarked.

The first trimester

66 Having a baby is one of the most exciting experiences
that you will ever have. 99

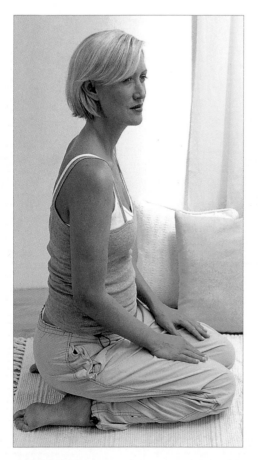

The first term of pregnancy, known as the first trimester, is roughly the first three months. This is an immensely thrilling time for a couple who have decided they want to start a family.

You and your partner will undoubtedly have many questions. Hopefully, this book will answer the majority of them but you should not hesitate to see your midwife or family doctor if you have any persistent worries. You will gain understanding, too, from your own experience. As every day passes, you will learn more about your body, your feelings about the pregnancy and the new life that you will soon be introducing into the world.

Pregnant women often experience minor physical disorders such as nausea and backache. There are often simple measures that you can take to relieve any discomfort that you may have, leaving you free to enjoy your pregnancy. In particular, complementary therapies can help to alleviate many pregnancy-related complaints and also enhance your well-being. The reference section on which

The first 12 or 13 weeks of pregnancy is known as the first trimester. Many women have hardly any visible signs at all, while others do start to 'show'.

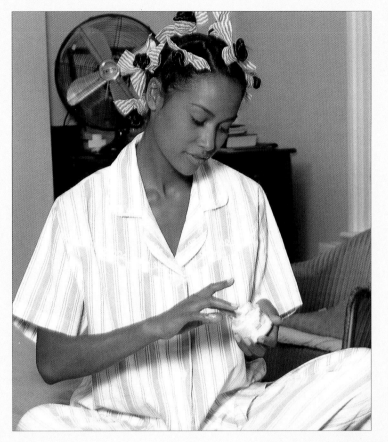

Don't stint on pampering yourself whenever you can, and get plenty of rest and relaxation.

What you eat and drink remains as important as ever in these early formative weeks. Make sure you get your five portions of fruit and vegetables each day. Freshly squeezed fruit and vegetable juices are an especially enjoyable way to include these in your daily diet.

therapy to choose will help you to select the therapy most suitable for you or for how you are feeling.

Having a baby is one of the most exciting experiences that you will ever have. These first few weeks are precious, not least because you and your partner will see your baby's heart beating on ultrasound for the first time. This is living proof of the new life within you.

Don't forget that your body needs at least the first 12 weeks to adjust to this new state, physically, mentally and emotionally. As your hormonal balance shifts and your body adapts to some massive changes, you will experience a whole new range of feelings. Look after yourself as much as possible – put yourself first and your baby will benefit too.

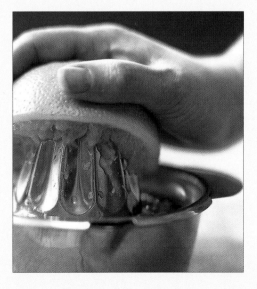

Am I really pregnant?

Some women believe that they sensed the conception of their babies: they did not need to wait for a missed period or other symptoms to know that they were pregnant. This feeling could simply be intuition, or it is possible that these women are able to detect tiny changes inside the body that are associated with the first secretions of the pregnancy hormones. However, most women cannot be sure that they are pregnant until they have had it confirmed by a pregnancy test.

EARLY SIGNS AND SYMPTOMS

The first definite sign of pregnancy is a missed period, known medically as amenorrhoea. Pregnancy is the most likely reason for a missed period, but it is not the only one – stress is another possible explanation. It is therefore best not to assume that you are pregnant just because you have missed your period. The following signs are other early indicators of pregnancy, some of which may occur before you miss a period. However, many women do not notice them until later in the pregnancy:

- Increased tiredness.
- Feeling nauseous, particularly in the mornings.
- Urinating more frequently than usual.
- Tenderness in the breasts.
- Changes in taste, such as a sudden craving for a particular food or a metallic taste in the mouth.

CONFIRMING A PREGNANCY

Most women do their first pregnancy test at home. Pregnancy-testing kits are available from any pharmacy, and they are very accurate. The tests work by measuring the amount of one of the pregnancy hormones, human chorionic gonadotrophin (HCG), in your urine. If enough HCG is present, it triggers a reaction in the test. This is

WHEN YOUR BABY IS DUE

If you know the date of your last period, you can work out your estimated date of delivery using the chart below. The delivery date is normally 40 weeks from the date of your last period but it can be up to two weeks earlier or later. A delivery outside those dates would be considered premature or post-mature.

MONTH	ESTIMATED DATE OF DELIVERY	MONTH
January	1 2 3 4 5 6 7 8 9 10 11 12 13 14 15 16 17 18 19 20 21 22 23 24 25 26 27 28 29 30 31	January
October	8 9 10 11 12 13 14 15 16 17 18 19 20 21 22 23 24 25 26 27 28 29 30 31 1 2 3 4 5 6 7	November
February	1 2 3 4 5 6 7 8 9 10 11 12 13 14 15 16 17 18 19 20 21 22 23 24 25 26 27 28	February
November	8 9 10 11 12 13 14 15 16 17 18 19 20 21 22 23 24 25 26 27 28 29 30 1 2 3 4 5	December
March	1 2 3 4 5 6 7 8 9 10 11 12 13 14 15 16 17 18 19 20 21 22 23 24 25 26 27 28 29 30 31	March
December	6 7 8 9 10 11 12 13 14 15 16 17 18 19 20 21 22 23 24 25 26 27 28 29 30 31 1 2 3 4 5	January
April	1 2 3 4 5 6 7 8 9 10 11 12 13 14 15 16 17 18 19 20 21 22 23 24 25 26 27 28 29 30	April
January	6 7 8 9 10 11 12 13 14 15 16 17 18 19 20 21 22 23 24 25 26 27 28 29 30 31 1 2 3 4	February
May	1 2 3 4 5 6 7 8 9 10 11 12 13 14 15 16 17 18 19 20 21 22 23 24 25 26 27 28 29 30 31	May
February	5 6 7 8 9 10 11 12 13 14 15 16 17 18 19 20 21 22 23 24 25 26 27 28 1 2 3 4 5 6 7	March
June	1 2 3 4 5 6 7 8 9 10 11 12 13 14 15 16 17 18 19 20 21 22 23 24 25 26 27 28 29 30	June
March	8 9 10 11 12 13 14 15 16 17 18 19 20 21 22 23 24 25 26 27 28 29 30 31 1 2 3 4 5 6	April
July	1 2 3 4 5 6 7 8 9 10 11 12 13 14 15 16 17 18 19 20 21 22 23 24 25 26 27 28 29 30 31	July
April	7 8 9 10 11 12 13 14 15 16 17 18 19 20 21 22 23 24 25 26 27 28 29 30 1 2 3 4 5 6 7	May
August	1 2 3 4 5 6 7 8 9 10 11 12 13 14 15 16 17 18 19 20 21 22 23 24 25 26 27 28 29 30 31	August
May	8 9 10 11 12 13 14 15 16 17 18 19 20 21 22 23 24 25 26 27 28 29 30 31 1 2 3 4 5 6 7	June
September	1 2 3 4 5 6 7 8 9 10 11 12 13 14 15 16 17 18 19 20 21 22 23 24 25 26 27 28 29 30	September
June	8 9 10 11 12 13 14 15 16 17 18 19 20 21 22 23 24 25 26 27 28 29 30 1 2 3 4 5 6 7	July
October	1 2 3 4 5 6 7 8 9 10 11 12 13 14 15 16 17 18 19 20 21 22 23 24 25 26 27 28 29 30 31	October
July	8 9 10 11 12 13 14 15 16 17 18 19 20 21 22 23 24 25 26 27 28 29 30 31 1 2 3 4 5 6 7	August
November	1 2 3 4 5 6 7 8 9 10 11 12 13 14 15 16 17 18 19 20 21 22 23 24 25 26 27 28 29 30	November
August	8 9 10 11 12 13 14 15 16 17 18 19 20 21 22 23 24 25 26 27 28 29 30 31 1 2 3 4 5 6	September
December	1 2 3 4 5 6 7 8 9 10 11 12 13 14 15 16 17 18 19 20 21 22 23 24 25 26 27 28 29 30 31	December
September	7 8 9 10 11 12 13 14 15 16 17 18 19 20 21 22 23 24 25 26 27 28 29 30 1 2 3 4 5 6 7	October

Find the first day of your last period on the pink band. The date on the lighter tint below is your estimated date of delivery (EDD).

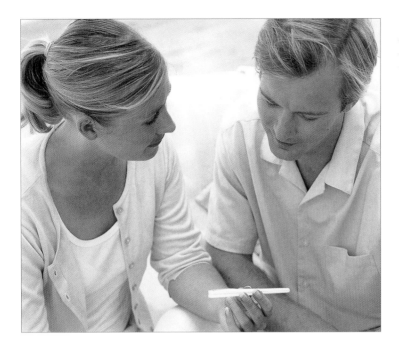

usually shown as a coloured line in the window of the testing strip. The colour may be quite faint, particularly if you are doing the test early on. However, this still counts as a positive result.

The amount of HCG in a woman's body doubles every two or three days during the first six weeks of pregnancy. If a test is negative but your period still does not start, it is worth repeating the test in another two or three days. If the second result is also negative, you are probably not pregnant. See your family doctor for confirmation if you are still unsure.

For optimum results, it can be helpful to do a pregnancy test early in the morning, when HCG is present in its greatest concentrations. However, most modern tests are very sensitive, and they should give an accurate reading at any time of day. You can do the test on the day that your period is due.

How reliable are pregnancy tests?

Pregnancy tests are extremely reliable – if you get a positive result you are almost certainly pregnant. However sometimes women make a mistake, and either do the test wrongly or read the result incorrectly. Very occasionally the test fails to work properly or there is not enough HCG to show a positive result. If you are unsure about a result, you can ask your doctor to do a test for you: you will need to provide a urine sample while you are at the surgery.

Finding out that you are not pregnant can be be very disappointing, especially if you have been trying for a while. It is important for you and your partner to take some time to recover from the disappointment and to talk about how you both feel.

A POSITIVE RESULT

If the result of your home test is positive, make an appointment to see your doctor so that you can start your antenatal care. If you are on any medication, it is important to see your doctor straight away – to ensure it does not interfere with the development of your baby.

What a doctor will do

Your doctor will confirm the pregnancy by doing another pregnancy test. He or she will check that you are taking folic acid and will also ask you about your general health.

You may be offered an ultrasound scan to date the pregnancy if you are not sure when your last period started. A scan through the abdominal wall will show the baby's heartbeat at seven weeks from the last period, so long as you are not overweight. If you are overweight or if the pregnancy is less than seven weeks, a scan through the vagina may be recommended. A vaginal scan can feel slightly uncomfortable, but it does not increase the risk of miscarriage nor does it cause any harm to the baby.

If you have symptoms such as bleeding or pelvic discomfort, a vaginal scan may be done to check that the pregnancy has not established itself outside the uterus (an ectopic pregnancy). This is important because an ectopic pregnancy can be life-threatening if left untreated.

Early development

By the fourth week of its life, your developing baby is showing the first beginnings of the human form that will develop over the months to come. The sex of your child, the colour of its hair and eyes, its build and potential height, and other genetic characteristics are already decided. The embryo is firmly embedded in the wall of your uterus. Soon, he or she will be floating in a protective sac of warm amniotic fluid.

At this stage, the tiny embryo consists of three layers of tissues, which will develop into different parts of the body. The outer layer of tissue (known as the ectoderm) will grow into the baby's skin and nervous system, as well as its ears and eyes. The middle layer (called the mesoderm) will form the cartilage, bones, connective tissues, muscles and the circulatory system, which includes the heart, the kidneys and the sex organs. The inner layer (the endoderm) will develop into your baby's intestinal tract and digestive system, the lungs and the bladder.

A CRUCIAL TIME

Many vital tissues and organs form between the fourth and eighth week, making this the most important period in the development of the baby. A harmful substance or an infection is more likely to cause a serious problem at

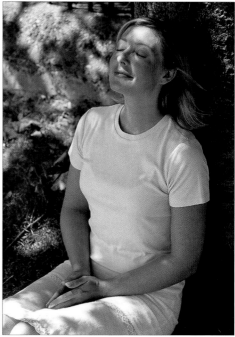

Your baby develops rapidly during the first few weeks of pregnancy, which is why women tend to feel so tired in the first trimester. To help your baby thrive, you need plenty of rest and early nights, as well as fresh air, regular exercise and a healthy diet.

this stage rather than later in the pregnancy, when the baby's organs are in place. This is why it is so important for women to look after their general health when they are trying to conceive – because they could already be carrying a baby and not be aware of it.

Weeks 5–8

Between the fourth and fifth week of its life, the embryo more than doubles in size. By week five, it measures 5–6mm (about ¼in) in length. Despite its tiny size, it has the beginnings of a brain and spinal cord. This develops

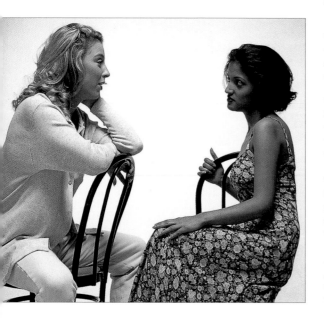

As soon as you know that you have conceived, your pregnancy may dominate your thoughts. Confiding in a close friend allows you to share your joy and also to voice any mixed feelings or anxieties.

EARLY DEVELOPMENT OF THE EMBRYO

Your baby's life starts from the moment that the sperm penetrates the egg – conception. At this point the egg is still in the Fallopian tube, but it will make its way to the uterus over the next few days. As it journeys towards the uterus, the fertilized egg is undergoing the first stages of its development.

WEEK 1
FERTILIZATION

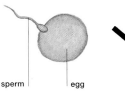

sperm | egg

Conception occurs when a sperm fertilizes the egg in the Fallopian tube. It will take four days for the fertilized egg to make its way to the uterus.

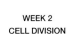

WEEK 2
CELL DIVISION

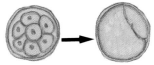

ball of eight cells | blastocyst

The fertilized egg divides again and again, forming a ball of cells. Eventually, there is a mass of 150 cells, arranged in two sections: the outer cells will develop into the placenta and amniotic sac, while the inner cells become the baby. The blastocyst, as it is now known, attaches itself to the uterus lining.

WEEK 4 +
DEVELOPING EMBRYO

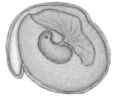

The tiny embryo begins to take shape. Its brain and spinal cord are starting to develop, and its heart is beating. It is attached to the placenta by a tiny stalk, which will develop into the umbilical cord.

WEEK 3
THREE LAYERS

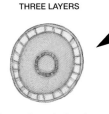

The inner cells are in three layers. The outer layer will become the baby's skin and nerves; the middle one will be the muscles, heart and skeleton; and the inner one develops into other organs.

from the neural tube, which has started to form. At this stage, the baby's heart has already started to beat, although it will not be detectable by ultrasound for another week or two. The heart has only two chambers rather than the four that will develop within another week or so.

The embryo is connected to the developing placenta by a thin stalk, which is the rudimentary beginning of the umbilical cord. Blood vessels are already forming here. From this lifeline, the baby will derive essential nutrients and oxygen, which are needed for its healthy development and growth. At this early stage the placenta is larger than the embryo.

WHAT THE DOCTORS SAY

Medically, your growing baby is known as an embryo until the eighth week of pregnancy, when all the internal organs are formed. It is then known as a fetus until the delivery.

Medical terms can sound baffling. Always ask about unfamiliar terms and abbreviations that you do not understand. Your doctors and midwife should be happy to explain what they mean.

Development from six weeks

The embryo develops rapidly from the sixth to eighth week of pregnancy. It passes through a number of phases that some theorists believe resemble the stages of human evolution – from 'tadpole' through a fish-like stage to primitive mammal and finally a tiny human being.

Week 6
During the sixth week, the baby's head forms, rapidly followed by the chest and abdominal cavities. Its rudimentary brain is completed and a spinal column, as well as a spinal cord, is properly formed. The circulation is about to begin functioning. The embryo's heart is now beating steadily, much faster than your own. The stomach is forming, the kidneys are maturing and the liver has grown so much that it almost fills the entire abdominal cavity.

It is also in the sixth week that the baby's face starts to take shape. This is a process that will take several more weeks to complete. Small depressions are appearing where the eyes and ears will be situated. The mouth and jaw are beginning to develop. The embryo is now, incredibly, 10,000 times larger than the fertilized cell from which it originated.

Week 7
The kidneys and lungs start to develop and the head continues to grow, forming a more recognizably human shape. The buds that will form arms and legs are apparent.

Week 8
All the internal organs are now formed, although they will continue to mature. The baby now measures 2.5cm (1in) in length. Doctors will now start referring to it as a fetus.

Weeks 10–11
The baby is moving about a great deal, although you will not yet be able to feel this. The fingers and toes are forming, but are still joined by webs of skin. The facial features are more distinct, and the baby now has eyes.

EARLY DEVELOPMENT, WEEKS 6–13
By week 7, the embryo can be seen on an ultrasound scan. The tiny heart is beating, and the major organs have started to develop. By week 12 or 13, the embryo is a tiny recognizable human with facial features.

6 WEEKS

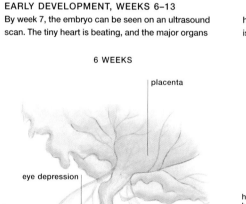

placenta

eye depression

head and face starting to form

umbilical cord

spine

arm bud starting to appear

7–8 WEEKS

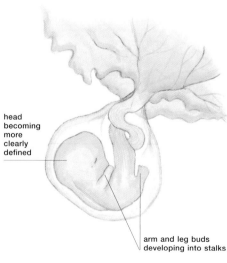

head becoming more clearly defined

arm and leg buds developing into stalks

Weeks 12–13

The external genitals have formed and all facial features are in place. Your baby measures about 7.5cm (3in) in length (roughly the size of an avocado). The muscles are getting stronger, so movements are more vigorous.

SEEING YOUR BABY

Ultrasound enables you to see your baby while it is in the uterus. Most people find this a very moving experience, and it can help to strengthen your feelings of connection with your developing baby.

An ultrasound is invaluable in determining the definite existence of a pregnancy as well as the age of the embryo or fetus. You will be offered an early scan to date the pregnancy if you do not know the day of your last period. Otherwise, most women have their first scan at 10–12 weeks. This scan is used to confirm that the baby is able to develop – in medical terms, whether the fetus is viable. The scan can also identify the existence of a multiple pregnancy, so you will know early on if you are carrying twins, triplets or more.

Another scan is usually carried out at about 18 weeks. This scan is used to identify any developmental and structural abnormalities that may not have been apparent at an earlier stage of the pregnancy.

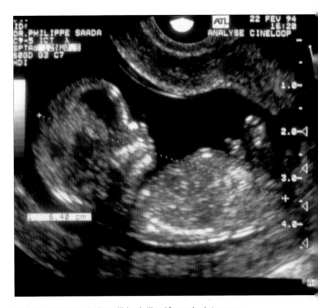

This is what your baby will look like 12 weeks into your pregnancy – you can see the face at the upper left of the picture. The baby weighs about 45g (1½oz).

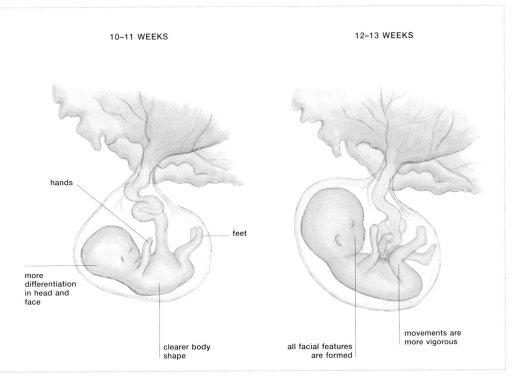

10–11 WEEKS

hands

more differentiation in head and face

feet

clearer body shape

12–13 WEEKS

all facial features are formed

movements are more vigorous

How your body is changing

Your baby grows rapidly during the first three months of pregnancy, and your body changes at the same time. However, most of these developments will go unnoticed by anyone except you and, to a lesser extent, your partner. Many women find it hard to believe that they look much the same as normal, but they do.

Your uterus grows to accommodate the developing baby, but by the end of the first trimester it is still no bigger than an avocado pear. Few people will see any difference in your outward appearance. However, when you are naked, you and your partner may notice that your breasts are fuller, and that your nipples have increased in size and darkened. Some women do fill out a little.

The most noticeable effects of your pregnancy, though, will be in the way you feel rather than in the way that you look. Your breasts may tingle. You may experience a feeling of fullness in your abdomen. You are likely to want to pass water more frequently, and you may feel nauseous some or perhaps all of the time. You will probably feel alternately anxious and excited as you come to terms with the fact that you are pregnant.

FATIGUE

The rapid development rate of the baby in the first weeks of pregnancy is bound to make you feel tired. To help yourself to cope – and to ensure that your baby thrives – you need early nights, regular exercise and a good, healthy diet. Some women feel energized during early

MEETING YOUR NEEDS

Your body will undergo various changes in the first trimester and you will almost certainly need extra sleep. You may also benefit from doing some of the following:

- Take a rest in the afternoon.
- Drink lots of fruit and vegetable juices.
- Go for a short walk every morning before you start work.
- Swim at lunchtime or after work, two or three times a week.
- Avoid doing any everyday tasks that are not vitally important – for example, ironing or dusting. Ask your partner or friends for help when you need it.
- Wear flat, comfortable shoes.
- Go to bed an hour earlier every night – read in bed for a bit if you don't feel sleepy immediately.
- Treat yourself to an aromatherapy massage or acupuncture session (always seek professional advice about such treatments).
- Buy some relaxing herbal bath preparations and pamper yourself.
- Show your partner that you love, respect and desire him.

pregnancy, but most feel very tired in a way that feels new. You may feel an overwhelming desire to nap in the afternoon, or to get to bed much earlier than usual. The best way to deal with this is to give in to it – rest as much as you can.

MORNING SICKNESS

Some women sail through their pregnancies without having any nausea, but most experience at least some morning sickness. There are various theories about why this nausea occurs, and some doctors maintain that it is purely psychological. However, most experts think that it is connected to the increased level of hormones circulating in the blood. Morning sickness most commonly affects women in the morning – hence its

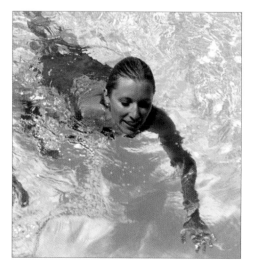

Swimming – say, two or three times a week – is one of the best forms of exercise in pregnancy. It works all your muscles, and increases flexibility and stamina.

> **❝** Your baby grows rapidly during the first three months, and your body changes at the same time. Most of these developments will go unnoticed. **❞**

name – but it can also occur at other times of day. Some women feel nauseous all day for the first few weeks. Morning sickness usually starts during the sixth week and continues until the twelfth or fourteenth. However, it sometimes continues throughout pregnancy.

Eating little and often can be helpful, and it is usually best to eat something to raise your blood sugar levels before you get up in the morning. A dry biscuit or piece of toast is ideal. Many women find drinking ginger tea or sucking on a piece of raw ginger can help. You should also make sure you drink plenty of fluids, particularly if you are vomiting.

Morning sickness may be exacerbated by kitchen smells, tobacco smoke and alcohol, so these should be avoided. It is not uncommon to notice flecks of blood in the vomit. This is because repeated vomiting may cause breakage of tiny blood vessels in the throat or gullet. The blood vessels will heal by themselves so there is no need to be alarmed by this. However, if your sickness is very severe, tell your doctor.

URINATION

One of the earliest signs of pregnancy is an increased frequency in urination. This is known medically as micturition. Some women notice they are passing water more often as early as one week after conception. The increase is due partly to the growing uterus pressing against the nearby bladder, and partly because alterations in hormone levels lead to changes in muscle tone. The increase in frequency of urination is often particularly pronounced in the first nine weeks. After this, the uterus tends to moves upwards, which relieves the pressure on the bladder until much later in the pregnancy.

Some women find that they need to pass water more often throughout their whole pregnancy. It is also quite common to pass a small amount of urine when you laugh or cough. Wearing well-fitting briefs with a light sanitary towel or incontinence pad will help.

TENDER BREASTS

Your breasts may feel heavy and tender, and they often increase in size early on so it is worth investing in a new bra. Your nipples may feel sore and sensitive. They are likely to become harder and may darken in colour. Small white spots may become more pronounced. Breast tenderness is usually relieved after the eighth week.

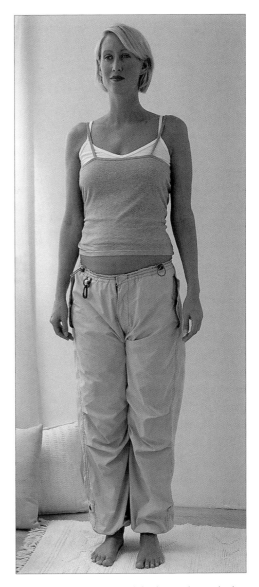

You will soon start to see subtle changes in your body shape as your baby grows and your uterus increases in size to accommodate him or her.

TASTE

Pregnant women often report experiencing a strange metallic taste in the mouth. You may also develop new preferences for certain foods and drinks, and go off others – particularly coffee, alcohol and fried foods. Try to resist any cravings for sugary or high-fat snacks since these are high in calories but low in nutrients.

Emotional changes

The first few months of pregnancy are a time when you and your partner will be discussing all sorts of practical as well as emotional issues. For example, should you stay in the same home or should you move somewhere bigger or closer to family? If you are staying put, do you need to make changes? Will you want to start decorating a nursery?

You need to consider whether you tell close family and friends straight away, or whether you keep the news to yourselves for a few weeks. Keeping quiet can give you a precious opportunity to enjoy and look forward to this very special journey together. Many couples wait until they are past the twelfth week, and they know that the pregnancy is well established, before sharing the news.

FEELING ANXIOUS

Almost everyone experiences anxiety at some stage of their pregnancy, and most women find that different worries crop up throughout. It is very common to have underlying fears about the health of the baby, particularly before you have gone through any of the antenatal tests. Many women feel anxious about how they will cope with the pregnancy, and how they will deal with the labour and delivery. In addition, couples often doubt their ability to be

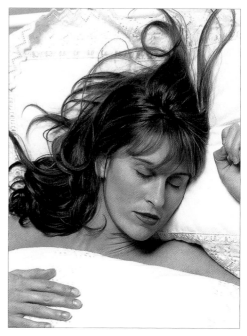

Most pregnant women find that they want to sleep more; dreams can be very important now, allowing your mind to adapt to the profound life changes ahead.

good parents and worry about how they will cope with all the practicalities of caring for a child. Concern about the impact that a child will have on your financial situation, sexual relationship, careers and social lives can all surface during pregnancy.

It is important to keep a sense of perspective, and to realize that doubts and worries are perfectly normal. After all, you are embarking on a life-changing event. However, if anxiety starts to dominate your thinking, it can be helpful to confide in a close friend or relative who has had a child, or to talk to your midwife.

You may also experience strange dreams about giving birth or becoming a mother. These dreams reflect the natural anxiety that you feel, and they are also a way of preparing psychologically for the new role ahead of you.

Fluctuating hormone levels may play havoc with your emotions and stability. Get plenty of rest and recognize any volatility for the biological phenomenon that it is.

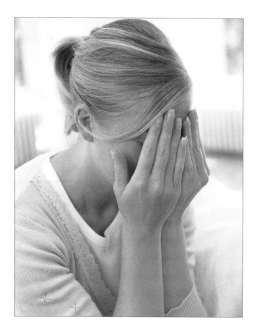

COMMUNICATING WITH YOUR BABY

Some women find that they do not experience a sense of connection with their baby until later in their pregnancy – and occasionally only after the birth. However, many women feel a bond with the growing baby early on, perhaps as soon as they know they are pregnant. This can be a very special feeling; suddenly the most important thing in the world is the health and well-being of the tiny baby inside you.

Fathers often do not feel a sense of bonding in the first months, when there is little outward sign of the baby's presence. This is understandable, but many women find it hard to accept their partner is not quite so fascinated with the pregnancy as they are. Both partners may need to exercise some tolerance about the different ways that they react to the pregnancy.

It usually helps if the father gets involved right from the start. Ideally he will attend any scans so that he can see the baby on screen. Some men like to talk to the baby through the mother's abdomen. Stroking the mother's

> 66 Suddenly the most important thing in the world is the health and well-being of the tiny baby inside you. 99

belly or playing music to the baby can also help fathers to feel more connected with the life they have created.

Nobody knows how much unborn babies can hear or feel in the uterus, but some research shows that they learn to recognize their parents' voices before they are born. The ears are formed by the seventh week, and it is known that external sounds filter through. Researchers have now found that unborn babies can also distinguish different intonation patterns – so they may be able to recognize the speech sounds you and your partner make.

Communicating with your baby can help you and your partner to bond with your unborn child, long before he or she comes into the world to be part of your family.

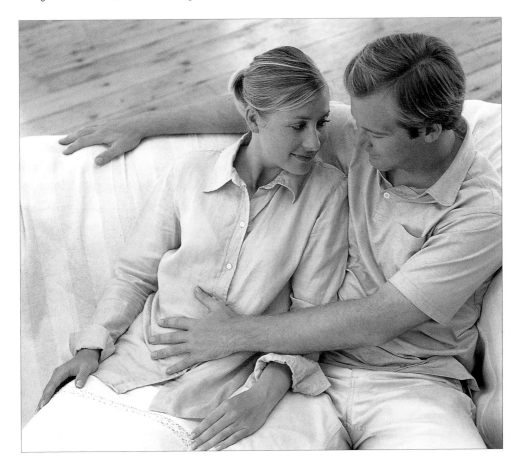

Pregnancy and eating

For the whole of your pregnancy, and longer if you are breastfeeding, your baby is dependent on you for essential nutrients such as protein, calcium, folic acid and water. These nutrients come either from your current diet or from the stores you built up before conception.

Providing for your own and your baby's needs is not complicated. All you need to do is eat a variety of wholesome foods that are fresh (or minimally processed) from the essential food groups. These are listed on pages 30–31. You also need to avoid a few potentially harmful foods, which are listed on pages 36–37.

The amount of food that you need to eat does not increase that much during pregnancy. However, make sure that you are eating enough to receive certain essential nutrients – especially plenty of fruit and vegetables, so that you get a wide range of vitamins. Other important nutrients for pregnancy are protein, calcium and iron.

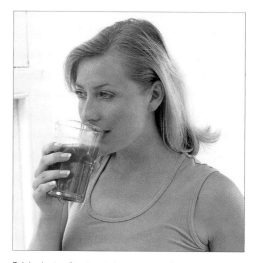

Drink plenty of water and unsweetened fruit juices. Cut out tea, coffee and alcohol for optimum health.

PROTEIN

You need 60–100g (2¼–3¾oz) protein per day, and high-protein foods should constitute about 25 per cent of your diet. Good sources of protein include vegetables, lean meat, chicken, fish, eggs, skimmed milk, nuts, cheese, dried peas, beans and grains.

IRON

Pregnancy results in a large increase in the volume of blood in the mother's body. This means that extra iron is needed to make haemoglobin, the oxygen-carrying pigment found in red blood cells. The more haemoglobin that blood contains, the more oxygen it can carry to the various tissues, including the placenta.

The recommended daily amount (RDA) of iron required during pregnancy is 27mg, and you may be prescribed a supplement. The need for iron increases particularly in the

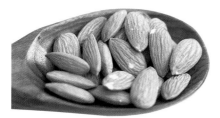

If you feel like a snack, take some healthy protein in the form of almonds or other whole nuts. Combine them with some dried fruit for extra nutrients.

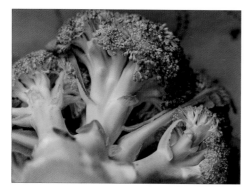

Iron is an important element of your diet, especially when you are pregnant. Broccoli is a good source, and it also contains essential folic acid.

WHEN NAUSEA STRIKES
If you are suffering from morning sickness, try eating little meals at frequent intervals rather than having one or two large meals. This will help to prevent indigestion and heartburn, too.

second and third trimester. Good food sources include breads, cereals, dried peas and beans, broccoli and green leafy vegetables.

CALCIUM

Your daily need for calcium is about 1200mg in pregnancy. Good food sources include milk, all other dairy products and green vegetables. Your growing baby needs calcium to build strong bones and teeth. If you do not take in sufficient from your diet, the baby will take calcium from your bones and teeth. You also need vitamin D – produced in the body after exposure to sunlight and also found in some foods – to help your body to process this mineral.

FOLIC ACID

Your folic acid requirement increases considerably in pregnancy, to 400mcg (or more in some high-risk categories). High intake before conception will also help reduce the risk of neural tube defects in your baby. You can make sure that you receive enough by taking a daily supplement of 400mcg. You should also try to eat at least one dark green leafy vegetable and two to three servings of fruit a day. Sprinkling wheatgerm on your food and not overcooking it will also help maximize your intake – overcooking food destroys any folic acid.

PROTECTING YOUR BABY

The baby will take the nutrients it needs from the mother's bloodstream through the placenta. Researchers are now learning that the developing baby is much more sensitive to the mother's nutritional status than previously thought. Occasional treats do no harm, but it makes sense to follow a healthy diet throughout your pregnancy. Poor intake of one or more essential nutrients during critical periods in an organ's growth can alter the structure, size and functions of that organ. Mothers who eat an excessive amount and who consume a diet high in saturated fat could be putting their unborn babies at greater risk of heart disease, diabetes and high blood pressure later in life.

AVOIDING CONSTIPATION

Pregnant women often suffer from constipation, which contributes to a general sense of lethargy and bloating. It is caused by hormonal changes, which make the muscles of the digestive and gastrointestinal systems less efficient.

Do not take any drugs for constipation. Instead drink eight to ten glasses of water every day and follow a healthy diet: make sure that you are eating five helpings of fruit and vegetables each day and that you include high-fibre wholegrain cereals in your diet. It can also be helpful to avoid bananas, hard-boiled eggs, Brussels sprouts and red meat for a few days.

ESSENTIAL VITAMINS AND MINERALS

Certain vitamins and minerals are vital for a healthy pregnancy. You may need a higher-than-average daily intake of some nutrients, such as vitamin B1. Use the following list to help you to plan your pregnancy diet:

- **Vitamin B1 or thiamine:** about 1.4mg a day – from enriched breads, cereals, grain products, seeds and nuts.
- **Vitamin B2 or riboflavin:** 1.4mg a day – from meat, dairy produce and cereals.
- **Vitamin B3 or niacin:** from fish, meat, nuts, and wholegrains.
- **Vitamin B6 or pyridoxine:** from chicken, fish, soya beans and oats.
- **Vitamin B12 or cobalamin:** from meat, fish, eggs and milk and also from enriched grain products.
- **Vitamin C:** 50mg – from citrus fruit, tomatoes, red and green peppers, broccoli, cauliflower, spinach and strawberries.
- **Vitamin D:** 10mg a day – from milk, eggs, butter and fortified margarine.
- **Vitamin E:** from margarine, vegetable oils, wholegrains and nuts.
- **Magnesium:** 300mg a day – from dairy products, vegetables and meat.
- **Zinc:** 7–15mg a day – from nuts, wholegrains, legumes and eggs.
- **Vitamin A:** 700mcg a day – from fortified milk, eggs, carrots and dark green leafy vegetables.

Plums and other fruits provide you with beneficial vitamins and help to combat constipation. They can also give you a quick boost when you feel tired.

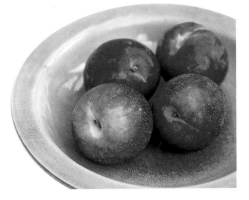

Your lifestyle checklist

Pregnancy is an exciting time, but it can also be stressful, too. Monitoring the different aspects of your lifestyle is an essential element of good antenatal care. By prioritizing your health, you can make the experience of pregnancy much easier. In particular, you need to be:

- Eating well.
- Sleeping well.
- De-stressing and relaxing.
- Exercising regularly.

YOUR EATING HABITS

Have regular meals and give yourself time to eat in a relaxed way. Avoid eating heavy, fatty foods late at night and do not go out on an empty stomach in the morning. Think about what you are eating and drinking and ask yourself if your daily diet is nurturing you and your baby. Are you providing yourself with sufficient nutrients to maintain your energy and well-being?

Try to cut out snacks that are high in sugar or saturated fat. In particular, avoid the following, or have them only as an occasional treat:

- Crisps.
- Cakes and biscuits.
- Coffee and tea.
- Sweetened drinks.
- Red meat (once a week is ample).
- Fried foods.
- Foods containing white sugar.
- White bread.
- Chocolate.
- Convenience foods and ready meals.
- Salt (particularly in snacks).
- Fast food takeaways.
- Sugar and sweets.

SLEEPING

You need to rest as much as possible to combat the fatigue that is typical of the first trimester. This will help to keep you in good shape for the pregnancy and the birth. Consider whether you are getting enough rest. Ask yourself if you are:

- Tired on waking up.
- Using chocolate or other high-calorie snacks to keep you going during the day.
- Sleepy in the middle of the afternoon.
- Exhausted by a day at work.
- Falling asleep in front of the television.
- Unable to sleep when you get to bed.

All these are signs that you need more sleep and more exercise. Try going to bed half an hour earlier for a week. In the second week, continue going to bed earlier than normal and then get up half an hour earlier every morning as well. Have a drink of water or juice and eat a slice or two of toast, then go for a short walk or practise some stretches at home.

FEEDING THE BODY WITH JUICES

Whip up your own juices or smoothies. Most of the body is made up of water, so it can quickly become dehydrated. The vitamins and minerals contained in fruit and uncooked vegetables, together with their high liquid content, make them the ideal food for you and your growing baby. And of course, they taste delicious . Try the following combinations:

- Cranberry, peach and mango.
- Papaya and melon.
- Gooseberry and apple.
- Radish and cucumber.
- Spinach and lemon.
- Carrot, apple and ginger.
- Pineapple and pink grapefruit.
- Strawberry and nectarine.
- Banana and lemon.
- Carrot and beetroot.
- Cucumber and celery.
- Banana and kiwi fruit.
- Red cabbage, apple and lemont.
- Pear, beetroot (beet) and pineapple

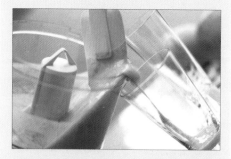

A juicer is a great investment, letting you prepare fresh, health-boosting drinks whenever you like.

DE-STRESSING

Stress is not good for you or the baby. Many women feel anxious about whether the baby is developing properly, about whether they are doing the right things to maintain the pregnancy, and about how they will cope with having a baby. In addition, you have to cope with all the normal demands of daily life – at a time when you may be feeling unwell or very tired.

If you are feeling unduly stressed or simply don't seem to be able to relax, then it may help to get some extra support from a complementary therapist. Acupuncture, aromatherapy massage, reflexology, shiatsu and homeopathy can all help to relieve anxiety and stress. It is also important to make sure that you have time to do things that you enjoy – whether that is going for a walk or

seeing a film. Try to earmark time for yourself each day. Use this for activities that you really enjoy, or just to sit quietly and rest.

EXERCISE

Gentle exercise helps to boost your circulation, which increases the oxygen and nutrients reaching your baby. It also helps to build muscular strength and stamina, which you need to cope with pregnancy and birth. Any form of exercise will help: walking, swimming and cycling are ideal because they are sustained and rhythmic, providing a workout for the heart and lungs. Exercise taken early in the day will set you up and get the circulation going for the rest of the day. Exercising in the evening will help you to unwind and may enhance sleep, so long as it is not too vigorous.

Chest opener

This Pilates-influenced chest stretch is good to practise if you are feeling stressed or tense during the day. It opens up the upper body, soothing tired muscles, making

breathing easier and promoting relaxation and a straight spine – very important for the expectant woman. It is especially helpful if you have been sitting at a desk all day.

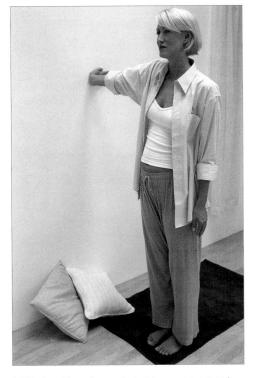

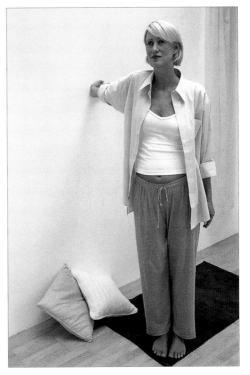

1 Standing side-on to a wall, stretch your arm out and place your hand against it as shown. If it feels more comfortable, place your hand so that the fingers are pointing towards the ceiling.

2 Now turn away from the wall, keeping your hand on the wall. This gives a gentle stretch to your chest. Do not force anything, and keep your shoulders relaxed as you turn. Repeat on the other side.

Good ways to exercise

The following forms of exercise can be of particular benefit during pregnancy:
- dancing
- swimming
- walking
- t'ai chi
- Pilates
- yoga

If you are not used to exercising, confine yourself to regular walking or swimming in the first three months. Thereafter, it should be fine to try a new form of exercise provided that you have not experienced any bleeding or other problems. Check with your midwife or doctor first, build up your fitness slowly, and do not to overstretch yourself. Seek out a professional instructor who is used to working with pregnant women.

SWIMMING

A few lengths at your local pool can be remarkably energizing. The water will take the weight of your body so that you can move freely. Swimming helps to improve your suppleness as well as your stamina. It also helps to stimulate blood flow around your body, and thus increases the delivery of oxygen to your growing baby.

You may like to consider taking swimming classes to improve your technique, and to ensure that you are not putting unnecessary strain on your body. The Shaw method is based on Alexander technique, and will help you to use your body in the most efficient way possible. Another great form of water exercise is aqua yoga – literally, yoga in water – and many local pools and leisure clubs offer classes in this.

WALKING

Like swimming, walking is a great form of exercise when you are pregnant. A brisk walk really helps to stimulate your respiratory and cardiovascular systems, which need to be in good form when you are carrying a baby and in preparation for the birth itself. Walking is also good for encouraging circulation in the legs – thus helping to prevent varicose veins – and it gets you out into the open air, which usually encourages good sleep and relaxation. Cycling offers many of the same benefits.

DANCE THERAPY

Going to dance classes is usually good fun, and a great way of socializing, making new friends and maintaining fitness at the same time. You will find a number of

Exercising in water

Doing simple exercises and stretches in water is an especially good idea when you are pregnant because the water is so supportive. The two steps shown below use the water's resistance to help tone your upper

arms, which can accumulate fat during pregnancy. This exercise will also open the chest, helping the heart to work faster as your baby grows, and strengthen the upper body in general, aiding your posture.

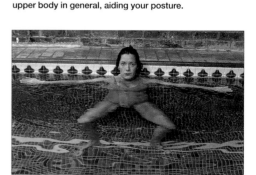

1 The water should come up to your neck, so stand with your knees slightly bent, if necessary, or kneel if the water is shallow. Now, with both palms touching, stretch your arms right out in front of you.

2 Turn your hands out and open your arms in a wide, circling movement. Take them as far back as possible, then return to the centre. Repeat several times. Inhale as you stretch out and exhale as you return to the centre.

different dance classes on offer at all kinds of places in your local area, and private classes may also be available – a good way to start if you are self-conscious.

One exciting way of keeping fit during pregnancy could be belly dancing. This gentle, rhythmic exercise promotes muscle strength and stamina, so it can help you to manage pregnancy and labour. Belly dancing originated from a combination of symbolic rituals and sexual display. The undulating movements of the pelvis and abdomen, which involve considerable muscular control, are thought by some to be symbolic of conception and birth. These are usually beneficial during a normal pregnancy, but check with your midwife or doctor first. Look out for classes aimed specifically at pregnant women.

PILATES

A gentle form of exercise that improves flexibility, strength and stamina, Pilates places a strong emphasis on posture and alignment. Pilates works on both mind and body, so it can induce deep relaxation and a sense of greater control over your body, which may be helpful during labour.

Exercises can be tailored to individual needs, so Pilates can be practised safely throughout pregnancy as long as you already understand the basic techniques and avoid certain postures. Seek advice from an experienced, qualified teacher, and be sure to tell them that you are pregnant. If you are new to Pilates, do not start in the first three months of pregnancy.

YOGA

Certain types of yoga are widely recommended for pregnancy, particularly the second and third trimesters. Practised regularly, it strengthens muscles, enhances suppleness and improves posture – all of which are helpful during pregnancy and labour. Yoga also involves breathing exercises, which can help with relaxation.

Specific yoga postures, such as squatting, are particularly helpful for pregnant women; others are not suitable and may be harmful. It is therefore best to attend special antenatal yoga classes, or ask your teacher how to adapt the poses. Do not go to general classes if you are new to yoga, particularly in the first trimester.

T'AI CHI

Sometimes described as 'meditation in motion', t'ai chi is a non-combative martial art that involves moving very slowly through a set routine of postures. You repeat the routine over and over again, producing a flowing, synchronized series of movements.

T'ai chi involves controlled, slow movements, which aim to improve the body's flow of energy. It helps mobilize the joints, improve posture and enhance well-being. T'ai chi aids relaxation and enhances body-awareness. It is generally considered safe in pregnancy.

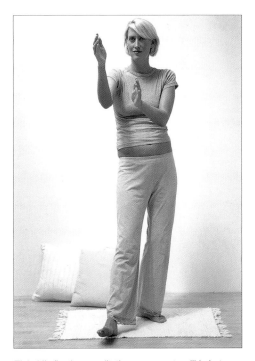

T'ai chi's flowing, meditative movements will help to enhance your awareness of what is happening to your body and mind during pregnancy.

EXERCISING DURING PREGNANCY

You should exercise regularly (ideally for at least 30 minutes, four times a week) in order to work the muscles and circulation, raise energy and endorphin levels and combat stress.

If you have an established exercise routine, it is safe to continue it provided that there are no problems with the pregnancy, but tell any instructors that you are pregnant. However, you may need to reduce the amount or the intensity of any exercise as you must not overexert or exhaust yourself when pregnant (so avoid long periods of aerobic exercise). Do not let yourself become overheated or dehydrated, as this can reduce blood flow and in turn the supply of oxygen to your baby (drink plenty of water as you exercise). If you experience problems with your pregnancy, such as bleeding or abdominal pain, ask your doctor about the advisability of exercising.

In general, it is not a good idea to start a new, unfamiliar form of exercise in the first months of pregnancy. This is because you can easily cause yourself harm if your technique is incorrect.

Keeping your joints mobile

It is important to keep your body open and flexible, in order to enjoy a pregnancy that is as free as possible from aches and pains, and to help pave the way towards a good, comfortable birth.

Releasing the head, neck and shoulders will help to get you into good posture habits, ease stress and minimize certain kinds of tension headache. It will also help to expand the chest, improving breathing and circulation and so making you feel more energetic and helping to bring plenty of nourishing, oxygen-rich blood to your developing baby. The beauty of the neck and shoulder exercises shown below is that they can be done virtually anywhere, any time, as you sit at your desk at work, watch television or sit on the bus, for example.

Loosening the joints

Anyone can do the following easy stretches, which will help to keep your joints mobile and flexible. They make a good short loosening-up routine for the morning, and can help you to warm up for more aerobic exercise, such as brisk walking on the spot or cycling. Work very gently and go only as far as feels comfortable to you.

RELEASING THE HEAD AND NECK

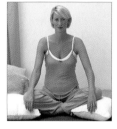 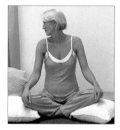 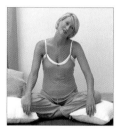 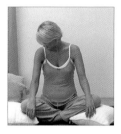

1 Sit comfortably on the floor, cross-legged or with one leg in front of the other. Place one cushion under your buttocks and another under each knee.

2 Slowly turn your head to the right and bring it back to the centre. Now turn it slowly to the left. Repeat several times, breathing normally as you do so.

3 Now slowly drop your head so that your ear is close to your right shoulder. Return it to the centre, then repeat on the left. Repeat several times.

4 Turn your head to the right, drop your chin close to your chest, then move over to the left. Repeat in the opposite direction. Repeat several times.

RELEASING THE SHOULDERS

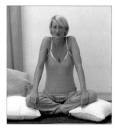 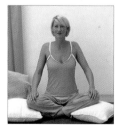 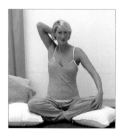 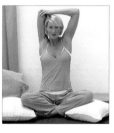

1 Bring your shoulders upwards and slightly forwards, until they are close to your ears. Keep breathing as you do so.

2 Then move the shoulders back and down, to make a rotating movement. Repeat this several times.

3 Raise your right arm, bending the elbow. Drop your forearm down so that you can place your palm in your upper back.

4 Hold the elbow with the left hand. Relax the shoulders, and hold for a few moments, breathing deeply. Repeat on the left.

Loosening up the spine helps to keep it strong and supple. A flexible spine is the lynchpin of good, upright posture, which can start to suffer with the weight of a growing baby. Correct posture brings these benefits:

- It holds the uterus in the correct position and opens up more space in the abdominal area, so making pregancy more comfortable for both you and your baby and ensuring that the blood supply to the uterus is not constricted.
- It opens up the chest cavity, which becomes more restricted as your baby grows in size, and so improves breathing and circulation, the benefits of which have been covered opposite.

- It makes you feel and look better and minimizes the backache, cramp and sciatica suffered by so many pregnant women.

Loosening up the hips and legs brings vital benefits. The exercise shown below helps to:

- Rest the lower back and legs, which often feel tired and achy during pregnancy.
- Open up your entire pelvic region, exercising and toning the all-important muscles of the pelvic floor area. Well-toned pelvic muscles help to: keep you comfortable when the baby is pressing against the pelvic floor; ease the baby's actual birth; prevent certain post-natal problems.

RELEASING THE SPINE

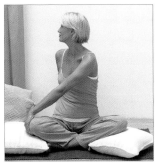

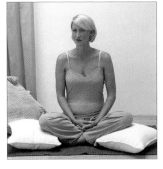

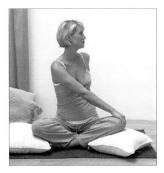

1 Place your left hand on your right knee, gently turn the upper body and look over your right shoulder.

2 Drop your shoulders, hold for a few moments, then return to the centre. Keep breathing deeply.

3 Repeat on the other side. Be very gentle, and take care not to push your body into a strong twist.

RELEASING THE HIPS AND LEGS

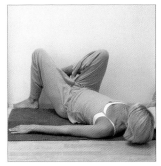

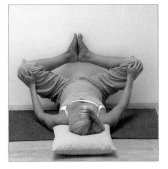

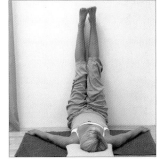

1 Sit next to a wall, so that the side of your body is facing it. Lie down, moving from your side to your back, and slowly swinging your legs up the wall as you do so. Your buttocks should touch the wall. Rest your head on a cushion and breathe.

2 Bend your knees, bringing the soles of your feet together. Place your hands on your knees and press gently towards the wall. Hold for a few moments, or longer if you like, then release. Do not force this: your flexibility will improve with practice.

3 Slide your legs back up the wall. Remain in this posture for a few minutes if you like, breathing deeply and letting any tension drain away. To come up, bend your knees again and then roll on to your side, before getting up slowly.

Yoga for the first trimester

These easy yoga exercises help to improve the posture, which can be adversely affected during pregnancy. Always take care when practising yoga poses, even simple ones like these. Go only as far as feels comfortable, and keep breathing evenly throughout. Lie down and relax for five minutes afterwards.

Grounding

Your hips, legs and feet take your weight, while the pelvis helps support the upper body. These important muscle groups can be strengthened by this grounding exercise, which allows your weight to pass through the legs and feet into the ground. Practised regularly, it will help you cope with the growing weight of your baby.

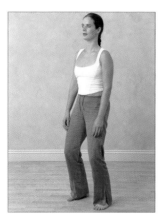

1 Stand with the feet apart and knees slightly bent. Keep an upright spine, tucking in your chin and tail bone, and keeping the head erect.

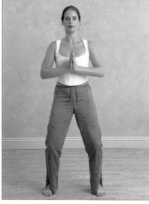

2 Bring your hands into a prayer position. Press your palms firmly together with elbows out to the sides. Do not tense the shoulders.

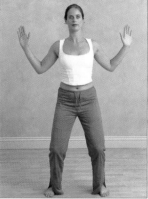

3 Now spread your hands wide, keeping your elbows bent and opening up your chest area. Breathe in deeply as you do this.

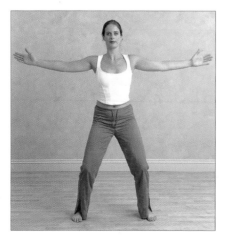

4 Left: Stretch your arms out to the sides and lower them to your sides, breathing out. Repeat steps 2 to 4 several times.

5 Right: For a stronger version of this exercise, place one foot on a low chair and bend the other knee. Change legs after a few breaths and repeat with the other foot on the chair.

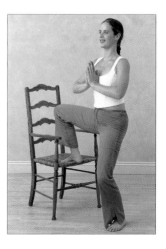

Standing stretches

By extending up from the hips and through the waist, you create space for the diaphragm, which helps you to take deeper breaths. Gently turn and sway rhythmically as if you are dancing, but do not go into a strong twist.

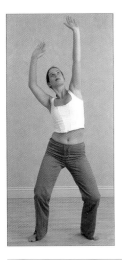

1 Left: Stand in an upright, relaxed posture with your knees loosely bent. Stretch your arms overhead, first one and then the other. Feel your ribs and waist opening and releasing.

2 Right: Now bring your arms out at shoulder level and swing round from the waist, first to one side and then the other, without changing your leg or arm position. Repeat both movements.

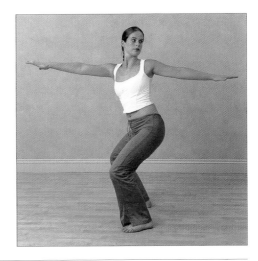

Adapted easy triangle sequence

This sequence works out your abdominal muscles and increases flexibility in the lower spine. This can help to prevent backache and tone up your muscles. However, make sure that you proceed very gently.

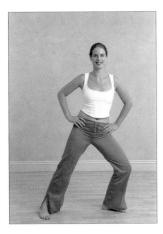

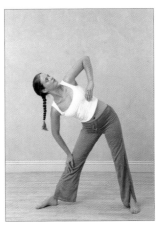

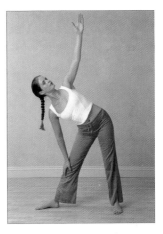

1 Stand tall with feet wide and knees bent. Place your hands on your hips. Sway from side to side, tipping your pelvis up to the right as you sway to the right and up to the left as you sway to the left in a rhythmical movement. Keep your spine erect, coccyx tucked under and chest lifted. Repeat several times.

2 Now bend to your right side without tipping forwards – keep your back straight and do not push yourself further than feels comfortable. Place your right hand along your leg and bring your left elbow back to open the left side of the waist and chest as you look up. Keep breathing rhythmically.

3 Without losing the extension in your back, stretch your left arm up and back to open the left side of your body. Keep your abdomen relaxed and do not tense the right shoulder. Breathe deeply. Now come up slowly and repeat the bend on your left side. Do the exercise several times on both sides.

Creating a balanced life

Being pregnant may mean that you have less energy than usual. It is very important to make time for relaxation and exercise, and this may mean that you have to make adjustments to your daily life.

Your list of priorities will probably run something like this:
- My health and my baby's health.
- My partner.
- My family and friends.
- Work commitments and any other must-do activities.
- Socializing.

Bear this list in mind if you are feeling overwhelmed. Decide what you are going to do – and remind yourself that you cannot do everything. Some things may need to be left undone, others may have to be delegated. Make the following your motto: prioritize, delegate, eliminate.

YOUR QUALITY TIME

You are likely to feel tired when you are pregnant and coping with all the demands of everyday life can sometimes be difficult. Make sure that you prioritize time for yourself, or your own needs are likely to be eclipsed by home and work.

Think about what you would most enjoy, and what would help you to relax most. This could be singing, walking, going for acupuncture treatment, joining a pottery class, salsa, swimming or having a facial. Make sure that you incorporate regular 'me time' into your week so that you can do what gives you pleasure. In addition, make sure you spend at least half an hour, and preferably more, relaxing at home every day.

SHORTCUTS AT HOME

Some things have to give when you are pregnant – and household chores are often a good place to compromise. Cut back so that you do the bare minimum. Ask your partner to do more, or consider hiring some extra help. Here are some good ways to reduce the time you spend.

Shopping

Don't fritter away your time by shopping for food every day or two. Keep shopping down to the minimum – if possible, do one big shop per week. Ask your partner or a friend to come with you, or to do the shopping for you. Wherever possible, get your groceries delivered: investigate local vegetable-box schemes and shop via the Internet for non-perishable items that you don't need to select yourself. Buying teabags, toilet paper, washing

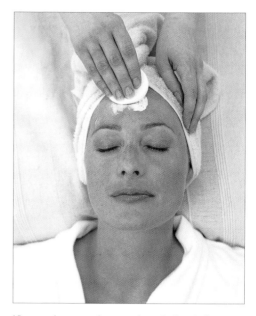

View regular pampering as an important part of your pregnancy care. Relaxing moments and treats help to lift your spirits and raise your energy levels.

powder, tins and other essential items in bulk can save you both time and money.

Cooking

If you can get a good lunch during the working day, you may need only a healthy snack and lots of liquid in the evening. When cooking at home, concentrate on quick and easy, nutritious dishes rather than complex meals. Try the following:
- Home-made soups with wholemeal bread.
- Baked potato and cottage cheese.
- Fish risotto.
- Grilled bacon and tomatoes on wholemeal toast.
- Baked potato with baked beans and poached egg.
- Spaghetti with pancetta and tomatoes.
- Poached salmon with salad and new potatoes.
- Poached chicken with tomatoes and red peppers.
- Fish pie (if made in advance) and vegetables.
- Grilled trout with salad and new potatoes.
- Casseroles (beef, lamb, chicken) or other dishes that you can make ahead of time.

If you feel like a dessert, have something healthy such as:
- Fresh fruit and natural yogurt.
- Bananas and crème fraîche.
- Baked apples.

When cooking dishes such as casseroles or pasta sauces, make double the quantity and freeze the rest for another day. That way, you cook less often and will always have a stock of nourishing food in the house.

Housework
- Wash clothes twice a week at most, and preferably only once.
- Change your bedlinen less often than usual. Once every 10–14 days is fine.
- Iron only what you really have to – don't worry about bedlinen, tea towels, hand towels, undersheets, duvet covers, underwear or T-shirts. If you take washing off the line or out of the dryer as soon as it is dry and fold it immediately, you should not have to iron.
- Remember that your home doesn't have to be pristine – a bit of dust won't harm you.

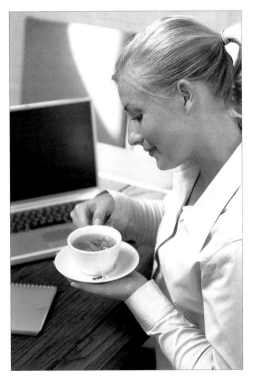

Take regular time out when you are working – an afternoon break with a cup of herbal tea and a cereal bar can help to refresh you for the rest of the day.

GETTING ON TOP OF WORK
Many women find work a struggle, particularly in the early months of pregnancy when they may be feeling exhausted and nauseous. Here are some ways that can help to make it easier.
- Get to work a little early so that you have some quiet time to yourself to get your breath back from the journey, and have a nutritious drink (chamomile tea, for example, or fresh fruit juice).
- If you control your workload, tackle the most demanding jobs early in the day if possible. Remember the first rule of management: 'Don't touch any piece of paper more than once'. Deal with it, file it or bin it straight away. Treat emails in the same way.
- Do not stand for long periods at work – sit down whenever you can. If you work sitting down, stand up and stretch at regular intervals.
- Take at least 45 minutes for your lunch break. Make this a time to eat and rest rather than an opportunity to go shopping. If you feel very tired, see if you can find a place to take a nap.
- Be sure to get some fresh air at lunchtime – just walking once round the block will really help to refresh you – so that you don't start to feel sleepy halfway through the afternoon.
- Counter a mid-afternoon energy dip with a healthy cereal bar and a cup of herbal tea (keep your favourite herbal tea bags at work). If possible, use this time to do any easier jobs, such as making routine phone calls.
- Take your holiday as and when you should. Don't allow your holiday allocation to slip over from one year to the next.
- Take some of your holiday as single days – say, one day every couple of weeks. Use this time to rest, not to rush around trying to catch up at home.
- Take sick days if you need them. Don't struggle into work if you are feeling poorly. Consider telling your manager why you are taking time off.
- If feasible, work from home at least one day a week, in order to give you a break from travelling.
- When you get home from work, try not to jump straight into your next task. Instead, sit down for half an hour and rest, relax with the newspaper or a book, have a bath, or go for a walk.

❝ Remind yourself that you cannot do everything. Some things may need to be left undone, others may have to be delegated. ❞

Bonding with your partner

It is important to share feelings and activities with your partner during the long weeks and months of pregnancy. Naturally, most of the attention – from your family doctor, hospital staff and midwives, and from family and friends – will be focused on you. You need to make sure that your partner is fully involved with the pregnancy, the birth itself and of course the baby.

Some men are less interested than women in the physical aspects of pregnancy and birth. However, most will not wish to be excluded from enjoying the growing life inside you – your baby has received the gift of life from both its parents, after all. Do not worry if your partner does seem less excited about the pregnancy than you – at the moment, the baby could seem very abstract to him. As time goes on, and the pregnancy becomes more visible, men tend to become more involved.

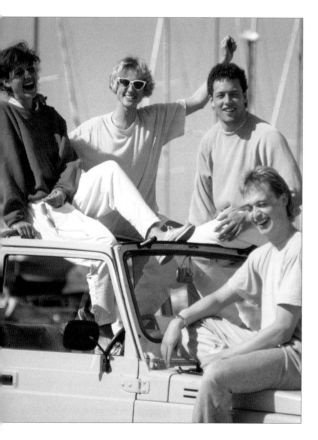

ENJOYING THE EARLY DAYS OF PREGNANCY

The baby at eight weeks is now the classic curled shape you see in pictures, with the ears starting to form and little hands that are at the moment webbed.

The highlights of early pregnancy will probably include the first pregnancy test, your doctor's confirmation of the test and then the first signs of the changes that your body is now undergoing.

Then comes the ultrasound scan. At 12 weeks you may not be able to discern a human form, but around 20 weeks you will probably be able to see the baby's head, perhaps in profile, and the shape of his or her body. Most men and women find these milestones completely fascinating. You may find that you study the ultrasound photograph and talk about it endlessly – Is it a boy or a girl? How much detail can you see clearly?

To outsiders, these kinds of intimate chats would seem trivial and pointless, but in fact they perform an important function for you as a couple. They allow you to get used to the idea that your life is about to change. They give you a chance to bring your imagination to bear on the transforming effect of having a baby in your life. They are, in other words, mental preparation.

YOUR PARTNER'S WORRIES

Men often have specific worries about childbirth and the early days of fatherhood. Some men, for example, are not sure in the early stages that they want to be present at the birth. It is not that they do not want to support their partner. Usually, any apprehension is centred on the fear of feeling helpless or useless at a time when their partner is in pain or distress.

This kind of anxiety is normal. It takes most men time to get used to the idea of seeing their child born, and most men are glad, after the event, that they were there.

Conversely, neither of you should forget that men are not in any sense obliged to be there, and should not be railroaded into something that they feel uncomfortable about. Although it is now considered normal for a man to attend the birth, it is not so long since this was considered completely out of the question.

Some men even now will find it less distressing to pace the corridors in the hospital than to hold your hand in the delivery room, and you may decide that this is the best

Remember that your life is not solely concerned with pregnancy. Make a point of going out with your friends and enjoying yourselves when you can.

way to do it for both of you. The main thing is that you and your partner should be able to discuss all of his anxieties frankly and openly. The chances are that, in the drama of it all, his reaction will be completely different from anything that you or he have anticipated.

LIFE OUTSIDE PREGNANCY

Things don't stop – for you or for your partner – just because you are having a baby. Continue to share your other interests, and to enjoy time together as a couple. Show your partner you are still interested in him by continuing to talk about his work, his ups and downs, and all the things that you used to chat about before you became pregnant.

Going for a walk or a swim together before or after work will benefit both of you and the baby, too. Make a point of doing things that are just for fun, and don't neglect your friends: you can still go out and enjoy yourselves. In fact, you should grab the chance, because in the first three months or so of parenthood your attention will focus solely on the baby and it may seem to your friends that you have dropped off the social radar.

> **“** Things don't stop – for you or for your partner – just because you are having a baby. **”**

CARING FOR YOUR PARTNER

Don't stop supporting your partner just because you are pregnant. It is tempting to put your own needs and emotions first, but remember that he may feel ill or depressed some days, and needs you as much as ever.

Think of ways to make your partner feel special: for example, take time to show a real interest in one of his hobbies; go to see the films he wants to see several times in a row and generally give in to him a little more than usual. Encourage him to share his feelings with you and share yours with him. Show him that you care about him all the more now that you are expecting a baby together.

Affection and companionship are the cement that binds a couple together. A good relationship helps us feel secure and strong, and ready for parenthood.

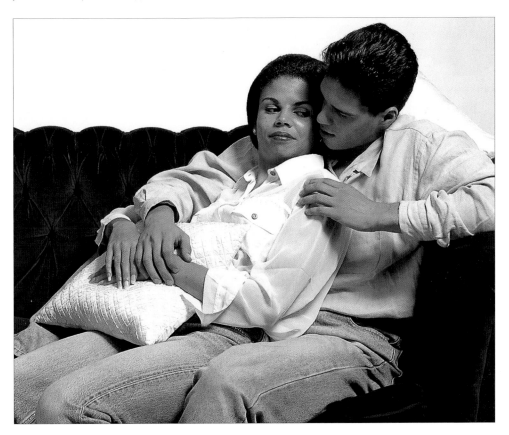

Routine antenatal care

By the eighth or ninth week of your pregnancy, you should have seen your family doctor and registered for antenatal care. If not, then make an appointment as soon as possible. Where you actually receive your antenatal care, and the type of care that you receive, is usually linked with where you ultimately want your baby to be delivered. The first consultation – commonly called the booking-in appointment – is usually held at the maternity unit of your local hospital, where you can discuss your future care. You will be referred here by your family doctor.

It is useful to have an idea of where you would like the baby to be born, and to have discussed this with your partner, before the first antenatal appointment. However, don't worry if you are not sure – there is plenty of time to make a decision and you can, of course, change your mind at a later date.

HOSPITAL-BASED CARE

If you have chosen to have your baby in hospital, then you will probably see hospital staff two or three times during your whole pregnancy. Your family doctor or community midwife will undertake the rest of the care. You will probably be seen at the hospital for a booking-in appointment at around 10 to 12 weeks, then again at about 34 or 36 weeks and once more when your baby is finally due.

If you prefer all the antenatal visits to be carried out at the hospital where you will have your baby, your family doctor can arrange this for you.

FAMILY DOCTOR OR COMMUNITY CARE

You may be able to have all your antenatal care in your family doctor's surgery or at the community midwives' office, particularly if you have decided to have your baby at home and so long as there are no problems with your pregnancy. You should discuss your preferences at the first booking appointment.

DOMINO SCHEME

The word Domino stands for Domiciliary In/Out. This is a scheme in which a community midwife shares your antenatal care with the hospital and your family doctor, sometimes visiting you at home to do the routine antenatal checks. The midwife will look after you at home, take you into hospital, deliver your baby and then arrange for you to return home within 48 hours of the birth.

MIDWIFE DELIVERY

You may choose to have a midwife be responsible for all your antenatal care and the delivery. In this case, you may not see a doctor during your pregnancy, except for the initial referral and unless the midwife becomes concerned about the pregnancy.

Your midwife or doctor should be happy to discuss any fears or questions that you have about your pregnancy.

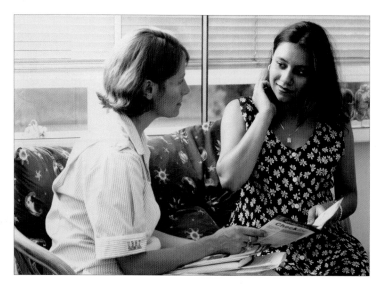

TESTS

By around 12 weeks, you will have an appointment at your antenatal clinic – probably the first of several. This first visit is intended to ascertain whether or not your pregnancy and delivery are likely to be normal. Routine checks will be done, including your weight, blood pressure, urine and blood. You may be offered an HIV test. The midwife will examine your abdomen to check the size of your uterus.

You can discuss screening procedures during this visit and are likely to be offered a routine ultrasound scan, usually done around weeks 10 to 12, to check the baby is developing normally. There are other diagnostic tests available, such as nuchal fold ultrasound, triple alphafetoprotein (AFP) and amniocentesis. You don't need to decide what tests, if any, you would like to go ahead with straight away: take time to consider the options.

YOUR FIRST ULTRASOUND

You will be asked to drink a pint of water before your appointment so that you have a full bladder for the ultrasound. This causes the uterus to be pushed outwards so that it – and the baby – can be clearly seen.

You lie down for the scan with your abdomen bared. Your skin is covered with a gel, because soundwaves cannot travel through air. The sensor or probe has to make direct airtight contact with your skin. The probe is placed on your abdomen and you will see an almost incomprehensible picture on a screen next to you.

The operator will explain what you can see. You should be able to see the baby moving and you will see its heart beating from the seventh week and hear it from the tenth week. Because the baby is so small, it is not possible to see if it is a boy or girl at this stage.

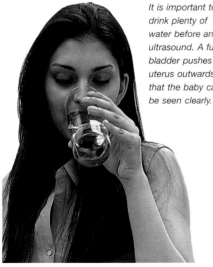

It is important to drink plenty of water before an ultrasound. A full bladder pushes the uterus outwards so that the baby can be seen clearly.

WHO'S WHO IN THE ANTENATAL TEAM

These are the people who may be involved in your pregnancy care:

- **Consultant obstetrician:** senior hospital specialist in charge of maternity care.

- **Consultant pediatrician:** senior hospital specialist in charge of newborn babies and children.

- **Registrar:** senior doctor who is junior to the consultant and resident in the hospital.

- **Senior house officer:** junior hospital doctor undertaking next level of training and able to call upon the registrar for advice if necessary.

- **Midwife:** nurse specializing in the management of normal pregnancy and labour.

- **Family doctor:** many family doctors undertake much of the antenatal work but few supervise delivery.

- **Health visitor:** about ten days after midwife care finishes, the health visitor takes over. She will advise on the care of your baby and help you deal with any problems.

- **Anaesthetist:** doctor specially trained in giving general and local anaesthesia, including epidurals.

- **Radiologist:** doctor who interprets pictures from imaging techniques, such as X-rays and ultrasounds.

- **Radiographer:** health professional, not a doctor, who performs imaging techniques.

- **Physiotherapist:** health professional who teaches antenatal care and exercises, helps to combat the pain of labour and is skilled in teaching muscle-strengthening exercises and dealing with other ligament and joint problems that occur during or after pregnancy.

- **Social worker:** assists with social problems that may occur during or after pregnancy. Social workers have special counselling skills for women who have emotional or social problems and bridge the gap between the family doctor and the health visitor.

- **Medical students:** may observe antenatal care, labour and delivery as part of their training. Students are required to undertake a certain number of normal deliveries under supervision and to learn certain procedures such as repairing an episiotomy. You have the right to ask for students not to be present.

Tests and specialist care

It is natural to worry about whether your baby is developing normally, but remind yourself that around 97 per cent of pregnancies end in the safe delivery of a healthy baby – and that your antenatal team is there to ensure that any problems are picked up quickly. As well as routine antenatal care, you will be offered diagnostic tests, used to identify serious problems with the baby.

SPECIALIST TESTS
Many women find it reassuring to have diagnostic tests done, but some do not. You are under no obligation to have any of the tests you are offered: you and your partner have the right to decide what is best for you. It is important to remember that no test is 100 per cent accurate, and tests cannot detect all abnormalities.

Chorionic villus sampling
This test is usually carried out between eleven and twelve weeks (can can be done later if necessary) and can be used to diagnose Down's syndrome. It can also detect the same chromosome abnormalities as amniocentesis and other genetic disorders such as sickle-cell anaemia and thalassaemia. It is also possible to detect the sex of

> **Around 97 per cent of pregnancies end in the safe delivery of a healthy baby.**

the fetus and this may be of value if there is a known sex-linked condition in the family.

A narrow plastic tube is passed into the uterus through the cervix and some cells from the developing placenta are drawn off. Some doctors may insert a needle through the abdominal wall rather like amniocentesis, using ultrasound to guide them. The results should be known after ten days. The risk of miscarriage after the test is one in 100, which is higher than with amniocentesis.

Nuchal fold ultrasound
The nuchal fold ultrasound is also known as the nuchal fold or the translucency scan. It is done at about 11–14 weeks, and it is used to predict Down's syndrome cases. The procedure is the same as that for a routine ultrasound, but the operator concentrates on getting a good image of the fetus's neck on the screen and then measures a layer of fluid at the back of the neck. The thicker this layer is, the greater the chance the baby will have Down's syndrome. The chance or risk is expressed as a probability such as a one in 10,000 chance or a one in 100 chance. Depending on the risk identified, you may be advised to have further tests such as amniocentesis.

Doppler ultrasound
This ultrasound is an advanced form of ultrasound imaging and is available only in some specialist hospitals. It can be used to diagnose more accurately the well-being of the baby if previous tests have shown that it is not growing sufficiently well.

The Doppler scanner can identify the veins and arteries through which blood flows and can detect the speed at which the blood is travelling. As this indicates how much oxygen the baby is receiving, it also predicts if a placenta is not functioning well. Colour Doppler is a more sophisticated technique than standard Doppler, and its benefits are still being evaluated.

Later tests
Amniocentesis or the alphafetoprotein test may also be offered as part of your antenatal care. These tests are carried out in the second trimester – see pages 138–141.

WHAT IS DOWN'S SYNDROME?
Normal babies have 23 pairs of chromosomes: 46 in total. In Down's syndrome, there is an extra chromosome – usually in the 21st pair. This causes various physical and mental abnormalities.

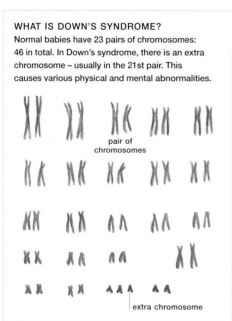

pair of chromosomes

extra chromosome

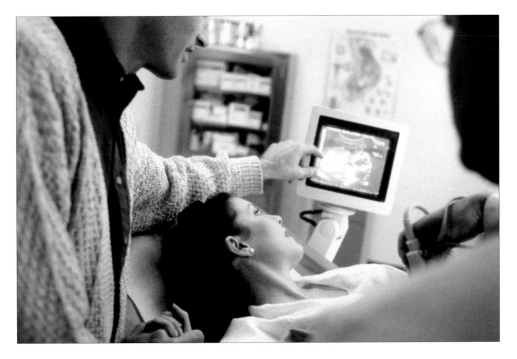

RISK FACTORS

Some women have a higher risk of carrying a baby with abnormalities than others. Doctors have identified certain risk factors, including the mother's age, her or her partner's medical history and the outcome of previous pregnancies. These factors do not mean that you will develop problems in this pregnancy, only that you have a statistically higher risk of doing so than women who are not affected by the same risk factors. Because of this, you may be monitored more closely by the medical team.

TWINS AND MULTIPLE PREGNANCIES

If you are expecting twins or more, you will be more closely monitored throughout your pregnancy. You will probably need more assistance during and after the delivery, so a home birth may not be advisable. Fatigue and nausea may be increased throughout the pregnancy. Twin or multiple pregnancies are usually shorter than the norm: about 37 weeks rather than 40.

INHERITED DISEASES

You should tell the doctor at your first antenatal check if any of the following or any inherited diseases are known in your family or in your partner's family:
- Single gene defects such as Huntington's chorea/disease, cystic fibrosis and sickle-cell anaemia.
- Disorders linked to damage on the X-chromosome such as haemophilia and muscular dystrophy.

During an ultrasound, the operator will explain what you can see on the screen. You will be able to ask any questions that you have and discuss the findings.

- Chromosomal defects such as Down's syndrome.
- Neural tube defects, which include anencephaly and spina bifida.

GENETIC COUNSELLING

You may be offered this to assess the likelihood of certain problems in your pregnancy. It is most often offered to:
- Women over the age of 35, because there is an greater risk of the baby being affected by Down's.
- Parents of a child with a genetic abnormality, a neural tube defect or other form of physical impairment.
- Women who have a tendency to miscarry.
- Couples with known chromosome abnormalities.
- Women who may be carriers of X-linked disorders (such as haemophilia).
- Couples whose family members have a high incidence of a certain disease.
- Couples whose ethnic or racial backgrounds increase the likelihood of a particular problem such as sickle-cell anaemia, thalassaemia or Tay-Sachs disease.

If you believe you need genetic counselling but you have not been offered it, discuss the reasons with your family doctor or consultant.

Checklist of common problems

The first trimester brings its own distinct symptoms. Many first-trimester complaints can be eased by complementary therapies, but always seek advice from a qualified therapist and check any therapies and remedies with your midwife or doctor.

If a complaint persists or troubles you, or you are not sure what it is, consult your family doctor. In any case, mention any problem at your next antenatal check. Do not take any over-the-counter drugs (or prescription drugs left over from pre-pregnancy) unless you have checked that they are safe in pregnancy with the pharmacist, your doctor or a consultant.

Anxiety There are many things that women worry about while pregnant, and anxiety is especially common during the early stages of pregnancy because the whole experience is new and unfamiliar and also because miscarriage is most common during the first trimester. Discuss particular worries or persistent anxiety with your doctor or midwife. You will also find that breathing exercises and meditation will lower general anxiety levels very effectively.

Bleeding Bleeding or spotting is not uncommon during the first three months. The cause may never be found or it may spring from a variety of causes, such as a minor infection. However, there may be more potentially dangerous reasons, so always get any bleeding or spotting checked out.

Breast soreness One of the classic early signs of pregnancy, sore, sensitive or unusually tender breasts can be relieved greatly by a professionally fitted maternity bra. You will find that this symptom usually eases after the first trimester.

Fainting You may feel slight faintness alongside morning sickness and a general feeling of being under par. However, if faintness is persistent or regular, or you actually faint or feel like you are going to, then you should drink plenty of water and consult your family doctor without delay.

Fatigue Tiredness is the frequent complaint of many pregnant women, particularly during the first trimester, when hormonal changes put the woman's body under unfamiliar strains. The simple answer is to make sure that you go to bed earlier and take naps whenever you

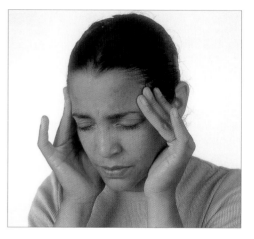

Headaches are a regular occurrence for many pregnant women, and may accompany the general feelings of being unwell that often occur in the first trimester. Acupressure can be especially helpful in esing symptoms, but always seek out professional advice about using this.

can. However, fatigue can be a symptom of anaemia, so extreme tiredness should be always be checked out properly by a doctor.

Headache Troublesome headaches are another symptom that can accompany general under-par feelings in early pregnancy, as hormonal changes make themselves felt. If headaches persist for more than two days, you must consult your family doctor without delay.

Acupuncture can be a useful therapeutic tool in relieving headaches. Massage can prove very effective, because it relieves the muscle tension that causes so many headaches and also improves blood circulation. Chamomile tea soothes headache symptoms, as can lavender oil – just three or four drops on a compress, applied to the temples. Good homeopathic remedies to try include calc carb, arsen alb, and nux vomica.

Insomnia Many women have problems sleeping during pregnancy – at first because of bodily changes and perhaps early anxiety, and then later because the increasing bulk of your growing baby can make it difficult to find a comfortable position. Perhaps the most important strategy here is to establish a regular nighttime routine – for example, have a warm bath and a milky drink at night and go to bed at the same time. Do not eat late at night and avoid salty, sugary, fatty and spicy foods. Do not drink tea or coffee at night, as the caffeine is over-stimulating; chamomile tea is a very soothing night-time drink. Getting into these good habits as early as possible during pregnancy will mean that you don't suddenly have to impose them later on.

Complementary therapies have much to offer where insomnia is concerned. Ask your partner to give you a gentle massage in the evening. Walk or swim regularly, early in the morning or during the day, perhaps at lunchtime. A medical herbalist, homeopath or acupuncturist may also be able to help.

Morning sickness This is the main symptom associated with the first trimester and includes general feelings of nausea and actual vomiting. Despite its name, this sickness is not confined to mornings – some women feel nauseous only in the evening, some only in the morning and some at intervals all through the day.

The precise cause of morning sickness is unknown, but is assumed to relate to hormonal changes. Start the day with dry toast and a cup of tea. Eat light meals and take small, frequent drinks. Avoid fats and fatty and spicy foods. Reiki may help, and you might also like to consult a medical herbalist or a homeopath – good homeopathic remedies include ipecac, nux vomica and pulsatilla (See also pages 88–89.)

Stretchmarks Marks caused by stretching of the skin as your baby grows are common during pregnancy, and may persist afterwards. Get into the habit of moisturizing this area as early on as possible, so that, when the skin starts to be stretched, it is supple and marking is minimal. To do this, massage the abdomen, thighs and buttocks regularly (and gently) with vitamin E oil.

Urinary infection This is common in pregnancy, but should always be treated without delay. Signs include the need to race to the lavatory, burning or stinging upon urination, a need to pass urine frequently, difficulty in passing urine or passing urine flecked with blood. See your doctor straight away if you have any of these symptoms or suspect the possibility of infection.

In order to allay infection, make sure that you always drink plenty of water. Cranberry juice is very effective at keeping the urinary tract healthy and able to stave off potential problems.

Urination, frequent This is something most women have to put up with in pregnancy and especially during the first trimester. It is typically caused by hormone changes and the growing uterus pushing on the bladder

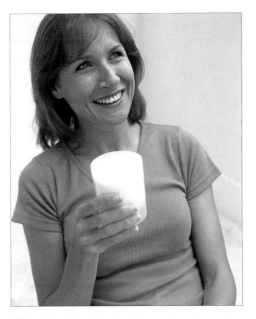

Milky drinks taken before bedtime may help to ease the insomnia that so often accompanies early pregnancy.

and decreasing its size. Do not drink less as this can lead to an infected urinary tract. In fact, the frequent urination may actually be caused by a urinary infection – tell your doctor if you have any signs of this (see above).

Vaginal discharge Consult your family doctor straight away if you notice unusual or heavy discharge.

This long list may make it seem as though pregnancy is fraught with problems. However, the great majority of women do not experience any serious difficulties. Many symptoms, including nausea, will not last long. They can be uncomfortable but most have no serious effects.

SEEKING ADVICE

If you are worried by any symptom, do not hesitate to call or visit your doctor.
See your doctor straight away if you have:
- A high temperature (38.5°C/101°F or above).
- Swelling of the hands and ankles.

Seek emergency assistance if you have:
- Vaginal bleeding other than spotting.
- Severe abdominal pain.
- Excessive vomiting.
- Sudden swelling of the hands and ankles or blurred vision with a severe headache.

Common Qs and As

Q: My partner and I are expecting our first baby in about six months' time, but he does not seem as excited as I am. Should I be worried?

A: Many men do not fully appreciate the wonder of new life until the baby is actually born and named: in other words when the baby has a tangible identity. This probably sounds awful to the newly pregnant woman, but don't despair. Once the baby is born, the man is usually fantastically proud, wanting to show off his little girl or little boy to everyone.

Q: My mother and my mother-in-law keep dropping broad hints about our starting a family – and we ourselves have wanted this for a long time. Now I am pregnant, but I am loath to tell anyone until I am absolutely sure everything is all right. Both of us are finding the pressure hard to take. What should we do?

A: Carry on fending off their enquiries as best you can. They will understand once you get to the 12th week and tell them the happy news. A word of warning, though: don't let them take over your pregnancy with lots of well-meaning advice. Tell them you that want to do things your own way and remind them that you are receiving good antenatal care. When the baby comes along, remind yourself that it is your child, not theirs, and set boundaries if you have to. Go with your own instincts about what to do – or seek professional advice.

Q: We had not intended to start a family quite so soon and my pregnancy has taken us both by surprise. Now the weeks seem to be whizzing by and I feel as if I cannot quite catch up. What can I do?

A: How lovely not to have to plan when to start your family. Don't worry, you and your partner will soon be rejoicing in your good fortune. In the meantime, make a list of all the things that you think you would like to do before the baby comes. Consider whether all these tasks are essential – if not, eliminate them. Work out how you will achieve these, month by month, making allowances for the fact that you will be feeling tired, especially in the latter months of pregnancy. Consider what you can delegate to others, and what you want to do yourself.

Q: I am not sure if I want all the tests to do with antenatal care but I don't know what to say to the doctor.

A: One of the benefits of having the tests is to receive confirmation that there is nothing wrong with the baby. Another benefit is that some problems can be treated in the uterus. Alternatively, hospital staff may arrange to have relevant specialists on hand at the delivery if they know of a potential problem. They will also arrange for the baby's well-being to be monitored through the hours of labour and delivery, and, if necessary, they will perform a Caesarean.

You are not obliged to have any test – and some women feel strongly that they do not want to do so. The best thing to do is to talk over your feelings with your midwife or family doctor so that he or she understands your perspective and can advise you accordingly. You can take your partner or a good friend to the appointment if you feel you need extra support. It can also be helpful to contact natural childbirth organizations for a different point of view.

Q: We are expecting twins and don't know how to tell our two-year-old the news. We are also worried how he will react when the twins arrive, since he will inevitably receive less attention in the future than he has been used to. What do you advise?

A: Children can become very excited about the birth of a brother or sister, even if they subsequently feel rather jealous of them. It's a good idea to tell children about a pregnancy when it is advanced enough to be visible. Show him your bump and let him touch it. Explain that there is a baby inside – he might like to try to talk to it. Show him any scan pictures you have as well. As your pregnancy progresses, your son will enjoy feeling the baby kick.

The fact that you have anticipated problems after the birth is half the battle. Your little boy may feel somewhat eclipsed because twins do demand a lot of attention, and they usually attract wonder and admiration from friends and family.

You need to keep in mind your little boy's need to be admired himself, and express daily your love for him. Perhaps you could arrange for someone else to look after the twins for a short period each day so that you can concentrate on your little boy.

Two is not an easy age in any case, when your little boy will, quite naturally, start to express his independence. Signs of temper and disobedience are all part of this and will not necessarily be related to the birth of the twins. Chat to your health visitor about this when the time comes so that she can give you useful tips for your individual situation.

Q: I have a hugely demanding job and cannot imagine how I can cope with pregnancy and then look after a small baby while I continue to work.

A: First, you will be on maternity leave – perhaps for as long as six months or a year. Second, someone else will be doing your job while you are away. Third, you will find that the pregnancy hormones will have the effect of slowing you down. While it may seem unthinkable at the moment, you will find ways of reducing the work demands made upon you as time goes on.

Ultimately, you will be compelled to make some difficult choices. Will you give up your job and stay at home? Could you job-share? Would working part-time be an option? Could you return to work full-time six weeks or so after the baby's birth and have a childminder or a nanny? Could you get help in the home to help you to cope?

You will not know what is really right for you until after the delivery of the baby. For the time being, concentrate on your work and your pregnancy, and deal with any problems only when and if they arise.

Q: I am self-employed and will need to return to work quite quickly after the birth. How can I keep my clients happy in the last month of my pregnancy and in those first few weeks?

A: You will need to cut down the hours that you work for a few weeks before the delivery, and you will not be able to return for a few weeks afterwards. Tell your clients your situation when you are about six months pregnant, so that you can prepare them for your absence. It may be worth employing someone to cover for you, or to take over essential administration. Avoid becoming overtired; stick to early nights and catnap in the afternoon if you can.

The second trimester

❝ Many women find that they are glowing with good health and vitality. **❞**

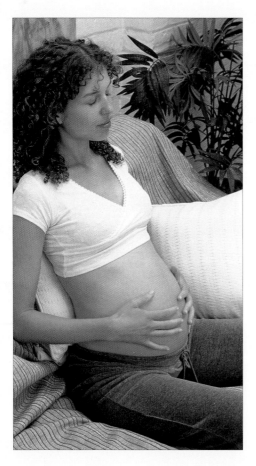

The second three months are often the best and the happiest stage of a woman's pregnancy. You are now past the early weeks in which the chance of miscarriage is high, and the 12-week scan is already behind you. This is the best stage at which to enjoy your pregnancy and start making plans for the birth.

By this time, most women are no longer suffering from sickness and the overwhelming fatigue that is often brought on by the hormonal changes of the first few weeks. Better still, many women find that they are glowing with good health and vitality. You will most likely experience a growing sensation of well-being during the second trimester, and you may well look as good as you feel. Your eyes may shine, your hair may become thicker and more lustrous, and your skin may be clearer, with a smoother texture and luminous look.

This is an exciting period, too. You and your partner can see your body changing from week to week, and with each week passing you are better

As the second trimester progresses, you can watch your baby growing week by week. The extra weight may cause tiredness, so rest whenever you can.

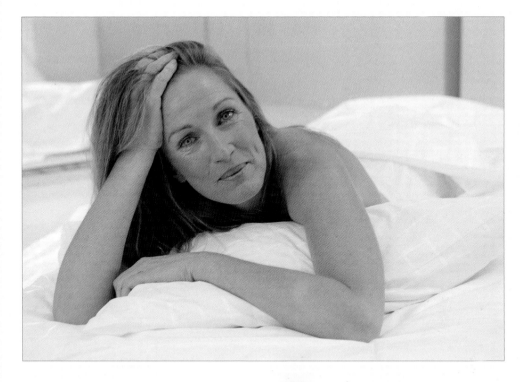

able to visualize your growing baby. You are likely to be very physically aware of your pregnancy, but as yet the baby is not big enough to slow you down too much and prevent you from doing the things that you want to do. Enjoy it.

Continue to look after yourself as much as you can. Be aware that the steadily increasing size of the baby inside you is starting to place pressure on your spine. This may lead to backache and extreme tiredness if you don't take preventative steps. Check your posture at all times, standing tall and sitting with your back firmly upright and supported. Yoga will help to strengthen your back at this stage, and this is also valuable preparation for labour. Similarly, Alexander technique classes can provide many tips for relaxed but upright postures and movement, and an osteopath can help with any muscle problems.

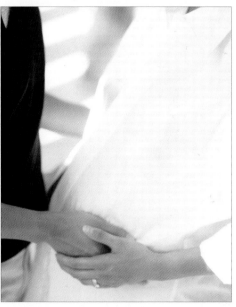

Top: For many women, the second trimester brings a wonderful sense of well-being, with morning sickness a thing of the past and a new lustre to skin and hair.

This is the time to enjoy your pregnancy to the full. Share the excitement and sensations of each new development with those closest to you.

Growth from twelve weeks

By the end of the third month of pregnancy (12 or 13 weeks), your baby has become a recognizable human being. All the body's structures and organs have formed. Your baby's arms and legs, fingers and toes have all developed, although they are still very small.

The baby's sexual characteristics are developing at this time. The boy's penis is emerging, while a girl's cervix, vagina, uterus and ovaries will already have formed. If the baby is a girl, she will at the moment have in her ovaries about 4-5 million eggs, a number that drops to 2–3 million by the time she is born.

The baby's heartbeat is stronger; it is not yet audible with a stethoscope, but it can be heard with a hand-held electronic device. The placenta has started to function, giving your baby the nourishment he or she needs. Your baby will start to practise breathing movements for the first time between weeks 12 and 16.

During the second trimester of your pregnancy, your baby will be developing at an astonishing rate. He or she will increase in weight from 10g to over 600g (¼oz to 1lb 5oz). This growth will be reflected in your growing size and in your continued need for rest.

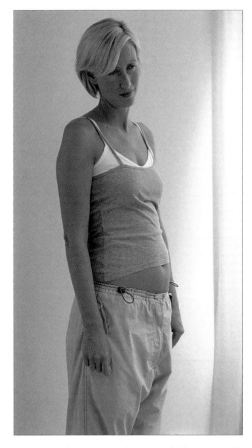

At the start of the second trimester – which spans weeks 13 or 14 to around week 26 – the baby is still tiny and so you probably won't have a bump.

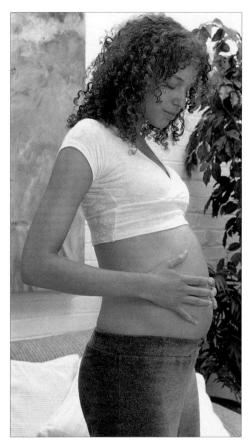

As your pregnancy develops, you will see your belly growing more noticeable. By the end of this second term, you will be quite obviously pregnant.

At week 12, your baby is about 60mm (2½in) long, measured from the crown of the head to the rump. He or she weighs about 9–13g (¼–½oz). He or she will have doubled in size in the last three weeks.

By now your baby is able to move his or her jaw and yawn. He or she can also suck and swallow – vital preparation for the life ahead. It is also around this time that the fingernails and toenails start to develop.

Week 13

The length of your baby, measured from crown to rump, will be about 65–80mm (2½–3¼in). If you include the legs as well, his or her length will be 100mm (4in). He or she will weigh about 14–20g (½–¾oz). The eyelids meet and fuse together. They will not now open again for several weeks. An ultrasound taken at this time may show that your baby now puts a thumb in his or her mouth. The baby's skin is transparent and rosy red in colour, because you can see the blood vessels beneath the skin. The skeleton is becoming stronger, hardening as cartilage gradually develops into bone.

Week 14

The baby now measures about 80–115mm (3¼–4¼in), crown to rump and weighs about 25g (1oz). The face is well developed with all the facial features recognizable. The cheeks and bridge of the nose appear, the ears move to a higher position on the head, and the eyes come closer together. As the baby develops more muscle tissue, he or she starts twisting and kicking and waving the arms within the amniotic sac. You are unlikely to feel your baby's movements because he or she still has plenty of space in which to splash around. A baby responds to gentle touch at this stage, and also moves away from threatening stimuli. During amniocentesis, babies have been seen to move away from the needle.

Week 15

Your baby is now a recognizable human being, but he or she is not yet capable of independent life. The baby weighs about 80g (2¾oz) and is 10cm (4in) long. His or her fingernails are developing.

GOING PUBLIC

Your pregnancy is bound to become obvious during the second trimester, not least because your bump is increasingly difficult to hide. You are past the most dangerous time for miscarriage, and will very probably have had the 12-week scan. This should give you the reassurance that your baby is growing normally. Now is the time to share your good news with family and friends, and to start making plans for the future.

EARLY SECOND TRIMESTER

The baby's rapid development is sustained by a constant supply of nutrients, drawn from the mother's blood supply via the umbilical cord, and a network of blood vessels in the placenta.

WEEK 14

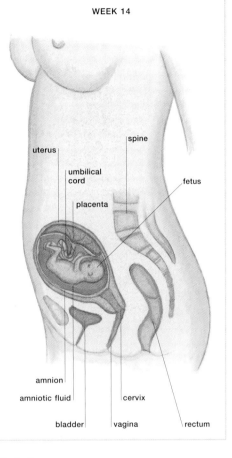

uterus
spine
umbilical cord
fetus
placenta
amnion
amniotic fluid
cervix
bladder
vagina
rectum

Week 16

Your baby is now growing and gaining weight very quickly, He or she has grown to about 16cm (6in) in length and weighs about 110g (3¾oz). The baby is now moving around a great deal, although you are still unable to feel these movements. The baby's head is able to turn, the mouth open and the chest and stomach move up and down as if he or she were breathing deeply. The baby can also yawn and stretch, and even frown.

There is a growth of fine hair, known as lanugo, all over the baby's body. The head still looks very large compared with the rest of the body. The placenta is now completely developed. The baby's tiny toenails are forming.

Week 17

A baby now weighs about 150g (5oz), and the reproductive organs are fully formed. The baby passes water containing waste products every 40–45 minutes. Much of this waste passes through the placenta and into your own circulation. You then excrete it through your urine and sweat.

Weeks 18-19

By now your baby weighs about 200g (11oz). Between now and the 20th week, you may become aware of the baby's movements, which will feel like soft ripples. The arms and legs are well formed, and he or she does a lot of kicking, bumping, twisting and turning within the amniotic sac. The baby is able to move quite freely within the sac, and is lying in salt water, which gives extra buoyancy. The wall of the uterus is springy, so the baby can push against it with the feet, hands or head, then bounce off it.

Many babies are especially energetic in the evening when their mothers are more relaxed. You are most likely to feel the first signs of life – a little kick – at this time.

One of the most exciting thoughts of all is the fact that your baby is now able to make simple facial expressions, such as pleasure and distaste. His or her tastebuds are starting to form.

Weeks 20-23

The baby now measures 25cm (10in) in length, and he or she weighs between 260g and 280g (9–10oz). His or her head is still large in proportion to the rest of the body: this signifies the brain's spectacular importance in all aspects of the baby's development. The teeth are beginning to form in the jawbone, and the hair is starting to grow.

By this stage, your baby will be completely covered in an oily layer known as vernix. The vernix comprises fatty

---

CONTINUING DEVELOPMENT

By the end of the second trimester, the baby is well developed, with hair, fingernails and eyelashes all in place. His or her movements have become increasingly energetic. The baby's eyes will open for short periods in the next month. He or she will be able to see light, and will be aware of different sounds.

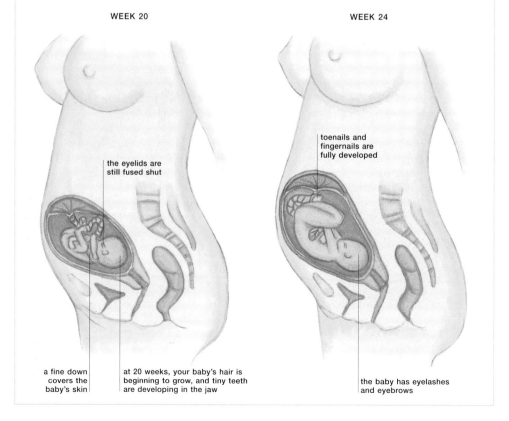

WEEK 20

the eyelids are still fused shut

a fine down covers the baby's skin

at 20 weeks, your baby's hair is beginning to grow, and tiny teeth are developing in the jaw

WEEK 24

toenails and fingernails are fully developed

the baby has eyelashes and eyebrows

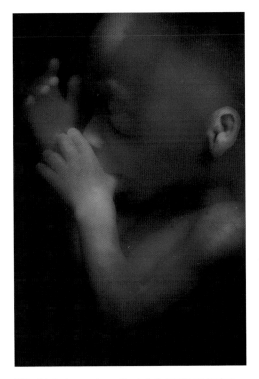

> **If your baby was to be born at 24 weeks, he or she would stand a reasonable chance of survival.**

The baby may be sucking his or her thumb and may be hiccuping a lot. He or she is learning to co-ordinate sucking and swallowing in preparation for feeding after delivery. The organs of balance inside the ears have developed and are the same size as an adult's. The baby will be able to hear sounds from within and outside your body from about week 21, although it is very unlikely that he or she will be able to make sense of those sounds yet.

The baby's eyes begin to open occasionally but they do not remain open until about week 27. He or she now has delicate eyelashes and eyebrows, and can perceive light through the abdominal wall. The baby is now about 33cm (13in) in length. He or she has been gaining in weight rapidly in the last few weeks. Now that you are six months' pregnant, your baby will weigh approximately 570g–630g (1lb 3oz–1lb 6oz).

Once the baby's weight starts to make itself felt, it can be all too tempting to slump, causing painful back problems. Always try to sit with your spine upright and your back properly supported.

This detailed scan shows the baby's hands up by her face. She may be sucking her thumb at this stage in an instinctive action that helps prepare for feeding later on.

material and dead skin cells. This acts as a protective coating (in a sense, waterproofing the skin against the amniotic fluid). It remains present until the birth, when it helps to protect the baby during his or her passage down the birth canal and delivery into the outside world.

You may now be very conscious of your baby's movements, which feel like fluttering. At around this 20-week point, the key ultrasound scan – the mid-pregnancy one – is done. Most hospitals recommend this so that they can be well prepared for any problems that may arise at delivery time.

Week 24

The baby is well developed in most respects by now, but his or her lungs are not capable of functioning fully. A baby born at this stage stands a reasonable chance of survival, but would need to remain in an intensive baby care unit and be given assistance with breathing.

The baby is getting longer and is still quite thin. Creases are visible on the palms and fingertips, and the skin is red and wrinkled. The fingernails have completely formed by now.

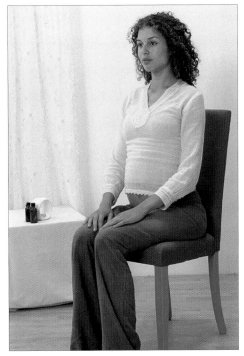

How your body is changing

In the early weeks of the second trimester, you will feel very aware of your pregnancy. It will become obvious to other people at this stage, but you can still disguise the small bump by wearing loose clothing if you wish. You may still be suffering with morning sickness but this will almost certainly wear off very soon.

Your body will undergo many complex changes during the second trimester. Some of the changes that started in the first three months of your pregnancy will also become much more noticeable in the next few weeks.

At the beginning of this trimester, your uterus is the size of a large grapefruit; the top of the uterus will be swelling out just above your navel by the time you reach the third trimester. Food takes longer to digest now – about twice as long as before you were pregnant – so you may feel congested or bloated.

STANDING TALL
You can alleviate backache to some extent by maintaining good posture. Keep your shoulders back but relaxed. Avoid jutting your head forwards; keep it back and tuck your jaw into your chin.

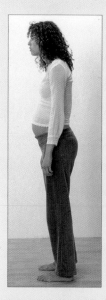
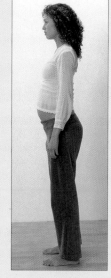

This posture increases pressure on the spine.   *Standing tall helps your back muscles.*

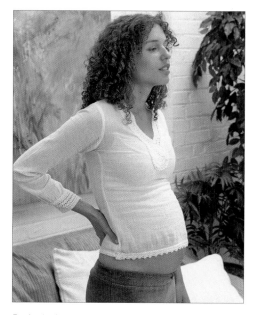

Backache is common during pregnancy, so make sure that your back is always well supported.

COMMON SIGNS AND SOLUTIONS
Your clothes may start to feel uncomfortable, so choose trousers and skirts with elasticated waists. Wear loose sweaters, T-shirts or tunics on top.

Because your uterus is pressing against the bladder, you will probably feel the need to pass water urgently and frequently. Some women may need to wear an ultra-thin panty liner to catch any leaks. Your breasts will be much larger. You should be professionally fitted with a good bra in a larger back size and larger cup size.

You may be suffering from backache. This is very common during pregnancy, and is a result of your increased weight and altered posture, combined with the effect of the pregnancy hormones upon the muscles of the back. It can be a good idea to invest in a pelvic belt to give your back increased support. Practising yoga or Pilates on a regular basis can also significantly alleviate back pain, and it can often prove helpful to visit a chiropractor or osteopath.

Your heart is beating more strongly and faster than usual in order to pump an increased volume of blood around your body and into the placenta to feed the growing baby. There are more blood vessels in the vagina than before, and it will gradually become darker and softer. The nipples and surrounding areolae will be noticeably darker because of a general increase of pigmentation in your body. This increased pigmentation affects pregnant women in varying degrees, depending on their skin type and natural colouring. Women with pale skin will probably see very little change, while olive-skinned women may notice that their skin goes several shades darker everywhere, particularly around the nipples and areolae.

A dark line down the centre of the abdomen, known as the linea nigra, usually appears around the 14th week. It may be up to 1cm (⅖in) wide, and may stretch from the pubic hair to the navel. In some women, it reaches as far up as the breastbone. The linea nigra usually fades after delivery. If you have any birthmarks, moles or freckles, these too may darken during pregnancy.

Some women develop blotchy brown patches, called chloasma, on the face and neck. These will be intensified by the sunlight, so it is best to avoid the sun if you are affected. Chloasma usually fades after delivery, and disappears completely within around three months of the delivery of the baby.

Because of the complex hormonal changes taking place within your body, your skin may develop a healthy bloom. You can enhance this by regular walking, which will also strengthen all your muscles in preparation for labour. You may also notice how shiny and luxuriant your hair looks: this, again, happens for hormonal reasons. Once you have given birth, you will shed a lot of hair, but this is nothing to worry about.

STRETCHMARKS

Some women develop stretchmarks on their breasts, abdomen, thighs and buttocks during pregnancy. These develop for two reasons. The extra weight and bulk you are gaining causes the collagen bundles of the skin to stretch so much that they tear. The increased levels of hormones in the blood disrupt the protein in the skin, making it thinner and more delicate than usual.

Stretchmarks show as pale wavy stripes on the skin. They tend to fade a little after the baby is delivered, but they will not disappear altogether. For this reason, it is best to do everything you can to prevent them: daily massage with vitamin E oil or essential oils, and care with your diet, may help.

Try to avoid excessive weight gain and make sure that your diet contains foods that are rich in vitamins B, C and E, as well as zinc and silica. Silica is found in wholegrains, green leafy vegetables, potatoes, nuts and seeds. A healthy diet that includes these foods will help to maintain the elasticity of your skin.

LOOKING AFTER YOUR FEET
Your feet enlarge during pregnancy, partly because of extra fluid in the body and partly because of the extra weight you are carrying. Some women find that they go up a shoe size. The following steps will help you to care for your feet:

- Do not wear tight, rubbing footwear.
- Avoid wearing shoes with high heels while you are pregnant. A laced almost-flat shoe is the ideal choice.
- Do not wear knee-high tights (pop socks) when you are pregnant.
- Put your feet up on a footstool in the evenings. This will improve the circulation and allow any swelling to subside.
- Walk as much as and whenever you can to boost the circulation in your legs and feet.
- Avoid standing completely still, for example, when in queues. If you have to stand, keep your circulation moving by walking on the spot, and by flexing and circling your ankles.
- Have a footrest for your feet if you work for long hours at a computer or bench.

If you work sitting down, support your legs by using a footrest; you can improvise by using a firm cushion or a pile of telephone directories.

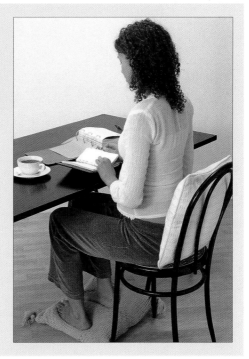

Emotional changes

As your pregnancy progresses, you will probably experience a mixture of emotions. Pregnancy hormones are likely to make you feel more emotional and excitable than normal.

You and your partner may be growing closer together as your pregnancy advances and you become more aware of the commitment now firmly established in your lives. You are likely to be making practical plans, such as where the baby will sleep, and deciding what you need to buy and what you need to do to your home.

By now you are likely to feel more confident about your pregnancy. The chances of miscarriage are greatly reduced and the early sickness and fatigue have almost certainly eased off, leaving most women with a sense of well-being and anticipation.

However, it is very common for women to feel happy one moment, and tearful the next. Many women run the entire spectrum of emotions, from confident, optimistic and relaxed to depressed, worried, irritable and weepy. Sometimes seemingly insignificant things may set you off.

Being pregnant and anticipating your future role as a parent can bring up difficult issues from your own childhood. You may have unresolved feelings, such as sadness, anger or guilt. At the same time, you may discover insights into your parents' feelings about you.

It is important that you express your emotions and work through any unresolved issues. Talking to your partner, a close friend or relative can often be all you need. Sometimes, it may be helpful to see a counsellor or visit a complementary therapist for extra support.

ENHANCING YOUR EMOTIONAL WELL-BEING

Most people will react positively when you tell them you are pregnant, but some may not. If someone shows a less than ecstatic response to your news, try not to let it affect you. A negative reaction is more likely to say something about that person than about your news. Some people have hidden issues about pregnancy or childbirth – for example, they may not be able to have children themselves – or they may simply not be that interested.

It can help you to deal with doubts and worries by imagining what a positive person would say if you were to ask for advice. For example, will I cope with childbirth? Well, hundreds upon thousands of women do. How will I

Holistic therapies such as t'ai chi and yoga emphasize the importance of relaxing the body. This can help you to carry the weight of your baby more easily.

manage without enough sleep? You will take catnaps and do less about the home than you have been used to doing. Will I be able to feed my baby? Breastfeeding does not always come naturally, but there will be people to help and advise you. At worst, the baby will not starve: you will simply bottle-feed her. There is not one problem that cannot be solved.

TIME TO THINK

During this time, it is good to allow yourself to relax and indulge in the dreams you and your partner have for your baby. You obviously want him or her to be happy and healthy, and we all hope for a world in which our children can grow up safely.

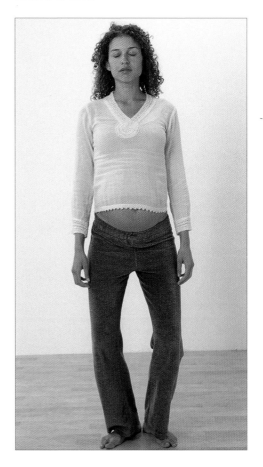

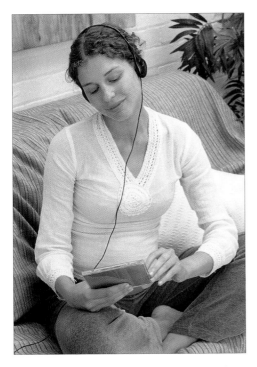

> **It is very common to feel happy one moment, and tearful the next. Many women run the entire spectrum of emotions during pregnancy.**

you rather than to him. He may even feel a little left out because of all the attention that you are attracting.

Your partner may harbour anxieties at the prospect of fatherhood, the changes it will mean for him and the changes that it will mean for your relationship. After all, you will soon be part of a family rather than a couple.

It is important that both of you have a chance to discuss your feelings, whether negative or positive. Left unspoken, they may lead to tensions in your relationship. You may be experiencing anxieties yourself about, say, the loss of freedom and your ability to accommodate both job and child. This puts you in a good position to show your partner understanding and support.

Many men do not express their feelings as freely as women. Do not worry if your partner seems to be preoccupied with readying the baby's bedroom, for example, rather than discussing his feelings with you. Be happy that actions speak louder than words.

Spend time alone, just relaxing, whenever you get the chance. Enjoy listening to music, reading or simply sitting quietly and experiencing your pregnancy.

Take some time each day to allow yourself to get in touch with your feelings. Visualization can be very helpful: close your eyes and imagine the baby developing inside you. Bring to mind, too, a picture of how your own body is nurturing your growing baby.

Many parents-to-be feel that their baby is very real at this stage and begin to talk to him or her. There is good evidence to suggest that babies can learn to recognize their mother's voice before they are born. Communication need not be limited to talking. Play music, sing or stroke your belly. This can help you to form a bond long before the birth. Even if little of your communication reaches your baby, it can still have a profound effect on your emotions and enhance your psychological readiness for the most important role of your life.

HELPING YOUR PARTNER BOND

Encourage your partner to feel your baby moving and kicking by laying his hand upon your growing abdomen. The first time that this happens can be a very exciting experience. However, it is not unusual for a father still to feel a little removed from the pregnancy at this time. Certainly all the big changes seem to be happening to

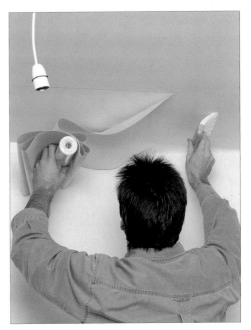

Your partner may not want to spend hours discussing the pregnancy, but may show his excitement by getting the nursery ready for your baby.

Aromatherapy for pregnancy

It is important to take time to pamper yourself during your pregnancy. This can help you to adjust to the changes in your body, and will also enhance your emotional well-being. Aromatherapy can be an excellent feel-good therapy for the second trimester. Earlier, only a few oils are considered safe (some people think that no oils should be used), and in any case, morning sickness may make you dislike strong aromas. By 16 weeks, however, any nausea is likely to have passed and most women can use a greater range of oils.

Essential oils can be used to help alleviate a number of pregnancy-related complaints, notably stress and insomnia. They also have powerful effects on your moods. This is because scents are processed by the part of the brain that also deals with emotion and memory – making smell the most evocative of all our senses.

It is especially important that you observe basic safety precautions when using essential oils during pregnancy. Only use pure oils that you know are safe, and dilute them in a carrier oil before massaging into the skin or adding to

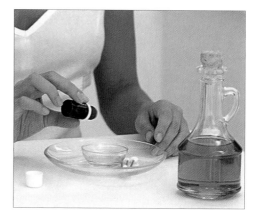

Always dilute aromatherapy oils before you apply to the skin. Choose a good-quality carrier oil such as almond, wheatgerm or sunflower.

the bath. Do not apply oils directly to the skin and never take them by mouth.

Many oils are not suitable for use during pregnancy; others should be used only at particular times or under the guidance of a qualified practitioner. Clary sage, for example, can be useful during labour but hazardous if used earlier. See page 212 for a list of the oils to be avoided during pregnancy. Seek professional advice if you are at all unsure about the safety of an oil.

DILUTING AROMATHERAPY OILS
Use a low dilution of essential oils during pregnancy – no more than 1 drop per 2 teaspoons (10ml) of base oil. Use a light vegetable oil, such as sunflower or wheatgerm, as a base. If using essential oils in the bath, dilute in oil or full-fat milk, then add to a warm (not hot) bath.

Do a patch test to check for sensitivity the first time you use any oil: apply a little of the diluted mixture to your inner wrist, then wait 24 hours, without washing. If no reaction occurs, the oil is safe to use. Your skin can become more sensitive during pregnancy, so do a patch test even if you have used the oil before conceiving. Stop using any oil if you develop a reaction to it.

USING OILS IN MASSAGE
You can use essential oils to enhance any of the massage sequences described over the following pages and elsewhere in this book. Experiment by blending different

---

SIX GOOD OILS

Essential oils are not suitable for everyone and it is a good idea to consult a professional aromatherapist for help on choosing oils, especially if you want to treat a particular problem. The following are generally considered safe for use during pregnancy.

ENERGIZING OILS
- **Mandarin** Refreshing, uplifting oil made from the ripe peel of the fruit.
- **Ginger** Warming, stimulating oil that can boost the immune system. It is good used in massages or footbaths, but should not be used in the bath.
- **Petitgrain** Uplifting, sweet-smelling oil made from the leaves of the bitter orange tree (neroli is made from the flowers).

RELAXING OILS
- **Ylang ylang** Exotic-smelling oil that has soothing properties. It is sometimes used to help to reduce high blood pressure.
- **Neroli** Soothing oil that also lifts the spirits. It has a rejuvenating effect on the skin.
- **Lavender** Versatile oil with calming and restorative properties, which is often used to treat insomnia and stress. Can be used from 16 weeks.

---

oils together: aromatherapists use up to five but as a novice, it is probably best to use no more than two or three at a time. Relaxing blends to try after 16 weeks include neroli and lavender, or ylang ylang and sandalwood. You may like to try rosewood, a gentle, calming oil that helps to steady the emotions.

Aromatherapy massage is often recommended as a means of preventing stretchmarks, although many doctors say that massage does not make an appreciable difference. If you want to try it, use a blend of mandarin and neroli diluted in wheatgerm oil. At the very least, this will have a moisturizing effect. Adding a little avocado oil to the mixture will increase its moisturizing properties.

OILS IN THE HOME

Use an aromatherapy oil burner to fill your home with relaxing or energizing scents. Fill the bowl with water, add a few drops of oil and heat. At night, try sandalwood, said to have aphrodisiac properties. Lavender is useful if you are having trouble sleeping (it also has antiseptic qualities). Lemon can be a good oil to burn if you are still suffering from nausea after 16 weeks.

For an aromatherapy room spray, add several drops of an essential oil to a spray gun filled with water, and spray several times around the room like an air freshener. Ylang ylang, mandarin and lavender make a refreshing blend that can help to relieve fatigue.

IN THE BATH

Aromatherapy baths can be a great way to relax at the end of the evening: add a few drops of diluted oil to a warm bath (do not add to running water).

For a quick booster when you come home from work, try soaking your feet in an aromatic footbath for ten minutes. Two drops each of ginger and mandarin makes

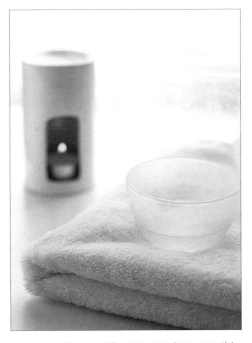

A vaporizer offers a subtle way to experience essential oils. Try burning oils in the bedroom before you go to sleep, or in the bathroom while you enjoy a long soak.

a warming blend, or try lavender and tea tree to soothe hot, tired feet. Add the oils, diluted in full-fat milk, to a large bowl of warm water.

To add another element to the footbath, add a large handful of marbles. As you soak your feet, roll them backwards and forwards for an easy mini-massage.

AROMATHERAPY FIRST AID

Most of the over-the-counter remedies for colds and stuffy noses are not suitable for pregnant women, but an aromatherapy inhalation can provide effective relief. Add a couple of drops of tea tree oil to a bowl of hot water, then place a towel over your head and breathe in the aromatic steam for a few moments.

Warm aromatherapy compresses are useful for soothing general aches and pains, while a cold compress can soothe a headache or any swelling. Dilute the essential oil in full-fat milk, then add to a bowl of hot or cold water (add a few ice cubes if using cold). Drench a clean cotton cloth in the water, wring it out and then apply to the affected area.

Try a cold lavender compress to relieve a headache, or a hot ginger compress for back pain.

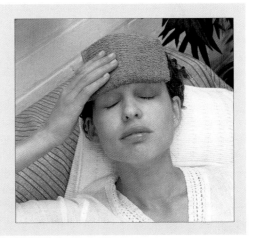

Massage relief

We instinctively use touch to connect with each other, to nurture and to express love. This is why even the simplest form of massage can be richly comforting. Positive, gentle touch can also have a profoundly beneficial effect on our health. It is known to improve circulation, it relaxes the muscles, it helps the digestion, and it regulates the nervous system.

Massage is especially beneficial during pregnancy, provided that deep pressure is not applied to the abdomen or lower back. The number-one aim of massage is to relax mind and body, and so it can help to relieve the stresses and strains of daily living while you are pregnant. It can also help to alleviate many pregnancy-related problems, such as insomnia, circulatory disorders, high blood pressure, swollen legs and headaches.

HAVING A PROFESSIONAL MASSAGE

A professional massage can be a real treat. Choose a qualified practitioner who is experienced in treating pregnant women (your midwife may be able to recommend someone).

Most therapists work from a consulting room, which may be in their home. Some will come to your home, particularly if you find it difficult to get around. If you are having the massage at home, make sure you heat the

> 66 Even the simplest form of massage can be richly comforting. 99

room well beforehand; your body temperature will drop after you have been lying still for some time. Your masseur should bring a massage couch and towels.

Before the massage, the masseuse will check whether you have any particular aches, pains or other health problems. He or she should also ask you for a basic medical history. It is important that you tell the masseuse

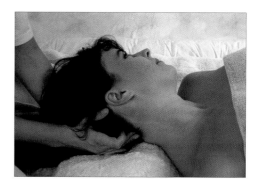

A head massage is particularly helpful for relieving tension commonly found in the upper back, shoulders and neck areas.

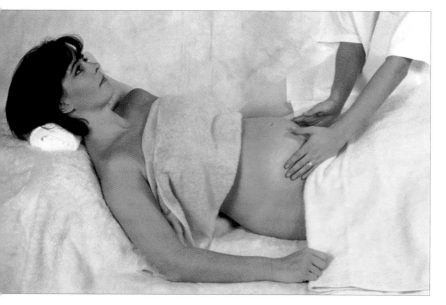

Go to a masseuse who specializes in pregnancy and antenatal massage so that you can relax in the knowledge that you are in good hands. Enjoy.

about your pregnancy and any health problems you have. You should tell the masseuse if you have varicose veins, since the skin over these should not be massaged.

You will be asked to undress and to lie on a massage couch, covered with a towel. You can keep your pants on if you prefer (although they may get covered in oil).

The masseuse will warm some oil in her hands and then spread it over the surface of your skin before starting the massage.

Most sessions include a full-body massage but your therapist may massage only certain areas of your body, depending on your needs. Each masseur will have a different way of combining the different massage techniques and of working around your body.

A full-body massage session usually lasts for an hour, but it may take an hour and a half if you are having a face and head massage at the same time. At the end of the session, you should be left to rest for a few minutes; close your eyes and relax. Don't plan to do anything strenuous afterwards – if possible, take the opportunity to put your feet up and relax for the rest of the day.

SEEING AN AROMATHERAPIST

Aromatherapists work in the same way as masseurs, but they add a blend of essential oils to the massage oil. Different oils will be chosen depending on your individual needs. It is important that you like the scent of any oils used so you will be asked to smell them before they are blended together. You can also ask your aromatherapist for advice on using essential oils at home. Check that any oils used are safe in pregnancy – you should therefore see an experienced practitioner who has experience of treating pregnant women because some oils can have a harmful effect.

MASSAGE AT HOME

You and your partner or a close friend can practise gentle massage at home. A simple massage can be a real help in soothing away general aches and in reducing tension.

Anyone can give a pleasurable massage. The key is to use slow, smooth strokes. Focus on what you are doing and ask the person you are massaging for feedback. You should not massage directly over a bone, and it is important not to apply deep pressure to the abdomen or lower back of a pregnant woman.

For a general massage, warm some oil in your hands; you want enough to give you a good slip, but not so much that your hands are dripping. Apply to the skin with plenty of smooth, stroking movements; these are very calming. Alternate between using your fingertips and whole hands. Then apply deeper pressure to release

Ask a friend or your partner to give you a quick massage to help relieve lower back pain.

areas of particular tension, making small circular movements with the tips of your thumbs.

It is often good to follow a back massage with a leg massage, but let your intuition guide you rather than following a set routine. Add a little more oil whenever you feel the skin starting to pull against your hands.

Back massage

Lower back pain is probably the most common complaint of pregnancy, but a massage can do a lot to relieve the discomfort. The best way of receiving a back massage when you are pregnant is to sit astride a chair, so that you are facing its back. Lean on a cushion and drop your shoulders to help release any tension.

As well as easing your backache, a massage can also give you a comforting sense of being lovingly cared for, which is in itself beneficial. You may like to have a shoulder massage at the same time – ask the person massaging you to adapt the self-massage routine described on the following pages.

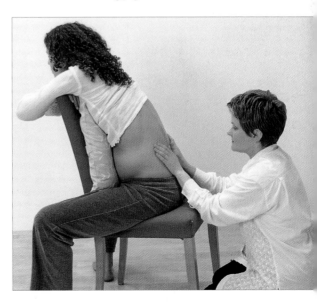

How to massage yourself

Self-massage can be very soothing and beneficial – and you can do it whenever you like. You can use it to energize yourself before an appointment during the day or to unwind in the evening before going to bed. Massage also feels good when performed in the bath. The following routines can also be adapted for partner massage.

Soothing tired legs

Massaging the legs is especially good if your legs ache after standing. It stimulates the circulation and soothes tiredness or swelling. Do not apply heavy pressure, and use very light movements on the inner leg.

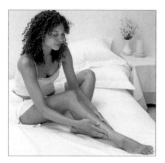

1 Rest the foot of the leg you are working on flat, and bend the knee slightly so you can reach the lower leg. Stroke the whole leg with alternate hands, one on each side of the leg. Work up from the foot to the top of the thigh. Repeat five or six times, then work on the other leg.

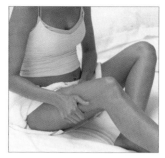

2 Now use alternate hands to knead the thigh. Squeeze and release the flesh, working in a rhythmic fashion from just above the knee to the top of the thigh. Repeat this two or three times, and then work on the thigh of the other leg.

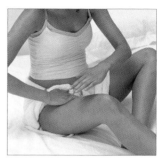

3 Stroke the thigh, working up the thigh from the knee and using both hands, with one hand following the other. You will enjoy the smooth, flowing strokes after the more energetic kneading. Now repeat on the other leg.

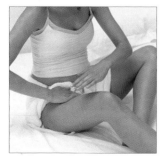

4 Make loose fists and lightly pummel the front and outside of the thigh. This movement will help to relieve any stiffness. Pummel up the thigh a few times, and then repeat on the other thigh.

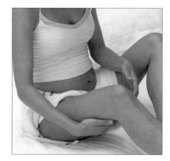

5 Using the tips of your fingers, stroke the area around the kneecap. Hold the thigh steady with your other hand. Now stroke gently behind the knee, then continue the action up your thigh. Repeat on the other leg.

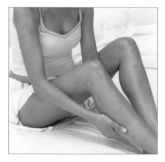

6 Knead the calf muscle using both hands, alternately squeezing it and releasing it. Then stroke the area gently, with one hand following the other one up the back of the leg. Repeat on the other leg.

Shoulder massage for tension-relief

Tension tends to accumulate in the shoulders, causing aching shoulders, stiff necks and headaches. This quick massage should help to relax your muscles. It is particularly beneficial if you work at a computer.

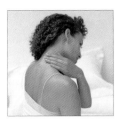 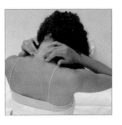 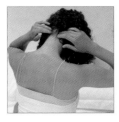 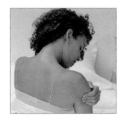

1 Stroke the left hand down the right shoulder, working from the neck to the elbow. Do three times. Repeat on the other side.

2 Use your fingertips to make small circles on either side of the top of the spine. Use firm but not painful pressure.

3 Making the same circular movements, work up the neck to the base of the skull. Keep the fingers either side of the spine.

4 Squeeze and release the flesh on your shoulder and at the top of your arm. Repeat the movements on the other shoulder.

Feel-good facial (self-massage)

A face massage can get rid of headaches, as well as relieving fatigue and anxiety. Use a good-quality face oil to prevent any dragging of the skin. Do all the movements at least two or three times – more if you like.

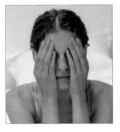 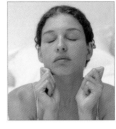 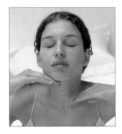

1 Put your hands over your face, fingers on forehead. Hold for a few moments, then slowly draw them towards your ears. Do not pull the skin.

2 Use your thumbs and the knuckles of your forefingers to inch gently along the jaw line. Begin just below the chin and work out to the ears. Pinch near the bone.

3 Slap the backs of alternate hands under the chin. This is a good stimulating movement, and it may help to prevent a double chin.

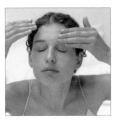 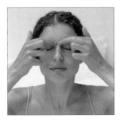 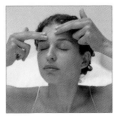 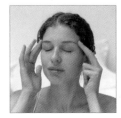

4 Stroke your hands, one after the other, up your forehead. Work from the bridge of the nose to your hairline. Close your eyes as you do this.

5 Place both index fingers on the bridge of your nose and stroke firmly upwards, then gently across. This may help to reduce any frown lines.

6 Using the fingertips of your index and middle fingers, make circular movements all over the forehead. Press firmly but do not drag the skin.

7 Using your fingertips, stroke your forehead gently, working from the centre to your temples. Finally, press them firmly against the temples.

Treating ailments at home

Some women glow with health throughout pregnancy, but most experience minor ailments at one time or another. The majority of these health problems are not a cause for concern, but they can cause considerable discomfort. Both indigestion and constipation, for example, can be painful and irritating.

You should avoid taking medication in pregnancy if at all possible. Some natural remedies offer a safe and gentle way of relieving discomfort. They can also help to balance mood swings and strengthen the emotions.

The following remedies are generally considered safe to take during pregnancy. Even so, not every treatment will suit every pregnant woman. It is therefore a good idea to seek advice from a qualified practitioner who is experienced in treating pregnant women. You should discuss health concerns with your doctor. Always tell your doctor about any natural remedies that you are considering taking.

HERBAL TEAS

Most herbal remedies should be taken only under the direction of a medical herbalist, but some are gentle enough to be used as self-help remedies. These include dandelion, lemon balm, meadowsweet, fennel and lime flower teas. They are available in tea-bag form from health food shops and some supermarkets, or you can make your own infusion (see box). However, do not drink herbal tea in excessive quantities – three cups a day is the usual recommended limit. Popular choices include:

- **Lemon balm or meadowsweet tea**. These can help to ease indigestion, which most pregnant women experience at some time or other. Sip a cupful after each meal. Lemon balm also helps to calm the emotions, so it can be also a useful tea if you are suffering from stress or anxiety.
- **Fennel**. This is a calming herb that also works on the digestive system and acts as a mild laxative, so it can be helpful if you suffer from constipation. Infuse 5ml (1 tsp) of crushed seeds in a cup of boiling water, strain, and drink at bedtime. Drinking a cup of hot water with a slice of lemon before breakfast can also ease constipation. You should also be drinking plenty of fluid – at least eight glasses of water a day.
- **Lime (linden) flower tea**. This can help to relieve anxiety and stress, which in turn can improve your sleep. It may be helpful for stuffy noses. Chamomile is another good stress-reliever and sleep promoter.
- **Dandelion tea**. This is useful if you are feeling bloated. It works as a diuretic, so it helps to remove excess fluid from the body. It is also a good source of iron, so it can be useful if you are anaemic.

TEAS TO AVOID

In general, do not drink one type of herbal tea repeatedly – a varied selection is key. Ask a herbalist which herbs to avoid or use in moderation during pregnancy as some encourage uterine contractions and should be avoided totally or taken only in the final stages and at the birth.

Always study the contents lists on bought teas and avoid any bought or home-made teas that contain the following: celery, cinnamon, cohosh, mugwort, nutmeg, pennyroyal and sage (sage is also to be avoided if breast-feeding). Raspberry leaf tea is a well-known uterine tonic and stimulant that helps to prepare the uterus for birth. As such, it must not be taken until the last six to eight weeks of pregnancy (one or two cups a day is a good dose) and during labour. There are many less common herbs that may be found in some teas, which is why expert advice should always be sought (see also page 210).

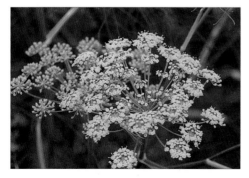

Fennel helps with digestive problems such as constipation and also exerts a calming effect.

MAKING AN INFUSION
Place about 5ml (1 tsp) of dried herb in a cup or ceramic teapot (do not use an aluminium or tin teapot). Add a cupful of boiling water and leave to infuse for five to ten minutes. Strain, then sip slowly. To save time, make up enough for three cups and store in a vacuum flask to drink that day. Or let cool, and store in the refrigerator.

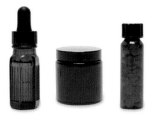

Homeopathic remedies are usually stored in dark bottles. This helps to prevent them deteriorating.

HOMEOPATHIC REMEDIES

Natural, usually plant-based medicines, homeopathic remedies are so highly diluted that only the minutest amount of the active ingredient remains. They are generally considered very safe in pregnancy but, like any remedy, they should be used with care.

Homeopathic remedies are widely available from pharmacies and health food shops, and they are commonly used for self-help. However, it can be very difficult to choose the correct remedy for your individual circumstances without specialist knowledge. It is therefore a good idea to seek advice from a qualified, professional homeopath – who will have trained for several years – rather than trying to diagnose and prescribe for yourself. Not all women require the same remedy, even when they are suffering from what seems to be the same problem. The homeopath will also bear in mind the fact that your unborn baby is receiving treatment as well as you.

Common homeopathic remedies for pregnancy-related ailments include:

- Nux vomica, carbo veg, pulsatilla or sulphur for indigestion and heartburn.
- Aconite, belladonna, natrum mur, bryonia or sepia for headaches.
- Bryonia, natrum mur, nux vomica or sepia for constipation.
- Nux vomica, hamamelis, aesculus or sulphur for haemorrhoids.
- Calc fluor or hamamelis for varicose veins.
- Calc fluor to improve the elasticity of the skin, thus helping to prevent stretch marks.

BACH FLOWER REMEDIES

These gentle flower- and plant-based remedies are highly diluted and are safe for use in pregnancy. They can be very helpful for dealing with difficult emotions, such as anxiety. Flower remedies are preserved in brandy, so you should take them in water. Simply add a couple of drops to a glass of water and sip throughout the day.

Bach Flower Remedies, like homeopathic ones, are highly diluted. Just add two or three drops of your chosen remedy to a glass of water, and take sips throughout the day.

There are 38 flower remedies to choose from. The following may be of greatest help in pregnancy:

- Olive to counteract lack of energy and fatigue.
- Walnut to help with adjusting to change.
- Red chestnut to relieve anxiety about your baby's well-being.
- Crab apple if you are feeling negative about the way that you look.
- Mimulus to help with anxiety about the birth or the effect that pregnancy is having on you.
- Rescue Remedy to use in moments of panic and general tearfulness.

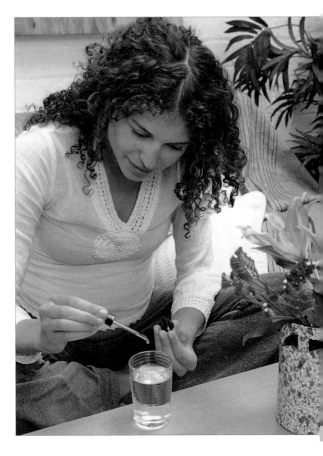

Yoga for the second trimester

Pregnant women tend to feel more energetic and healthy in the second trimester, but the baby's increasing weight can alter your sense of balance and lead to poor posture. Yoga encourages you to stand correctly and also works to strengthen the back muscles, preventing backache. Yoga also encourages good breathing and improves the circulation, so that fresh nutritious blood reaches your baby. It is a good idea to attend specialist classes for pregnant women during the second trimester. You can also practise simple postures at home.

Centring down

Getting your legs, rather than your lower back, to support your increasing weight and bulk is probably the most important postural adjustment that you can make during your pregnancy because it will save you from backache. Stand tall with your head erect and chin tucked in naturally. Tuck in your tail bone (coccyx). Now extend up through the spine, relaxing the tension from your upper body. At the same time, bend the knees and imagine your weight dropping downwards through the legs.

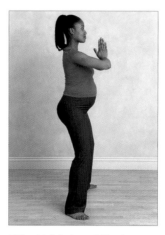

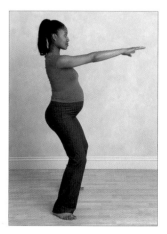

1 Stand tall, feet apart. Bend your knees to take your weight down. Press your palms together at throat level, elbows out. Inhale, opening up your back ribs as you do so.

2 As you breathe out, stretch your arms forwards and bend deeply in the knees. Keep your upper body erect. Hold a moment, then breathe in again. Repeat several times.

Tiger stretch and relax

This exercise is a good way to relieve lower backache. It also helps sciatica, in which back pain extends down the leg. You will need to balance firmly on strong wrists and hands as you raise your leg parallel to the floor.

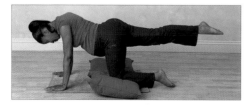

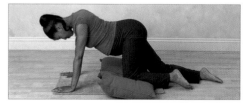

1 Go on to all fours, with hands below your shoulders and a cushion under the knees. Extend the spine (do not dip your back). Slowly lift your right leg parallel to the floor and extend it back to release any tension. Point your toes.

2 Let your leg sink to the floor and relax it. Maintain your balance and the strength in your spine, but drop your right hip. Shake your leg loosely from hip to toes to release pressure on the sciatic nerve. Repeat on the left.

Swing and release

In this vigorous exercise, the palms are pressed firmly together to strengthen the arm muscles and the muscles by the upper spine. Strength in these areas makes it easier to maintain a good upright posture.

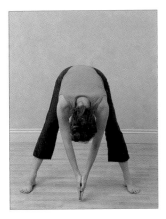 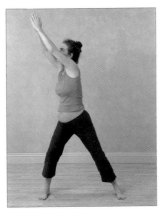 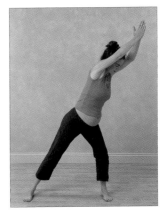

1 Stand with your feet a comfortable width apart and your knees bent. Bring your palms together and bend forwards from the hips so that your fingertips touch the floor. Breathe out in this position.

2 Stretch the arms forwards, pushing the palms together. Breathe in deeply, raising your head, arms and trunk up and to your right, and turning the upper body gently to your right. Hold this for a few seconds, pressing your palms together and feeling your muscles engaging along the arms and upper spine.

3 Breathe out through the mouth, making a 'HAH' sound, and drop back to the starting position with your knees bent. Keep your hands together and strong. Breathe in and out to relax in the starting position. Then breathe in again deeply to repeat the upward stretch and turn to the left. Repeat a few times.

Modified positions for deep relaxation

It is important to relax after doing any yoga routine. As your baby grows, lying on your back will no longer be comfortable. It will also restrict circulation, so it is not a good idea, particularly from 30 weeks onwards. Instead of lying flat on your back, either bend your knees and place a cushion or blankets under your hips, lie on your side or lean forwards over a bean bag. You can even relax deeply while sitting up, as long as you are well supported and your legs are not hanging down. Take time to find a comfortable pose for you.

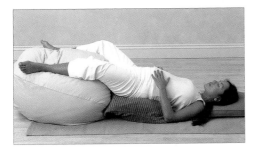

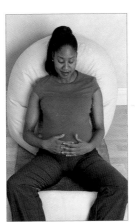

2 Push the bean bag against a wall for extra support and recline against it so that you are as comfortable as possible. Sit with your knees bent and out to the sides and add cushions underneath to open up your hips and expand the whole pelvic area.

1 Place a bean bag underneath your legs and a cushion under your hips. Your raised legs will improve the blood flow to your heart and should also reduce swelling and aching in the legs. Raising up the hips helps to take strain off the lower back.

Pregnancy and your sex life

The most commonly asked question about making love in pregnancy is whether or not it is safe. Experts say that it is – and there is no evidence to suggest that it might not be. A pregnancy is actually much more robust than some of us believe. Some consultants even say that it is safe to go riding – something that women are usually advised to avoid. They maintain that if the pregnancy were to be lost in this way then it was going to be lost in any case; in other words, that the pregnancy was frail. So, one need not fear causing miscarriage through the act of lovemaking.

The next big question is whether or not both you and your partner feel like making love. Some women go off sex during their pregnancy while others enjoy sex more than ever before. Similarly, some men find that their partner seems even more attractive when she is pregnant. Others are nervous of making love once their partner is visibly pregnant and prefer to wait until after the baby has arrived. However, for many couples the frequency of lovemaking does not change substantially whether or not the woman is pregnant.

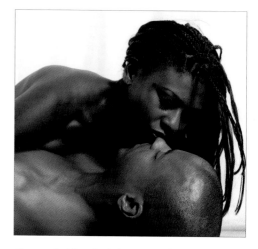

You may find it easier to be on top when you make love with your partner, so that pressure on the abdomen is reduced and you have better control.

If you lost interest in sex early on in your pregnancy, as many women who suffer with morning sickness do, your sex drive will probably return later on. Some women find arousal easier and orgasm more intense during pregnancy. It may be that the pregnancy hormones are responsible for this, but general feelings of well-being and happiness may also be a factor.

GOOD POSITIONS IN PREGNANCY

Now that you are getting larger, you will probably need to experiment with different positions in which to make love. Lying on your back will probably not feel comfortable. Experiment with different positions until you find some that work well for you and your partner.

One good position to try is the spoons position, in which both partners lie on their sides. You lie with your back to your partner, who lies curled around you and facing your back. He can then enter you from behind without putting any pressure on your abdomen. You may also find it easier to use the doggy position, with you on

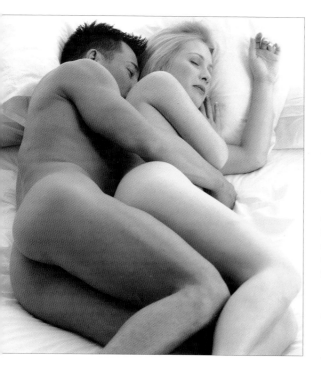

Pregnancy can often have an impact on your sex life, but it is not necessarily a negative one. This is the time to experiment with different positions to find the most comfortable. The spoons position, where you lie with your back to your partner, is a good option.

your hands and knees and your partner behind you. Another good position is with the woman on top, when again there is no pressure on her abdomen.

IF YOU GO OFF SEX

If your sex drive has diminished, try to show your partner love and affection in other ways. Of course, your partner will respect your wishes but he may feel rejected or alienated all the same. Showing that you love him is all the more important at this time. Reassure him of your feelings in thoughtful ways. Give him a glorious pampering massage, cook deliciously for him, send him a card, email him during the day if he is at work.

IF HE GOES OFF SEX

Lovemaking necessarily involves respecting one another's wishes. You may naturally find it disturbing if your partner rejects you sexually while you are pregnant, particularly if your sex life was very active beforehand. Try talking to him when he is neither tired nor busy and explain how you feel. Ask him to talk about he feels, too.

Show your partner that you cherish him in ways that are unrelated to sex. For a start, make sure that you are paying him as much attention as you are paying your pregnancy and your unborn baby. It may be that your partner has started to feel a little left out while you are, inevitably, receiving a lot of attention.

It may help if you cast your mind back to what your partner found attractive about you when you first met. Find ways to subtly recreate that picture – what did you wear? where did you go? what did you eat? You may find that focusing on your partner and his needs helps to rekindle the sexual attraction between you.

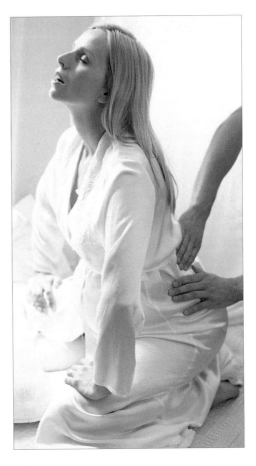

Massage can be a wonderful way of achieving physical closeness, and relaxing together.

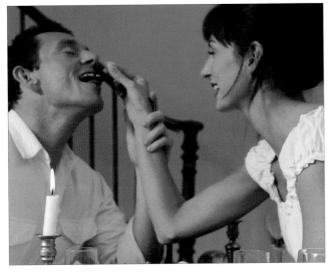

Show your partner that you are as interested in him as ever. Make time for him and have fun together.

Routine antenatal care

Many pregnant women find that the regular monitoring and tests carried out during pregnancy cause anxiety. Sometimes the anxiety can be so great that it can outweigh the benefits of good antenatal care.

It is important to remember that antenatal care is a well-established and thoroughly researched form of preventative health, with the interests of the mother and the baby at the fore. It is now more than ten times safer to have a baby than it was 100 years ago. However, you always have the right to veto any test or procedure that you do not feel is appropriate for you.

Most women find it helpful to be fully informed and to take time to think through the significance of each test, the possible consequences and any associated risks. Make sure that you discuss any medical concerns with your family doctor or hospital consultant. You may find it useful to take notes at such consultations and discuss the matter further with your partner, a close friend or relative. If you feel unsure about any test, ask for more information and for more time in which to consider your options.

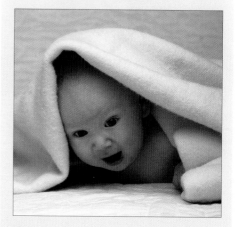

MEDICAL TERMS
Doctors may use the following terms when talking about your baby:
- **Fetus:** 8 weeks to birth (before 8 weeks, the term is an embryo).
- **Neonate:** from birth to 4 weeks.
- **Baby:** from birth to two years.
- **Infant:** first year of life.

The arrival of your baby may still seem a long way off, but you will soon be able to greet him or her.

ROUTINE MONITORING

Your weight, blood pressure, urine and blood-sugar level will be checked at antenatal appointments – changes here can give early indications of common problems.

Weight

Your weight may be monitored throughout the pregnancy in order to judge the baby's growth, the estimated delivery date, and the amount of amniotic fluid, although very regular weight checks are now less common at many clinics as some doctors feel they are not so important. There are known disadvantages to starting a pregnancy overweight: for example, there is a stronger likelihood of pregnancy-related diabetes and high blood pressure as well as the increased risk of a difficult labour and

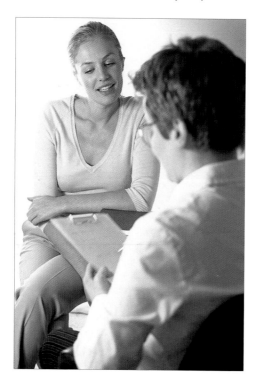

Antenatal check-ups are a good opportunity to discuss any anxieties you may have, however small they seem.

> **❝ It is now more than ten times safer to have a baby than it was 100 years ago. ❞**

delivering a large baby. In addition, anaesthetic complications associated with a Caesarean section are increased. These complications can sometimes occur if you gain excessive weight during your pregnancy.

Blood pressure

Your blood pressure is checked regularly. If it is too high, it is easily brought down with medication that does not harm the developing baby. High blood pressure is a typical sign of pre-eclampsia. If left untreated, it can develop into eclampsia, which can be life-threatening to the pregnant woman and the baby. In its fully developed stage, eclampsia is characterized by high blood pressure, severe headaches and fits. The symptoms of pre-eclampsia are high blood pressure, swelling of the ankles and hands, protein in the urine and sudden weight gain.

Urine

You will be asked to provide a urine sample at antenatal appointments. This will be checked for various substances: protein, sugar, bile, salts and blood. Urine tests are used to detect a number of conditions that could adversely affect your pregnancy, such as kidney disease, diabetes and infections in the urinary tract, such as cystitis.

For this test to be performed as efficiently as possible, you need to provide the hospital with a 'mid-stream' urine sample. To obtain this, first pass a little urine into the lavatory in the normal way, then contract your muscles to halt the flow for a couple of seconds. Resume the flow, allowing some of the urine to pass into the specimen bottle. Then remove the bottle and finish passing water.

Blood

Your blood sugar levels are checked to see whether pregnancy diabetes has developed. Your blood may also be checked for a number of other conditions, depending upon your individual medical history.

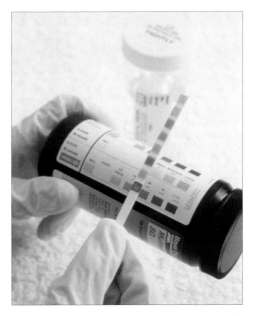

A multiple test stick is used to check your urine at each antenatal appointment. The colour of each pad is held against a colour chart to ensure that levels of protein, blood, bilirubin, glucose, ketones and acidity are normal.

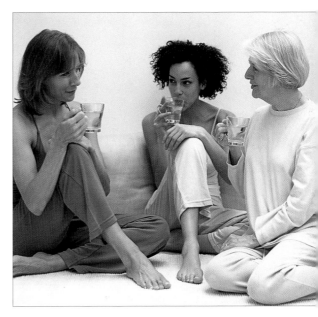

Talking to your mother or another older woman about your pregnancy can help allay doubts and fears. However, be wary of following out-of-date advice.

CHECK IT OUT

As soon as you tell people that you are pregnant, you are likely to find yourself on the receiving end of a lot of advice, particularly from women who have already had children. It can be very helpful to talk to women who have experienced pregnancy. However, do bear in mind that antenatal procedures and our understanding of what constitutes good pregnancy care are continually changing and developing. Always check any advice with your midwife.

Tests and procedures

As part of your antenatal care, you will be offered various tests to check that your baby is healthy. Some tests are standard and offered to all women; others are recommended only if the risk of a problem is higher than average. No test is compulsory: it is entirely up to you whether or not you have any procedure. However, most hospitals recommend the routine tests.

Ultrasound

Pregnant women are usually offered their second routine ultrasound scan at around 20 weeks. This important scan is used to assess the baby's growth, to confirm the estimated date of delivery and also to check that the baby is developing in a normal way.

At the scan, the baby's head can be seen clearly in outline and its diameter can be measured on the ultrasound screen and correlated with the known average. Earlier in the pregnancy, it may be difficult to measure the head and later on, each baby will develop its own shape and size. At this point, though, most babies' heads are roughly the same size. Once the diameter of the head is measured it is plotted on a graph and equated to a known value so that an accurate estimate of the delivery date can be made.

The baby is checked in all respects including the heart, the limbs, the spine and the head, which provides the opportunity to look for any abnormalities such as spina bifida, kidney, brain and heart defects. Some defects detected at this time can be treated *in utero* (in the womb) before the baby is born. Others may require medication or surgery after the baby has been born.

Nuchal screening

This more detailed ultrasound scan is carried out between about 11 and 14 weeks, and can indicate the likelihood of a Down's baby. It is described on page 108.

Chorionic villus sampling

This test is usually performed within the first twelve or so weeks of pregnancy. It is a way of detecting the likelihood of the baby being affected by Down's. See page 108.

Alphafetoprotein test

The substance alphafetoprotein (AFP) appears in your blood in varying levels throughout the pregnancy. Between about 15 and 18 weeks the level is fairly constant in most women (before or after this time the level is very variable). A higher than normal level at this time can indicate that the baby could be suffering from a defect of the spine, such as spina bifida, or another abnormality of brain development. A low level of AFP may be found in Down's syndrome babies.

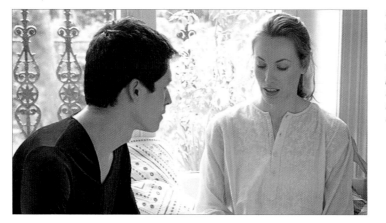

People often have strong feelings about amniocentesis, and it is important to discuss these fully, with your partner and with the hospital consultant, before you come to a decision about the test.

The non-invasive AFP test may be done before amniocentesis: if AFP gives a good result, you may feel that amniocentesis is unnecessary. However, AFP tests are being done less often as ultrasound can be more accurate.

Bart's test

This test – known as the 'triple screen' in the US – involves taking a blood sample from the mother at about 16 to 18 weeks and measuring three hormones that are commonly secreted in pregnancy. The hormones are AFP, oestriol (which indicates how much oestrogen is circulating in the blood; spelled estriol in the US) and HCG (human chorionic gonadotrophin, present in high levels in pregnancy).

The Bart's test is essentially a screening test for fetal abnormality, the commonest of which is Down's. A very high result indicates the risk of a Down's child but it does not absolutely diagnose a Down's baby. The advantage with this test, like the AFP, is that it is non-invasive and you may feel it renders amniocentesis unnecessary.

Amniocentesis

This test is usually carried out around 16 weeks. It involves a sample of fluid being drawn from the amniotic sac using a needle. Ultrasound is used to guide the needle to the correct place. The fluid is then analysed to determine the likelihood of Down's syndrome and other fetal abnormalities. The test and its implications are described in detail over the following pages.

Fetal blood sampling (cordocentesis)

This procedure (called PUBS or Percutaneous Umbilical Blood Sampling in the US) involves taking blood from the umbilical cord and analysing the baby's blood cells. Like amniocentesis, it makes use of ultrasound to guide the needle to the correct location. Cordocentesis can be performed from the 18th week to determine the baby's condition and to identify inherited disorders such as those detected by amniocentesis.

The advantage of cordocentesis is that results are available within a week, while amniocentesis usually means a wait of up to three weeks. Cordocentesis may be used if a late ultrasound scan indicates a problem or if the alphafetoprotein test reveals a level of protein that is too low or too high. It is also useful when it is vital to know the baby's blood group before birth, as in cases of congenital forms of anaemia, or if the baby's blood needs to be tested to determine whether he or she has developed an infection – for example, of the toxoplasmosis organism.

Like amniocentesis, cordocentesis carries a small chance of causing miscarriage (it may be 1–2 per cent) – discuss this with your consultant. Rhesus-negative women will be given a protective injection of anti-D immunoglobulin after this test in case any fetal cells are disturbed, which would increase the risk of antibodies developing.

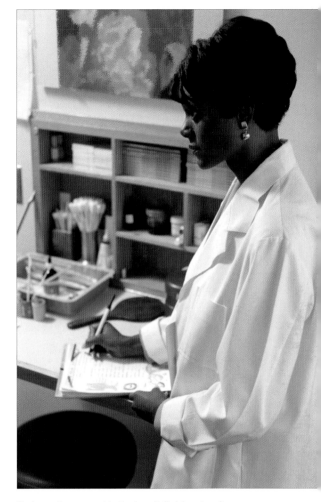

Test samples are sent to the hospital's laboratory for analysis and interpretation. You may have to wait several weeks for some results.

Fetoscopy

This procedure is used only rarely and involves inserting a fibre-optic tube into the uterus through a cut in the abdomen. A microscope camera can be attached to the end of the tube so the fetus can be photographed. The fetoscope can also be used to take a sample of tissue, which enables diagnosis of several blood and skin diseases that amniocentesis cannot detect. In some centres, certain fetal conditions can be treated before delivery by means of fetoscopy. For example, babies with excess fluid of the brain can have a shunt inserted to drain the fluid. Other conditions, such as urinary tract obstruction, can be treated, too.

Amniocentesis in perspective

Amniocentesis is an antenatal procedure that may be offered to women who have a higher than average risk of carrying a baby with an abnormality. It may be offered, for example, to women who have been in contact with the rubella virus in the first three months of their pregnancy. Amniocentesis may be offered to women in their late thirties, and will usually be offered to women over the age of forty as a matter of course.

WHAT AMNIOCENTESIS INVOLVES

Amniocentesis is normally performed at around 16 weeks, although it can be done a little earlier and up to a few weeks later. Ultrasound is usually used to locate the amniotic sac, the placenta and the baby. It is best not to have amniocentesis without ultrasound since this increases the risk of miscarriage. In addition, the test may not be successful if insufficient liquid is obtained.

You will need to have a full bladder to have ultrasound and you will therefore be asked to drink a pint of water an hour before your appointment (and not to go to the lavatory). A local anaesthetic may be applied to your abdomen and a fine needle is then inserted through it. You may feel some discomfort at this point.

The ultrasound picture is used to locate the best pool of liquid in the amniotic sac and to make the sure that the needle does not pierce either the placenta or the baby. This is particularly important in women who are rhesus-negative as the procedure may cause the fetal and maternal blood to mix, which will sensitize the mother in future pregnancies. A protective injection of anti-D immunoglobulin is given at the time of amniocentesis to a woman who has a rhesus-negative blood group.

“ The vast majority of people are given good news after amniocentesis. ”

The needle is used to draw some of the amniotic fluid. The growing baby is not harmed by the needle because it swims around in fluid and tends to move away from any object that approaches it.

After the test, it is advisable to rest for the remainder of the day in order not to irritate the uterus and to prevent leakage of fluid from the tiny hole made by the needle.

The amniotic fluid is then analysed in a number of different ways to detect fetal abnormalities. The levels of AFP hormone will also be measured. The cells will be grown (cultured) in a laboratory and their chromosomes subsequently analysed.

AFP analysis results from amniocentesis come within a couple of days but the chromosomal results of an amniocentesis normally take up to four weeks, as it takes some time to culture cells.

IS AMNIOCENTESIS SAFE?

The main disadvantage with amniocentesis is that it carries a risk of causing miscarriage. Withdrawing the fluid can sometimes cause trauma to the uterus, which may then start contracting. Twenty years ago the risk of miscarrying a healthy baby through amniocentesis was one in 100. Improved procedures mean that it has now fallen to about one in 200.

The degree of risk depends to a certain extent on how experienced the doctor is in carrying out the technique: some doctors are more skillful than others. It also

---

WHO IS OFFERED AMNIOCENTESIS?

It is up to each individual woman, in consultation with her partner, whether or not she decides to have an amniocentesis. The test will usually be offered to the following women:

- All women over the age of 37, because there is an increased risk of Down's syndrome.
- Women with a history of a child born with Down's syndrome or with certain other chromosome abnormalities.
- Women in whom a Down's blood test has shown an increased likelihood of chromosome abnormalities.

- Sometimes, women who have had a previous child affected by spina bifida or hydrocephalus. However, sophisticated ultrasound techniques may mean that an amniocentesis is not necessarily recommended in such cases.
- Women whose medical history includes having a child affected by certain sex-linked diseases, such as haemophilia.
- Certain women with a family history of rare abnormality, following genetic counselling and possibly genetic testing of several or all family members.

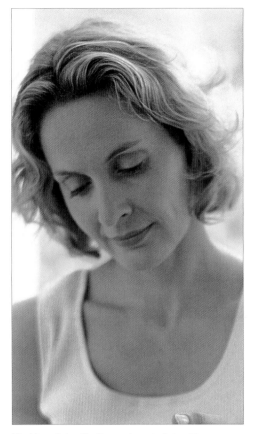

Most hospitals will offer amniocentesis to older women, sometimes to the over-35s and usually as a matter of course to women over the age of 40.

depends on whether or not ultrasound is used to help guide the needle. If you are considering amniocentesis, you should ask your consultant the following questions before deciding to go ahead:

- Is ultrasound going to be used?
- Who is going to carry out the test: will it be the consultant or senior registrar or another doctor?
- What is the practitioner's personal rate of miscarriage? Is it higher than the average?

When deciding whether to have the test, weigh up the risk of miscarriage against the value of the information ascertained. A 20-year-old woman has a one in 2000 chance of bearing a Down's syndrome child and a one in 200 chance of miscarriage as a direct result of amniocentesis. She is thus likely to feel that the test is not worth the risk. On the other hand, a 41-year-old woman has the same risk of miscarriage from the test, but a one in

50 risk of carrying a Down's baby. She is therefore four times as likely to have a Down's child as she is to miscarry through having amniocentesis. In this situation, many women decide that they do want to take the risk.

THINKING AMNIOCENTESIS THROUGH

Amniocentesis is a useful test, which can offer you the peace of mind necessary to enjoy the rest of your pregnancy. It also provides valuable information for medical and nursing staff, so that they are more likely to know what, if any, abnormalities they are dealing with, and to be better prepared. The difficulties surrounding amniocentesis are:

- It could cause miscarriage and the unnecessary loss of a healthy baby.
- It could lead to a further dilemma – whether or not to terminate the pregnancy if the baby should be affected by Down's syndrome or another problem.

It is important that you and your partner share any concerns with your consultant, and ask any questions that you have before you come to a decision. Ideally, you will make a decision that all of you are happy with.

YOUR OPTIONS

The choices you have are as follows:

- Not to have amniocentesis.
- To have amniocentesis for information, even if you are certain that you would not terminate the pregnancy if you were carrying a Down's baby.
- To have amniocentesis, having already decided that you would terminate the pregnancy in the case of a serious abnormality.
- To have amniocentesis for information, although you are uncertain as to how you would proceed in the case of an abnormality.
- To have other tests that carry a lower chance of miscarriage, in order to assess the chance of carrying a child with an abnormality. You then have the option of proceeding to amniocentesis if the risk appears to be high. Other useful tests include nuchal screening, the alphafetoprotein test and Bart's test.

THE RESULTS

The vast majority of people are given good news after amniocentesis. The test shows that there is something wrong in about 3 per cent of cases. Nearly half of these concern Down's syndrome babies.

A termination may be recommended if the amniocentesis shows that something is severely wrong with your baby and his or her quality of life would be strongly affected. If amniocentesis identifies a less severe disability or an operable deformity, many women will continue with the pregnancy.

When something is wrong

If tests show that something is seriously wrong with the baby you are carrying, then you will be asked if you want to end the pregnancy. Terminating a wanted pregnancy is obviously a very difficult and complex decision to make. Only you and your partner can know what is the right choice for you.

Some people feel strongly that they would not terminate a pregnancy under any circumstances. For example, people who hold profound religious or humanitarian beliefs would probably decide against termination even if there was a serious problem with the baby. Women who believe that this pregnancy is their last chance of having a child may also be reluctant to terminate the pregnancy. Some parents feel that they are able and willing to care for a disabled child, whatever the extent of his or her problems.

Many couples would, however, consider termination the most feasible option if a test such as amniocentesis or chorionic villus sampling (CVS) showed that the baby was not developing normally. There are many reasons why a pregnancy may be terminated. These are just some of the common ones:

- The parents may know that they could not cope with a disabled child.
- The parents may believe it to be wrong to bring a child into the world if she or he would develop an incurable, untreatable disease.
- The mother's physical and mental well-being may be at risk. If the child is so severely handicapped that he or she will inevitably die later in the uterus or shortly after birth, the mother, and the father, may be saved some suffering by opting for a termination.
- The likely effect on the parents and other children in the family may seem too great. A severely handicapped child can exert a profound influence upon its family. He or she will need full-time care and this may strain the emotional, physical and financial resources of the family to a great degree.
- The child may suffer needlessly and die either in childhood or in early adulthood.

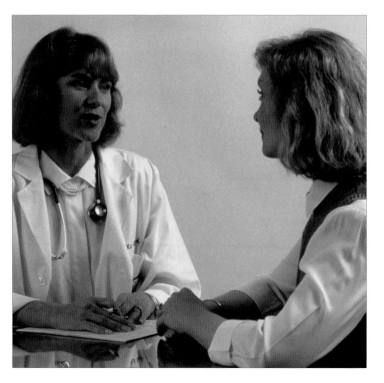

Everyone involved in maternity care knows that choosing to have a termination is the most distressing decision a woman can make. You will be given all the support that you need.

You may want to talk to your family doctor, the hospital consultant or your midwife more than once if you are contemplating a termination. Healthcare staff will understand only too well that you need to gather as much information as possible, and that you need to take time to make your decision. Rest assured that nobody will try to persuade you to have a termination if you really do not wish to do so.

TERMINATING A PREGNANCY

The procedure for terminating a pregnancy varies depending on whether it is performed before the end of the 13th week or after it. If you are considering having a termination after an amniocentesis, you will need to have a late termination.

Early termination

A termination performed at 13 weeks or earlier is a simple and quick operation, with minimal risks to the woman's physical health. It may be done following a test carried out early in the pregnancy, such as CVS.

Early terminations are carried out under a local or general anaesthetic. The woman's cervix is dilated (expanded) so that the fetus can be removed by suction. You will usually be able to go home on the same day as the operation, but you will be advised to rest for 24 hours.

Late termination

A late termination is available to those women who wish to end a pregnancy after amniocentesis or other tests. At this stage of pregnancy, it is not possible to dilate the woman's cervix to the required degree without risking permanent damage to it. Because of this, many doctors prefer to use the technique in which the natural process of birth is imitated.

The woman is given synthetic prostaglandin in the form of a vaginal gel or pessary, or in the form of an infusion directly into her uterus, at regular intervals. This process is known as prostaglandin induction, and causes the woman to go through what is, in effect, a mini-labour. Her uterus starts contracting to expel the fetus, and in response to this, the cervix dilates. If the pregnancy is being terminated after 20 weeks, then an irritant substance may be injected directly into the amniotic sac around the fetus.

It may be some hours before the fetus is expelled, just as it is during labour and birth. The fetus is usually born dead. The woman then normally undergoes a procedure called dilatation and curettage (D and C) in which all the contents of the uterus are removed. This is done to ensure that no part of the placenta or anything else relating to the pregnancy remains.

You will probably have to stay in hospital overnight, and should rest at home over the days that follow.

THE RISKS

There are certain risks attached to terminating a pregnancy, and these risks are higher the later the abortion. Your doctor will explain these to you in detail, but they include:

- Infection in about 3 in 100 women.
- Prolonged bleeding in 4 in 100 women.
- Abnormal blood clotting in one in 200 women.
- Operative trauma, such as tissue damage or perforation of the uterus. This occurs in less than one in 100 women.
- Feelings of regret for what might have been. Most women will need time to come to terms with the end of a wanted pregnancy.

FEELINGS OF REGRET

In cases where the developing baby has, or is likely to have, severe abnormalities, having a termination may be the best choice for everyone. However, this does not mean that you will not mourn your baby. Ultimately, this may prove to be an event in your life that is never completely forgotten, never completely accepted.

It is extremely important that, immediately after the event, you give yourself whatever time you need to grieve and to fully explore and express your emotions. Talk to your partner about how you feel, and also encourage him to share his feelings.

You may wish to carry out some kind of closing ceremony or ritual to help you say goodbye. How you choose to do this is a personal matter, but you could visit a local church or religious centre of some kind, or simply go somewhere beautiful and say goodbye in your own way. Making a donation to a children's charity or perhaps planting a tree that will live for many years may feel like a positive and helpful thing to do.

FINDING SUPPORT

You and your partner may well need support from other people – don't feel that you have to sort out your feelings between just the two of you. Friends and relatives can be a great source of comfort, although they may be too close to the two of you and to the situation. If you prefer to see a counsellor, your family doctor will be able to refer you. There are centres you can contact direct that offer specialist post-termination counselling and also confidential helplines. Remember that such counsellors are happy to discuss your feelings about a termination even if it is years after the event.

A complementary therapist may also be able to offer support. Acupuncture and zero balancing – a therapy in which gentle touch is used to release difficult emotions – may go some way towards helping you to deal with what has happened to you. Reiki is another gentle and non-intrusive method of healing that might prove helpful.

Checklist of common problems

By the second trimester, women usually feel healthier and more confident about their pregnancies. You are likely to have more energy, and morning sickness has usually passed. However, you may still be affected by ailments such as constipation and indigestion.

The following solutions should help to relieve any discomfort, but also check the relevant safety advice in Section Four.

Some treatments may work better for you than others and you may need to experiment to find one that suits you. If any complaint persists, or if it troubles you, or you are not sure what it is, you should consult your family doctor. In any case, tell your midwife about the problem at your next antenatal check.

Back pain Many women suffer from back pain during pregnancy (and almost everyone is affected in the last months). However, there is a lot you can do to minimize the pain. First of all, make sure that you have a good, supportive mattress; if you do not, consider buying a new one. Be aware of your posture: check how you are holding yourself at regular intervals, and change your position if you are sitting awkwardly. Try yoga or Pilates, which can help to strengthen the muscles in your back and improve your posture.

For persistent back pain, see an osteopath, Alexander technique teacher or chiropractor. Flotation therapy, which allows you to relax in a supported position, can be a pleasing way to relieve back pain. Reiki, massage and acupuncture can also be good therapies to try.

Varicose veins Eat a healthy diet, that includes plenty of foods that are rich in vitamin E, such as wheatgerm, wholegrains, sunflower seeds and cold-pressed vegetable oils. Avoid standing still for long periods: walk on the spot or flex and rotate your ankles. Walk daily to help the circulation, and rest with your feet up twice a day, for 20 minutes a time. Brushing the skin daily with a soft-bristled brush can help – use long, upward strokes.

For temporary relief, apply commercially prepared witch hazel or aloe vera compresses to the affected area. Ask your doctor about wearing support stockings. Homeopathy, acupuncture and aromatherapy can be helpful. You may also draw comfort from the fact that varicose veins often subside after the birth.

Stretchmarks Eating a healthy, balanced diet that is rich in vitamin E, silica and other nutrients can help to

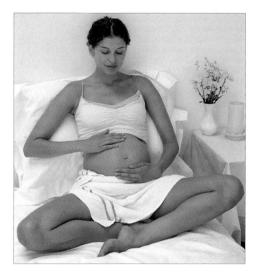

Massaging oil into the skin of your abdomen, using a circular clockwise motion, may help to prevent the formation of stretchmarks.

prevent stretchmarks (see also page 121). Massage the skin gently with a good-quality oil enriched with vitamin E to help maintain suppleness. Add a few drops of an essential oil such as neroli or mandarin to your massage oil. Marigold or lavender flowers can also be used. Soak the flowers in wheatgerm oil for two weeks, then strain. Apply the oil daily, rubbing it gently into the skin in a circular motion. A homeopath may prescribe calc fluor as a preventative measure.

Constipation Start the day with a glass of hot water with a little fresh lemon juice. Include plenty of wholegrains, fruit and vegetables in your diet, and drink lots of water. Avoid bananas and hard-boiled eggs, and do not eat late at night. Take more exercise, particularly walking, and try yoga – some yoga postures specifically work on the digestion.

For temporary relief, try massaging the abdomen with essential oil of ginger diluted in wheatgerm oil (see pages 124–7): use a smooth circular movement, starting on the lower left-hand side and working clockwise (apply light pressure only). Herbal medicine, homeopathy, acupuncture, chiropractic and osteopathy can all be helpful.

Haemorrhoids Piles are often caused by constipation, so follow the steps given. Try resting on your left side regularly; this can relieve pressure on the pelvic veins. Keep the area clean, washing with unperfumed soap after emptying your bowels. Cold, witch hazel compresses can help relieve itching. However, be sure to tell your doctor or midwife about the problem.

Headaches and migraines Eat regularly and make sure that you are drinking enough water – low blood sugar and dehydration can lead to headaches. Try to identify any migraine triggers, such as cheese, chocolate, citrus fruits and caffeine, and avoid them. Watch your posture: relax your shoulders regularly since tension here can cause headaches. A shoulder massage can provide temporary relief, as can applying a lavender-oil compress to your temples. Consider seeing an Alexander technique teacher, chiropractor, osteopath or cranial osteopath. Reiki, reflexology and acupuncture can also help.

Cystitis Urinary infections require immediate treatment: see your doctor if you have an increased need to pass urine, and burning or pain when you do so. Drinking plenty of water and two glasses of cranberry juice a day will help prevent and ease cystitis. Tea tree and lavender oils have a healing effect: dilute two drops of each in a base oil or full-fat milk and add to a warm bath. Do not use lavender if you are less than 16 weeks pregnant.

A homeopath may recommend remedies such as cantharis or apis mel, which can be taken alongside antibiotics. Reflexology and herbal medicine can also be useful as an adjunct to medical treatment.

Thrush See your doctor to check the diagnosis, even if you have had thrush before (other vaginal infections may also cause itching, redness and discharge). Many women

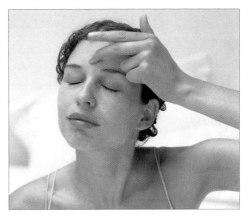

You may be able to relieve a headache by massaging the acupuncture points just above the bridge of the nose and at the external tip of each eyebrow.

find that it helps to avoid sugar and yeast, and to eat plenty of vegetables. You should make sure that you use unscented soap and bath products.

Live yogurt is a soothing natural remedy: apply to the affected area every two hours. Tea tree and lavender essential oils may help: try diluting two drops of each in a base oil or full-fat milk, and add to a warm bath. If you are less than 16 weeks pregnant, use tea tree oil only.

Indigestion Eat little and often rather than having two large meals a day. Limit fluid intake at mealtimes, and eat slowly. Do not bend or lie down afterwards, and make sure that you eat your evening meal at least two hours before bedtime. If indigestion persists at night, use more pillows to keep your upper body elevated. Try drinking lemon balm tea after meals, and ask your doctor about taking calcium-based indigestion tablets. Homeopathy, acupuncture, osteopathy, Alexander technique and chiropractic can all be beneficial.

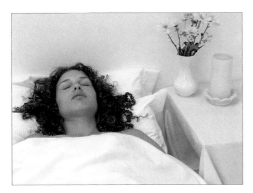

If you suffer from heartburn at night, do not sleep on your back; sleep on your side propped up with pillows. Do not eat less than two hours before bedtime.

WHEN TO CALL A DOCTOR
Seek emergency assistance if you have:
- Vaginal bleeding other than spotting.
- Severe abdominal pain or vomiting.
- Sudden swelling of hands and ankles or blurred vision with severe headache.
- From week 22, no fetal movements for more than 12 hours.
- Breaking of the waters.

See your doctor if you have:
- A high temperature (101°F/38.5°C +).
- Swollen hands or ankles.
- Pain on urination.

Common Qs and As

Q: I am getting irritated by all the advice that I am receiving from anyone and everyone, and by all the tests that one is given during antenatal care. Is all this fuss necessary?

A: It is important to distinguish between well-meant advice from friends and family, and that from your doctor and midwife. Remember that friends and family may not be up to date – some of what you are told may not be correct. Antenatal care, however, is valuable. Today, it is the expectation of most women in the West that they will have a safe and successful pregnancy leading to the delivery of a healthy baby. This is in stark contrast to our grandmothers and great-grandmothers. Before 1935, one in every 200-250 pregnancies resulted in the death of the mother, most commonly from infection. These days you almost never hear of women dying in childbirth – thanks largely to regular antenatal monitoring and improved delivery procedures.

Q: My sister has been trying for a baby for three years. Now that I am pregnant she is avoiding me. What can I do?

A: This is a very difficult situation, particularly for your sister. It may help to be open about what is happening; perhaps you could tell her that you fully realize how painful it is for her to be around you while you are pregnant and that you understand how she is behaving. You could also reassure her that many couples do conceive after several years of trying, and encourage her to see her doctor for investigations if she has not already done so.

You may want and need your sister's support at this eventful time in your life, but it is probably best to let her decide how much she wants to be involved with your pregnancy. If she does remain distant, you may find that the situation changes when the baby is born, and your sister can enjoy her niece or nephew.

Q: How would I know if there was anything wrong with my baby?

A: The chief way of checking that everything is progressing well is through your regular antenatal checks: this is why it is so important that you attend them. If anything should be amiss, it can be quickly identified and treated.

If there were anything seriously wrong, your body would soon tell you. Be alert to the chief danger signs and symptoms, which are listed on page 145. Be aware, too, of your baby's movements. Should these stop for a period of 24 hours or more, you should consult a doctor without delay.

Q: I am five months pregnant and have only a very small bump. Is something wrong?

A: Women do vary in the size of their bump, and if you are of a slight build you are more likely to give birth to a baby who also has a slighter build. However, if you are worried, the best thing for you to do is to talk about your concerns with your antenatal team. They should be able to reassure you that everything is fine.

One of the great advantages of antenatal care and all the research that has gone before is that the hospital consultants will almost certainly know if anything is wrong. They will be able to tell if you are carrying what is known as a 'small for dates' baby. They will also know from blood and urine tests, as well as from the scans, if the pregnancy is not progressing as it should do.

Q: I feel uncomfortable about the whole idea of making love now that I am well into the pregnancy, and worry that some damage may be done. Am I being ridiculous? Exactly how safe is it?

A: There are certain circumstances under which sex must be avoided – in certain high-risk pregnancies or in the last trimester when expecting more than one baby, for example. Your doctor will advise and warn about this. However, in the majority of cases, experts feel that there is no danger at all in making love at any stage of the pregnancy, as long as you are not overly athletic.

You will find that you need to explore different positions as your size increases, in order to be as comfortable as possible. Also, be prepared for some loss of libido at certain stages due to hormonal changes or fatigue. Take time to explore non-penetrative options and always keep loving lines of communication open with your partner.

Q: I cannot decide whether or not to have an amniocentesis. I would be devastated if I lost the baby through having the test.

A: This is without doubt an extraordinarily difficult decision to make. You should discuss with your hospital consultant the risks of your particular case, bearing in mind your medical history and your age. Then give yourself and your partner time to consider how much you are personally at risk of carrying a baby with a serious problem such as Down's syndrome. If the risk is slight, you may be well advised not to have amniocentesis. If the risk is thought to be high or very high, you may prefer to have the test. However, if you knew that you would be devastated at the loss of any baby, whether or not he or she was impaired with a condition such as Down's, clearly it would be better if you did not have the test.

Q: If I had to terminate a pregnancy, how long would I have to wait before we started trying for another baby?

A: Medical opinion remains divided on this issue. The minimum wait is naturally until your periods return to normal or at least return to what was normal for you. After that, the general consensus is that you should wait for three or four months before attempting to conceive again. If you wait a little longer than that, both you and your partner will have that little extra time in which to recover both physically and emotionally after the termination. Some consultants advise six months but this is not strictly necessary.

Q: My doctor says that I need a course of antibiotics to clear up a severe attack of sinusitis. I am worried about taking medication when I am pregnant. Do you think that it is okay to take them?

A: You should obviously avoid taking any unnecessary medication during pregnancy. However, if the infection is severe, clearly it needs to be treated before it starts to affect your general health and energy levels. Any medication prescribed during your pregnancy will be given in the knowledge that you are pregnant and will be chosen accordingly. Always remind any prescribing doctor that you are pregnant, just in case he or she fails to refer to your notes and especially if you are not yet big enough for it to be obvious.

The third trimester

❝ It is important for you to make rest and relaxation a priority by taking a rest every day ❞

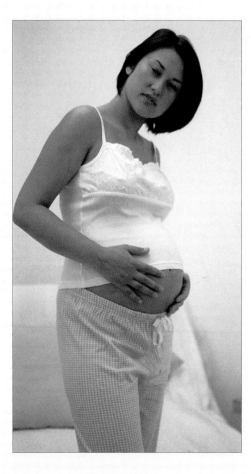

You are now embarking on the third and final trimester of your pregnancy, week 27 onwards. This is a tumultuous, exciting time for you and your partner. Now that your baby is fully formed, you may more easily be able to imagine him or her as a little person.

The normal length of time for a pregnancy is 40 weeks, but yours may last just 38 – less if the baby is premature – or it may run to 42. Once a pregnancy goes beyond 42 weeks, medical intervention may be recommended. If you are pregnant with twins (or more), you will almost certainly deliver early, usually at about 37 weeks.

During these last weeks, you may feel that you have been pregnant forever. You may feel slightly breathless when bending down. Your sleep may be interrupted when you turn over, by frequent trips to the lavatory, and by kicks from your baby. Your stomach will have less space to expand in when you are eating, and so you might find it easier to have smaller meals more often than three times a day.

You may feel a greater bond with your baby in these last weeks. Now you can start looking forward to getting to know him or her in person.

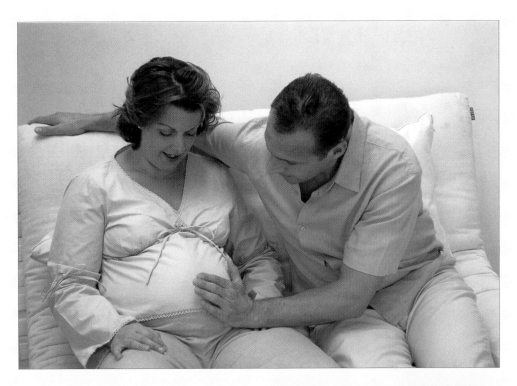

It is important for you to make rest and relaxation a priority, by taking a rest every day, and perhaps chat to your baby or play music as you do so. Complementary therapies can be particularly beneficial during the last three months. Good ones to try include reiki, yoga, massage, aromatherapy and Alexander technique. These will encourage you to relax, improve your posture and help relieve any backache that you may be experiencing.

Do not attempt to do any more than you feel comfortable with, but remember the value of exercise. A short walk each day will improve muscular fitness and at the same time boost your energy and prepare you for labour and the birth.

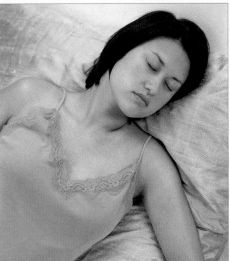

Top: Talking to the baby regularly will help him or her to become familiar with the voices of both parents. You may even feel your baby respond with a little kick when you start speaking.

Sleep may become more fitful in later months. Get as much relaxation as you can, and take an afternoon nap to compensate if possible.

How your baby is developing

During these last months of your pregnancy, the baby will continue to mature, and he or she will also become much fatter.

Weeks 26–27
The eyelids open briefly for the first time at the end of the second trimester; they start to remain open from week 27. The iris of the eye is blue at this stage, and will remain so until a few months after delivery. The baby looks quite lean, and at 26 weeks weighs about 500g (1lb 2oz). Over the next few weeks, his or her body weight will more than double as more muscle and fat develops.

Weeks 28–31
At 28 weeks the baby measures 36cm (14in), and weighs about 900g (2lb). You will feel a good deal of kicking and fluttering at this stage. Your baby's breathing movements will have become rhythmic by week 30, but he or she may experience hiccups – which you will feel as small jerks – when amniotic fluid goes down the wrong passage.

If your baby were to be born at this point, there is a fair chance that he or she would survive. However, the lack of body fat means that the baby would have difficulty in regulating his or her body temperature. He or she would also experience breathing difficulties and would need to be placed in an incubator with a ventilator attached. The baby's immune system and liver functioning would still be weak, rendering him or her particularly susceptible to infection. Specialist care would be needed for several more weeks while the baby continued his or her development outside the uterus.

Week 32
Your baby is perfectly formed, with fully developed lungs. It has been shown experimentally that the baby can now focus on external stimuli – a needle, for example. From now until week 34, your baby is likely to turn so that he or she is head down, in preparation for the birth. Before this time most babies are in the breech position, with the head facing up. The baby weighs about 1.8kg (4lb).

THE FINAL STAGES
You will become much larger in the last trimester as your baby is growing rapidly. Your expanding uterus will press against your intestines and stomach, impeding your digestion, and on the lungs, causing slight breathlessness. The baby is fully formed at 36 weeks but needs to put on weight before birth.

WEEKS 27–31

WEEKS 32–36

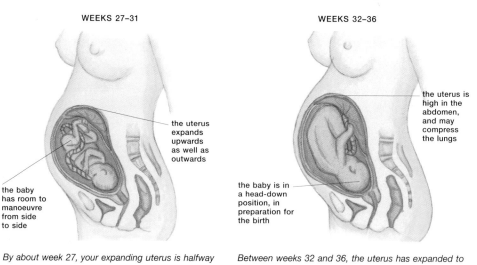

the uterus expands upwards as well as outwards

the baby has room to manoeuvre from side to side

the uterus is high in the abdomen, and may compress the lungs

the baby is in a head-down position, in preparation for the birth

By about week 27, your expanding uterus is halfway between your navel and ribs.

Between weeks 32 and 36, the uterus has expanded to fill the abdomen, extending almost up to the ribs.

Weeks 33–36

The baby is becoming plumper and gaining about 14g (½oz) of fat each day. Fat ensures that a baby can regulate heat and cold once they leave the controlled environment of the uterus. The fingers and toes have soft nails, which reach right to the ends. The hair on the baby's head may be as long as 2.5cm (1in) long and is very slippery to aid the baby's passage during birth. By week 36, the baby's skull is firm but not hard, because it will need to compress as the baby squeezes down the birth canal.

The baby is about 46cm (18in) long and weighs about 2.75kg (6lb). If this is your first baby, the head will soon engage – drop downwards into the upper pelvis – in preparation for the birth. If you have given birth before, the baby may not engage for several more weeks, and sometimes not until just before the labour.

Weeks 37–39

Your baby's nervous system is maturing, ready for birth. The layer of fat under the skin is now ready to regulate body temperature when the baby is born. The lungs are lined with surfactant, which resembles bubbles of foam. This keeps the lungs partially inflated each time the baby breathes out after she is born; without surfactant the lungs would collapse. The baby's heartbeat is about twice as fast as yours, about 110–150 beats per minute.

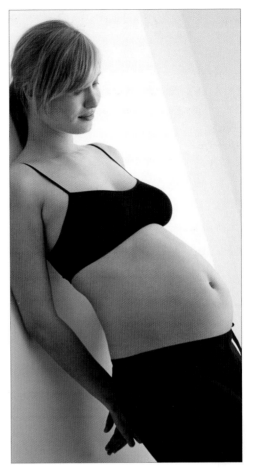

During these final weeks, you will feel a variety of movements as your baby turns over, moves his or her hands and feet, and even hiccups. These movements are often felt more when you are resting.

Other people may now be able to hear the baby's heartbeat simply by putting their ear to your abdomen. The baby will weigh about 3.1kg (almost 7lb).

Week 40

The baby's movements decrease from now on, because there is less space in the uterus for him or her to move around. You may miss these movements, although you may still feel strong kicks from the baby's hands and feet. When the baby is awake, his or her eyes are open a good deal of the time. In a boy, the testicles will almost certainly have descended. The baby may now measure about 51cm (20in) in length and he or she weighs about 3.5kg (7lb 8oz).

WEEKS 37–40

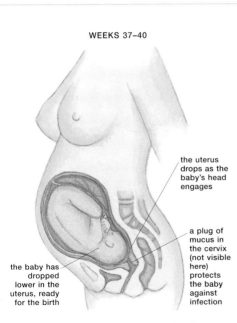

the uterus drops as the baby's head engages

a plug of mucus in the cervix (not visible here) protects the baby against infection

the baby has dropped lower in the uterus, ready for the birth

Some time from week 36 onwards, the head engages. The uterus drops lower, easing pressure on the lungs.

What the baby hears and feels

As recently as the 1970s, some people believed that babies were born both deaf and blind. However, we now know that babies learn to recognize the sound of the mother's voice several weeks before they are born.

The uterus is neither completely dark nor silent: babies discern light through the uterine wall, and they can also feel vibrations made by music and voices. They may learn to associate certain sounds with the mood of the mother, and may even develop preferences for particular sounds.

TOUCH

The unborn baby's sense of touch starts to function before the other senses. Experiments have shown that the fetus responds to touch on the lips as early as seven weeks. This responsiveness then spreads to the cheeks, the forehead and the palms, followed by the arms. By week 14–15, most of the body responds to touch.

It is difficult to assess whether or not an unborn baby can feel pain. However, increases in heart rate have been observed in fetuses following invasive tests such as fetal scalp blood sampling, and increases in movements have been observed during amniocentesis.

HEARING

Research has shown that a baby's sense of hearing begins to function before the birth. What a baby hears is a jumble of sound – perhaps a low rumble and the distant beating of the mother's heart – as well as the mother's voice, which the baby will recognize and respond to once he or she is born.

Your baby's ears begin to develop in the fourth week of pregnancy and they are reasonably well formed by the end of the seventh week. It is known that external sounds filter through to the baby, although they are likely to be changed in quality. The rhythms of the sounds, however, remain unchanged. Ultrasound pictures have shown that an unborn baby of 24–25 weeks will respond to a noise

> **"** The uterus is neither completely dark nor silent: babies discern light through the uterine wall, and they can feel vibrations made by music and voices. **"**

applied to the mother's abdomen. However, the external noise has to be quite loud to be audible over the noise of the mother's digestive and cardiovascular system.

In the last few months of your pregnancy, your baby will learn to register your voice, becoming familiar with the vibrations of your speech. The unborn baby's experience of speech patterns and vibrations may actually begin the process of acquiring language.

VISION

Experiments have shown that the visual sense is functioning in the uterus from 26 weeks. Babies will blink or close their eyes if a light is shone on the mother's abdomen. They will also train their vision by focusing on their own hands and feet, and on the umbilical cord.

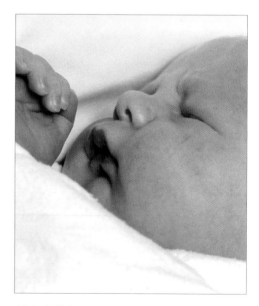

A baby is likely to recognize the sound of the mother's voice as soon as he or she is born. It seems that babies start to learn while they are still in the uterus.

HOW MUCH DO WE KNOW?
New technology has given us great insight into how babies develop physically. However, we can only speculate about how much they perceive. One leading expert, Professor Peter G. Helpert, says that 98 per cent of what is said about fetal perception is guesswork and 2 per cent is proven fact.

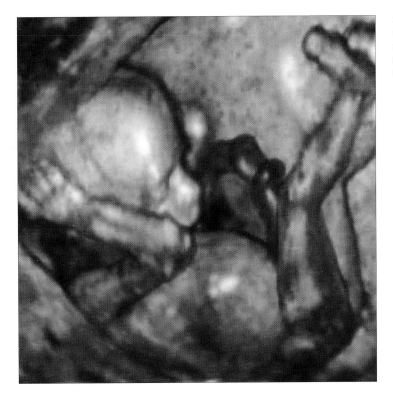

Researchers have discovered that babies can remember sounds and tastes that they experienced in the uterus.

TASTE AND SMELL

It is impossible to distinguish between a baby's sense of taste and smell in the uterus, since both may be stimulated by chemical stimuli in the amniotic fluid. For this reason, researchers tend to investigate them together. We know that babies practise sucking movements in the uterus, in preparation for feeding after the birth, and it seems that they have a preference for sweet tastes. When saccharin is added to the amniotic fluid, an increase in swallowing is observed.

One study found that a newborn responded to an odour previously experienced only in the uterus. In this experiment, a mother was given capsules of cumin with meals for the last 12 days of pregnancy. After the birth, the newborn baby was exposed to cumin, lemon and clean air while his heart rate was measured to assess his responses. The greatest change in heart rate was noted when the baby was presented with cumin. Thus there is some evidence that the sense of smell starts to function before a baby is born.

LEARNING IN THE WOMB

Studies have provided some evidence that learning ability is present at about 22 or 23 weeks. It is thought that the sensory system develops sufficiently in the uterus to allow a developing baby to discriminate between different stimuli, and that the baby's memory is good enough to retain this information.

One study looked at the babies of women who regularly watched a well-known television serial, screened five times a week, during their pregnancies. Researchers found that these babies seemed to recognize the programme's theme tune. This suggests that an unborn baby is able to learn and remember familiar auditory stimuli in the uterus and retain this information over the birth period. Other later studies have confirmed the ability of the unborn baby to learn familiar auditory stimuli *in utero*.

The continuing study of fetal behaviour may in the future make significant contributions to the understanding of the development of mind.

DO BABIES THINK?

There is little doubt that babies' sensory systems are functioning, to a certain extent, while they are still in the uterus. The big question now is whether babies also have powers of perception. In other words, do they attach meaning to what they hear, smell, taste or feel? As yet, there is no way that we can know the answer to this question.

How your body is changing

You will experience both physical and emotional changes in the last three months. The often powerful emotions are nature's way of preparing you for all the changes and challenges ahead. Heightened sensitivity and the ease with which tears often flow are all signs that you are in an emotional state that will make you peculiarly responsive to your newborn baby. In this way nature ensures that you look after your baby, that you respond to cries, that you feed him or her, and that you keep the baby with you and protect him or her from others.

You and your partner may watch, curiously, as your body steadily changes in shape and size. During the third trimester, the changes become much more pronounced.

There are five principal signs that help to indicate that your baby is well and progressing normally towards delivery. These signs are:

The baby's kicks

You will feel a lot of kicking. Many babies are lively at certain times of day, suggesting that they develop a regular pattern of sleep and activity. Babies are often most active when the mother is resting.

Breathlessness

It is common to be out of breath in pregnancy, particularly in the last few weeks. You may feel quite short of breath

Towards the end of your pregnancy, Braxton Hicks contractions can cause discomfort, but they do not last long. Unlike labour contractions, they are irregular and do not increase in intensity. Putting your hands on your belly and breathing deeply may help to relieve them, and they usually stop if you have a bath or lie down.

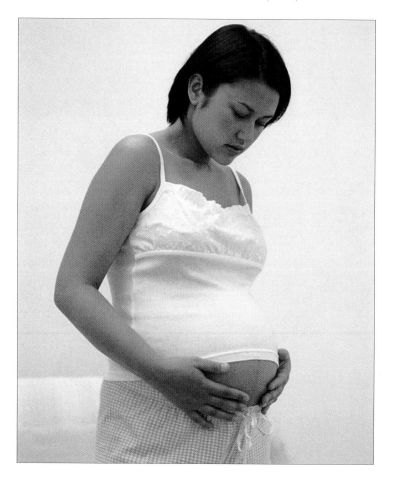

during even relatively minor exertion. This happens for two reasons. Your lungs are working twice as hard as usual in order to supply both you and the baby with oxygen, and the work of the lungs has been made harder because the baby is now so large that he or she is pressing up against your lungs. Rest assured that the baby will receive enough oxygen, even though you may sometimes find yourself panting with the effort.

Increased urine frequency
You will probably want to pass water often, and you may be caught short now and again. This happens partly because the baby is pressing upon all your internal organs, including your bladder, and partly because your muscles have become smoother and softer, in preparation for the birth, when they will be required to stretch to the limit. When you urinate normally, you relax your muscles. When you are pregnant, these muscles tend to relax of their own accord whether you want them to or not. That's what causes the feeling that you need to pass water, and what can cause slight incontinence, too.

Small and irregular contractions
'False labour' contractions can start from week 23, or even earlier, although some women do not experience them at all. They feel like a tightening in the abdominal area. Towards the end of pregnancy, these contractions are known as Braxton Hicks contractions and they become more pronounced, although they are still nothing like the contractions for labour. These 'false labour' contractions last for no more than 20 seconds or so.

When you go into labour, contractions will be more powerful and last for 40 seconds or more. Some specialists maintain that contractions occur throughout pregnancy in order to encourage the blood flow in the placenta, which brings oxygen to the baby.

Engagement
The baby's head becomes engaged in the upper part of the pelvis, usually after the 36th week. All through pregnancy, your uterus expands upwards in your body in order to accommodate the baby's increasing size. The baby is quite low down in your body during the first trimester; after this, he or she rises steadily upwards until week 36. Then, the lower part of the uterus expands, in preparation for the baby's birth, and the baby moves downwards a little.

The baby's head engages in the upper part of the pelvis ready for delivery just a few weeks later. You will experience this as pressure against the cervix (the neck of the uterus). Women who have had babies before may find that their baby's head does not engage so soon, not until the final week of the pregnancy or even as late as the start of labour.

Your increasing size and the frequent activity of the baby mean that you may need extra support to keep you feeling well. Natural therapies can be really helpful in relieving any sleeplessness, stress, tension, fatigue and anxiety that you might be experiencing. They can also help you to feel good about yourself, encouraging you to revel in your swelling size – after all, this is a sure sign that your baby is progressing well.

SUPPORTIVE NATURAL THERAPIES
A weekly session with an experienced therapist may help you cope better with the ups and downs that are often part of pregnancy. Acupuncture, aromatherapy massage and reflexology can all help you to maintain a sense of balance and well-being.

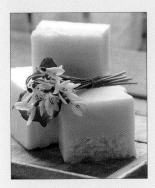

Small feel-good treats – such as soaps scented with essential oils, or gentle herbal home treatments – can lift your mood and relieve tension in the last weeks.

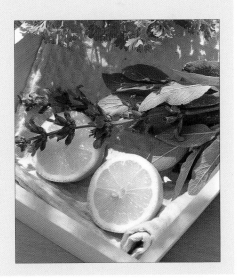

Emotional changes

The last few months of pregnancy are a time of great anticipation and preparation. Both emotionally and mentally, you are readying yourself to become a parent. Physically, your body is gearing up for the birth as well as meeting the needs of your rapidly growing baby. On a practical level, you are likely to feel a strong urge to create a welcoming home for your child.

Not surprisingly, many women find that they become more inward-looking during the third trimester. You may feel absent-minded or forgetful, or rather detached from the world. Work, family and socializing may become less important to you as your focus turns towards the birth.

However keen you are to have your baby, you may experience a real sense of boredom about the pregnancy, particularly in the last weeks. It may feel as though you have been pregnant forever. Now that the birth is near, you may long to get it over with, and start your new life.

> " It is important that you allow yourself to express any recurrent emotions, doubts or anxieties that you have, so that you can deal with them and release the tension they create. "

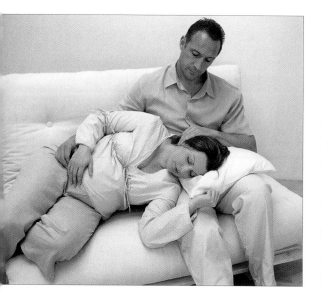

A LIFE TRANSITION

The strong and fluctuating emotions associated with pregnancy may intensify in the final months, although many women find that they start to feel much calmer as the birth approaches.

Some women feel sad about the loss of freedom having a first baby entails, even if the baby is very much wanted. Many women find themselves worrying about something quite minor – such as where they will put the baby clothes or how they will find time to exercise after the delivery. Almost every pregnant woman feels anxious about the pain of labour and worries that she will not achieve the birth she is expecting.

All these feelings are normal and natural. However, it is important that you allow yourself to express any recurrent emotions, doubts or anxieties that you have, so that you can deal with them and release the tension they create.

Talk to your partner so that he can understand what you are going through and offer you support. This may encourage him to share any ambivalent or difficult emotions that he is experiencing. If you are on your own, talk to a close friend or relative. It can also be invaluable to share your experiences with other pregnant women or with mothers. Your midwife is another good source of support and reassurance.

YOUR RELATIONSHIP

Pregnancy is bound to affect your relationship. For many couples, a new closeness and tenderness emerges. Your partner may develop a new protectiveness towards you. At the same time, you may become aware of a new feeling of vulnerability and dependency – something that can feel very strange to you both.

The emotional turbulence of pregnancy can put pressure on the relationship, too. Your partner may miss the companionship you used to share and find it difficult to cope with mood swings; you may have unreasonable expectations of how much others can do for you, or feel disappointed that your partner does not seem as interested in your pregnancy as you are.

As with most aspects of pregnancy, it is helpful to cultivate a sense of acceptance and enjoyment about these changes. Continue to spend time alone together and to talk about your feelings.

Couples often draw closer in the later stages of pregnancy, and men commonly feel a new sense of protectiveness towards their partner.

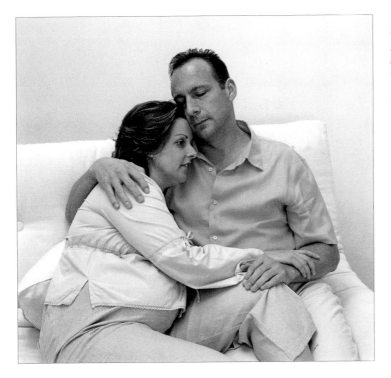

You may feel increasingly disinclined to go out as your pregnancy progresses. Spending quiet evenings at home with your partner can seem far more appealing.

Physical closeness is also important. Massage can be a wonderfully sensuous way of retaining intimacy. Of course, making love will help you to explore any new feelings towards each other. Pregnant women often worry that their partner no longer finds them attractive, particularly in the later stages of pregnancy. However, you may find that your partner enjoys your new curves and voluptuousness. Some couples find that the tenderness pregnancy can evoke – as well as the need to experiment with new positions – brings a new element to their love-making. Other couples find it hard to contemplate the idea of having sex late in pregnancy.

There are no rights and wrongs here – and it is best to do what you feel most comfortable with. But if you both want to make love, sex can usually continue until the waters have broken, as long as the pregnancy is progressing normally. Check with your midwife or doctor if you are not sure.

THE FATHER-TO-BE

The third trimester can be an exciting time for fathers. The baby is becoming more and more visible and active, and may respond at the sound of the father's voice.

However, late pregnancy also has its challenges. Inevitably the attention is on the pregnant women and some men can feel rather isolated and redundant. This is a false impression: the woman needs their support and love more than anyone else's.

New fathers do have a lot to contend with – and this is something that is rarely recognized. If they are to be the main breadwinners for a while, they may well worry about how they will cope with the extra burden. In addition, men often grow nervous about how the baby will affect their lives. They might find themselves wondering if they will ever again be able to go out for a quiet drink once the baby has arrived.

Becoming a parent is a huge event and it is natural for fathers to have anxieties. Expressing these fears will make them seem more manageable, and will help fathers to support their partners.

As well as talking to their partners, father could try seeking out other fathers. It can really help to talk to someone who has been in the same situation. Another man is likely to have a similar perspective and may have dealt with the same feelings.

COUNSELLING
You may want to consider seeking help from a counsellor if your emotions become overwhelming and you feel that you cannot cope alone.

Rest, rest and more rest

You are bound to feel tired during pregnancy. The extra weight you are carrying – which can be as much as 13.5kg (about 2¼ stone) – means not only that fatigue sets in more quickly, but also that your muscles have to put more effort into making even small movements. Your body is also working harder than usual – your heart, for example, is pumping 25 per cent more blood around your system in order to meet the baby's needs.

Despite the fact that you need a lot of rest, you are likely to suffer from disturbed sleep. Your size can make it hard to find a comfortable sleeping position, while increased urination means you are likely to be getting up several times during the night.

It is important that you respond to your body's needs and relax as much as possible during the day. Relaxation helps you to maintain good health, and makes you better able to cope with mood swings. Your baby needs you to relax, too. When the muscles around your uterus are at rest, more blood and oxygen gets through to the baby – which helps him or her to grow.

BOOSTING YOUR RELAXATION QUOTA

If you are suffering from insomnia, herbal teas, gentle homeopathic remedies or aromatherapy oils can help. However, even if you are sleeping well at night, you still need to rest during the day. Doing the following may help.

- Have a nap whenever you are feeling tired. Don't be embarrassed if you need a short sleep if you are visiting friends or relatives. Most people understand that pregnant women need extra care and will be happy to accommodate you.
- Make sure that you have a sleep each afternoon. Be aware of when your energy dips – often between 2pm and 4pm – and set this time aside for a rest.

- Go to bed early. Cutting out television and late-night telephone calls can help you to prepare for sleep.
- Get up late at the weekend or any other day that you can. If you have had a restless night, eat breakfast in bed and try to doze afterwards.
- Make a point of getting out into the fresh air every day. Breathe deeply as you walk to increase the supply of oxygen around your body.
- Put your feet up whenever you can. Always sit rather than stand up.
- At regular points during the day, stop whatever you are doing and check how you are standing or sitting. Notice any awkwardness in your posture and move if necessary to adopt a more comfortable position. In particular, drop your shoulders down and slightly back, and relax any tension in your face by smiling a little. Take a few deep breaths.
- Don't push yourself in any activity, whether it is socializing, exercising or housework. Respect your body's limitations and be prepared to leave jobs unfinished if you need to.

QUICK RELAXER

A short relaxation or breathing exercise can be as energizing as a nap. This quick abdominal breathing exercise can be done anywhere – including on public transport or at work.

Rest your hands on your abdomen and breathe deeply, allowing your abdomen to rise on the in-breath and fall on the out-breath. Focus on your hands rising and falling to help you to concentrate. Continue for about ten breaths.

It can be hard to find a comfortable sleeping position when you are pregnant. Avoid lying on your back as this can put pressure on the spine, and can also impede the supply of blood to the baby. Try lying on your side, with your bump supported with pillows.

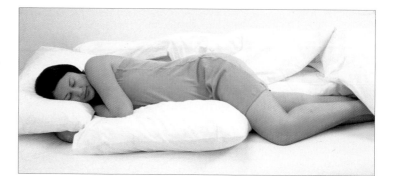

WORK AND REST

How long you continue to work obviously depends on financial considerations as well as on how you are feeling. Many women work during the last months of pregnancy, which can make it difficult for them to get enough rest. Finding a place to nap in your lunch hour, working at home sometimes, or changing your hours to avoid rush-hour traffic can all help.

Consider taking occasional days off sick: don't struggle into work if you are feeling poorly. Talk to your doctor if you do work that involves standing up for long periods, bending down or carrying things, or if you do shift work, which can disrupt your sleep patterns; you may need to change the way that you work.

All other things being equal, you should give up work as soon as it becomes too difficult to manage both your work and your pregnancy – your baby is more important than your job, after all. Ideally, you should stop working four to six weeks before your due date at the latest. This gives you time to prepare for birth and, who knows, the baby might come early.

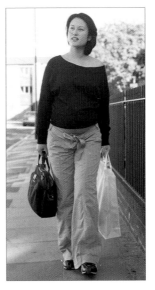

Adopt a sense of moderation and balance in all that you do. For example, if you have to carry shopping and work files, spread the load between two bags.

Deep relaxation exercise

The starting point of this exercise is to tense the muscles in your body one by one. As you relax them, the psychological tension will dissipate and flow out of you, like water down a drain. You can do this in bed at night or whenever you feel you need to relax.

1 Lie down in a comfortable position (on your side or propped up against a pile of cushions). Breathe deeply a few times, letting your body sink downwards. Try to release any obvious tension from your body – in particular, drop your shoulders.

2 Squeeze your toes so that they are pointing inwards. Hold the tension for a few seconds, then release it. Press your heels downwards until you feel the stretch working the muscles in your calves. Hold, then release. Clench your thigh muscles, hold, then relax. Do the same with your buttock muscles.

3 Bring your focus to your abdomen. Take a few deep breaths, letting your abdomen sink downwards as you do so. Your middle area should feel heavy and warm.

4 Move on to your upper body. Draw your shoulders back and, breathing deeply, feel your ribcage expand. Release the tension as you breathe out. Make fists, then let go, and repeat. Hunch your shoulders, hold tight, release, then repeat until your shoulders feel relaxed. Pull your chin down towards your chest, hold, and then release.

5 Now work on your face. Purse your lips, hold, and relax. Grin, hold, and relax. Make a deep frown, hold, and relax.

6 Your body should be feeling soft and heavy. In this state, continue to breathe deeply and regularly for 10 or 15 minutes. If you like, you can practise some visualization at this point – imagine you are lying on the grass under a warm sun as you breathe.

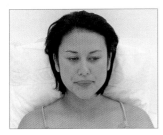

Purse your lips for a few moments.

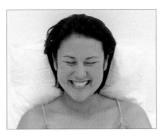

Grin like a Cheshire cat.

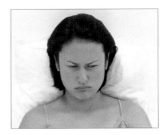

Make a deep frown, then relax.

Feel-good treats and therapies

Many women revel in the changes that late pregnancy brings, enjoying their new voluptuousness. However, others dislike becoming so much larger and heavier, particularly if their weight has been an issue before conceiving.

Pregnancy can certainly be a challenge to your self-image, and many women find it hard to cope with stretch marks, varicose veins and other visible ailments. However, it is important to develop a sense of acceptance and appreciation of your body in these last months. This will not only help you to enjoy pregnancy, but it will enhance your general feeling of well-being.

Touch is one of the best ways to maintain a sense of connection with your physical self. Try regular self-massage or enjoy massage with your partner. Gentle exercise, particularly walking, swimming and yoga will help you to feel good. Above all – treat yourself. Incorporating indulgent moments into every day and looking after yourself physically will help you to embrace your growing body. This, in turn, will help you to enjoy the journey towards motherhood.

LOOK GOOD, FEEL GOOD

Making an effort to look good can often improve the way you feel. Try these quick fixes.
- Get your hair cut. Having a good haircut is one of the quickest ways to make yourself feel attractive. This is probably not the time to go for a radical style – choose something that you know suits you.
- Have a manicure. Even if you don't usually worry about how your hands look, late pregnancy can be a great time to spoil yourself.
- Buy something new to wear. By now, you are probably heartily sick of all the maternity clothes you

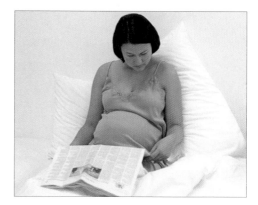

Late pregnancy is one time when you can enjoy being lazy without feeling guilty – after all, your baby needs you to rest. Go to bed for the afternoon with a glossy magazine or paper, and indulge yourself.

have bought so far. Women often feel guilty about spending money on clothes they are going to wear for only a few months, with the result that they make do with two or three outfits throughout their pregnancy. However, one new outfit can lift your self-esteem and help you to feel happy about the way you look.
- Wear clothes in natural fabrics, which are softer and more comfortable than manmade materials. Colour therapists often recommend green or blue as good colours to wear during pregnancy because they have a calming effect. Yellow can also be a good choice since it can lift the spirits. But, most importantly, choose clothes in a colour that you feel good in.

PAMPER YOURSELF

Late pregnancy is a good time to indulge yourself. Set some time aside to do things that you really enjoy – such as meeting a friend for a long catching-up session, reading a novel, going for a walk in the park, or one of the following:
- Buy yourself a large bunch of flowers and put them somewhere you will see them often.
- Book a meal in a favourite restaurant for you and your partner. Enjoy spending a romantic evening together as a couple. Book the table for the earlier part of the evening so that you can still get a good night's rest.

Enjoy small extravagances, such as buying yourself a bouquet of beautiful fresh flowers.

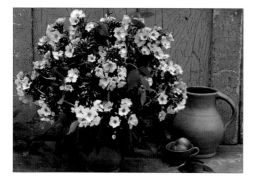

- Spend an afternoon or a whole day in bed. Forget about chores, preparing for the baby or working. Enjoy getting up late, reading the papers or a book or just dozing for a day.
- Go to the cinema, theatre, opera or ballet. It will be much more difficult to organize nights out once the baby is born, so make the most of these last weeks. Go to an afternoon or an early-evening show if you usually feel tired later in the evening.

NATURAL THERAPIES

A treatment with a qualified complementary therapist can boost your energy and help to relieve some of the discomforts of late pregnancy. The following can also be deeply pleasurable to receive:

- **Reflexology** Few things are more relaxing than a foot treatment. Find a professional reflexologist who specializes in treating pregnant women – some points can stimulate contractions of the uterus.
- **Reiki** You can receive reiki sitting up and fully clothed. It is gentle, soothing and non-invasive. The practitioner places his or her hands on or just above different areas of your body. You may feel a warm or tingling sensation as healing energy flows through the practitioner's hands to wherever it is needed.
- **Shiatsu** This Japanese massage is given on the floor, and you remain clothed. It can be deeply relaxing,

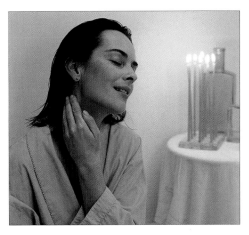

Take the time to look after yourself in the evening: have a warm bath, wrap yourself in a robe and apply a mask or deep moisturizer to your face.

and acupressure points may be used to relieve common symptoms such as fatigue. See a practitioner who is experienced with pregnancy. Tell them if you have any varicose veins, as direct pressure should not be applied to them. Abdominal work and heavy pressure on the legs should also be avoided.

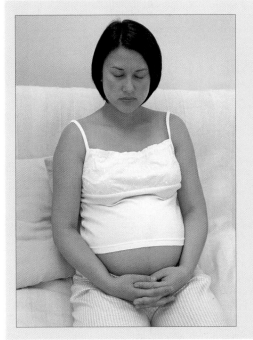

POSITIVE THINKING

If you are finding it hard to embrace the physical changes of pregnancy, try doing this exercise for five or ten minutes. It will work best if you do it daily.

Sit in a comfortable position, ideally with your back straight. If you have back problems or are feeling tired, prop yourself up against a pile of cushions. Take a few deep breaths, allowing your body to release any tension.

Silently focus on an affirmative phrase about the physical changes you are experiencing. Your affirmation should be a short, positive phrase in the present tense. Make up your own or try one of the following:

I am growing more and more beautiful every day. I welcome and embrace the changes in my body.

Continue to breathe deeply as you repeat the affirmation over and over. Don't worry if you don't feel what you are saying is true – just keep on silently repeating yourself. Eventually, the message will sink in.

When you are ready to finish, bring your attention back to your breathing. Now, slowly open your eyes. Remain sitting quietly for a minute before you get up.

Positive affirmations can shift negative feelings about yourself and help you to enjoy your pregnancy more.

Perineal and breast massage

Massage of the perineum and breasts is both pleasant and beneficial during the last trimester. Regular massage of the perineum, the area between the vagina and rectum, may help to reduce the chance of tearing during the birth. Massaging your breasts will help to prepare them for breastfeeding. You need not use oil to massage these areas, although you may well find it easier to do so. Use pure, plain oils such as wheatgerm, olive or almond oils, avoiding any that are contraindicated during pregnancy. If you want to use any oils not mentioned below, then consult an aromatherapist first.

PERINEAL MASSAGE

The perineum has to be strong to support the contents of the abdomen, especially as your baby grows heavier. At the same time, however, the perineum will also have to yield and stretch in order to let your baby pass down the birth canal. Nature provides for this change in texture by releasing 'loosening' hormones that soften the ligaments. You can also help to improve elasticity in this area by self-massage. Massaging gently can greatly increase the comfort and ease with which you give birth, and possibly prevent a tear or the need for a surgical cut (episiotomy).

It is truly amazing just how quickly the normally tight tissues in the perineum and vagina will stretch with regular massage. The more that you are able to pre-stretch these tissues before the birth, the better you will return to your original shape after it.

During the last weeks of pregnancy (starting around 36 weeks), massage the perineal area once a day for around five or ten minutes, always doing so with great care and sensitivity. Ideally, perform the massage after soaking in a warm (not hot) bath, to soften the area, and when your bladder is empty. If using oil, wheatgerm is a good choice, and aromatherapists recommend adding a few drops of lavender to the oil.

HOW TO MASSAGE THE PERINEUM

When you start practising perineal massage, use two fingers, oiled if you wish. Insert the two fingers into your vagina up to the first knuckle, progressing to the second

For massage of the perineal and vaginal areas, make sure you are in a relaxed and comfortable position. Lying on your side against a bed or beanbag is a good position, as is squatting or half-kneeling with one leg up.

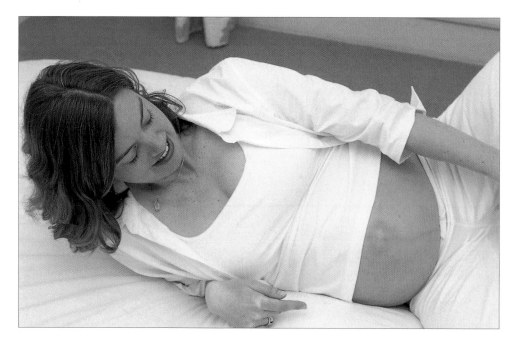

knuckle with practice. You may like to use three or four fingers, and apply a little more pressure, once you are used to the technique. Now use a light touch to explore the layers of tissues along the back wall of your vagina and the skin that separates your vagina and anus. It is this area that will be most stretched during the birth of your baby and is most prone to tearing.

As you press against the back wall of the vagina, against the spine, breathe deeply. You will experience a tingling sensation and will feel the muscles under your fingers as they engage on the breath out. As space is gradually created, move in further and exert a little more pressure, using your breath to help you, but you should never take this kind of massage any further than feels totally comfortable.

You will probably find that nothing much seems to happen at first, but soon your perineal tissue starts to give and then begins to stretch. You will be amazed how much you can stretch it, simply by breathing out into the areas under your fingers.

MASSAGING THE BREASTS

Up to around 36 weeks, regular massage of the breasts is a wonderful way of bringing a combination of tone, strength and elasticity to the tissues here, in readiness for breastfeeding. Remember to avoid the nipple area. If you decide to use oil then almond oil is a good choice. Calendula cream is also gentle and safe. Like perineal massage, breast massage is best done after a warm and relaxing bath.

To massage the breasts, use your entire hand, with your fingers kept together. With each stroke, start with the heel of your hand and take the stroke through your fingers. Keep the pressure even and smooth; do not jab or press harshly.

In order to understand the technique, you need to imagine the ducts that carry breast milk rather like the spokes of a wheel, radiating out from the central spoke – your nipple. The milk travels down these ducts to the

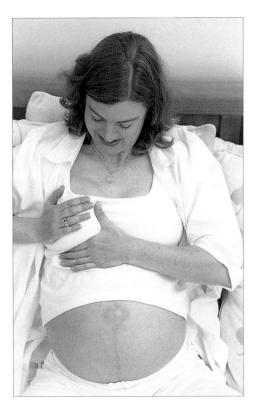

When massaging the breasts, either massage through clothes or directly on to the skin. As well as massage, you may find that exposing your breasts to the elements from time to time will feel especially pleasant.

nipple, and your massage should also work from the outside of the breast towards the nipple. Do this slowly around the whole of each breast, working in a clockwise direction. Many pregnancy books compare the breast to a clockface, and recommend starting at 1 o'clock, working from the outside in to the nipple, then repeating this at 2 o'clock and so on.

MASSAGING OTHER AREAS

While you are in a relaxed mood, with suitable oils at the ready, it is a good idea to extend your massage to other areas of the body. A facial massage is always enjoyable (see page 129) and you could also try gentle massage of the abdomen, in order to help prevent stretch marks. During the latter weeks of pregnancy, massage down the sides of your belly. Work from the ribs to your navel, with both hands and using circular strokes, and continue down over your hips and thighs. Using plenty of oil feels especially pleasant when massaging the abdomen.

SAFETY POINTS

Take great care with perineal or vaginal massage, and never deliberately stretch out or pull these very delicate tissues.

Do not perform breast massage after about 36 weeks. When massaging the breasts, always proceed gently and avoid massaging the nipples themselves. However, a very gentle tweaking of the nipples can be appropriate once your due date has arrived. This tweaking is said to stimulate production of the hormone oxytocin and so may help to bring on labour.

Yoga for the third trimester

You will find that your baby is sensitive to your moods, shares your enjoyment and joins in with many of your activities. So the more that you dance around and stretch, and open and tone your body, the better he or she will like it. Your centre of gravity lies deep within your pelvis. The opening up of your hips and pelvic area, plus all the activity, will encourage your baby to find the very best position to be in as birth approaches. Putting aside time each day for a few minutes of energetic yoga dance, followed by a perineal stretch, is a great way to prepare for labour with your baby and it will also help release tension. Don't forget that all these rotating, twisting and opening movements of the hips should be done with knees bent. Keep breathing deeply all the time.

Knee circles

This is a balancing exercise that shakes out your hips and legs as you get into a knee-swinging stride. It is a loosening and strengthening movement, which helps to boost the circulation and is also good for lifting your mood. If you feel wary about trusting your balance, try placing one hand against a wall for support. Keep your arms, shoulders and neck relaxed. The raised leg is also kept as loose as possible throughout, and the knee circles should be done smoothly and lightly. Before you start, stand erect and breathe deeply for a few moments.

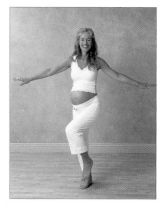

1 Raise your left leg, bending the knee. Stand on your right leg, with your arms spread out to the sides to help your balance, and your spine erect. Now swing your left knee up in front of you as high as is comfortable.

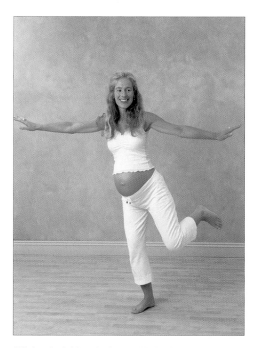

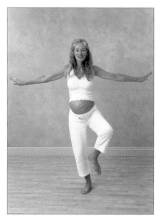

2 Bring your left knee to the side to open your left hip and so make more room in the abdomen and pelvis.

3 Swing the left leg slowly round behind you and kick back with your left foot. Finally, swing your knee forward, then straighten your left leg and place your left foot firmly on the floor. Repeat the exercise with the right knee.

Pushing the sky

In this empowering pose, you are pushing your palms up into the sky. The aim is to lift and strengthen your upper body, and to make space in your lower body as you flex your thigh muscles. Use your diaphragm and breathe deeply, so that you involve all your abdominal muscles in the action.

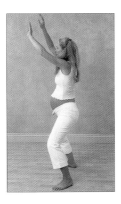

1 Stand with feet wide and toes pointing outwards so that you can bend your knees deeply and hold this position comfortably. Keeping the spine erect and coccyx tucked in, raise your arms. Push up further with first one palm and then the other. Turn your palm upwards if you can. Feel a lengthening stretch up through each side of your body in turn.

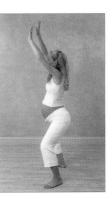

2 Keep your arms raised directly over your head. Push both hands upwards while bending the knees further and dropping into a semi-squat. Do this on an outbreath, feeling a lengthening stretch through your middle as you do so.

Standing twist

This is a good position for easing tension in the neck and shoulders, and it also acts as a counter-pose to the strong sideways stretch of the Knee circles. Breathe deeply and twist through the whole torso.

Seated perineal stretch

A low stool and several cushions are useful props for this gentle perineal stretch, which is good preparation for the birth. Place one cushion on the stool and the others under your dropped knee as required in Step 2. The breath is very important when you are stretching the yogic way – otherwise nothing happens, or you simply stretch a little in the groin area. Remember to move gently and slowly.

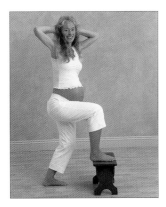

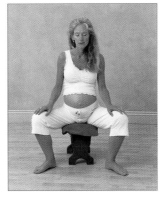

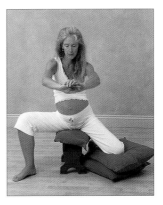

Place your right foot on a low stool, thigh parallel to the floor. Raise your arms and open the elbows to expand the chest. Place your palms behind your head, neck erect. Breathe in. As you breathe out, turn the head and shoulders to the right. Let your chest follow, but keep your lower body steady. Come back to the centre, change legs and repeat on the left.

1 Place a cushion on a low stool and sit astride it, with your knees wide and feet firmly planted on the floor. Stretch up through your spine by pressing the palms of your hands against your spread thighs. Breathe normally but evenly as you do this.

2 Press into your right foot and drop the left knee back and down on to two firm cushions. This is a good stretch for the perineum and the left groin. Clasp your hands. Inhale as you push the palms away, pressing further into your right foot. Push out further as you exhale and lift through the spine as you inhale. Do this several times. Change legs and repeat.

Hip-openers in water

Here are some good yoga exercises to do in the swimming pool. The buoyant water supports your weight, making it much easier to stretch and move around. In these exercises one leg is raised to rotate and open the hip, involving all the lower back muscles on that side as well as the pelvic muscles. They both prevent and relieve lower backache, particularly sciatica or inflammation. Start with the small knee circles, then proceed to the wider hip circles. Do them very slowly, with your leg moving as much water as possible.

Knee circles

For this exercise, face the wall and hold on to the bar or edge of the pool, or face the pool and rest your arms on a woggle (long float) in front of you. The same exercise can be done facing the pool and supporting yourself on the bar or edge from behind, or on a woggle under your arms and behind your back. While facing the wall, the main stretch is in the lower back; facing the pool a greater emphasis is placed on opening the pelvis.

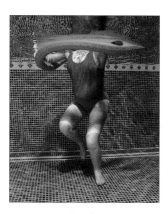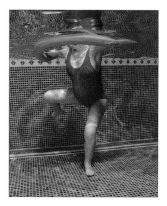

1 Start in a standing position. Bend the knee of your standing leg slightly. Lift your other leg up from the pool floor, bending your knee as you do so. Keep your upper body relaxed.

2 Move your knee to make small smooth circles in the water. Keep your whole body relaxed and feel the resistance of the water. Change legs and repeat the exercise.

Hip circles

Start in a standing position, facing the wall and holding on to the bar or the edge of the pool, or resting your arms on a woggle in front of you. Keep your standing leg a little more bent than for the knee circles, to allow for a wider opening of your other leg as you engage your hip in the rotating movement.

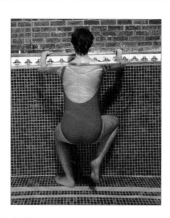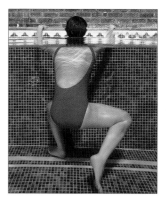

1 Lift one leg, bending the knee. Slowly circle the hip and knee, feeling the resistance of the water as you do so. Make small circles at first.

2 Gradually increase the size of the circles by pushing your raised knee back. Exhale each time you open out the knee. Repeat on the other side.

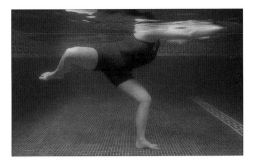

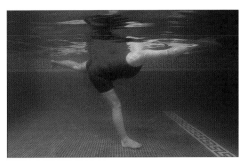

3 Move away from the side of the pool. Make larger circles, stretching the leg out to the side, then bending it again to come back to the centre. Do this a few times. Breathe deeply, using your abdominal muscles.

4 Now extend your raised leg back behind you before bringing it back. As you become fitter, extend your leg higher towards the surface of the water, straightening your standing leg.

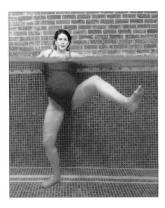

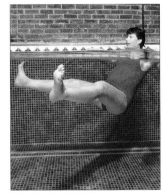

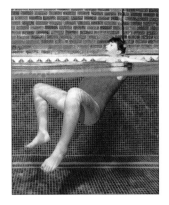

5 Move so your back is facing the side of the pool or place a woggle under your arms for support. Make circles with your leg, opening the hips wide on each side while keeping your back straight.

6 Supporting your extended arms on the bar, pool edge or a woggle, work both your hips at the same time, using a wide backstroke movement with your legs.

7 Now stretch the legs out in front of you, inhaling as you do so. Bend the legs in as you exhale. Keep the upper part of your body as relaxed as possible.

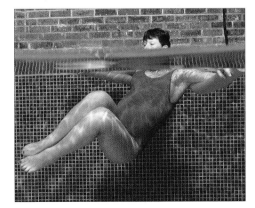

8 Complete the routine by bringing both legs together and making a rotating movement. Do small circles at first, then gradually increase the size of the circle, breathing deeply all the time. With practice, your circling will start to become smoother and more regular.

Antenatal care

The three cornerstones of antenatal care at this stage of your pregnancy are: attending antenatal checks; going to antenatal classes; and looking after your general health.

ANTENATAL CHECKS
Most women attend their antenatal clinic every month until about the 28th week, fortnightly until about week 36 and then weekly until the birth. During your antenatal visits, the following routine checks will be carried out:
- Weight.
- Blood pressure, to detect pre-eclampsia.
- Urine, to detect signs of pre-eclampsia and diabetes.
- The baby's heartbeat.
- The size of your abdomen, in order to monitor the baby's continuing growth.
- Your hands and legs for any sign of swelling, which could indicate pre-eclampsia.

Your blood pressure
Pregnancy brings about enormous changes in blood volume and pressure, partly because your heart is beating much faster and more frequently than usual and partly because of hormonal changes in the blood vessels. Your blood pressure will usually return to normal within a few days of the birth.

High blood pressure early in pregnancy can indicate a number of conditions, including kidney disease and diabetes. In later pregnancy, raised blood pressure alone does not usually signify problems, but high blood pressure combined with swelling of the ankles or feet, pronounced weight gain and the appearance of protein in the urine are signs of pre-eclampsia, which develops in about one in every 20 pregnancies.

What is pre-eclampsia?
Pre-eclampsia is not yet fully understood, but it is believed to be due to abnormalities of hormone secretion, kidney secretion, or the production of abnormal substances by the placenta. Mild pre-eclampsia is usually simple to treat: rest may be all that is needed. Left untreated, it can progress to eclampsia, which is a dangerous complication of pregnancy.

An eclamptic fit dramatically reduces the oxygen supply to the unborn baby, and can also be life-threatening to the mother. If a fit occurs, the baby will be delivered immediately either by induction or by emergency Caesarean. You may not notice any symptoms if you have pre-eclampsia, which is one reason why

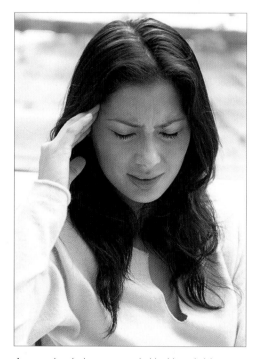

A severe headache accompanied by blurred vision or flashing lights could be a sign of pre-eclampsia.

antenatal checks are so vital. The symptoms of this condition can include:
- Severe headache.
- Visual disturbances such as flashing lights or blurring.
- Vomiting.
- Severe pain in the upper abdomen.
- Feet, ankles or hands swelling up suddenly.

Seek immediate medical advice if you develop any of the symptoms listed above during your pregnancy; you must call an ambulance if any of them are severe.

> ❝ If you or your partner are in any doubt about an aspect of your health, your baby's health or your antenatal health care, seek professional advice. ❞

The 32-week scan

You will probably have had a scan around week 20 of your pregnancy. If you are receiving specialist antenatal care because of an identified risk factor in your pregnancy, you may have another scan at about 32 weeks. This allows the accurate measurement of the baby's head and abdomen. The information obtained from the scan at this stage of development is more precise than that obtained from a physical examination.

LOOKING AFTER YOUR HEALTH

During the third trimester, you should still be eating healthily every day, taking some exercise and avoiding smoky atmospheres and alcohol. It is especially important at this stage that you make every effort to keep stress at bay and make sure that you get plenty of relaxation, rest and sleep each day. This will stand you in good stead not only for the birth itself, but also for dealing with your newborn baby once he or she arrives.

If you or your partner are in any doubt about an aspect of your health, your baby's health or your antenatal health care, never hesitate to seek professional advice. The family doctor, your midwife, your hospital, and your antenatal class teacher are there to answer any questions that you may have.

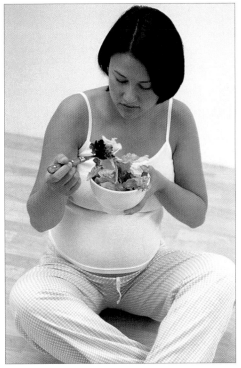

Look after yourself and your baby by continuing with a healthy lifestyle – the food you eat and the amount of exercise and relaxation you get are all important.

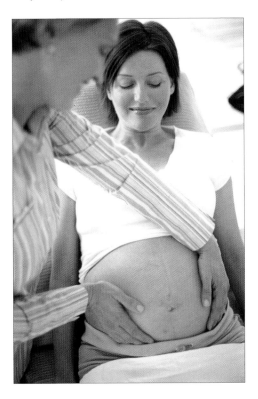

WHEN THE BABY COMES EARLY

A pre-term baby is one that arrives or has to be delivered for medical reasons up to three weeks before the estimated date of delivery. A premature baby is one that has arrived more than three weeks early. He or she has an increased chance of respiratory problems in the first few days, and may need special care. Drugs can be given to activate the baby's lungs artificially to speed them towards maturity. These work only if administered early in the third trimester (about weeks 29–33), and are given only if doctors are about to deliver the baby. Once the baby is born, he or she can be put on a ventilator to assist with breathing. The baby also needs to be kept very warm while he or she builds up the fat reserves that would normally have built up by delivery.

During each antenatal visit, the midwife will feel your abdomen to check the increase in the size of your uterus, and therefore the growth of your baby.

Antenatal classes

The various kinds of antenatal classes are quite distinct from antenatal care, which you receive in an antenatal clinic. While the clinics concentrate mainly on your health and that of your baby, antenatal classes cover the practical and emotional aspects of pregnancy and labour. Classes usually cover a wide range of topics, from sex during pregnancy to pain relief at the birth.

Many women find antenatal classes helpful. You are not only given valuable information, but the classes also provide an opportunity for you to ask any questions that you may have and to swap experiences with other women at the same stage of pregnancy as you. Women often forge friendships at antenatal classes that continue long after the birth of their babies. These can be a good source of support during the first months of motherhood.

Antenatal classes are known by various names: for example, parentcraft, childbirth education classes or preparation for parenthood. Active birth classes – which encourage the use of yoga – may also be available. Classes are run by different organizations, such as the health authority, charities and independent teachers. Your doctor or midwife will tell you about the different classes on offer, and you can choose a system that suits you.

The classes usually run weekly for five to six weeks, perhaps eight weeks, and you attend them during the last couple of months of pregnancy. Most classes actively encourage male partners to come along, and offer specific advice for them. However, you can also go on your own or take a friend or relative along with you.

Antenatal classes help you understand exactly what happens during pregnancy and childbirth. Here a teacher uses models of a baby and a pelvis to demonstrate the breech (feet or buttocks first) position.

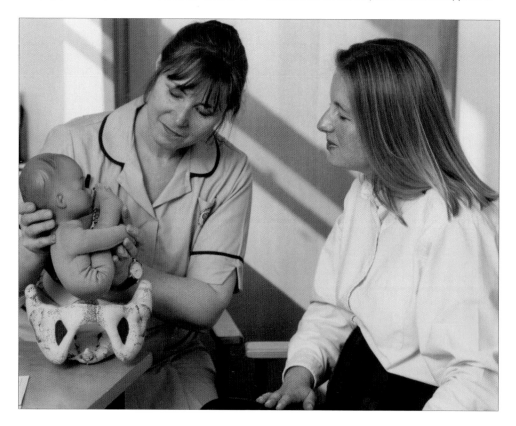

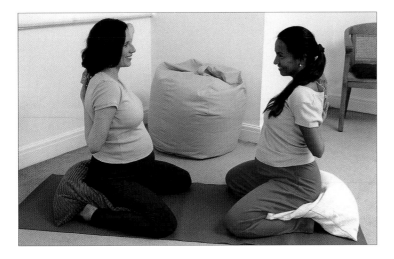

You will learn simple exercises to relieve backache and to prepare your body for the birth. You can then practise these regularly at home with a friend.

WHAT ANTENATAL CLASSES COVER

Antenatal classes will always include an opportunity for you and your partner to ask any questions that you may have. The classes will usually also cover set topics each week, which will include all or most of the following:

Pregnancy

- Diet, health and fitness in pregnancy.
- Caring for your teeth and gums.
- Bathing in pregnancy.
- Posture and back problems.
- Maternity clothing.
- Relationships and sex during pregnancy.
- Talks for partners covering pregnancy, the birth and fatherhood.
- How the baby grows – the developmental milestones of the unborn baby.
- Coping with common discomforts such as piles, constipation and back pain.
- Exercises, including pelvic floor exercises, to help you prepare for the birth and to prevent problems such as stress incontinence.

The birth

- Breathing exercises for labour. In antenatal classes, you are taught how to change your breathing deliberately during labour, adjusting to the changing characteristics of the contractions. This can help you to manage your labour and cope better with the pain. Synchronizing the breathing with the signals that are received from the uterus demands total concentration and it is important to practise the techniques regularly beforehand.

Many classes will include special advice for your partner or a friend, who will then be able to assist you and provide support in labour.

- A visit to the maternity ward and labour ward. This will help you to understand the technology of birth: medical terms will be explained and you'll have an opportunity to see some of the equipment. You'll also get a chance to see what options are available in your particular unit (for example, water births), and to become familiar with the wards and labour suite.
- What you will need for a home birth.
- How to recognize the signs of labour.
- What happens during labour.
- Options for pain relief during labour.
- Breech births.
- Medical intervention, such as induction, Caesarean section and assisted deliveries.

After the birth

- Breast and bottle-feeding.
- Caring for the nipples when breastfeeding; coping with other associated problems, such as mastitis.
- What you will need after the birth for yourself – maternity bras and other clothing.
- What you will need for the baby – equipment and clothing.
- Basic baby-care skills – including how to change a nappy and how to bath a baby.
- How to recognize postnatal depression.
- Advice on contraception after delivery, because you can become pregnant quite quickly after the arrival of your baby. It is best to delay conceiving again for at least nine months after the birth.

Checklist of common problems

Your baby almost doubles in size during the third trimester, and your body has to stretch and grow to accommodate it. Not surprisingly, most women feel heavy and uncomfortable during this stage of pregnancy.

It can be difficult to find a comfortable sleeping position, so you may feel very tired. You may also suffer from breathlessness, since the expanding uterus presses up against the lungs, or from circulation problems, such as swollen ankles.

Make sure that you get plenty of rest during the day, especially if you are sleeping badly at night, and put your feet up regularly. If you are suffering from other minor ailments, complementary therapies can often help to relieve them. However, always check the relevant safety advice in Section Four, and talk to your midwife or doctor before using any remedy.

You should report any symptoms you are experiencing to your midwife during your antenatal visits. See your doctor beforehand if symptoms are severe, persistent or concern you in any way.

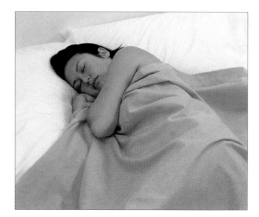

Sleep is an excellent restorative. Make sure you get as much as possible in these last weeks of pregnancy. You need to be well rested for the labour.

Cramp Leg cramps often occur in late pregnancy. They may be caused by deficiencies of calcium and magnesium, so try eating more dairy products, sardines and green leafy vegetables (for calcium) and plenty of nuts and seeds (for magnesium). Vitamin B2, which is found in yogurt, lean meat and fortified breakfast cereals, may help. You should make sure that you drink plenty of water and take regular exercise. If you do get cramp, rub your calf briskly. Try flexing your foot at the same time so that the toes point upwards.

Stress incontinence Leaking urine can be an embarrassing problem, but it is one that many pregnant women experience. It is usually caused by weakness of the pelvic floor, which supports the neck of the bladder. To prevent stress incontinence, practise pelvic floor exercises several times a day: tighten the ring of muscles around your vagina and anus, as though you were stopping yourself from urinating mid-flow. Hold for a count of five, then release. Repeat five times or more.

You are most likely to leak urine when you are lifting, laughing, coughing or sneezing, so pull up the pelvic floor whenever you are about to do so. Regular exercise and yoga can also help to strengthen the pelvic floor.

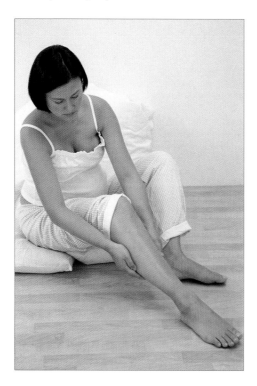

If you get cramp in the calf, rub briskly, then massage using a squeezing action. Make sure you get some gentle exercise – such as a half-hour walk – each day.

Backache Almost all pregnant women suffer from backache in the third trimester, and often earlier, too. The growing weight of the baby in your uterus alters your centre of gravity, and you may sit or stand awkwardly to compensate. An Alexander technique teacher can help you to adjust your posture, and chiropractic and osteopathy can also be very beneficial. Regularly practising yoga and Pilates often helps; ask your teacher to recommend specific exercises to do at home. A gentle massage should help to relieve discomfort. Chiropractic and osteopathy are also useful.

Pubic joint pain The pubic joint (symphysis pubis) softens in preparation for childbirth, which places strain on the spine and pelvis. This can cause pain in the pubic area, and sometimes in the lower back and groin as well. Tell your doctor if you are affected; he or she may refer you to a physiotherapist to be fitted with a support belt. Otherwise regular chiropractic or osteopathy sessions can be very helpful. Other therapies that may be useful include acupuncture, reiki, reflexology and the Alexander technique.

Shortness of breath As your uterus expands, it presses against your lungs, which can cause breathlessness or exacerbate respiratory problems such as asthma. Practising abdominal breathing will help to improve your breath control, as will yoga, Pilates and the Alexander technique. If the problem gets worse when you lie down, use pillows to prop yourself up. If you suffer from asthma, try eating more oily fish; fish oils seem to protect against attacks. Homeopathy, aromatherapy, acupuncture, reflexology and reiki may help with both asthma and shortness of breath.

Indigestion and heartburn These problems can get worse in the third trimester, when the growing uterus presses on the stomach. Eating little, often and slowly is the simplest way to prevent them, and you should avoid eating spicy foods. Sipping a cup of lemonbalm or meadowsweet tea after meals may help. If you suffer from heartburn, make sure that you do not bend or lie down for at least an hour after eating.

Itchy skin Hormonal changes during pregnancy can lead to skin problems, particularly during the third trimester. If you have dry, itchy skin, try eating more oily fish, nuts and seeds. Moisturizing your skin with an evening primrose lotion can help, or you may like to use essential oil of lavender or chamomile well-diluted in a carrier cream or base oil. Herbal medicine or homeopathy may also be useful – a homeopath may prescribe sulphur or kali arsenicum. See your doctor if the itching becomes severe.

Water retention Pregnant women often experience mild swelling (oedema) of the ankles, especially during the third trimester. If you have swollen ankles, rest with your feet up for at least 15 minutes twice a day. Regular leg massage – working up the leg – and drinking dandelion tea can be useful. You may also find acupuncture helpful. If you have severe swelling and a headache, see your doctor at once.

High blood pressure Your blood pressure will be checked at every antenatal visit; high blood pressure accompanied by fluid retention and protein in the urine indicates pre-eclampsia. This condition can affect your pregnancy so it is important that you follow any advice given by your doctor. You can help to maintain a healthy blood pressure by taking regular exercise and eating a nutritious diet that includes oily fish and plenty of raw fruits and vegetables; you should also follow a low-salt diet. Reducing stress and practising relaxation techniques, meditation, yoga or t'ai chi is often helpful. You may also like to try herbal medicine, aromatherapy, colour therapy, reiki or reflexology.

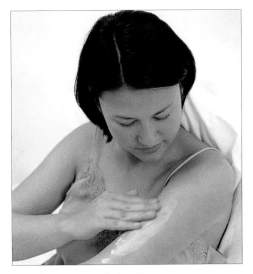

For immediate relief of itchy skin, use a cream containing evening primrose oil. Increasing the amount of oily fish that you eat should also help.

WHEN TO CALL A DOCTOR
If you experience sudden or severe symptoms, you should contact your doctor or the emergency services without delay. See page 145 for a list of danger signs in pregnancy.

Common Qs and As

Q: If I have a row with my partner or my mother, will my baby be affected or harmed by that? Will he or she know?

A: Your baby certainly won't 'know' that you are having an argument in any real sense of the word. He or she will have no means of placing what is said in a meaningful context and assessing it. However, your increasing heart rate and anxiety level will transmit to your baby in some way.

It is best to try to avoid becoming very stressed when you are pregnant, and it will help all of you if you can learn to handle disagreements calmly, through discussion and negotiation and compromise. Once your child is born, he or she will certainly be upset by rows, long before he or she is able to speak.

Q: I am so huge now, I feel quite otherworldly – as if this is not me – I just want it to be over and see my baby.

A: Many women feel like this towards the last few weeks of their pregnancy, and you are probably experiencing entirely normal feelings. However, it is worth discussing these feelings with your doctor just in case your feelings of depersonalization are associated with depression or acute anxiety. Depression can happen before the birth as well as after it, and it is best treated sooner rather than later.

Q: I don't know whether I will be able to handle the loss of privacy that giving birth entails. I am a very private person and am worried about the pain, the unknown nature of it all. All my friends seem to have coped better than I think I would.

A: Your question raises a number of issues. First, it would be a good idea to confide your fears and feelings to your family doctor and to the midwife in charge of you so that they can appreciate how you will feel in any given situation. They may well reassure you that many women feel this way. You will also be able to choose not have medical students present for the delivery.

Second, you may well imagine that all your friends have coped better than you think you would. However, this may be supposition on your part. Have you talked to them? Have you asked them if they felt nervous? You may find it helpful to discuss with them how they coped with the pain and loss of privacy.

Third, your own self-esteem may be an issue here. Are you usually confident? Do you often suffer from feelings of lack of confidence or low self-esteem? Experiencing the birth of your baby is without doubt something you can do. It does not matter if you scream or weep – medical staff will have seen other women do the same thing. You should also remember that people will be there to help and comfort you. Rest assured that you will receive the professional assistance and support you need.

Fourth, remember that this is just one day of your life, and you will get through it. Try to see the labour and delivery as a means to an end... seeing your very own gorgeous baby.

Q : I am seven months pregnant but I don't feel the emotional bond with my baby that other women talk about. Am I abnormal?

A : Not at all. Some women do feel rather detached from their pregnancy, almost as if the baby is growing within them irrespective of the woman herself as a person. Fathers-to-be also often do not bond with their baby until the actual delivery.

However, most parents do feel a surge of love for the baby once he or she is born. The hormones take over and allow you to feel the nurturing, protective love that is normal in parenthood.

If you have any remaining worries after the birth of your baby, be sure to discuss them with your family doctor or your health visitor.

Q : Now that I am pregnant, everyone seems to think they can touch my stomach. I really hate being stroked and prodded by strangers but don't know how to stop this happening. What can I do?

A : This is an entirely understandable reaction on your part and something expressed by many pregnant women – it is as if people believe that the bump is public property rather than part of your body. Short of staying at home, there is not a lot you can do, except to explain gently that your pregnancy is very personal to you and that you would prefer not to be touched.

Q : How will I know when to go to hospital?

A : Memorize the warning signs for labour and get your partner or best friend to do the same. They are:
- Breaking of the waters.
- A pinkish show of mucus tinged with blood.
- Contractions becoming regular and pronounced and lasting for some 40 seconds or more. (False labour is characterized by irregular contractions lasting less than 20–30 seconds.)

Ring your midwife if you are in any doubt about whether or not labour has started.

Q : What happens if I am caught short – say, if I am on a train or bus – when labour starts? Should I be taking any measures now?

A : Labour usually takes some time – and remember that even trains stop. Babies have been delivered in cars, buses, planes and on ships, but obviously one would prefer this not to happen. So, have a fully charged mobile phone with you at all times. From week 38, try to avoid any long journeys away from home and the place where you have chosen to have the delivery. If you are expecting twins, be cautious from week 35 onwards.

Q : I have started to worry that my partner may be away when the baby comes – he travels a lot, at short notice, for work – and am feeling panicky about what to do if he is.

A : In this situation, you may prefer to have a close friend or relative staying with you, or on stand-by, for the final stages, so make sure you have someone lined up now. If you do not have a friend or relative living close by, talk to your neighbours, who will probably be helpful, and alert your family doctor and midwife to the situation. They may be able to tell you of local back-up services.

Countdown to birth

" The most important thing to do is to focus on, and prepare yourself for, the labour. "

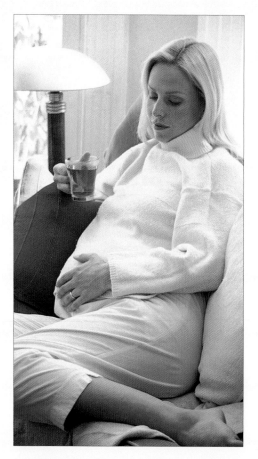

Seeing your new baby for the first time is an entirely magical, joyful and breathtaking moment, an event that you will remember for the rest of your life. Now this moment is just a few weeks away.

As you wait, the most important thing you can do is to focus on, and prepare yourself as much as possible for, the labour and delivery, and for the first weeks of your baby's life. All other considerations – work, socializing, doing the housework – should take second place to this.

You are much larger now and may feel constantly tired. It is more important than ever to focus on rest and relaxation. Avoid becoming overtired because it will be difficult to catch up – once the baby has arrived, your sleep is likely to be repeatedly interrupted. Take a rest in the early afternoon if you can. Drink plenty of water every day in order to expel the toxins from your body and help to reduce general feelings of fatigue.

Set aside some time each day to sit and relax and be with your unborn child. This can help the mother-child bonding process, and will help you to conserve your energy levels for the birth. It can also be a valuable time to start thinking of your first few days as a mother.

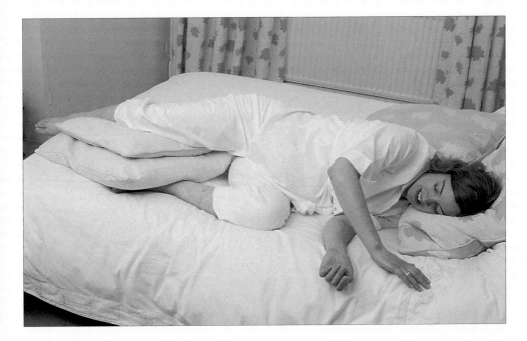

Feed yourself well, regularly and healthily. This will stand you in good stead for the demanding hours of labour and the delivery itself. Gentle activity and antenatal exercises are important in these last few weeks – try to get at least some exercise every day. It is also helpful to prepare mentally for the birth – through breathing, relaxation exercises and visualization, as well as enjoying periods of quiet contemplation each day.

On a practical level, you will probably already have decided on a room or space for your baby. You may be enjoying decorating it and providing for the baby's needs. Creating a welcoming physical space dedicated to your child can be a thrilling experience, and doing it together is a real opportunity for you and your partner to share in the preparations in a practical way.

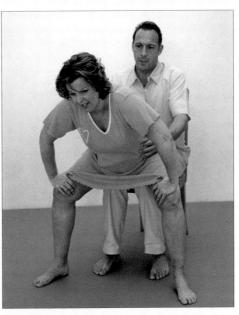

Top: You may find that this is a particularly comfortable resting position during the very late stages of your pregnancy. Place some padding, such as a pillow or two, under your upper leg in order to relieve pressure on the abdominal blood vessels.

Practice makes perfect. Experiment together with different positions for the labour – standing, squatting or kneeling – so you know what to try when the time comes. As you practise, make sure you don't push or exert any downward pressure.

Your birth plan

Giving birth is the most personal and intense experience of a woman's life. It is natural that you will want to make it as comfortable and stress-free as possible. Women often have different approaches to giving birth, and midwives and hospitals are now happy to accommodate your preferences where possible.

A birth plan is a note of exactly what you want to happen during and after the birth. Your plan will include details on the type of pain relief you want and who you want to be present. It will also specify whether you want to have your baby at home or in hospital.

Birth plans are highly individual: what suits one woman is not necessarily right for another. It is easy to become overwhelmed by all the options that are open to you, but writing a birth plan can help to clarify your thoughts and preferences. It will also help to highlight any areas where you are unclear about what is possible. You will be able to discuss every aspect of the birth with your midwife. Remember that your midwife is there to help you make the right decisions for you.

Discuss your birth plan with your partner or anyone else you wish to be present at the birth, so that everyone is aware of your wishes. However, bear in mind that circumstances can change. Maintaining a flexible attitude will help you cope if your labour doesn't quite go to plan.

WHAT IS ON A BIRTH PLAN?

Birth plans vary from country to country and from hospital to hospital, but your plan is likely to include:
• Where you want to give birth.

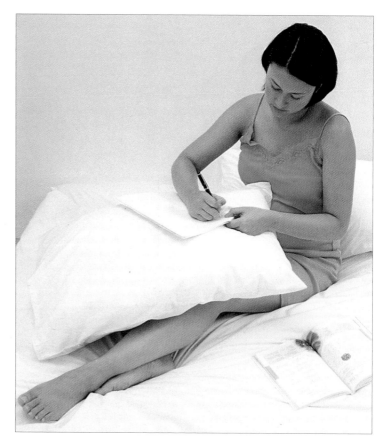

Writing a birth plan encourages you to think seriously about all the options available. This can help you to identify what is really important to you – for example, having your aromatherapist present and ensuring that you have access to an epidural if you need one.

- A note of who you would like to be present (partner, friend, family member, acupuncturist, hypnotherapist).
- What position or positions you hope to adopt for labour and delivery.
- Your feelings about monitoring the baby.
- Your feelings about induction.
- Your feelings about episiotomy.
- Details of what pain relief you want, if any.
- Whether you want the baby put to your chest straight after delivery and before he or she is cleaned up.
- Whether you intend to feed by breast or by bottle.
- How you feel about staying in hospital after the birth.

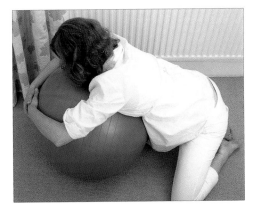

A FLEXIBLE PLAN

Remember that a birth plan is a list of your preferences rather than an agenda of what is actually going to happen. Labour and delivery can take a different direction in individual cases, acquiring a momentum of their own. Whether or not your birth plan is followed will depend on what happens before, during and after the birth.

Some women prefer not to write a birth plan at all – and it is fine to turn up at the hospital without one. Equally, many women change their mind about certain things. For example, most women would wish to avoid an episiotomy. However, if the baby becomes severely distressed (short of oxygen) and needs to be delivered quickly with forceps, an episiotomy may have to be performed. Equally, some women decide they want to give birth with no pain relief at all. However, it is not possible to predict the degree of pain that may occur nor how easily you will be able to cope with it. In some cases, the woman changes her mind and asks for pain relief.

The birth plan, then, is provisional. It does not commit you to a particular course of action: you may deviate from it if you wish to do so. Medical and nursing staff will also be prepared to deviate from the plan if necessary to preserve your health and the health of the baby.

Include on the birth plan details of anything that you wish to take into the delivery room – from a birthing ball to soothing chamomile oil or homeopathic tablets.

WHO TO HAVE AT YOUR BIRTH

Most women want someone who they know well to be at the birth – this is usually, but not necessarily, the father. Your birth partner can offer valuable emotional support, act as an advocate with medical staff, and also do simple things to enhance your well-being, such as rub your back or pour you a glass of water when you need one.

Think carefully about who you want to be at the birth, and discuss this with your partner. Most men want to be at the birth of their baby, but a few do not feel able to support their partner in this way. It is usually better to ask a friend or relative to come with you rather than trying to press-gang an unwilling partner.

You may also like to consider asking a complementary therapist to be present for part of your labour. An acupuncturist, for example, may be able to stimulate certain points to ease labour pains, while a homeopath could prescribe remedies for weak contractions or distress.

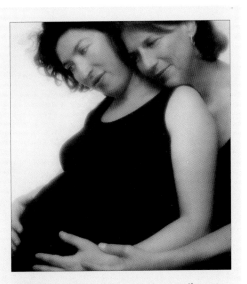

If you are having the baby on your own or if your partner is unable to be present, take a close friend or relative to support you during the birth.

Where to have your baby

The first decision you have to make when planning your birth is where to have your baby – at home or in hospital. Your personal feelings are very important, but you also need to consider any medical issues, as well as your facilities if you want to have a home birth.

You should discuss the issue of where to have your baby with your partner, who may have strong opinions either way. In particular, if you want to have your baby at home, it is important that you have your partner's support.

HAVING A HOSPITAL BIRTH

The majority of women prefer to give birth in hospital, where there are the medical resources available to deal with any complications that may arise. You will also have access to the complete range of pain relief if you give birth in hospital, and advice and support will be on hand after the birth. The norm is to have a natural (vaginal) delivery, attended by a midwife rather than by a doctor.

However, doctors will be available should you need medical assistance to deliver the baby.

If you deliver normally, you may be encouraged to go home between six and 48 hours later. Women and babies who are unwell after delivery often need to stay longer. The community midwives will continue your care at home for up to ten days, extending to 28 days if necessary.

HOME BIRTHS

Some women feel more relaxed about the prospect of giving birth in their own environment. One of the advantages of having your baby at home is, of course, that you are the boss. You can watch television in the early stages of labour. You don't have to see anyone that you don't want to see. You can eat when and what you wish. You can have the music and the lighting of your choice. In addition, you can have as many people in the room as you wish.

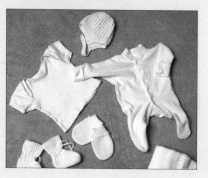

BEING PREPARED FOR HOSPITAL

Have a small case or bag packed a few weeks before your estimated date of delivery, so that you are well prepared should the baby come earlier than expected. Have the bag packed at 35 weeks if you are expecting twins or more. You will need most or all of the following:

- Dressing gown.
- Slippers.
- Two nightdresses (which open down the front if you plan to breastfeed).
- Comfortable loose clothes, such as big T-shirts, track pants, skirts.
- Underclothes, including socks and a nursing bra if you want to breastfeed.

- Sanitary towels for after the birth.
- Something to read.
- Sponge bag, containing toothbrush and toothpaste, deodorant, flannel, soap, shampoo, cosmetics, tissues, skin cleanser, moisturizer, cotton wool, scent, wet wipes, nail varnish remover, comb.
- Essential aromatic oils plus electric vaporizer, flower remedies and homeopathic remedies.
- Herbal teas (for example, chamomile or raspberry leaf tea for the labour).
- Facial water spray.
- Address and telephone book.
- Phone card and coins for the telephone (you are often not able to use a mobile phone in a hospital).
- Music and portable stereo.
- Bottled water.
- Snack foods to eat during labour (dried fruit, nuts and raisins, bananas, grapes, carrot sticks, crackers, cheese, yeast extract, cereal bars).
- Sleep suits for your baby.
- Lightweight blanket or shawl.
- Mittens, woolly hat and outdoor suit for the baby.
- A correctly fitted new car seat for your baby to travel home safely.

Don't forget to take one or two outfits to the hospital for your new baby to wear.

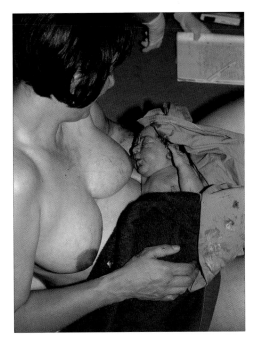

Giving birth at home gives you greater control over your environment. It also means the first sights, sounds and smells a baby encounters are those of his or her home.

However, there are disadvantages to home births. The biggest drawback is that you will not have immediate access to specialist medical care if something goes wrong. This is the main reason that many doctors are uncomfortable about the idea of a home birth.

Another consideration may be any other children who live with you. It may prove difficult or distressing for them to hear you in labour, although there is no doubt they will be thrilled when they see the newborn baby. You may wish to arrange for your children to be looked after by a relative or a close friend while you are in labour.

If you give birth at home, it can be more difficult to let go of responsibility for household chores. Make sure that there is someone to look after you who will take over the running of the home. You will not want to answer the telephone or the doorbell within a few hours of giving birth to your baby. There will also have to be someone to clear up and change the bed linen.

DOCTORS AND HOME BIRTHS

Many doctors understand some women would prefer their baby to be delivered at home. However, they often discourage home births, particularly if there has been any indication that complications may ensue or if you are in a higher-than-average risk category.

If there is a problem during a home birth, valuable time will be lost while arrangements are made for an ambulance to collect the woman and drive her to the hospital. If the complications are serious, this delay could prove life-threatening to either you or your baby.

You may find that your own family doctor will not accept you for antenatal care if you choose to have a home birth. If this is the case, your midwife should be able to put you in touch with another doctor. The delivery will be undertaken by one or two midwives.

Can you have a home birth?

You have the right to give birth at home. However, if this is your first child or if you are in a high-risk group, a hospital birth will be recommended. The following women are actively discouraged from giving birth at home:

- Women over 35.
- Women expecting twins or more.
- Women expecting their first child.
- Women who had a difficult labour with their first child.
- Women who have had a Caesarean delivery, a stillborn baby, or one who died shortly after birth.
- Anyone who has a serious medical condition that could affect the outcome of the pregnancy and delivery, such as high blood pressure, heart disease, diabetes, significant heart murmur or kidney disease.

WHAT YOU WILL NEED AT HOME

You don't need a lot for a home birth, but the following are essential:

- Adequate heating – the room should be around 20°C (under 70°F).
- Telephone – so that help can be summoned in an emergency.
- Anglepoise lamp so the midwife can see in a dim light.
- Sheets and towels – these should be clean but preferably old so that it doesn't matter if they are stained.
- Clean nightdress for after the birth.
- Sanitary towels.

These items will be helpful:

- Chair and a low stool.
- Several cushions and a large bean bag.
- Natural sponge.
- Mineral water and fruit juice.
- Essential aromatic oils and vaporizer, flower remedies, homeopathic remedies.
- Herbal teas.
- Snack foods to eat during labour (dried fruit, nuts, bananas, grapes, carrot sticks, crackers, cheese, yeast extract, cereal bars).

Giving birth in water

Whether you are planning to give birth at home or in a hospital, you may wish to opt for a water birth. Midwives have long known that taking a bath can help with relaxation and pain control in early labour. Since the 1980s, an increasing number of women have chosen to spend long periods of their labour in water and to give birth in it. Water births account for approximately one in every 200 births in the UK, and they are also growing in popularity in the United States.

Supporters say that women who spend their labour immersed in warm water benefit in many ways.

- Warm water is naturally soothing and comforting. The pool also provides a private space for the labour.
- Water's buoyancy supports a woman's weight, making it easier for her to relax and change position.
- Water helps to support the pelvic floor and soften the perineum, making women less likely to tear or to require an episiotomy.
- Contractions are less painful because the body is less tense – your body releases pain-killing endorphins when it is in a relaxed state.
- When pain is reduced, women find it easier to concentrate on their breathing, which can help to shorten the labour.
- The father can get in the pool too, making the birth more of a shared experience.

Babies are usually lifted out of the water as soon as they are born, either by the mother, father, midwife or doctor, so that they can breathe. However, the family can usually stay in the water after the birth in order to bond.

ARE WATER BIRTHS SAFE?
Water births are controversial, and many doctors do not approve of them. However, the *British Medical Journal* conducted a study of all the water births that took place in the UK between 1994 and 1996. It found that the mortality rate for the babies was no greater than that associated with conventional births. In the USA, water births are strongly disapproved of by the American Congress of Obstetricians and Gynecologists (ACOG) and the American Academy of Pediatrics (AAP) but supported by two major midwife associations and the American Association of Birth Centres.

There has been only limited research into water births, so it is impossible to be entirely sure of the risks. One problem is that it is difficult to maintain the water temperature: if it is too hot, it may cause the baby's heart

> **" Midwives have long known that taking a bath can help with relaxation and pain control in early labour. "**

beat to increase. Another concern is that the baby may be at risk of drowning. Supporters of water births say this is not possible because the baby does not breathe until he or she comes into contact with the air. However, one report from New Zealand suggested that a few babies have suffered respiratory problems as a result of inhaling water. Many women choose to get out of the water for the actual delivery because of this concern.

If you are considering a water birth, you need to discuss the benefits and risks with your midwife early on. You may find it helpful to seek out other women who have given birth in this way. Ask your antenatal teacher, search the Internet and look for local support groups.

CAN I HAVE A WATER BIRTH?
You should be able to have a water birth if your pregnancy has been straightforward and so long as no complications are envisaged. Many hospitals and birthing centres have birthing pools, so water births should be possible in most areas. In practice, however, the pool may not be available when you need it. For example, it may be being cleaned or in use by another woman. It may be available only if your labour coincides with the shifts of a specific midwife.

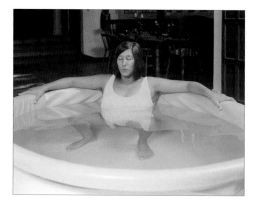

If you are having a water birth at home, hire the pool a few weeks before your due date. It is a good idea to fill the pool for a trial run beforehand.

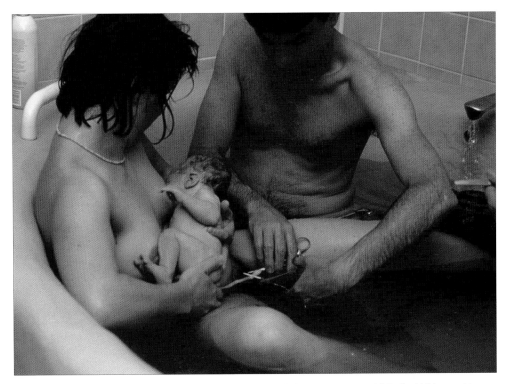

Some hospitals actively discourage women from having a water birth, even if they have the facilities to provide one. Asking these questions should let you see how likely it is that you will be able to have a water birth at your hospital:

- How many women use the birthing pool each year?
- How many women actually give birth in the pool?
- How many midwives are trained to attend water births?
- Will the pool be available when I go into labour?

If you feel that staff are not keen on facilitating a water birth, talk to your midwife. There may be good reasons for this, and it may be that the hospital does not support the practice. If so, you may want to consider having the birth elsewhere. However, make sure you will be assisted by a qualified midwife who is experienced with water births.

WATER BIRTHS AT HOME

If you are having a home birth, you can hire your own pool. Ask your midwife for details of local companies who rent out pools. Make sure your midwife is happy and confident about facilitating a water birth. If not, ask for a referral to someone who is.

You will need to hire the pool for several weeks, so that you can be sure that you have it when you go into labour. Make sure that your floor can take the weight, and that there is plenty of space around the pool.

The father may want to get into the birthing pool to share the first moments of his baby's life, or even to cut the umbilical cord, under instruction from the midwife.

WHEN WATER BIRTHS ARE UNSUITABLE

Water births are not recommended if the baby is in the breech position; if you are expecting twins; if the baby is more than two weeks early; if you have an infection or other medical condition, or if there is meconium (the baby's first bowel movement) in the amniotic fluid.

It is also important that women do not get into the pool too early in their labour. You should wait until you are at least 5cm (2in) dilated, otherwise the relaxing effects of the water can slow labour down.

STAY FLEXIBLE

If you are planning a water birth, remember that labour does not always go to plan. If complications occur, you will need to get out of the pool so that medical assistance can be given. Also, bear in mind that the main aim of a water birth is to facilitate relaxation and well-being: don't turn getting one into a stressful event.

Preparing for the birth

Many women feel a growing sense of confidence and ease as the due date approaches. However, there can still be moments of anxiety about the birth ahead. You may also have times when you feel very bored – these last few weeks can seem to last forever. Fluctuating emotions are normal in pregnancy. However, it will help you to cope with the birth if you are feeling as emotionally strong as possible. Try to deal with any fears you have now so that you can concentrate on your labour when the time comes.

If you have specific worries, get as much information as you can about what lies ahead. If you are not sure how you will cope with the pain, for example, look into the different methods of pain relief that you can have. Don't rule anything out – even if you are keen to have a natural birth, it can be reassuring to know that you have access to medication if you need it.

MENTAL PREPARATION

Take some time each day to contemplate the birth. Visualization can be very helpful: try to picture yourself in labour, adopting your preferred positions. Imagine yourself coping with the contractions – you may like to think of them as hurdles that you are leaping over or as powerful surges that are bringing you and your baby closer together. Think of your pelvic area opening and expanding, so that the baby passes more easily down the birth canal. Imagine your baby's arrival, and the joy that you will feel on seeing him or her. Think of the birth as an empowering rather than a worrying experience.

PHYSICAL PREPARATION

In general, you want to feel as fit and healthy as possible. Get plenty of sleep and relaxation, so you start your labour feeling rested and mentally alert. If you are still working, consider starting your maternity leave (ideally you should leave work by week 34-36 so that you have time to prepare for the birth). Drink plenty of water to help your body expel any toxins. Eat healthily and regularly; you will find it easier to digest your food if you eat little and often. Eat plenty of complex carbohydrates, such as wholegrain bread and rice, in order to stock up your energy reserves. Make sure you eat iron-rich foods and protein each day, and include a wide range of different fruit and vegetables, to be sure that you are getting a full spectrum of nutrients.

Practising yoga or Pilates will help to enhance your suppleness and general health. It is also a good idea to practise your preferred positions for the labour, and to take a short walk each day to maintain your fitness.

BREATHING EXERCISES

Controlling your breathing will help enormously at the birth. You will be taught breathing techniques at your antenatal classes, and you should practise these in advance. What you are aiming to avoid is the 'over-breathing' that results when we are tense and panicky – sucking air into our lungs and letting out short, sharp gasps. This will soon exhaust you, and fail to give yourself and your baby plenty of oxygen to cope with the birth.

Any breathing exercises you are given will focus on keeping your breathing steady and rhythmic. The in-breath should not be longer than the out breath; if anything, aim for the reverse. Try these simple exercises:
- Breathe in through your nose and out through your mouth, keeping your mouth soft. Try making a noise such as "Aaaaaaah" as you breathe out.
- As you breathe in, count slowly to three or four. Then do the same as you breathe out.

When it comes to pushing the baby out, you may automatically hold your breath as you push. This can hurt

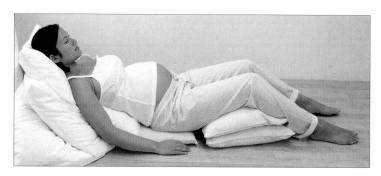

Do not lie flat on your back at this stage of pregnancy. Prop yourself up on plenty of cushions and place another pillow or two under your knees. Alternatively, lie on your side with your uppermost leg resting on a cushion.

your throat, and you should never hold your breath and push for as long as possible, which is sometimes advised, as this is tiring and oxygen-depleting. The better option is to take a deep breath as you feel a contraction starting, then breathe or blow out slowly as you push down.

If you feel the urge to push before the cervix is fully dilated, help to stop yourself from doing this as follows: give four short pants as a contraction arrives, then a quick in-breath, followed by four more pants. Breathe normally between contractions.

NATURAL THERAPIES FOR THE LAST WEEKS

A traditional herbal preparation for labour is raspberry leaf tea (see page 130), while perineal massage helps to improve the stretchability of the skin (see pages 162–63). It can be very helpful to see an acupuncturist who specializes in pregnancy. Specific points can be used to strengthen the emotions and help you to prepare for the birth. Your acupuncturist may also be willing to teach you and your partner about acupressure points to press during labour.

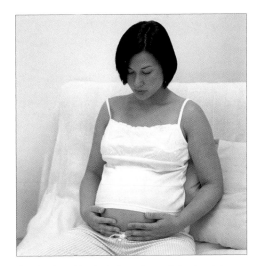

Practise breathing techniques learned at antenatal classes every day, so that they become automatic.

NATURAL REMEDY BIRTH KIT

The following natural remedies may be helpful to you during labour. Check with a qualified practitioner to ensure that you take remedies that are suitable for your individual needs. You should also discuss with your midwife any remedies you wish to bring into the delivery room, and they should be incorporated into your birth plan.

Essential oils

A mixture of 10 drops clary sage, 10 drops lavender and 5 drops jasmine in 100ml (3½fl oz) base oil makes a good massage oil for the lower back during labour; it can help to promote strong contractions as well as encouraging you to stay calm. Useful oils to burn in a vaporizer may include frankincense (for pain and hyperventilation), lavender (for anxiety), rose (for fear and doubt), ginger (for weariness) and chamomile (for irritability).

Herbal teas

Teas that may be helpful during labour include raspberry leaf (to promote regular contractions), chamomile, lime flowers or lemon balm (to induce relaxation), cramp bark (to release tension) and ginseng (to boost energy). Check that there are tea-making facilities in the delivery suite; if not, take two flasks of hot water and a cup.

Flower remedies

Gentle flower remedies can be very comforting: place a few drops in a glass of water and sip at intervals. Try Rescue Remedy for fear and panic; olive for exhaustion; or cherry plum if you start to feel that you cannot carry on with the labour.

Homeopathic remedies

See a homeopath for advice about remedies that may be helpful to take before, during and after labour. He or she may recommend arnica (for bruising), caulophyllum (to encourage regular contractions), nux vomica (for backache) or hypericum (to promote healing).

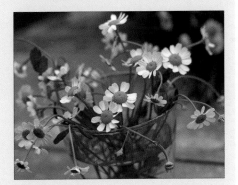

Chamomile flowers are used to make calming tea or oil.

Your baby's room

One of the best ways that you and your partner can prepare for the arrival of your new baby is to get the nursery ready. Ideally, the baby will have a room of his or her own. However, if you are short of space, don't worry. You can create a welcoming area for your baby in a corner of your own bedroom.

Creating a nursery can help you to adjust to the idea that you are bringing a new life into the world – something you may still find difficult to believe. Sharing this process with your partner will help you to prepare together for the new baby who is to share your lives.

Many women worry that they will not be ready in time. If this is the case, remember that preparing a room is more for your benefit than the baby's. Your baby will not mind if your home is disorganized, as long as he or she is with you. In any case, he or she should sleep in your bedroom for the first few weeks.

A RESTFUL NURSERY

First and foremost, your baby's room should be a clean and light place to be. Enlist your partner or a friend to help you clean it thoroughly (or ask them to do it for you). Don't

> **❝ Creating a nursery can help you to adjust to the idea that you are bringing a new life into the world. ❞**

forget to clean the windows inside and out. This will let more light into the room, which will make it feel cheerier. Make sure curtains or blinds are in a simple, non-fussy style, and do not obscure natural sunlight.

It is worth installing a dimmer switch or including a low-wattage lamp in the room. This will allow you to tend to the baby at night, without flooding the room with so much light that he or she becomes wakeful. A dim light will help to convey the message that it is still time for sleep: the sooner your baby is able to associate darkness with rest, the better for everyone.

Use child-friendly, non-toxic paint to decorate the room; matt paint gives a softer effect than gloss. Nurseries are often painted in primary colours, but it's probably better to use a soothing, sleep-inducing hue, such as lavender or pale blue.

Your baby is not going to care about great interior design. But he or she will probably thrive best in a room that is light, airy and restful. You could hang a mobile over the cot: this will provide something interesting for the baby to focus upon in the months to come.

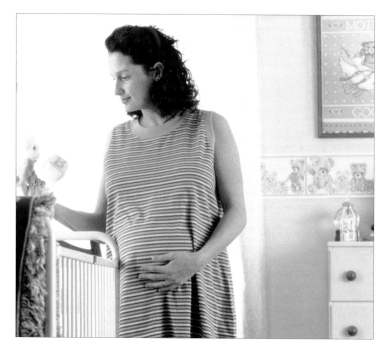

A rose quartz crystal is a beautiful addition to your baby's room. It is said to evoke a sense of comfort and love, and to promote restful sleep.

Consider having light-coloured wood flooring rather than carpet; it is much easier to keep clean. However, place a rug under the cot, just in case the baby has a fall. You'll also want a larger rug (with a non-slip underlay) for when your child starts to walk.

Keep the room as uncluttered as possible: a cot, a chair for you, a changing table and a storage unit is all you really need. A rocking chair is a great investment: it can help you to soothe the baby. Wherever possible, choose natural materials such as wood and cotton for your baby's room.

Position your baby's cot against a wall. Ideally, the cot should be in a position where you can see it easily from the door – this is so that you can readily check on your baby while he or she is sleeping. You should not place a cot directly under a window, since this may expose the baby to draughts.

FENG SHUI FOR NURSERIES

The Eastern art of feng shui is used to bring health and happiness to the occupants of a home. It involves promoting the flow of beneficial energy (chi) around each room, by removing any blockages and by adding enhancements ('cures'). Try the following to create a good atmosphere in your baby's room:

- Clean windows regularly. Open them for at least 10 minutes each day to allow fresh energy to enter.
- Keep the nursery free of clutter, which impedes the flow of chi (and can be a hazard).
- Cover up sharp corners, which cause an excess of chi. Incorporate soft, curving shapes into the room wherever possible.
- Include a few splashes of bright colour, such as red or orange, especially in dark corners.
- Hang a mobile over the cot – moving objects are said to promote the flow of chi, and this will also give your baby something to look at when he or she is lying in the cot.
- Plant a window box with healing herbs, such as lavender, basil or catnip. You could also place a green pot plant in the room (move it out of reach when the child gets older). Care for all plants well and replace them if they become unhealthy.
- Include a lucky charm in the form of an animal motif: bears and dogs both signify protection, the stork is a classic symbol of birth, and swallows represent joy and playfulness.
- Place a crystal in the child's room – rose quartz is associated with love and comfort (crystal healers sometimes use it to help cure sleeplessness).

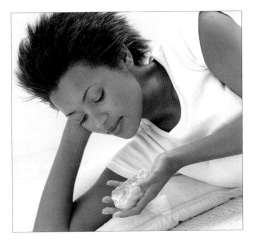

CLEARING THE SPACE

In China, a nursery is usually cleared of stale energy before it is decorated, and again just before the baby arrives. If you want to do this:

- Clean the room thoroughly and open all the windows on a sunny day; this brings fresh energy into the room.
- Stand or sit in the middle of the room. Spend a few moments quietly breathing and focusing.
- Go to each corner of the room in turn. Ring a bell or clap your hands there – as you do so, imagine you are clearing out old, stagnant energy and making room for the new. Follow your instincts and repeat a few times if necessary.
- To finish, stand in the centre of the room again for a few moments. You may like to practise some meditation or visualization, or to say a little prayer for the well-being and happiness of your baby.

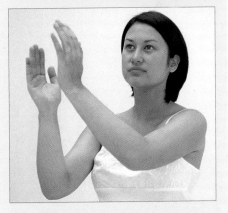

Clap your hands to drive out stale energy.

What your baby will need

Shopping is all part of the fun of expecting a baby. Unless you have already had a baby, you will need equipment for the nursery – a cot, a changing mat, a chest of drawers. You will also need a stock of clothes (remember that the baby will grow very quickly, so don't buy too many), nappies, toiletries and other items for the first few weeks. There are now plenty of natural and organic options available, so look out for these.

WHAT TO BUY FOR...

The nursery

- Cot with a drop-down side – make sure that you can drop down the side with one hand only (you may be holding your baby with your other arm).
- You may like to buy a Moses basket for the first four months or so. This is transportable so you will be able to move it around easily. It is a good idea to buy a stand to put the basket on at night. This means that you won't have to stoop to pick up the baby.
- Well-fitting new mattress for the cot and basket.
- Two cotton cellular blankets – these keep the baby warm, but not overheated.
- Linen, including cotton, fitted bottom sheets. Note that the baby will not need a pillow and must not have a duvet before the age of 12 months.
- Thick, dark curtains for daytime naps.
- Nursery thermometer – to monitor the temperature.
- A chair for you or your partner, or a small sofa.
- Changing table.
- A chest of drawers for clothes and nappies.
- Smoke alarm in or just outside the baby's room.
- Nightlight and baby monitor – check you have enough sockets.

The kitchen or utility room

- Kitchen paper and disinfectant spray and wipes for cleaning surfaces.
- Check that washing machine, tumble dryer, washing line, clotheshorse and pulley are working properly. There will be a lot more washing than you are used to once the baby arrives. Make sure that you do not use biological washing powders since these may irritate a baby's sensitive skin.

Feeding your baby

- Breast pads to catch leaks.
- Herbal nipple cream.
- Breast pump for expressing milk; for when you are somewhere where it would be difficult to breastfeed; this also allows your partner to feed the baby.
- Formula milk (organic varieties are available) and feeding bottles as standby.
- Bottle brush and teat brush.
- Sterilizing equipment (unless you are planning to just use boiling water).
- Bottle holders and carriers.
- Old towels to protect your clothes while feeding.

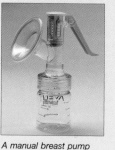

A manual breast pump   *Sterilizing tank and tablets*

Your baby's clothes

- Vests, body suits and sleep suits.
- Dungarees.
- Dresses.

- Cardigans – easier to put on than sweaters.
- Socks or booties.
- Mittens, if winter.

- Warm hat or sun hat, depending on the season.
- Muslin squares.

- An all-in-one suit for outdoor wear.
- Small lightweight blanket.

Playtime
- Music.
- Rattles and soft toys.
- A ball.
- Mobile (to hang above cot).

Bathing your baby
- Baby bath (choose from options that are used on or in an adult bath, and others that have their own stand).
- Natural baby soap, shampoo, lotion and oil, free from any harsh perfumes or colourings.
- Baby wipes for when you are out only (otherwise use water or lotion as the gentle, eco-friendly option).
- Cotton wool.
- Large tissues.
- Nappies, whichever kind you decide to use, and related accessories.
- Gentle herbal creams and oils for dealing with nappy rash (avoid using talc).
- Baby scissors or nail clippers.

Your baby's health
- Forehead strip thermometer.
- Basic first-aid kit and book.
- Gripe water.
- Herbal, homeopathic or conventional treatment for colic.
- Infant paracetamol syrup.
- Infant medicine spoon.
- Cough and cold treatments for infants.

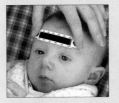

A strip thermometer

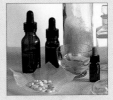

Homeopathic remedies

Going out and about
- Car seat – this must be correctly fitted; do not buy second-hand.
- Travel cot (or you can use a Moses basket).
- Lie-down baby buggy with transparent rain cover, or a pram (some are fitted with a removable carrycot to use as a bed, initially).
- Pram or buggy accessories, such as linen, cellular blankets, rain cover, parasol.
- Bag that is large enough to contain everything you need for feeding and changing your baby.
- A changing mat that you can put down anywhere on a table or on a floor.
- List of useful telephone numbers, such as your doctor's and health visitor's.

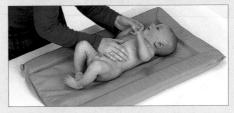

Changing mat

Sources for everything you need
Getting ready for a baby can be expensive, but there is no need to buy everything new. Shop around, and consider all the following sources:
- Friends and relatives.
- Charity shops and good second-hand shops.
- Magazines and direct-mail catalogues.
- The Internet.
- Large pharmacies and supermarkets (which often sell baby items more cheaply).

Remember that you are likely to be given outfits by friends and relatives. A close friend or relative who has recently had a baby may offer to pass on clothes and equipment that are no longer needed, especially if they are not planning another child.

REMEMBER
- Do not buy second-hand electrical equipment.
- If you are given or buy second-hand goods, make sure that they have been painted recently and do not contain leaded paint.
- Check catches, locks and hooks for safety.
- All clothes and linen should be washable and suitable for a tumble dryer.
- Cotton and light soft wools are kinder to the skin than synthetics.
- Avoid lots of buttons.
- Make sure that clothes are big enough to contain a nappy (diaper).

Before the birth

As the birth approaches, your baby will be monitored as part of your continuing antenatal care. During the last month of your pregnancy, you will probably visit your antenatal clinic once a week for the usual blood and urine tests and weight check. In addition, your baby's heartbeat will be checked at each visit, and he or she will also be checked over to ensure that growth and movement are progressing normally.

You and your baby will be assessed for labour by the following criteria:

- Just how well the baby is likely to stand up to the testing rigours of labour and delivery – this is assessed by checking the baby's general well-being and heartbeat.
- Whether or not the baby is in the right position for a normal vaginal delivery.
- Whether or not the baby will be able to negotiate the birth canal – this is determined by assessing both the size of the baby's head and the size of the mother-to-be's pelvis.

A Caesarean section will be considered:

- If the baby's head is thought to be too large in relation to your pelvis.
- If he or she is in a position that will make it hard to navigate the birth canal.
- If there are likely to be any other complications during the delivery.

THE POSITION FOR BIRTH

When discussing the baby's position for birth, medical staff will talk about the lie, the presentation and the position. These all mean different things.

The baby's 'lie'

When doctors and midwives use the term 'lie', they are referring to the way that the baby is lying in the mother's body. This term describes the relationship between the spine of the baby and the spine of the mother – the north-south axis. The baby may be lying in a longitudinal (vertical) lie with the head up or head down, or across the mother's body in a transverse (horizontal) lie.

Nearly all babies before the 32nd week change the way they are facing frequently, so yours may be in the breech position when you have your antenatal check-ups: this is a longitudinal lie with the head uppermost and the buttocks down. After the 32nd week, most babies turn to the head-down position. About 3 per cent of babies,

however, remain in the breech position. Another 1 per cent of babies assume a transverse lie, in which the baby lies across the uterus. You can see all of these positions clearly in the illustrations.

Babies who are in a breech position or transverse lie may suffer some difficulties during a vaginal delivery, so special checks are made beforehand. In particular, it needs to be established whether or not the mother's pelvis is large enough to accommodate the baby comfortably. If the pelvis is not large enough, then a Caesarean delivery is advised. This is always the case with a transverse lie, but it may be that a breech baby is able to be delivered vaginally.

It is important to know if there is an underlying reason for the baby assuming the wrong lie. For example, the placenta may be in a position that makes it impossible for the baby to assume a head-down position, or there may be some other obstruction – such as a fibroid, for example – in the mother's uterus. In these cases, a Caesarean delivery will be carried out.

The baby's presentation

This describes what part of the baby is at the pelvic brim before the delivery – that is, the part of the baby to be born first. Most babies adopt what is known as the vertex presentation. In this posture, the baby's head is well flexed, with the chin on the chest. This means that the vertex (crown) of the head is the part touching the cervix and will be born first.

A tiny number of babies – no more than 0.3 per cent – present their face or brow first. These presentations are known as face presentation or brow presentation. Face presentations are able to be delivered vaginally, but only if the back of the baby's head is facing the mother's spine. Brow presentations, however, are always delivered by Caesarean section because the baby cannot fit into the birth canal.

The baby's position

A baby's position describes the way the baby is facing as birth approaches. If he or she is facing towards the mother's spine, the position is said to be anterior and labour is likely to be easier, although that is not always the case. If the baby is facing outwards, with the back of its head to the mother's spine, the position is said to be posterior. In this case, labour may be slower, and the mother is more likely to experience severe backache during labour.

YOUR BABY'S POSITION

It can be hard to visualize the difference between a breech, transverse and face presentation. These illustrations show the various positions that a baby can adopt within the uterus in the last days before birth. All of them are perfectly comfortable for the baby, and none should cause undue discomfort to the mother.

NORMAL POSITION

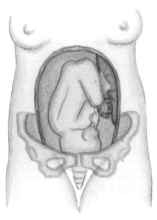

Here the baby is in the normal 'head-first' position, ready for the delivery. He or she is lying slightly to the right and is facing the mother's spine. The baby's chin is tucked into the chest, so that the narrowest part of the head will be born first.

BREECH POSITION

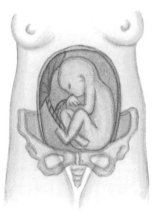

This baby is in the full, bottom-first breech position, with head up and legs crossed in front. Breech babies can have their legs extended up, so that their feet are in front of the face, or have one or both legs dropping down.

TRANSVERSE LIE

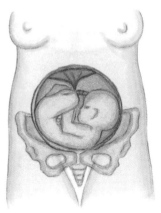

In a transverse lie, the baby is across the uterus. This means that his shoulder would come out first if a vaginal delivery were attempted. A baby can sometimes be encouraged to shift position, but, if this fails, a Caesarean section will be needed.

FACE-DOWN PRESENTATION

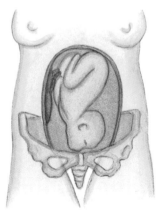

Here the baby is in the head-first position, but the neck is not tucked into the chest as in the normal position. Instead, the neck is extended so that the face is presented first. A midwife will assess whether or not a vaginal delivery is possible.

Going into labour

There are three main stages of labour: the cervix dilating (opening up) to let the baby through; the actual birth itself; and the delivery of the placenta. Much more about these stages is explained over the following pages.

Women can find it hard to judge whether or not they have gone into labour. If you are in any doubt, you can contact your midwife at any time. You can also ring the hospital if you are not sure whether or not you should go in. There are three signs that indicate that labour is imminent or has started:

- A pinkish 'show' of mucus.
- The breaking of the waters.
- Contractions that last for 40 seconds or more, becoming more regular and pronounced.

A 'SHOW'

The first sign that labour is imminent is usually the show. This occurs when the plug of mucus sealing the cervix is released. The show appears as a mucous vaginal discharge, which may be tinged with blood. It can happen several days before contractions start, or it may coincide with the breaking of the waters. It often goes unnoticed.

THE BREAKING OF THE WATERS

The membranes surrounding the baby can rupture at the start of labour, shortly before it or at the end of the first stage. This is known as the breaking of the waters, and it is painless. Once this happens, you should go to hospital, or call your midwife if you are having a home birth.

Normally, waters break with an unmistakable gush of liquid. Sometimes there is a less obvious breaking that may be confused with the incontinence that is common in late pregnancy. Contact your midwife if you are unsure. In some cases, the waters break spontaneously but labour does not start. Most hospitals will admit you if this happens because the baby is no longer protected from infection and labour needs to be induced. Occasionally, however, the hole in the membrane seals itself over and the pregnancy continues. Sometimes the waters may be ruptured by the obstetrician using a probe. This may be done when the birth is being induced, as it can encourage contractions to start.

Women may mistake the breaking of the waters for incontinence. Call your midwife if you think that you are in labour but cannot tell for certain.

THE WATERS

The term 'waters' refers to the liquid contained within the membranes. This amniotic fluid is a clear, yellowish liquid that contains the baby's urine and dead skin cells. Breaking the waters means breaking the membranes that surround and protect the baby in the uterus.

The baby depends for his or her well-being on the amniotic fluid. It has several functions:

- It enables the baby to turn and move his or her limbs easily.
- It serves to extend the uterus so that the walls do not exert any pressure upon the growing baby.
- It guarantees a constant temperature for the baby, which is the mother's body temperature.
- It absorbs the baby's waste products.
- It acts as a shock absorber, and so protects the baby from the impact if the mother falls or receives a jarring blow to the abdomen.

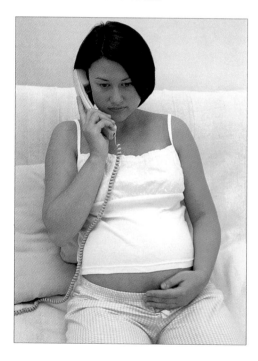

CONTRACTIONS

Many women experience small, irregular contractions throughout pregnancy. Towards the end of pregnancy these become more pronounced, when they are known as Braxton Hicks contractions. They can be painful but are irregular and do not cause the cervix to dilate – so you are not in labour. With Braxton Hicks contractions, the uterus may contract every 20 minutes or so for about 20–30 seconds. By contrast, the birth contractions felt during the first stage of labour last for 40–60 seconds, and become more powerful. This is the time to telephone the hospital to tell them that you are on your way. It will help if you have noted down the frequency and length of the contractions.

GOING TO HOSPITAL

Take your notes, birth plan and overnight bag with you. When you arrive at hospital, you will go through the normal admissions procedure and will then be taken to the labour ward, where your pulse, temperature and blood pressure will be checked and you will be examined externally and internally in order to judge the baby's position and see how far the cervix has dilated.

HOW LONG DOES LABOUR LAST?

	First birth	Subsequent births
1st stage	4–24 hours	2–12 hours
2nd stage	½–2 hours	10 minutes–1½ hours
3rd stage	10 minutes–1½ hours	10 minutes–1½ hours

When you go to the delivery room depends on how dilated you are, the baby's condition, and what space there is in the hospital. You may be allowed to make the delivery room a little more personal if you have arranged this beforehand – for example, plugging in a portable stereo or setting up an electric aromatherapy burner. These things should have been noted on your birth plan after discussion with the midwife, though there may not be time to carry this out if you are admitted as an emergency.

A team of midwives will provide all your medical care during labour, and will deliver your baby and check you are both well after delivery. Doctors are on duty for much of the day and night to assist if complications occur.

THE SIGNS AND STAGES OF LABOUR

As already explained, there are three signs that herald the start of labour, and three stages to labour itself. The three warning signs may occur separately or in combination. So, you may be in the first stage of labour, with strong contractions lasting 40 seconds or more, even though the waters have not broken. The artworks below show how the cervix widens during labour. Shortly before labour begins, the cervix starts to shorten in response to the contractions. A partially dilated cervix, encouraged by the pressure of the baby's head, indicates that labour is well under way. By the time the cervix has dilated enough to allow the baby's head through into the vagina, the second stage of labour has been reached – this stage lasts from when the cervix is fully dilated until the birth of the baby. The third stage of labour is the delivery of the placenta.

WHAT HAPPENS TO THE CERVIX BEFORE AND DURING LABOUR

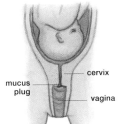

cervix

mucus plug

vagina

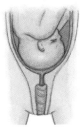

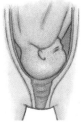

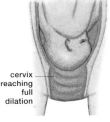

cervix reaching full dilation

Here the neck of the uterus – the cervix – remains closed. It is sealed by a plug of mucus, which protects the baby from infection. When this is released, labour is near.

The mucus plug is released before labour – this is the 'show', one of the early signs that labour is near or has started. When the contractions begin, the cervix becomes shorter.

The cervix now starts to dilate (open). This is the first stage of labour, which can last many hours. A normal rate of dilation is judged to be about 1cm (⅖in) an hour, but this varies.

As the cervix reaches full dilation (10cm/4in), ready for the baby to pass down into the vagina, you are in a brief period called the transitional stage, just prior to the second stage of labour – the birth.

Pain relief and monitoring

The key to having as fulfilling a labour experience as possible is to keep an open mind and to be well informed beforehand about the signs of impending labour, how your labour is likely to be managed, the type of pain relief you would ideally like and all the options available.

COMPLEMENTARY PAIN RELIEF

There are many natural, drug-free methods that can help to ease the pain of labour and birth. Some of these work by stimulating the release of endorphins, the body's natural painkillers. To use some of these methods, you may need to have a complementary therapist with you in the delivery room. If you do, then this should be noted on your birth plan, along with details of any natural remedies you want to use.

Make sure that any therapist treating or helping you in the delivery room is fully experienced in dealing with labour and birth. Also, any therapies that you use must be ones that you are already familiar with and have had some success with before, so you know what to expect

ORTHODOX PAIN RELIEF

Method	Stage of labour	How given	Does it work?	Side effects
Gas and air	1st, 2nd	You breathe in from a mouthpiece	Up to a point – gives only limited relief from pain	May make you feel light-headed or drowsy. It is difficult to put your breathing techniques into practice while using mask
Pethidine	1st	Injection either into a vein in the arm or into a muscle in the buttock	Timing is crucial – if given too early, effects may wear off; if too late, can prevent you pushing and can affect baby	May necessitate forceps delivery if it affects your ability to push. May make you feel drowsy and/or sick. The baby may be drowsy and slow to breathe
Epidural	1st, and if Caesarean delivery	Injected into epidural space between spinal cord and backbone of lumbar region	Usually very effective but occasionally does not work	Chances of forceps delivery and episiotomy are higher if you have an epidural. Necessitates continuous fetal monitoring. You may feel numbness in legs for some time after delivery. May cause headache
Pudendal nerve block	2nd, if forceps delivery is indicated	Injection through wall of vagina	Not always	None
Transcutaneous Electrical Nerve Stimulation (TENS)	1st, 2nd	Electrodes attached to back, and a low-frequency current directed by mother	Not always	None – often recommended by complementary therapists
General anaesthetic	If Caesarean delivery	Injection	Yes	Recovery is often slow

and are confident that they may have some effect. Below is a list of some common drug-free approaches:

- **Positions** Moving around and trying different positions – leaning against your partner or a wall, for example – will often bring relief (see also pages 196-199).
- **Water** Immersion in warm water is often relaxing, as the warmth is soothing and the water helps to take the body's weight. Find out well in advance about birthing pool options in your chosen place of delivery.
- **Massage** Effective for relieving discomfort and promoting calm, massage can easily be done by your birth partner. Massaging the lower back can be especially effective. To promote relaxation, stroke gently but firmly with the flat of the hand, working towards the heart. Using lavender oil will help to ease pain, while mandarin will lift the spirits.
- **Visualization/meditation** Practise well in advance. Simple approaches include imagining a scene such as a peaceful, sunny beach as contractions begin.
- **Acupuncture** This can be used to control various aspects of labour, from calming fears to easing backache. For the latter, needles can be inserted at points in the lower back. Needles can also be attached to an electrical device called an acutens machine, letting you control the stimulation level yourself.
- **TENS** (Transcutaneous Electrical Nerve Stimulation). This straddles orthodox and natural approaches (see table opposite). It uses a small electronic device attached to electrodes placed either side of the spine. Electric current is used to block pain impulses travelling along nerves and to stimulate endorphins.

MONITORING THE BABY

With each contraction, the blood vessels supplying your baby with oxygen narrow, forcing the baby to hold its breath. Some babies cannot hold their breath for long and will become short of oxygen (distressed). If this happens for too long, they could suffer permanent damage or die.

During labour, the baby's heartbeat is monitored by the midwife, to detect any distress. In a low-risk pregnancy, a baby may be monitored for short spells by placing a Pinard stethoscope or an electronic ultrasound device on the mother's abdomen. In high-risk pregnancies, doctors may recommend continuous fetal monitoring during the latter part of the first stage of labour. There are two methods of continuous heart monitoring: external and internal.

In external monitoring, two belts are placed around the mother's abdomen. One holds the instrument that records the tightness and stretch of the abdomen during contractions, allowing the length and frequency of contractions to be measured. The other belt holds a transducer, which records the baby's heart rate. The belts are attached to a monitor, which records details of the baby's heartbeat and the mother's contractions.

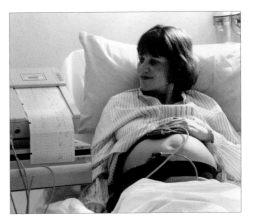

Here, an ultrasound scanner has been strapped to the mother's abdomen to monitor her baby's heartbeat.

With internal monitoring, once the cervix has dilated, a fetal scalp electrode is passed up through the woman's vagina and the end-point (a probe with a clip on the end) is fixed under the skin of the baby's scalp or buttocks. This allows a continuous read-out of the baby's heartbeat. If it slows for more than a minute or two, medical intervention may be needed.

If there is any sign of distress, a blood specimen can be obtained through a prick in the baby's scalp – fetal scalp sampling. The specimen's acidity reveals the degree of distress. If it is extreme, then immediate delivery, probably by Caesarean, will be carried out.

DEALING WITH MONITORING

While monitoring is highly advantageous for the baby's health, the machinery needed can create a clinical atmosphere. It may also mean that the mother cannot move about freely during labour and often requires her to lie down at an angle that is somewhat unnatural and difficult for childbirth. Always tell medical staff how you feel about the monitoring process so that the most satisfactory compromise can be reached.

However, there are active birth positions that you may be able to get into when attached to a monitor. Adjust the bed head to a comfortable sitting position, usually around a 25° angle. Bend your legs alternately for about 10 minutes, placing the sole of the foot of the bent leg against the inner thigh of the straight leg. You could also kneel on the bed and lean against the angled bed head, using pillows for support. Another position is resting on your side with one bent leg above the other and a pillow between your knees. If possible, swap between these positions every half hour or so, to create a rhythm that helps to relieve contraction pain.

The first stage of labour

During the first stage of labour, you should feel free to follow your instincts and do whatever feels right for you. You may find yourself rocking or swaying during contractions. Many women like to take a bath, finding the sensation of water to be pleasantly soothing.

Move around and try out new positions until you find the one or two that seem most comfortable. Any of the positions shown here may be right for you.

A lot of women like to keep moving around during the first stage of labour, getting into their favourite position each time a new contraction starts. Take one contraction at a time, and breathe your way through it, perhaps using imagery to help you. For example, you could try to visualize your cervix opening out like a flower.

THE TRANSITIONAL STAGE

This is the term for the short period of time at the end of the first stage of labour, just before moving into the second stage. It is the shortest part of labour, but it can be very intense and contractions can feel even more painful and seem to be absolutely relentless.

You may feel discouraged and find yourself not wanting to go on for much longer without additional pain relief. You may also be very emotional and perhaps irritable or bad-tempered. Your legs may start shaking and you might shiver; you may even need to vomit.

You may also get an urge to push, or bear down, though you shouldn't do this until the midwife has examined you and has confirmed that your cervix is fully dilated. Panting a little may help you resist the urge.

Whenever you feel that you just can't go on, remember that your baby will be born soon. Keep telling yourself to hang on, stay calm, and all will be well.

GOOD POSITIONS IN TRANSITION

It is difficult to find a comfortable position when you are in transition. Any position that you have found helpful up to this point is suitable for use now. You may like to kneel forward over a pile of cushions, or you may prefer to stand, sit, squat, or be held in a supported squat.

If the cervix has not yet fully dilated and you feel the urge to bear down, try kneeling on all fours: put your head down against the floor and your bottom up in the air. This position uses the force of gravity to help slow the baby down, while the cervix continues to dilate. This position also takes pressure off your lower back.

HELPING SOMEONE GIVE BIRTH
Remember that labour can be a traumatic and difficult time for a woman, so be prepared to deal with any strange or aggressive behaviour without getting offended. If she tells you to go away, stand aside, but do not go too far away. However useless you feel, you do have an important role.

Simple actions such as sponging your partner's face and holding her hand can help a lot. Don't be surprised if she shouts at you – and at anyone else around.

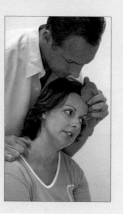

- Try to help her to relax, especially between the contractions.
- Help her to cool down with a water spray or moist sponge if she's hot.
- Wipe away perspiration from her face.
- Encourage her by telling her she's doing fine, never criticize her.
- Be alert to her moods and adapt to them.
- If she feels sick and says that she wants to throw up, get her a bowl quickly.
- If her legs begin to tremble, hold her legs firmly and offer her a pair of socks in order to keep them warm and so help her circulation.
- If she has backache, massage her lower back and offer her a hot-water bottle.
- If she says she wants to push or she starts to grunt and make pushing motions, tell the midwife immediately.
- Once the midwife has told her that she is fully dilated and she can push, let the midwife guide her through the pushing stage. Always do what the midwife tells you.
- Drink lots of water to keep yourself hydrated.

SIT

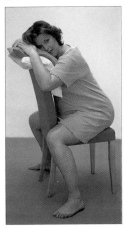

Sit astride a chair, facing its back, with knees apart and your back straight. Put a cushion against the back of the chair and lean against it. In this position, your body is vertical yet completely supported, and your pelvis is kept open.

STAND

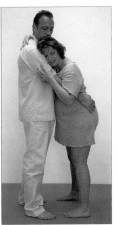

Stay upright and lean slightly forwards against your birth assistant. The downward force of gravity stimulates contractions and encourages the baby's descent. You may find it helpful to circle your hips. Your birth assistant can massage your lower back in this position, or rock you gently.

KNEEL

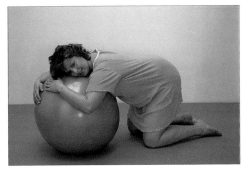

Kneel down and support yourself by leaning forwards against a nearby piece of sturdy furniture, over a pile of cushions or a big bean bag. You can also use a birthing ball for this.

SQUAT

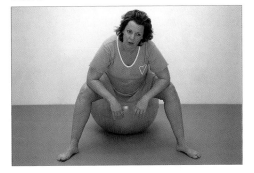

Squat on a low stool or birthing ball. This position tends to intensify contractions, as well as allowing the pelvis to open widely. It also encourages the baby's descent.

KNEEL ON ALL FOURS

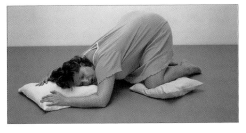

Kneel on all fours and rock back and forth during contractions. If they are very intense, kneel with your head against the floor and bottom in the air. Try moving your hips around, too.

LIE DOWN

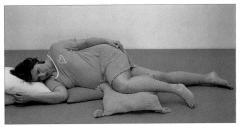

You may feel like lying down, particularly if you are getting tired. Try lying on your side, with your 'bump' well supported on cushions. It is not a good idea to lie on your back for any length of time, although this is fine for when you are being examined.

The second and third stages

When the cervix is fully dilated (about 10cm/4in), you have entered the second stage of labour. The second stage can be over in minutes or it may take up to two hours. It ends with the birth of the baby. Second-stage contractions are typically very strong, with the whole body engaged in a massive involuntary urge to bear down. This is a reflex, caused by the baby's head pressing on the pelvic floor and the rectum. Even if you had read nothing about the birth, you would know instinctively when to take a deep breath, thus lowering your diaphragm and exerting pressure on the uterus, which helps to push the baby out. Some women find the second stage easier than the first, although it may be difficult, especially if the baby is large or there are worries about tearing.

BEST POSITIONS FOR BIRTH

Pushing is harder work if you are lying on your back, because you are pushing the baby uphill. An upright, or semi-upright, position is therefore best for delivery, as gravity will help your efforts. Your pelvis should be open, and your pelvic floor and vaginal opening needs to be relaxed. Many women move about and change position throughout the second stage of labour, eventually finding the best position for them for birth. The following positions, shown opposite, are all suitable for the delivery:

- **Lying down** This position is good if you are feeling exhausted. Lie on your side with your head resting on a couple of pillows. Keep your legs open by holding the knee – your birth assistant can do this for you.

- **Sitting** Here, the woman sits propped up with plenty of bulky cushions, with her knees bent and apart, and her head dropped forwards towards her chest. This position lets her see the baby being born. However, it is an unnatural position for birth and unhelpful for the baby, so it is not the best one to use.

- **Kneeling** Many women choose to give birth in this position. Kneel on all fours, leaning over a bean bag or large cushion. The midwife receives the baby from behind. A kneeling position eases pressure on the perineum, allowing the soft tissues to expand and stretch as the baby is born.

- **Squatting** This is often found to be a good position. You can squat either while being supported from behind by one helper, or while being supported on either side by two helpers. Squatting opens up the pelvis to its maximum, relaxes the pelvic floor and uses the force of gravity. If squatting with one helper, your helper should stand, or preferably sit, behind you in a firm and stable stance. He should support you by taking your weight on his arms. Surrender completely to the contraction, bending your knees and spreading your feet apart so that the pelvis opens. This position usually encourages a rapid birth and is particularly suitable if there is any reason to speed up delivery, as in cases of fetal distress or a long labour. It is also helpful in a breech birth.

YOUR BABY EMERGES

Pushing a baby out is hard work. Try to do so smoothly and gradually, so all the vaginal muscles and tissues have the chance to stretch in order to allow the baby's head through without tearing or necessitating an episiotomy.

The first sign that the baby is entering the world is a bulging of the perineum and the anus. More and more of the baby's head then appears at the vaginal opening, which is known as crowning, at which point you may feel a stinging sensation as the baby pushes against your vagina. This sensation can be eased by deep breathing, or if an attendant holds a warm compress against the perineum, helping the tissues to stretch. Sometimes the baby will be born very quickly at this stage, with its head and body coming out in one contraction. The birth may also take place more slowly, over a number of contractions. Typically, as the baby's head emerges, it will turn its head to one side. Your contractions may cease briefly here, giving those attending you the chance to check that the umbilical cord is not wrapped around the baby's neck and, if it is, to reposition the cord more safely.

Your next contraction should see the baby's shoulders emerging, and once these are out, the rest of the baby's body will follow on swiftly, usually followed by gushing amniotic fluid.

SPEED OF DELIVERY

How fast delivery occurs depends on your position and that of the baby's head, as well as its size. If it is slow and you are in a lot of pain, medical staff will help you breathe the baby out gently in order to avoid a tear. If it is felt that you are likely to tear badly, the doctor will perform an episiotomy.

LYING

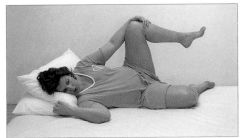

SITTING

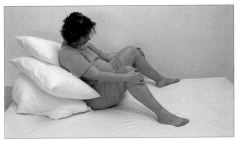

KNEELING

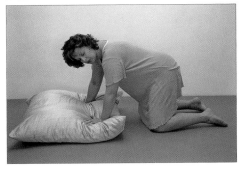

A SUPPORTED SQUAT

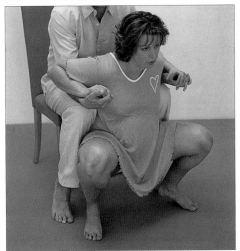

These pictures show four principal positions commonly adopted during the second stage of labour and delivery. The woman should be made as comfortable as possible with supportive cushions and allowed to swap between positions – she needs to find what is best and most comfortable for her.

YOUR BABY HAS ARRIVED

Caregivers will typically wrap the baby up and let you hold her immediately. Your baby may be breathing and crying as soon as he or she emerges, and may start to suckle virtually straight away.

If you are delivering twins, the procedures are the same. However, a twin delivery is more risky and complex, for the babies and the mother. There is an increased risk of fetal distress, and the likelihood of a Caesarean is higher with a twin delivery than with a single baby.

THE THIRD STAGE OF LABOUR

This stage occurs after delivery of the baby and is simply the expulsion of the placenta. When the baby is born, the uterus rests, but about 15 minutes later it starts to contract again, relatively painlessly, to expel the placenta and its membranes. You can help to push out the

Be prepared for a turbulent mix of emotions once the birth is over – relief, joy, shock, exhaustion and tearfulness are all perfectly normal reactions.

placenta yourself, both by squatting and also by putting the baby to the breast, which helps the uterus to contract. Medical staff will now carefully examine the placenta to make sure that absolutely all of it has been expelled, as leaving bits behind may lead to internal bleeding. Checks are then made for any large tears around the vulva area, which will have to be stitched.

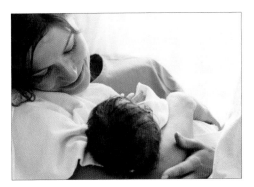

Medical interventions

Sometimes births go slowly or other problems develop. Medical staff may intervene to hasten the birth if they think there is any danger to the mother or baby.

DELIVERY BY FORCEPS

Forceps can be used to facilitate a speedier delivery. They look rather like big salad servers and are sometimes used to help the baby out in the second stage of labour, when the cervix is fully dilated and the baby's head has come down into the mother's pelvis but is not descending any further. They may also be used in cases of fetal or maternal distress. The forceps are easy to apply and cause no harm to the baby if applied properly, although the baby's head may be marked.

Your legs will be put in stirrups and a local anaesthetic injected into the perineum. An episiotomy (cut) is then done, and forceps inserted into the vagina and the blades cupped round the sides of the baby's head. The idea is that the mother then pushes, while the doctor pulls. Once the head is delivered, the forceps are removed and you can push the baby out normally.

VENTOUSE EXTRACTION

More than one in ten deliveries now involve the use of ventouse ('vacuum extraction' in the US). Like forceps, it is used to help speed the delivery. A suction cap is attached to the baby's head and suction is used to pull the baby out gently with each contraction as you push.

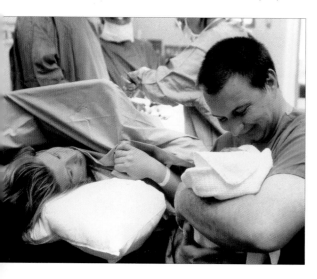

There are no risks to the baby and no drugs need to be used. The advantages of this method over forceps delivery is that the cervix does not need to be fully dilated, and it is perceived as a lesser intervention. The mother still has to do a fair measure of the pushing so she does not feel quite so outmanoeuvred by technology.

The disadvantage is that it can take time to apply enough suction. The baby may have a small bump on its head rather like a large bruised blister, which subsides after a day or two.

INDUCTION OF LABOUR

Sometimes, labour may need to be artificially induced. This is done by breaking of the waters and by giving the mother drugs, vaginally or intravenously. An induction may be done for the following reasons:
- The baby is overdue and the placenta is becoming less able to supply his or her needs.
- Raised blood pressure in the mother.
- Pre-eclampsia.
- Rhesus incompatibility.
- Bleeding in late pregnancy.
- Diabetes.
- The baby has stopped growing.

EPISIOTOMY

An episiotomy is a cut in the perineum. A local anaesthetic is given first, and then a cut is made – using scissors – into the skin and muscle at the lower end of the woman's vagina. After the birth, the cut is stitched up. Some people believe that a natural tear heals faster than a cut. An episiotomy may be needed in an assisted delivery, or if the woman is likely to be severely torn.

Getting into a good delivery position will help minimize the chances of episiotomy. If you would like to avoid having one, you should discuss this well in advance with the medical staff who are taking care of you and include it in your birth plan.

CAESAREAN SECTION

A Caesarean is a major surgical procedure whereby both baby and placenta are delivered through a cut in the mother's abdomen rather than through the vagina. It may be done under general anaesthetic or after an epidural, in

A delighted father holds his baby after birth by caesarian section. It takes a mother a little time to recover from this operation – as with any major surgery.

which case the mother will be awake when her baby is delivered. It is possible to have your labour companion with you during this operation if you have an epidural, but not if you have a general anaesthetic.

There are two types of Caesarean section: elective (by choice) and emergency.

- **Elective Caesareans** These are planned during pregnancy, usually because there is a medical or obstetric complication which means that a vaginal delivery is considered unsafe. Occasionally, women choose to have their baby delivered by Caesarean because of a personal preference.
- **Emergency Caesareans** A Caesarean may need to be done following complications that occur during labour, when your baby has become distressed and needs to be delivered speedily and safely.

Reasons for a Caesarean

There are many reasons why a Caesarean may be done. They include the following:

- If the baby is large and the mother's pelvis is small, making normal delivery virtually impossible.
- If the baby is premature, small or particularly vulnerable to distress.
- Pregnancies in which there is more than one baby.
- Babies who are in a position – such as a transverse lie – that makes normal delivery impossible.
- Inefficient contractions – which mean that the labour does not progress.
- Placental abruption, in which the placenta detaches itself from the wall of the uterus. This usually causes pain and bleeding, and necessitates the immediate delivery of the baby.
- Placenta praevia, in which the placenta is lying across the cervix and would be ruptured if labour were allowed to continue, causing dangerous bleeding, (known as antepartum haemorrhage).
- When the mother has a condition such as high blood pressure, pre-eclampsia or diabetes.
- When the umbilical cord has prolapsed and is presenting before the baby, obstructing the delivery.
- When an induction has not worked.
- If there are tumours such as fibroids or ovarian cysts, which will obstruct the baby's delivery.
- If the mother has had a pregnancy that ended in stillbirth, or if she has experienced a previous complicated and difficult delivery.
- If the baby becomes severely distressed.

WHEN DOCTORS INTERVENE

Medical intervention in labour is becoming more common: more than one in five births in the UK is by Caesarean delivery and about one in three in the USA. Some experts are concerned that medical staff can be too quick to intervene, and that some problems may resolve themselves naturally if allowed to do so. However, there is no doubt that intervention has saved the lives of many babies.

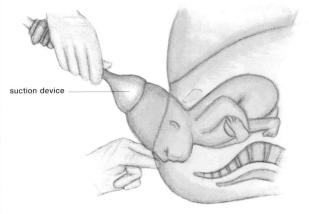

suction device

Assisted delivery may be necessary if the labour is progressing very slowly, if the baby becomes distressed or if the mother becomes so exhausted that she can no longer push. Here, a ventouse attached to the baby's head is used to help bring it out of the birth canal.

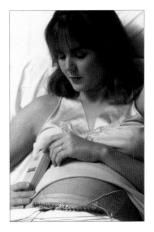

This woman is using a TENS pain-relief machine to cope with post-Caesarean discomfort. The stitched scar is from the operation.

Checklist of common problems

The last few weeks of pregnancy can be quite uncomfortable, and you may long to get the birth over with. Just remember that each day is bringing you a day closer to holding your baby. You may still be suffering from minor ailments, such as haemorrhoids or backache, at this stage. Natural therapies can often alleviate the worst of your symptoms and can also help you to cope with any tension. They may also help your baby to be better prepared for the birth – by virtue of you yourself being more relaxed.

Always discuss any natural remedies that you wish to take with your midwife – you will see her every week during the last month of pregnancy, so you will have plenty of opportunity to discuss any plans, anxieties or problems. If you decide to consult a complementary practitioner, make sure that you see only qualified therapists who are experienced in treating pregnant women. If you have any symptoms that are severe, prolonged or concern you, contact your midwife or doctor straight away. See page 145 for a list of emergency warning symptoms.

Breech baby   Most babies are in the buttocks-down (breech) position before 32 weeks but most will turn so that they are head-down for the birth. If your baby is in the breech position after 32 weeks, he or she may well turn spontaneously before the birth. There are also several natural methods that may help to encourage a breech or transverse baby to turn. Do not try any natural therapies if you are having twins or if you are ill.

- Take an hour-long walk each day. This may encourage your baby to move to the head-down position. Practising some yoga positions – such as 'the cat' – may also encourage the baby to move.
- Spend some time each day visualizing your baby moving into the right position. Make sure that you are feeling relaxed and comfortable when you do this – slow your breathing down and let go of any tension in your body first.
- The homeopathic remedy pulsatilla is sometimes used to encourage a baby to turn. Do not be tempted to self-prescribe; see a qualified homeopath to ensure that the remedy is suitable for you and that you take the correct dosage, and so that the homeopath can monitor the outcome.
- Moxibustion is a traditional Chinese method for turning breech babies. It is supported today by a variety of complementary practitioners, although it should be noted that doctors now do not attempt to

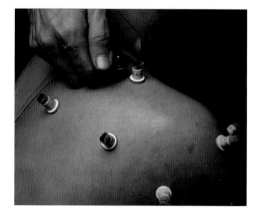

In moxibustion, a tiny amount of burning moxa is placed on different energy points on the body. In pregnancy, the points most typically used are located on the toes.

turn babies, as complications can result. Moxibustion involves lighting a stick of the herb moxa and holding it near acupuncture points on the outer corner of each little toe, or burning small amounts of the herb on the skin. The heat is said to stimulate the bladder energy channel, which is connected to the uterus. Moxibustion also has a general soothing effect. If you wish to try out moxibustion treatment, then you must seek the assistance of an experienced acupuncturist who is used to treating pregnant women, and do not attempt to do the treatment to yourself, or at home.

Late baby   Babies that are more than two weeks overdue are usually induced in hospital; induction may also be advised if your waters break early or you have high blood pressure. There are a number of natural methods that you can try if you have advance warning of an induction, but always talk to your midwife beforehand.

- Keep upright and keep moving around – activity can sometimes bring on contractions, but you should not overdo it.

> 66 Natural therapies can often alleviate the worst of your symptoms and can also help you to cope with any tension you are feeling. 99

- Make love. Having an orgasm can sometimes help to stimulate uterine contractions.
- Consult an acupuncturist: various points on the back can be stimulated, sometimes with electricity, in order to bring on contractions. You may need several treatments over the course of a week.
- See a reflexologist, who will work on various points on your feet.
- The homeopathic remedy caulophyllum is sometimes used to encourage contractions. However, you will need to see a qualified homeopath to ensure that this remedy is right for you, and so that your progress can be monitored.
- Try practising breathing techniques for relaxation, then visualize yourself going into labour. It can be helpful to do this daily.

Fear and anxiety Anxiety is a very common emotion for mothers-to-be. It is important that you discuss any specific worries that you have with your midwife. She may be able to put your mind at rest or advise you on any practical steps you can take. You might like to try the following suggestions:
- Practise relaxation techniques, such as yoga, Pilates, meditation or visualization. You may find it helps calm fears if you regularly visualize yourself and your baby surrounded by healing golden light.
- Consider complementary therapies, such as reiki, acupuncture or reflexology, all of which may help with stress or worry.

- Try Bach Flower Remedies, which are very gentle. Mimulus is good if you have specific, named fears, such as anxiety about the labour, while aspen is used for vague, unspecific fears. Red chestnut can be taken for excessive concern about the baby's well-being, and Rescue Remedy is excellent if you have moments of panic and tearfulness.
- Use essential oils such as lavender or rosewood, which can be very soothing in late pregnancy: use them in a burner or diluted in the bath or in a relaxing massage oil.

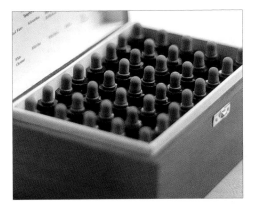

Bach Flower Remedies can be an effective natural way to relieve anxiety and fear. Keep them in a special box, separated out so each one retains its healing properties.

Instant calm

If you are feeling anxious or fearful, try this simple exercise to release tension and calm yourself down.

It serves to activate the energy channel of the heart, and it can feel very soothing and loving.

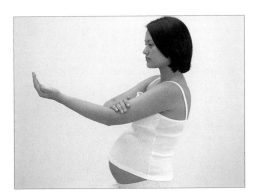

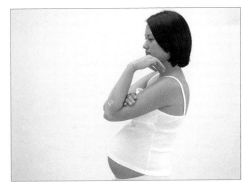

1 Hold your left arm straight out in front of you. Keep it loose rather than taut, and drop your shoulders to release tension here. Gently cup your right hand around the upper arm, just above the elbow.

2 Now, bring your forearm slowly towards your shoulder, until it rests upon your other hand. Breathe quietly for a few moments, focusing on your heart area, and feel a sense of release here.

Common Qs and As

Q: I felt my contractions starting and my partner took me to the hospital but they sent me home again, saying I wasn't ready yet. How could that happen?

A: It is possible to have contractions that mimic those of labour but are shorter and less pronounced. Once the hospital checks you out, they can tell immediately by how dilated your cervix is whether or not you have started true labour.

Q: I was planning a natural, drug-free birth but now my baby is going to be induced as I am two weeks overdue. I have heard that the contractions are more intense after an induction. Is that true?

A: Not necessarily. It depends on the individual woman, the reasons for the induction, how overdue she is, the drugs used, and how your particular hospital manages labour in respect of pain relief. It is better to induce a birth than to let the baby stay too long in the uterus, because there comes a point when the placenta can no longer nourish the baby.

Q: I had a very drawn-out, painful birth with my first child. My consultant has offered me an elective Caesarean. Do you think that this is a good idea?

A: It depends on the reasons why this has been offered. If the consultant knows that you are facing another lengthy and painful delivery, clearly it is sensible to elect for a Caesarean. If, for example, your pelvis and birth canal are too narrow to deliver a baby vaginally, the baby must be born by Caesarean. If, on the other hand, you are being offered a Caesarean to put your mind at rest, it may be better to try for a natural delivery first and only then to go for a Caesarean if there appears to be no other alternative. So, ask your consultant exactly why you have been offered a Caesarean, think it over, and base your decision on his or her advice.

Q: I am keen to give birth naturally and without pain relief. To me, it will not be a real birth if the doctors take control. How can I make sure that that this does not happen?

A: If everything goes well, you will not need medical intervention. You can give yourself the best possible chance of a natural birth by preparing well, practising your breathing exercises regularly, and by stating your wishes on a birth plan.

However, you cannot guarantee that your delivery will be straightforward. If anything does go wrong, you would be well advised to take advantage of all the skills and technology that modern medicine can offer. In the end, it is more important that your baby comes into the world safe and healthy than that you have the childbirth experience you hoped for.

Q: My underlying fears about coping with the financial aspects of having a baby are really crowding in on me now that the birth is imminent. How on earth are we going to pay for everything that the baby will need?

A: First of all, it is natural to start obsessing over certain worries once the baby is due, as this is a vulnerable time for you. Just focus on the fact that the most important thing for your baby is that he or she is with you. Your baby does not need much: just to be warm, fed and looked after. Think of positive solutions to any worries, such as asking your midwife if there are any outlets in your area where you can buy decent second-hand items.

Q: My partner seems quite relaxed about giving birth, but she has said she wants me to be there. I am not sure if I can handle this.

A: Many men feel this way. Some men really cannot cope and it would be unwise to try to persuade them. A few men have said that they never felt the same way about their partners once they had seen them giving birth. For other men, however, seeing their partner give birth is an absolute highlight of their life.

Explain exactly how you feel to your partner. It may be that when the time comes, you do feel able to be there. Alternatively, you could promise to be nearby during her labour, even if you feel unable to be in the room. You should also suggest that she takes someone else to support her through the labour. This will take the pressure off you, and you may then feel able to be there for some of the time.

Q: I have just broken up with my partner even though I am 36 weeks pregnant. I know that our decision to split is right for both of us but I am dreading giving birth alone.

A: You do not have to be alone. You can elect for one of your friends, a sister or another member of your family to be there with you. You could investigate the possibility and cost of a private room after giving birth for you and your new baby.

Try to arrange for extra help at home after the birth. Is there anybody who could come to help you for a couple of weeks after the birth? If not, it is a good idea to have at least one visit a day from friends or relatives. You should also tell your midwife your situation, as she may be able to arrange extra help.

Q: I have been asked to take part in a research project during my pregnancy and labour. Do I have to agree to this?

A: Many maternity units are committed to ongoing research projects to improve standards of clinical care. You may be asked to take part, but you do not have to. Many units are responsible for training doctors and midwives who need to conduct normal deliveries under close supervision by experienced midwives. You may refuse this option, but many women welcome the support that students can give them during labour.

Q: I am a single mother who is expecting my second child. I am worried that there will be prejudice about this from some of the other women on the delivery ward and from the nurses. How can I best cope with this?

A: Many women now have children when they are single: you are unlikely to be an unusual case. Nobody will be surprised if your birth partner is a friend or relative rather than the father.

You may find it helpful to discuss your anxieties with your midwife, and to note on your birth plan that you would like as much privacy as possible. Take a friend or relative to support you through the labour. Above all, remember it is your life and your baby: be happy and proud of the decisions you have made.

section three

natural therapies

Natural remedies may aid conception, alleviate ailments in pregnancy and speed recovery after the birth. However, they should be used with caution: many therapies need to be adapted for pregnant women, and others are not suitable in the first weeks. It is important to seek out a qualified practitioner who is used to working with pregnant women. Always tell the therapist if you are trying to conceive or are pregnant. Tell your doctor about any therapy you are receiving, and about any recommendations made to you.

Which therapy?

❝ A lovely way to revive spirits, lift your energy levels, help to reduce stress and irritability and promote a general feeling of well-being. ❞

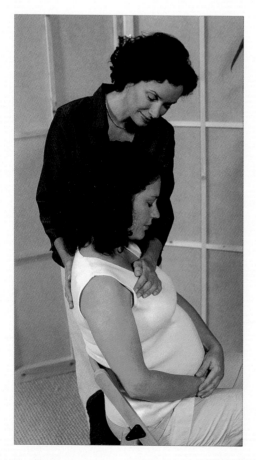

The following chapter brings together the various natural therapies that can be helpful during pregnancy. Herbalism uses the potency of plants to provide a natural way to treat illness and improve health. Many of the herbal remedies suggested for use in pregnancy have been used for centuries. Homeopathy is often used before pregnancy as a way to improve fertility and increase the chances of conception. Homeopathic treatments are also considered to be safe during pregnancy and can help to relieve some of the less pleasant symptoms such as morning sickness. Aromatherapy is another natural therapy that can help with morning sickness, and indigestion. Using essential oils as part of your daily routine, in the bath or in massage oils, is also a lovely way to revive spirits, lift your energy levels, help to reduce stress and irritability and promote a general feeling of well-being.

The physical natural therapies are also covered in this chapter. Massage is an ancient art that helps to

During a reiki session, healing energy is transmitted through the hands of the practitioner and into the recipient. It is a non-invasive therapy, and you remain clothed to receive treatment.

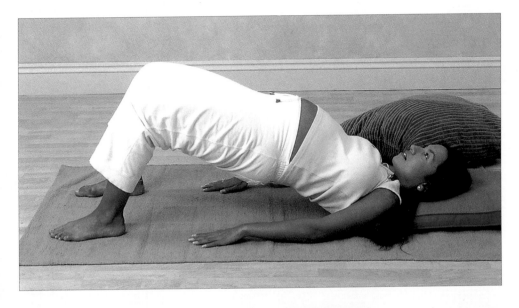

give comfort and to relieve pain, and is not only enjoyable and beneficial through pregnancy, it can also help in the delivery room. Shiatsu and reflexology use pressure points to improve the immune system, and can help to promote a high level of health and well-being that can help to support a woman through pregnancy, while acupuncture, osteopathy and chiropratic are thought to be able to also help with the new pressures on your organs, bones and muscles that your body is adapting to.

Gentle exercise or stretching routines, such as yoga, t'ai chi, pilates and Alexander technique help to keep your body fit and supple and keep your bone sturcture aligned for the birth, while hypnotherapy, reiki and meditation can help keep your spirits soothed and positive.

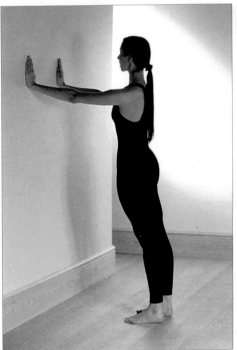

Top: Doctors and midwives commonly recommend yoga to pregnant women. This ancient form of exercise is known to foster general good health and improve posture and flexibility. Gentle lifts can help to extend the spine and release tension in the lower back. Place a flat cushion or block under your head for comfort. Yoga can also help to prevent or relieve common ailments such as backache, constipation and headaches.

Some Pilates exercises are similar to yoga postures, but they are repeated to create a flowing sequence. Like yoga, Pilates can help alleviate back pain and other problems common in pregnancy.

Herbalism

Many plants have therapeutic properties, which can be used to improve health and treat illness. Researchers are currently substantiating many of the claims made for herbal remedies. For the mother-to-be, herbs can offer support in all kinds of ways, from alleviating morning sickness to easing varicose veins.

Many modern medicines are derived from plants. Science has made it possible to isolate the active ingredients or recreate entirely synthetic versions. So, pharmaceutical drugs are now far removed from their natural origins. By contrast, herbal remedies use parts of the whole plant – roots, seeds, petals or leaves. Herbalists say that the subtle interaction of all the herb's ingredients promotes healing in a holistic (whole body) way rather than merely attacking a single symptom or disease as many laboratory-produced drugs do.

HERBAL MEDICINE AND PREGNANCY

Women have long used herbal remedies to alleviate the discomforts of pregnancy, prepare the body for childbirth, and aid recovery afterwards. Herbalists say that remedies can also be used to enhance fertility.

Herbal medicines are usually gentler than chemical ones, but this is not always the case. It is important to bear in mind that herbal remedies can have powerful effects. This is very important during pregnancy, when many herbs should not be used. It is not a good idea to self-prescribe herbal remedies, particularly if you are trying to conceive or are pregnant. See a qualified medical herbalist for advice.

SEEING A HERBALIST

When you see a herbalist, a medical history will be taken and you will be given a physical examination. You should tell your practitioner about any drugs you are taking since they may interact badly with natural remedies; for the same reason, tell your doctor about any remedies you are given. A medical herbalist will advise you on your diet and lifestyle

SAFETY REMINDERS
- Never take a herbal remedy unless you are sure that it is safe. Consult a qualified herbalist for advice.
- Talk to your doctor or midwife before taking any herbal remedies or supplements in pregnancy.
- Do not exceed the recommended dosage.
- Contact your practitioner or doctor immediately if you suffer any ill effects.

as well as prescribing remedies for your individual needs. You will usually have at least one follow-up appointment; often several sessions will be necessary.

SELF-HELP HERBAL REMEDIES

A few herbs are gentle enough to be used in infusion form during pregnancy. In the first trimester, ginger tea may alleviate morning sickness and aid the digestion. Later on, dandelion, meadowsweet, lime flower and nettle can be helpful. Drink no more than three cups of herbal tea a day.

Herbal ointments, compresses and poultices can ease symptoms relating to pregnancy, birth and breastfeeding. For example, calendula cream is often recommended for cracked nipples, and witch hazel can help promote healing of the perineum. Some plants are used whole: cabbage leaves are often used to soothe sore breasts.

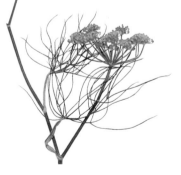

Fennel is a good remedy for indigestion, but like many herbs it can be harmful if taken in large quantities during pregnancy.

SOME COMMON HERBS TO AVOID

• aloe vera	• cottonroot	• pennyroyal
• angelica	• devil's claw	• pokeroot
• arbor vitae	• feverfew	• pulsatilla
• barberry	• golden seal	• rue
• black cohosh	• greater celandine	• sassafras
• bloodroot	• juniper	• shepherd's purse
• blue cohosh	• lady's mantle	• tansy
• broom	• mistletoe	• wild yam
• bugleweed	• mugwort	• wormwood
• comfrey		• thyme

Homeopathy

This gentle therapy can help with many of the physical symptoms and difficult emotions experienced while trying to conceive and during pregnancy. The remedies are derived from natural substances, and aim to stimulate the body's capacity for healing and restore well-being.

Homeopathy is based on the idea that 'like cures like': so a substance that causes illness can also be used to cure it. The remedies have been so diluted that only the merest trace of the active ingredient remains. In this state, they are far too weak to cause harm, but homeopaths believe that the minute dose can promote self-healing and cure the very symptoms that it may cause if taken in large amounts. Some doctors are sceptical about homeopathic remedies, but others accept that they can have good results. Some have trained in this therapy and offer it to patients as an adjunct to orthodox medical care.

Homeopathic remedies are considered very safe in pregnancy. They can help to relieve many ailments, such as morning sickness, and to speed recovery after the birth. Self-help remedies are available from many pharmacies, but it can be difficult to choose exactly the right one for you. For this reason, it is much better to consult a homeopath.

SEEING A HOMEOPATH

A homeopath will take a full personal and medical history during the first session, which can last two hours. People are often surprised by the number and type of questions they are asked. However, the homeopath needs to build up a picture of your habits and preferences as well as your mental, physical and emotional make-up. This information enables him or her to assess your 'constitutional type'.

Homeopaths consider both the patient's constitution and symptoms when choosing from the 2000 remedies at their disposal. You will be given instructions on how to take the remedies, and may also be given advice about your diet and lifestyle. A follow-up appointment is usually arranged; often several sessions are necessary.

EFFECTIVE HOMEOPATHY

- See a homeopath who is experienced in treating pregnant women; tell him or her if you are pregnant or are trying to conceive.
- Follow the homeopath's instructions when taking the remedy: peppermint, coffee and tea can nullify the effect, and you should avoid drinking or eating for 15 minutes after taking a remedy.
- Contact your homeopath if your symptoms worsen (this may be part of the healing process).
- Tell your doctor about any remedies you take, and report any unusual symptoms.

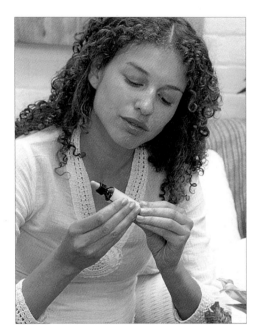

Flower remedies are a useful 'instant cure', and can be used to help resolve uncomfortable emotions, such as self-doubt, anxiety or low spirits.

BACH FLOWER REMEDIES

The Bach Flower Remedies are homeopathic remedies preserved in grape alcohol. Plant based, they are designed to help with negative feelings or states of mind. The most popular is Rescue Remedy, which is used for panic, tearfulness or shock. The remedies are available from health-food shops and pharmacies, and are usually self-prescribed.

To take a flower remedy, place a few drops in a glass of water and sip. Repeat several times a day if you are struggling with a recurring emotion. Flower remedies are preserved in alcohol, but you take only a tiny amount so they are safe for use in pregnancy. See your doctor if you are at all unsure about whether or not you should use them.

Aromatherapy

Aromatherapists use aromatic oils extracted from herbs and flowers to promote well-being. Certain oils have a wonderfully relaxing effect, which is very helpful throughout pregnancy. Others can help to relieve conditions such as the indigestion that is common in pregnancy, or lift spirits during labour.

Aromatherapy oils have wonderful aromas, and they are very pleasurable to use. They can be a gentle and effective way of boosting general health and treating minor ailments.

We do not know exactly how essential oils work, but it is thought that the scents trigger a reaction in smell receptors in the nostrils, which send messages to the brain. When the oils are used in massage, they also penetrate the skin and have a direct effect on the nerve endings here.

Some of the oils have proven medicinal qualities: tea tree, for example, is an antiseptic, antifungal and antibacterial agent, while chamomile has antispasmodic and antidepressant properties. Lavender is one of the most versatile oils: it helps with stress, insomnia, migraine and headaches, and it can also promote healing after a burn.

BENEFITS OF AROMATHERAPY

Aromatherapy is believed to be most helpful in treating long-term conditions, or recurring illnesses. Practitioners say that it can help to alleviate stress and related problems, including depression, headaches and insomnia. It may also relieve the pain of long-term conditions such as arthritis and may help skin problems such as eczema.

Most people find that aromatherapy's main benefit is relaxation. It can also help to induce general feelings of well-being, reduce fatigue and relieve backache.

In pregnancy, essential oils can be used to help the circulation, and so reduce the likelihood of varicose veins and haemorrhoids. Aromatherapy massage helps to

SOME OILS TO AVOID IN PREGNANCY		
• aniseed	• fennel	• pennyroyal
• basil	• hyssop	• peppermint
• birch	• juniper	• rosemary
• bitter almond	• marjoram	• sage
• camphor	• mugwort	• savory
• cedarwood	• myrrh	• tansy
• cinnamon bark	• nutmeg	• thyme
• clary sage	• oregano	• wormwood
• cypress	• parsley	• wintergreen

maintain the elasticity of the skin, thus helping to prevent stretchmarks. Minor ailments such as constipation and heartburn may also be helped by essential oils.

However, many essential oils are not suitable for use during pregnancy, because they may stimulate the uterus, causing miscarriage. Never use an oil unless you have checked that it is safe in pregnancy; the oils listed in the box above should definitely be avoided. It may be safest to avoid using essential oils entirely in the first trimester; see page 124 for good oils to use in the second trimester.

SEEING AN AROMATHERAPIST

Aromatherapists are usually trained masseurs. During the first session, a practitioner will ask you about your medical history and any problems you are experiencing. You should say if you are trying to conceive, or are already pregnant. If this is the case, it is probably best to see an aromatherapist who regularly works with conceiving or pregnant women.

The therapist will select which oils to use, and ask you to smell them to check that you like the aromas. Up to five oils may be used, and they will be blended in a carrier, such as almond oil. You will be asked to undress and lie on a massage couch. The therapist will then massage your whole body, smoothing the oils into your skin. The massage usually lasts an hour, and you should be given a few minutes to rest at the end. Your therapist may give you advice on using oils at home.

SELF-HELP AROMATHERAPY

Essential oils are widely available, and they can easily be used at home to enhance general well-being. To treat particular disorders (in conjunction with conventional

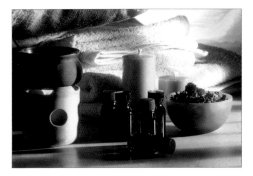

One of the gentlest ways to use essential oils is to heat them in a vaporizer. Their scent will fill a room and have an uplifting or relaxing effect upon everyone in it.

medical treatment), you may need to consult a professional aromatherapist. The following methods can be used for self-help at home.

BATHS

Aromatherapy baths are wonderfully relaxing, and can help to ease tension, and relieve backache and aching muscles. A warm bath with a soothing oil such as Roman chamomile before bedtime can promote restful sleep. Medicinal oils such as sandalwood and lavender can be used to ease cystitis and thrush (if pregnant, use only after 16 weeks).

Mix four to six drops of essential oil with a carrier oil or whole milk, then add to a full bath (not to running water). Lie back in the bath and breathe deeply, for 10–15 minutes.

FOOT AND HAND BATHS

An aromatic footbath can be a relaxing end to the day. You can also use a hand or foot bath to treat localized aches and pains, foot problems and swelling.

Mix eight to ten drops of essential oil in a carrier, then add to a large bowl of hand-hot water. Soak the feet or hands for 10–15 minutes; have a boiled kettle to hand so that you can top up with more hot water. Dry thoroughly. Smooth diluted essential oils over the skin, then wrap in a towel for 15 minutes, for a superb moisturizing treatment.

MASSAGE

Self-massage is a great way of applying essential oils, and can help with stress, skin complaints and fluid retention. It is often recommended in later pregnancy as a way of preventing stretchmarks. An essential oil should always be well-diluted in a vegetable oil, such as jojoba, sesame or almond: use a dilution of one drop per 5ml (1 tsp) base oil (or per 10ml (2 tsp) if you are pregnant).

COMPRESSES

Aromatherapy compresses can be used as to treat bruises, varicose veins, haemorrhoids, sprains, burns and scalds: lavender is often a good oil to use here. Use a warm

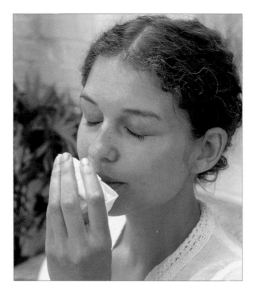

For instant relief, put a couple of drops of essential oil on a tissue and inhale. Tea tree is good for easing cold symptoms; sandalwood may alleviate anxiety.

compress for aching and pain, and a cold one if there is any heat or swelling. Dilute about eight drops of essential oil in a carrier, then add to a bowl of warm or ice-cold water. Drop in a small towel or flannel and soak for a few moments. Wring it out and hold over the affected area.

INHALATION

Another good way of treating stress, insomnia and colds is by inhalation. The simplest method is to put two drops of essential oil on to a tissue, and inhale. Slip a tissue with Roman chamomile on it under your pillowcase at night if you are finding it hard to sleep. For a steam inhalation, put five drops of essential oil into a bowl of hot water. Cover your head and bowl with a towel, and breathe (eyes closed).

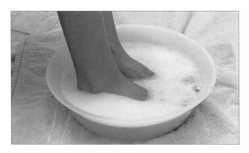

A footbath is a lovely treat at the end of the day: add your favourite essential oils to warm water, then relax. Try ginger and mandarin for a warming, reviving combination.

> **SAFE AROMATHERAPY**
> - Never apply an essential oil directly to your skin – always dilute it in a carrier first: use one drop per 5ml (1 tsp) carrier; one drop per 10 ml (2 tsp) if you are pregnant.
> - Only use oils that you know to be safe – if you are not sure, check with a professional aromatherapist.
> - Do a patch test before use: apply diluted oil to a small area on the inside of your wrist, then wait 24 hours without washing it to check you have no reaction. Women may be more sensitive when pregnant, so repeat a patch test at this time.

Massage

Touch has been used to enhance health for thousands of years and is a powerful way of giving comfort and relieving pain: we instinctively hug a friend in distress or rub an aching limb. Massage is a leading touch therapy that can be especially helpful as a pain-relief tool in the delivery room.

The term 'massage' covers many different therapies. On the one hand, there is purely physical Western massage, which works on the muscles. On the other, there are forms of Eastern pressure massage, which seek to enhance energy flow along invisible pathways in the body. These include shiatsu and acupressure. Massage techniques also form an important element of therapies such as osteopathy, aromatherapy and reflexology.

SWEDISH MASSAGE

In the West, most therapists practise Swedish massage. This system was devised by a Swedish gymnast, Per Henrik Ling, in the late 18th century. The techniques include:

- **Stroking** (effleurage) to relax. Firmer strokes are used to stimulate the circulation and release muscular tension.
- **Kneading** (petrissage) which soothes tense muscles and increases blood flow to particular areas. It can be used to relax deep muscles, such as those of the shoulders.
- **Friction** in which small, circular movements are made with the pads of the thumbs. It is used to break down areas of muscular spasm.
- **Percussion** in which fast, rhythmic movements are performed with the sides of the hands on fleshy parts of the body. It should be avoided during pregnancy.

RECEIVING A MASSAGE

To receive a Swedish massage, you'll be asked to undress and lie on a special couch. However, you can keep your underwear on if you wish. Towels will be placed over any areas of your body not being massaged. The therapist will usually massage your whole body, but may spend longer on some areas and leave out others. He or she will use oil or cream to prevent any dragging of the skin. The session typically lasts an hour, and you will usually be left to relax for a few minutes at the end.

Benefits of Swedish massage

There has been a great deal of research into massage, and most doctors accept that it promotes general good health. In pregnancy, it is good for backache and joint pain, and its relaxing effects mean it can help with anxiety, depression, blood pressure and digestive problems, as well as stress-related complaints such as headaches or insomnia. Stroking the lower back during labour can help to soothe pain and aid relaxation.

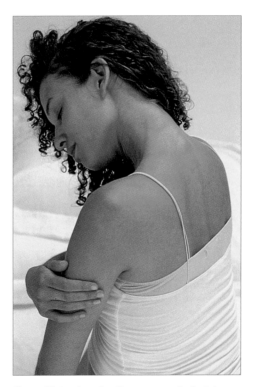

Pleasurable touch on the skin encourages the body to release endorphins, natural pain-killing chemicals. These help to induce feelings of happiness and well-being, and are one reason why massage can be helpful during labour.

Effective massage in pregnancy

Check with your doctor or midwife before having massage in pregnancy. Seek out a therapist who is experienced in treating pregnant women.

- Always tell the therapist that you are pregnant.
- You should not have deep pressure on the abdomen or lower back.
- Varicose veins, bruises or lumps must not be massaged.
- Do not have a massage if you have an infection or fever or if you feel unwell.
- Drink plenty of water and avoid strenuous activity afterwards. If possible, rest.

Shiatsu

The term shiatsu is Japanese for 'finger pressure'. Practitioners work to stimulate pressure points associated with the vital organs, in order to encourage a good flow of chi (energy) around the body and promote better health. Uses in pregnancy include dealing with backache and raised blood pressure, and pain-relief during labour.

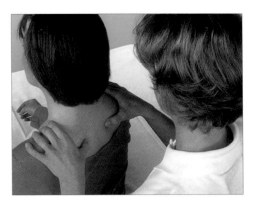

Many Japanese people undergo regular shiatsu treatment, sometimes as often as once a week. They believe that it can help to prevent illness as well as detect and treat any symptoms early on. Shiatsu is a holistic system of healing, meaning that the whole person – mind, body and spirit – is treated at once. However, it can also be used to treat problems such as back pain, digestive problems, insomnia, depression, migraine and toothache, and to help strengthen the immune system.

Shiatsu should generally be kept simple and non-specific during the first three months of pregnancy, when all the baby's organ systems are developing. To be safe, you should see a practitioner who specializes in working with pregnant women. A shiatsu practitioner can attend the birth to help with pain relief, or can teach the father or another birth assistant some simple pain-relief techniques with which to support the mother during her labour.

SEEING A PRACTITIONER

At the first consultation, a shiatsu practitioner should take a detailed medical and lifestyle history from you. He or she will take your pulses: there are six at each wrist, each associated with a vital organ. He or she may also feel your abdomen, which can give clues to problems elsewhere. The sound of your voice, your appearance and posture will also be observed.

To receive treatment, you keep your clothes on and lie on a mat on the floor. The practitioner will apply pressure to points all over the body using a variety of techniques. Sometimes the bulb of the thumb is used, sometimes the fingertips, and sometimes the palm or the heel of the hand. An elbow may also be used or perhaps a forearm or a knee. The practitioner may also perform gentle stretching or rocking movements.

How hard the therapist applies pressure depends on many things, including the part of the body being treated, how you react and whether you require a tonic or a sedating effect. Pressure is applied for a few seconds at a time and is repeated several times at each spot.

You can learn how to apply finger pressure at home after learning the techniques from a trained shiatsu practitioner.

Shiatsu practitioners often use finger pressure (above) to activate an energy point, but they also use the whole hand, the forearm (below), the elbows or the feet.

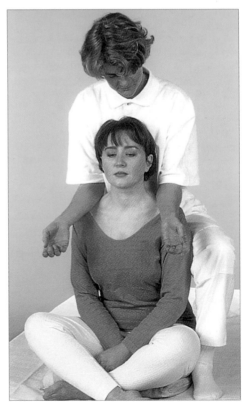

Acupuncture
Practised for centuries in China as a means of promoting good health and treating illness, acupuncture is now widely available in the West, and most doctors accept that it has positive effects. Acupuncture can help with fertility problems and with many pregnancy-related disorders.

Acupuncture is based on the idea that chi (energy) flows along invisible pathways – known as meridians – in the body. When this energy flows freely, good health and well-being are maintained. Illness and emotional upset are said to be a result of blockages or imbalances in the circulation of this energy.

In acupuncture, fine needles are inserted into certain points on the meridians to correct imbalances and improve the flow of chi. Acupuncture is usually practised holistically, so its ultimate aim is to bring the body back to its natural state of equilibrium. However, it can be used to treat specific complaints, such as back pain and digestion problems.

PREGNANCY AND ACUPUNCTURE
Acupuncture can relieve many pregnancy-related ailments, including morning sickness, constipation and poor circulation. It may also help with fertility problems or recurrent miscarriage. It is very important that you tell your practitioner that you are pregnant or trying to conceive, since some points should not be stimulated in that case. For this reason, it is best to choose a qualified practitioner who is experienced in working with pregnant women.

SEEING AN ACUPUNCTURIST
On your first visit, a full medical and personal history will be taken: your practitioner will ask you many questions about, for example, your appetite, bowel movements, sleep and energy levels. Your pulses will be taken and your tongue will be checked. Your practitioner will also observe other details, such as the sound of your voice and the colour of your skin.

THE ACUPUNCTURE MERIDIANS
There are 14 major meridians in the body, and most of them are linked to specific organs. Points on the meridians can be used to treat problems in different areas of the body. For example, the kidney, stomach and spleen meridians serve to nourish the uterus and the baby during pregnancy.

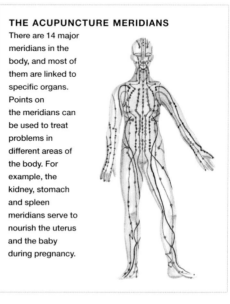

You lie on a massage couch to receive treatment. The acupuncturist will insert needles into different points on your body – this is swift and painless. Sometimes, the needles will be left in place for several minutes.

Most people have weekly or fortnightly sessions to start with, but you may need only occasional sessions once treatment has been established.

OTHER ACUPUNCTURE TECHNIQUES
Finger pressure can be used instead of needles to stimulate acupoints. Acupressure is less invasive than needling, and it can be used for self-help. Some acupuncturists will advise you and your partner on which points to stimulate during labour.

Another technique is moxibustion, where the herb moxa (mugwort) is burned on energy points. This can exert a profoundly soothing effect.

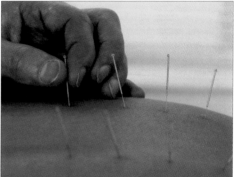

You may feel a slight tingling when an acupuncture needle is inserted, but it should not hurt.

Reflexology

Reflexologists believe that every body part is linked by an energy pathway to a specific point on the foot, and that finger pressure on the feet can detect and treat health problems. A range of pregnancy-related problems can be tackled, from backache to relieving pubic joint discomfort prior to the birth.

Reflexology is good for promoting general well-being and relaxation. It can also help alleviate complaints such as back pain, digestive problems and constipation. Some midwives use the techniques to promote regular contractions and for pain relief during labour. One study found that reflexology could reduce a woman's need for pain relief, and cut the length of labour by as much as half.

Many women enjoy reflexology during pregnancy, but it should be used only after the first 12 weeks. Some areas – the heels, Achilles tendons and ankles – should not be worked on at all because this can induce contractions. For this reason, it is important to see a practitioner who understands the needs of pregnant women.

SEEING A REFLEXOLOGIST

On your first visit, your practitioner will ask about your medical history, symptoms, diet, lifestyle and any other therapies you are receiving. You will be asked to take off your footwear and sit on a chair or couch. The reflexologist will massage your feet to relax them – which can be deeply pleasurable. After the initial massage, every area of your foot will be pressed and massaged in turn.

Some areas may feel very sensitive – this is said to be a sign of imbalance. Tender points will receive extra massage

WHAT THE DOCTORS SAY

Many doctors accept that reflexology can have a deeply relaxing effect. This may be the result of pressure on the nerve endings, of which there are more than 7000 in the feet. In addition, massage helps to stimulate the circulation of blood, which improves the delivery of oxygen and nutrients to different areas of the body.

If you are having reflexology treatment, you should let your doctor know. It is also important that you continue to report any unusual symptoms.

in order to stimulate energy flow to the corresponding area of the body. This can sometimes be painful, but tenderness should ease as the massage continues. The reflexologist will adjust the pressure, depending on your sensitivity.

Your reflexologist may show you some techniques that you can practise at home. The hands also contain a 'map' of the body, and these are often recommended for self-help because they are easier to treat than the feet.

Like most complementary therapists, reflexologists seek to help the body to heal itself. Regular sessions are often recommended in order to maintain well-being.

FOOT REFLEXES

Reflexologists work systematically round the foot, and they always treat both feet. Tender or sensitive points may receive extra massage to encourage healing in the related part of the body.

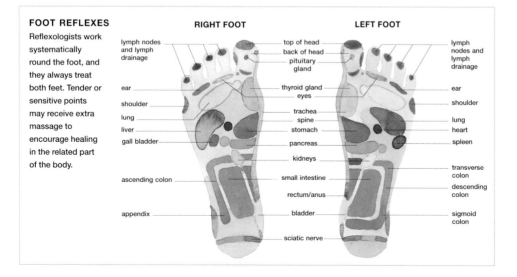

RIGHT FOOT

lymph nodes and lymph drainage
ear
shoulder
lung
liver
gall bladder
ascending colon
appendix

LEFT FOOT

top of head
back of head
pituitary gland
thyroid gland
eyes
trachea
spine
stomach
pancreas
kidneys
small intestine
rectum/anus
bladder
sciatic nerve

lymph nodes and lymph drainage
ear
shoulder
lung
heart
spleen
transverse colon
descending colon
sigmoid colon

Osteopathy

Osteopaths believe that good health depends on the proper functioning of our muscles and joints. They use manipulation and massage to correct imbalances caused by injury, poor posture and stress. Their approach can be especially helpful in easing the digestive problems often experienced in pregnancy.

Most people see an osteopath because of backache, but the therapy can also help with other physical problems, such as headaches, digestive disorders and breathing difficulties. Osteopathy is safe in pregnancy, but you should be sure to choose a qualified practitioner with experience in treating pregnant women: osteopathic techniques can be dangerous if performed by an untrained practitioner.

You should always tell your osteopath that you are pregnant, or if you are trying to conceive, and let your doctor know that you are having treatment. Some doctors will be able to recommend an osteopath to you.

WHAT TO EXPECT

An osteopath will take a full medical and lifestyle history on your first visit, and he or she will also give you a physical examination. People are usually asked to undress to their underwear so that the osteopath can observe the body's framework.

The practitioner will use gentle touch – palpation – to detect any areas of weakness or strain in your body. You may be asked to perform simple exercises while standing, sitting and lying on a couch so that your osteopath can check your posture, muscle tone and breathing technique. Sometimes other medical tests – such as blood tests – will be carried out to help with diagnosis.

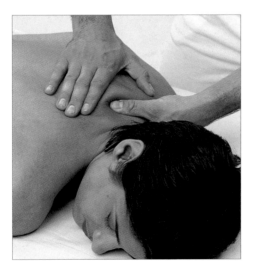

CRANIAL OSTEOPATHY

Some osteopaths practise cranial osteopathy. This gentle technique focuses on the delicate manipulation of the bones of the skull in order to improve the circulation of blood and fluid in the head. It is said to help many of the same conditions as conventional osteopathy, and it is often used to help babies who are suffering from sleeplessness, colic or birth trauma.

In cranial-sacral therapy, subtle pressure is applied to the head and the base of the spine. Therapists are aiming to regulate the flow of cerebrospinal fluid, which affects the whole nervous system and thus the functioning of the body. Many people find this therapy deeply relaxing, and it can help with insomnia, backache and headaches.

Doctors tend to be more sceptical of these gentle techniques than of conventional osteopathy, but many patients report good results. Some cranial-sacral therapists may not have undergone the rigorous training of an osteopath. Seek treatment only from qualified osteopaths or chiropractors with experience in dealing with pregnant women and babies.

You lie on a massage couch for treatment. The osteopath will then carry out a series of manipulations, which are tailored to your individual needs. The techniques used include massage, limb stretches and sharp thrusts. You may hear a clicking sound as a joint slips back into alignment, but you should not feel any pain.

The first session can last an hour but subsequent treatments are usually 20–30 minutes long. Most people need several sessions, and you may also be given instructions on exercises to do at home.

Pregnant women are often advised to have regular sessions to help them adjust to changes in their posture as the baby grows. This is a good way of preventing and treating lower back pain. Some osteopaths say that regular treatment during pregnancy can help to make the birth easier.

Many people are nervous of the clicking sound that occurs when an osteopath pops a joint back into place. However, this should not be painful. Treatment also includes gentle massage and stretches, which are very relaxing.

Chiropractic

Chiropractors use their hands to work on the spine, believing that a well-aligned spine is vital in maintaining good health because it supports the rest of the body and houses the central nervous system. Its main use for pregnant women is to ease back problems caused by carrying a growing baby.

Chiropractic is mainly used to help with back and neck problems. Gentle manipulation of the spine is performed to improve posture, and to correct any kinks caused by injury or stress. Regular sessions of chiropractic can help pregnant women to adjust their posture so that they cope better with the strain of carrying a growing baby. It may also alleviate pelvic problems and make childbirth easier.

Chiropractics say that working on the spine can also help seemingly unrelated problems. This is because nerve pathways branch off the spine at different levels and travel to all areas of the body. Distortions in the spine can affect nerve function, and may therefore be the cause of problems elsewhere. Fatigue, indigestion, constipation and headaches may all be helped by chiropractic treatment.

SEEING A CHIROPRACTOR

Your first session will focus mainly on the diagnosis of your problem. A full medical history will be taken and you will also be asked questions about your work, lifestyle and diet, and any exercise that you do.

You will be asked to undress to your underwear so that the chiropractor can observe your closely. If you feel embarrassed, you may be able to wear a gown. The chiropractor will observe your posture as you sit, stand and

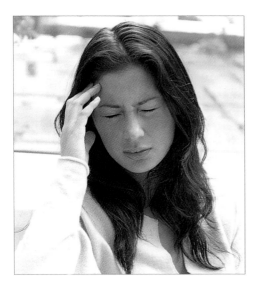

THE ORTHODOX VIEW

Chiropractic is widely accepted as a useful technique for many back problems. However, many doctors are sceptical about claims that it can help with problems such as digestive disorders.

OTHER FORMS OF CHIROPRACTIC THERAPY

Practitioners of McTimoney or McTimoney-Corley chiropractic use many of the same techniques as conventional chiropractors, but they tend to work in a more gentle way.

McTimoney chiropractors agree that the distortions in the spine are the principle cause of ill health but they think that all other joints should be treated as well. They examine and work on the whole musculoskeletal system in each treatment session. McTimoney-Corley chiropractic is different again: practitioners manipulate the vertebrae using their fingertips, and they do not practise the more vigorous techniques of chiropractic. They emphasize the importance of self-help exercises.

lie down, and you will be asked to perform some simple exercises. The chiropractor may check the mobility of your joints by asking you to perform a few stretches. He or she will then examine your spine to detect any misalignments or areas of stiffness, as well as the source of any pain you may have. Other checks, such as blood pressure or reflex tests, may also be performed.

You will be asked to lie on a massage couch for treatment. The chiropractor will use a variety of techniques to realign the vertebrae: these include gentle stretches, precise thrusts and massage. You may ache or feel rather stiff afterwards, but the treatment should not hurt.

Most people need several sessions of chiropractic, but you may start to see some improvement in your condition after just one treatment.

Chiropractors are able to treat much more than just back problems. For example, regular headaches and bouts of indigestion may also be relieved by releasing built-up tension in the spine.

The Alexander technique

In this therapy, gentle posture-improving exercises show clients how to stand, sit and move. This eases pressure on muscles and joints and is held to relieve all kinds of mental and physical problems, the main one in pregnancy being back strain from carrying a heavy 'bump'.

As children, we have naturally good posture. However, as we grow up we tend to develop bad habits: we may slouch or cross our legs when we sit, stand with our weight pushed on to one leg, and twist the back when lifting. Our mental state, too, can affect our posture: when stressed we may lift the shoulders and hold them in a state of tension, for example, and the problem may be compounded by poor sitting technique and by working at a computer.

Eventually, these habits, known as 'patterns of misuse', become ingrained. Poor posture becomes the norm, and we no longer notice when we are placing the body under strain. Over time, poor posture causes damage to our muscles and joints, and our digestive, respiratory and circulatory systems may also be affected.

The Alexander technique helps you to get in touch with your body and to become more sensitive to the demands you are placing upon it.

HOW THE ALEXANDER TECHNIQUE WORKS

The Alexander technique is a way of training people to become aware of bad habits, so that they can start to stand and move in a naturally better way. It emphasizes aligning the head with the spine, so that the neck remains free of strain. The technique is best taught on a one-to-one basis. During the first session, you will be asked to adopt various positions and perform simple movements, while the teacher observes how you stand, sit and move.

You will be asked to lie down, and the teacher will make subtle adjustments to your limbs, head, pelvis and so on, so that you can experience good posture for yourself.

During the classes, the teacher will show you how to perform a whole range of everyday tasks in the Alexander way – such as answering the telephone, getting in and out of a chair, writing a letter, answering the phone, carrying a bag, and walking. The lessons will combine gentle manipulations with verbal instructions. The aim is to build your awareness of how to move correctly – called 'thought in action'. Eventually, you will be able to bring this awareness into daily life, and maintain good posture.

Sessions are usually given once or twice a week for several months; thereafter top-up sessions may be needed.

HOW IT HELPS

The Alexander technique is accepted as an effective way of treating many back and neck problems. Practitioners say that posture work can also help people to become more resistant to stress. Other conditions that may be helped by the technique include depression, anxiety, headaches, high blood pressure, infertility, breathing problems, fatigue, arthritis, back pain and digestive disorders.

PREGNANCY AND THE ALEXANDER TECHNIQUE

The Alexander technique can help pregnant women adapt to their changing shape as the baby grows. This may prevent the backache that is commonly associated with pregnancy.

It will also help you to prepare for the birth. The Alexander technique teaches women to stay upright during labour – in a squatting position – so that the force of gravity can assist the baby's passage. An Alexander teacher will help you to learn how to cope with contractions without tensing the body. This can make childbirth easier, since tension increases pain.

Pilates

This is an effective form of body conditioning, which also develops mental awareness and an effective breathing technique. Some Pilates exercises are similar to yoga postures, but they are repeated to create a flowing sequence. Like yoga, Pilates can help alleviate back pain and other problems common in pregnancy.

Pilates aims to bring the body back to its natural alignment. The exercises encourage you to work to your maximum capability, without placing undue strain on the body. As a result, regular practice helps to improve your posture and flexibility, as well as toning the muscles. Pilates is particularly good for developing 'core' strength in the lower back and abdomen. It aims to work the mind as well as the body, and many practitioners find it deeply relaxing.

Pilates was originally developed in the First World War as a means of helping injured soldiers regain their mobility. It is still often recommended as a form of rehabilitation. Teachers say that almost anyone can practise Pilates because the exercises involved can be adapted to suit the individual's needs.

Pilates is safe for pregnant women because it uses carefully controlled movements and encourages you to work within your body's limitations. Advocates say that it can help to reduce backache, ease delivery and hasten recovery after the birth. However, it is important that the exercises are done correctly. Seek out a specialist qualified teacher who regularly works with pregnant women.

LEARNING PILATES

There are many books on Pilates, but it is best to learn the exercise from a qualified and experienced instructor. Pilates can be learned on a one-to-one basis or in a small class.

Some exercises are practised on a mat and others are done on specialized apparatus. The teacher demonstrates the exercises, and then guides the students through each series of movements. You should receive individual attention, even in a group class, and be shown how to adapt exercises where necessary. Blocks and supports may be used to help you to do this.

Classes usually last an hour. However, once you have learned the techniques, mat exercises can be done at home. Pilates teachers say that it is important to practise three or four times a week in order to obtain the most benefit from this therapy.

SAFE PILATES

- If you are pregnant and new to Pilates, do not start classes until after the first trimester. Try to find special pregnancy classes. Otherwise, go for individual instruction with an experienced teacher.
- Do not push your body further than is comfortable: you will build up flexibility and strength with practice.
- If you feel uncomfortable at any point, stop and rest.
- Do not do any exercises that require you to lie flat on your back after 30 weeks.
- Build up slowly – it will take time for you to increase your flexibility and strength.

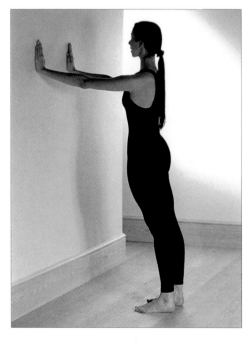

Many Pilates exercises are seemingly easy stretches like this one. When done correctly, they quickly build strength and muscle tone.

CHOOSING A TEACHER
Anyone can call themselves a Pilates teacher – even if they have had just a few days' training. It is important that you check that your teacher has completed a reputable training course and that he or she has been practising Pilates for several years. All Pilates teachers should have insurance.

Yoga

Doctors and midwives now commonly recommend yoga to pregnant women. This ancient form of exercise is known to foster general good health and improve posture and flexibility. It can also help to prevent or relieve common ailments such as backache, constipation and headaches.

Yoga is proven to help people relax, which makes it highly beneficial for women who are trying to conceive or who are already pregnant. Relaxation helps to improve the flow of blood, and so increases the supply of oxygen and nutrients to the baby. Yoga relaxation and breathing techniques can be very helpful during labour. A regular practice can help to strengthen the body and loosen up the pelvis in preparation for the birth; it can also aid recovery afterwards.

Yoga has been practised for thousands of years in India and is now widely taught in the West. Most yoga practised by Westerners is a form of hatha yoga. This means that it involves physical postures (asanas) as well as breath-control techniques, meditation and relaxation exercises. General classes are usually advertised simply as hatha yoga. There are also some very particular styles, such as Iyengar, which emphasizes precise alignment of the body.

Certain yoga poses, such as the spinal twists and headstands, should be avoided in pregnancy: so it is best to attend a class aimed specifically at pregnant women. Antenatal yoga classes are available in many areas for women in their second and third trimesters.

If you are pregnant and want to take up yoga for the first time, it is best to wait until you are past the 12-week mark before starting classes. If you already practise a regular, well-established yoga routine, it should be safe to continue in the first trimester, as long as you work gently and avoid unsuitable postures. However, tell your teacher that you are pregnant so that he or she can help you to practise safely.

CHOOSING A YOGA TEACHER
Anyone can teach yoga, and standards do vary. Before committing to a class, ask your yoga teacher about his or her experience and training – reputable teachers should be happy to discuss this. Your teacher should also be insured. Pregnant women should only attend 'yoga for pregnancy' classes.

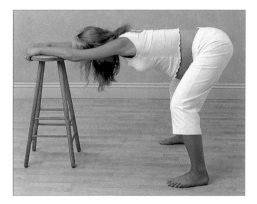

Many yoga asanas need to be adapted for pregnancy. This woman is doing modified dog pose; the standard position would place a strain on her uterus.

YOUR YOGA PRACTICE
In yoga, everyone works to his or her own capacity. So, although a class of students may be shown the same exercise, they may perform it in many different ways. Some people are flexible and can get into advanced postures quite easily; others are very stiff and need to work with a simplified version of the pose.

It is important that you do not push yourself any further than you are naturally able to go. With practice, your body will become stronger and more flexible. In many yoga classes, specialist equipment is available to help you work with the postures.

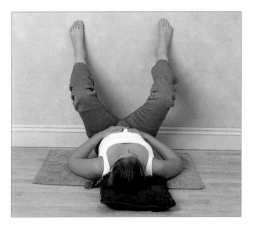

This is a version of shoulder-stand that is suitable for pregnancy. It helps blood to drain from the legs and may help to prevent varicose veins if done daily.

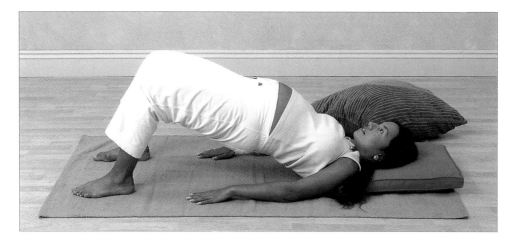

YOUR YOGA CLASS

Yoga classes can vary widely, depending on the form being taught and the particular teacher's training and interest. They usually last 1–1½ hours. Generally, you will start with easy postures, which serve to warm up the body, and then move on to more advanced ones. Usually, sitting, standing, reclining and some inversions (adapted if you are pregnant) will be covered.

The teacher will demonstrate each posture, then talk the class through the series of movements needed to get into it. He or she will also explain and demonstrate simplified versions of the postures where necessary. You may be given individual attention – and sometimes gentle physical

Gentle lifts can help to extend the spine and release tension in the lower back. Place a flat cushion or block under your head for comfort.

adjustment – in order to improve your alignment. All the postures should be done on a non-slip mat.

The class will end with simple breathing exercises and relaxation. It is very important that you complete the relaxation since it gives the body a chance to cool down. It also helps to calm the mind. People often like to cover themselves with a light blanket for this part of the class.

Yoga is most effective if you do it regularly. Your teacher will give you advice on which postures to do at home.

GETTING THE MOST FROM YOGA

- Always tell your yoga teacher that you are pregnant. Mention any health problems that you have.
- Do not eat or drink a large amount of water for an hour before the class; avoid eating a large meal in the three hours beforehand.
- Wear loose, comfortable clothing – a T-shirt and light tracksuit pants are ideal. You should always do the poses in bare feet, but you can put socks on for the relaxation if you wish.
- If you are practising at home, make sure that any postures you do are suitable for pregnancy. Do not do any postures that involve lying flat on your back after 30 weeks.
- Never strain or over-extend your body.
- Breathe freely: do not hold your breath when getting in or out of a posture.
- If you feel faint or uncomfortable, stop and rest on your left side for a few minutes.
- Always end a yoga session with at least ten minutes of relaxation time.

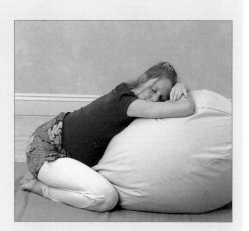

You'll need to adapt the relaxation pose in later months, when you should not lie flat on your back. Lie on your side, or place a bean bag in front of you and relax into it.

T'ai chi

The gentleness of t'ai chi exercise makes it ideal in pregnancy. It is a stylized form of martial art, performed in a controlled way so that you look as if you are dancing in slow motion. Regular practice is said to promote good health, strength, flexibility, balance and the breath control that is vital during labour.

T'ai chi is based on the idea that our well-being depends on the circulation of energy through invisible channels (meridians) in the body – the same theory that is behind acupuncture. The movements combine with breathing techniques to enhance this energy flow.

T'ai chi can be done by anyone. It improves posture and balance and also helps to keep the joints flexible. Researchers have found that it can lower blood pressure and improve breathing technique. Once learned, it is very relaxing, and can be an effective method of relieving stress.

The practice of T'ai chi can be beneficial for women who are trying to conceive or who are already pregnant, especially because it is such a calming influence and a gentle type of exercise. It may help with ailments such as backache, breathing problems, digestive problems and constipation. Its ability to develop physical and mental control can be of immense benefit when it comes to labour and birth. You should seek out a t'ai chi teacher who is used to dealing with pregnant women, as some stances may not be suitable.

LEARNING T'AI CHI

There are many aspects to t'ai chi, so it is difficult to learn more than the basics from a book or video. It is taught in classes of up to 30 people, but you can also learn it on a one-to-one basis. There are several forms of t'ai chi. The type most commonly taught in the West is Yang style, short form. This consists of 24 linked movements, which take about five minutes to perform.

Learning the movements properly takes time – you may spend a whole class on only one or two of them. The teacher will demonstrate each movement and then talk the class through it. There are many things to bear in mind, including the position of your hands, your leg movements, posture and breathing.

Only when each movement has been practised many times can you start to synchronize all the different elements. t'ai chi masters say that it takes years of practice to perform the movements perfectly. The movements are linked together to create a single flowing sequence. You practise the same sequence every day. This element of repetition, as well as the need to focus mind and body, make t'ai chi deeply relaxing, so that it is commonly described as 'meditation in motion'.

A t'ai chi class usually lasts an hour. Wear comfortable clothing that does not restrict your movements. Ideally, you should wear flat shoes with flexible soles (t'ai chi shoes are sold in Chinese supermarkets), but you can also do t'ai chi in bare feet. Most teachers will ask you to practise at home as well as attend classes – a daily practice session achieves the greatest benefits.

T'ai chi trains the mind as well as the body. You have to concentrate on your posture in order to keep your movements smooth and co-ordinated.

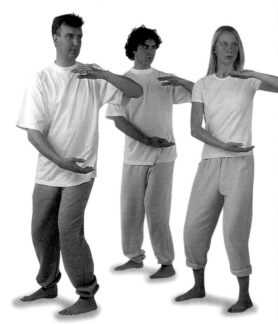

SAFE T'AI CHI
Few people suffer ill effects from practising t'ai chi. However, it is important to tell your teacher that you are pregnant, and to mention any health problems.

One problem associated with t'ai chi practice is sore knees, caused by incorrect posture. To avoid this, do not move the knee further forwards than your toes, nor allow it to collapse inwards or outwards.

Meditation

This is a form of mental exercise that can lead to greater inner harmony and awareness, making it the ideal way to relax and deal with the stresses of conception and pregnancy. It developed as a spiritual practice, but you do not have to subscribe to any particular philosophy to enjoy its benefits.

Many doctors believe that relaxation is an important part of general health care, and recommend meditation to their patients. Research has shown that regular meditation can reverse the effects of stress and help to alleviate ailments such as insomnia and digestive problems.

Meditation can soothe the emotions and help people to gain a wider perspective. Spending a few minutes each day in quiet contemplation can help women to cope with the disappointments that can be part of trying to conceive, as well as the challenges of pregnancy and new motherhood.

PRACTISING MEDITATION

Meditation practices vary, but they can often involve concentrating on a single object. The simplest way of practising meditation is probably to focus on your own breathing. You can also choose to focus on a physical object such as a flower or a candle flame, or on a sound that you repeat over and over again (known as a mantra). These concentration practices help to still the mind and have a relaxing effect on the body.

LEARNING MEDITATION

You can learn basic meditative techniques from a book or tape, and there are some simple exercises to try in this book. Most people find that it is much easier to learn and to concentrate when they are in a group. An experienced teacher will be able to answer any questions that you have.

Classes vary widely and it is important that you choose one you feel comfortable with. Talk to the teacher beforehand about what is involved.

SAFETY POINT
Check with your doctor before starting meditation if you have suffered from any form of psychiatric illness in the past. Sometimes meditation can bring up disturbing thoughts and images.

VISUALIZATION
This is a form of meditation that involves picturing an object, a happy event or a relaxing, beautiful scene in your mind's eye. It is a recognized technique for self-help and is much used by sportsmen with an athletic goal or achievement in mind.

Visualization can be used to promote well-being; in pregnancy, it may be helpful for easing anxiety and promoting bonding. For example, you can imagine your baby developing healthy and strong, or visualize healing pink or golden light surrounding you and your child. It can also be a good way of preparing for the birth, by imagining the birth canal opening and expanding.

Meditation takes time to learn – like, for example, mastering a musical instrument. However, its advocates say that perserverance can bring life-long benefits. Some people find that they prefer to practise meditation in conjunction with an alternative practice based on physical movement, such as yoga or t'ai chi.

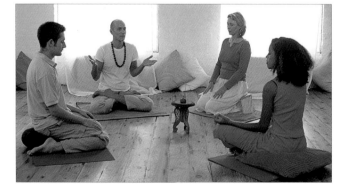

Meditation is best learned from an experienced practitioner. Classes vary widely: some may be based on Buddhist, Hindu, Christian or New Age philosophies; others may simply focus on relaxation in general.

Hypnotherapy

Hypnotherapists work by inducing a relaxed, trance-like state in their clients – a state in which clients are highly receptive to any suggestions, including suggestions for self-healing. This can be particularly helpful in dealing with the hopes and fears surrounding conception and childbirth.

Practitioners say hypnopsis can be used to help a person overcome addiction, combat anxiety, dispel a phobia or release negative states of mind, such as lack of confidence. It works by implanting positive suggestions that will help the person change ways of thinking or behaviour patterns that are contributing to their difficulties.

Hypnosis can be an effective way of relieving chronic pain and alleviating the symptoms of stress. The therapy usually works best if the subject is taught to use the techniques for self-hypnosis to control his or her symptoms.

Hypnotherapy is relaxing, and it may help some women who are trying to conceive. Practitioners say that they can help women to prepare for childbirth, particularly if they are fearful or anxious about the labour. Some hypnotherapists may attend the birth to assist with pain relief.

Hypnotherapy does not work for everyone, but nine out of ten people can apparently achieve a trance-like state. Practitioners maintain that it is impossible to hypnotize a person who does not wish it, claiming that the mind can always repel an unwanted hypnotic suggestion, although many people would dispute this. It is very important to find a reputable and experienced practitioner. Your doctor may be able to recommend somebody to you.

SEEING A HYPNOTHERAPIST

Hypnotherapy usually requires several sessions to show results. During the first session, the practitioner will discuss your reasons for seeking treatment and will take a full medical history, including any current mental or physical symptoms you may be experiencing. You should have an opportunity to ask about how hypnotherapy works and about the effects it may have on you.

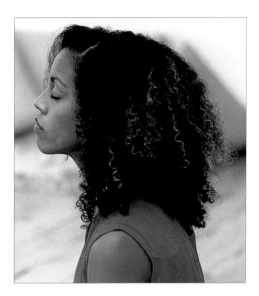

Self-hypnosis is a gentle healing technique that can help you to manage anxiety and stress-related symptoms. Some women find it a helpful way of preparing for childbirth.

You may sit on a comfortable chair or lie down for treatment. The practitioner then induces a trance by talking to you in a slow, soothing voice. You may be asked to look at a pendulum or a spot on a wall to help you relax. Imagery is often used: for example, you may be asked to picture yourself walking down a staircase. When people go into a trance, they usually feel deeply relaxed, but they are still aware of what is happening around them.

The practitioner will ask you questions in an attempt to discover the cause of the problem – sometimes deep-rooted anxieties and fears can be uncovered. He or she will also seek to implant positive thoughts or instructions that will help you to use the power of your mind to manage your particular problem.

At the end of the session, you will be slowly brought back to full consciousness. There should be an opportunity for you to discuss what has happened at this point. Most hypnotherapists will give you advice on using self-hypnosis and will ask you to practise the techniques in between sessions.

SAFE HYPNOSIS

There has been considerable research into hypnotherapy, and many doctors believe that it can be helpful. However, they stress it should be used as an adjunct to medical treatment, not as a substitute.

Choose a serious, qualified practitioner you trust, and check that he or she belongs to a reputable professional association. You should not have hypnosis if you suffer from epilepsy or if you have suffered severe depression in the past.

Reiki
This form of hands-on healing was developed by a Japanese scholar, Dr. Mikao Usui. It is based on the idea that there is a life-force energy – *rei* means 'universal' and *ki* (like *chi*) means 'life force' – that we can access for healing. This gentle therapy is often used to relieve mild depression during and after pregnancy.

Practitioners of reiki say that they act as channels for the healing energy (ki/chi) that flows through the universe and all things in it. In the course of a treatment, they lay their hands on or just above a person's body, so that this energy can be directed to wherever it is most needed. Neither the practitioner nor the person being treated need know exactly what the problem is in order for the healing to work.

BENEFITS
Many people find reiki deeply relaxing, and it may be helpful for stress, anxiety, depression and minor ailments such as backache or constipation. Most doctors are sceptical about the claims made for reiki, but usually see it as harmless so long as it is not used as a substitute for medical treatment. It is quite safe in pregnancy.

SAFE REIKI
- Choose a well-established reiki practitioner.
- Avoid practitioners who promise miracle cures or dramatic transformations.
- Continue to report any symptoms to your doctor.

HAVING A REIKI TREATMENT
Reiki sessions take about an hour. You lie fully clothed on a massage couch. If you are pregnant, it may be more comfortable to sit in a chair. In any case, you should not lie flat on your back after 30 weeks.

The practitioner will place his or her hands on different parts of your body for several minutes at a time. Twelve basic positions are used: four on the head, four on the back and four on the front. These are said to relate to different centres of energy in the body.

You may feel a sensation of tingling or heat emanating from the practitioner's hands. This is said to be a sign of the healing energy being drawn into your body, and it can feel very pleasurable. After a treatment, some people feel relaxed and sleepy; others feel energized. Practitioners recommend that you go home and rest afterwards. Regular sessions are usually recommended to maintain well-being.

SELF-TREATMENT AND TRAINING
Reiki practitioners believe that everyone has the capacity to access life-force energy and use it for healing. You can learn basic reiki in a weekend; the course usually includes instruction on using your hands for healing, ethical guidelines and 'attunement', a ceremony in which your healing channels are said to be cleared. After the course, you can practise healing on yourself and those close to you.

Practitioners have usually done further training; however, this is not regulated in any way, and can involve no more than a weekend workshop. Anyone can set up as a reiki therapist, and so it may be wise to find a practitioner who has completed the longer, more rigorous training that confers the accreditation of Master reiki teacher.

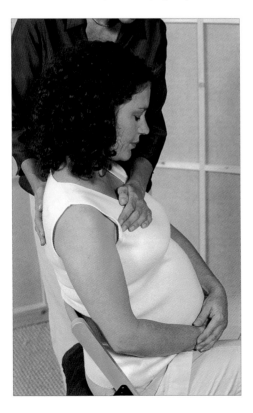

During a reiki session, healing energy is transmitted through the hands of the practitioner and into the recipient. It is a non-invasive therapy, and you remain clothed to receive treatment.

Feng shui

The Chinese art of feng shui is based on the idea that a life-force exists within everything and that buildings and rooms also contain this force. Feng shui aims to direct this energy to bring us spiritual and material benefits. One of the uses for parents-to-be is to create an harmonious nursery for their baby.

Feng shui is the art of arranging your home in order to harness positive energy, and using it to improve your health, relationships, career, fertility or other aspects of your life.

There are different schools of feng shui. The traditional form incorporates Chinese astrology and the use of a special compass (the lo pan). Some practitioners use a tool called a bagua to determine which areas of your home relate to different aspects of your life. Many Western practitioners work intuitively, preferring to sense which areas of your home are lacking in chi (energy).

Some aspects of feng shui can be used for self-help. However, much of the theory is complicated and using a practitioner is recommended if you want to ensure that your home is organized according to feng shui principles.

It is a good idea to talk to a practitioner on the telephone before arranging a consultation. As with any complementary therapy, choose someone you feel comfortable with, in order to benefit fully from the advice given.

WHAT A CONSULTATION INVOLVES

A feng shui practitioner will usually visit your home, but some practitioners work by post, using a floor plan. You should mention any difficulties you have experienced since living there – such as relationship or fertility problems.

During the visit, the practitioner will assess the surrounding environment to see whether there are negative influences: these could include a large tree that casts a shadow on your home, or a prison or hospital nearby.

Each room will be assessed to determine whether it has a positive or negative influence on your life. Some aspects

DOES IT WORK?
Feng shui experts believe that your environment is only one of several influences on your life – your birth date, birth place and personal character are others. There is no proof that feng shui works, but it is widely practised in China and it does include common-sense ideas that will enhance the atmosphere of your home.

of feng shui may seem strange: for example, it is considered to be bad luck to place your bed so that your feet face the doorway. Others may feel like common sense: feng shui says that your home should be clutter-free.

The practitioner may suggest that you use the rooms differently – sometimes people are recommended to site their bedroom elsewhere. You will be advised on the arrangement of the furniture, the decoration and lighting and the placement of any ornaments and pictures. A written report is usually sent, so that you can consider these recommendations at your leisure.

FENG SHUI SELF-HELP

- Keep doorways and outside pathways clear, to encourage chi into your home. Clean windows regularly.
- Repair or discard broken or damaged items.
- Remove clutter so that chi can circulate freely.
- Leave space around each item of furniture, and do not store anything underneath.
- Brighten up a dull corner with a lamp or colourful picture.

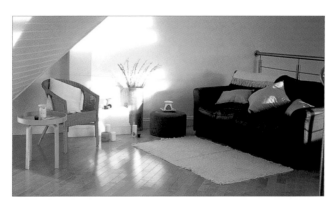

A bright and airy room like this one is said to be full of positive chi. However, the sharp edge of the sloping roof would be considered inauspicious. A feng shui practitioner may recommend 'cures' to counteract any bad luck that this could bring.

Colour therapy and crystal healing

Therapists say that colours and crystals give out positive vibrations that can have a beneficial effect on the mind and body. For the parent-to-be, they offer a pleasant way to deal with fluctuating moods and to promote a calm state of well-being.

COLOUR THERAPY

Colour therapists vary widely in what they believe and how they work: some draw on Western psychological research; others adhere to Eastern mysticism. All of them believe that colours transmit healing vibrations, and that these vibrations can be used to treat illness and improve well-being. Colour is an important aspect of feng shui, and some complementary therapists use elements of colour therapy in their work.

Most doctors are sceptical about the health claims made by colour therapists, but research has shown that colours can have a powerful effect on our mood. For example, blue can be very calming, while yellow can help to enhance learning ability. You can use the characteristics of colour for self-help – for example, by decorating a room in a particular hue – or you can consult a therapist for specific treatment.

Colours and their qualities

- **Red** is the colour of vitality, creativity and passion.
- **Yellow** lifts the spirits and promotes mental clarity.
- **Orange** increases your sense of happiness and joy.
- **Green** works to harmonize, balance and heal.
- **Violet** is associated with self-esteem and also with self-empowerment.
- **Pink** can be soothing, loving and supportive.
- **Blue** helps to quieten the mind and promote restful sleep.
- **Turquoise** serves to cleanse, calm and purify.

Seeing a colour therapist

Colour therapists work in a variety of different ways. Some may diagnose your problem by 'sensing' what colours you need; others ask clients carry out a simple exercise, such as ranking a set of colour cards in order of preference.

You may be asked to lie draped in coloured silks or to sit in front of a machine that directs coloured light at you. The therapist may advise you on visualization and meditation techniques, and may suggest that you wear particular colours and include foods of the same hue in your diet.

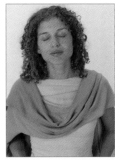

If you suffer from anxiety, a colour therapist may recommend you wear soothing blue.

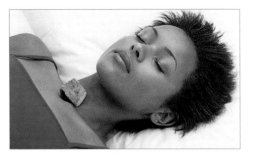

The crystal chrysocolla can be placed over the throat chakra to promote good communication – essential for coping with the many challenges of pregnancy, childbirth and parenthood.

CRYSTAL HEALING

Crystals are often used in feng shui, and healers say that they can be used to help a wide range of symptoms and emotional disturbances. If you visit a crystal healer, several crystals may be placed on different parts of your body – often over the body's energy centres (chakras) – to encourage healing. You may also be given a crystal to wear, carry or place in your home. These are some of the crystals used to foster well-being:

- **Amethyst** encourages peace and tranquillity and can help to promote restful sleep.
- **Rose quartz** has gentle, loving qualities and is associated with the heart.
- **Jade** soothes the emotion and promotes balance. It is said to encourage healing and recovery.
- **Coral** is a protective stone that may be used to ward off any negative energy.
- **Garnet** lifts the spirits and is a source of positive energy. It is associated with sexuality and fertility.
- **Smoky quartz** is said to be good for mood swings.

> **COMPLEMENTARY HEALING**
> Colour therapy or crystal healing may help some people with stress-related conditions and emotional problems. However, you should still report any symptoms to your doctor. Avoid practitioners who offer miracle cures.

section four

your
new
baby

Becoming a parent is a great adventure – one
that most people embark on at some point in
their lives, but one that is also unique to each
person: no one's baby, no one's family, is quite
like anyone else's. The arrival of a baby entails a
fundamental shift in the way you look at the
world: you are no longer the centre of your own
universe and in a strange sense you can now
never be entirely alone. Soon you will find it hard
to remember what it was like not to be the
father or mother of another human being.

The first days and weeks

> ❝ No two babies, not even twins, are the same, and yours will have likes and dislikes right from the start. ❞

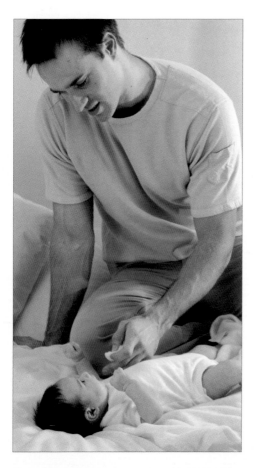

The most important thing that a new father can do is to spend time with his baby and partner. Most hospitals will leave the family alone to facilitate bonding.

The weeks after a child is born are a time of great transformation for your family. If this is your first baby, you and your partner have stepped over the threshold of parenthood. Here at last is the baby you have been looking forward to for so long. Your life – wonderfully and irreversibly – will never be the same again.

It will help you to enjoy and appreciate this special time if you can give it the importance it deserves. Spend as much time as you can together as a family, limit your visitors to those who will help and support you, and try to let go of other anxieties and concerns – work, money, family problems and so on. Above all, rest and recuperate as much as you can.

There will inevitably be moments – or even long interludes – when you feel you have taken on an almost impossible task. It is entirely normal and extremely common to struggle with fatigue and disorientation at first. You may have feelings of confusion or even despair when, say, your baby is crying and you don't know why. All new parents

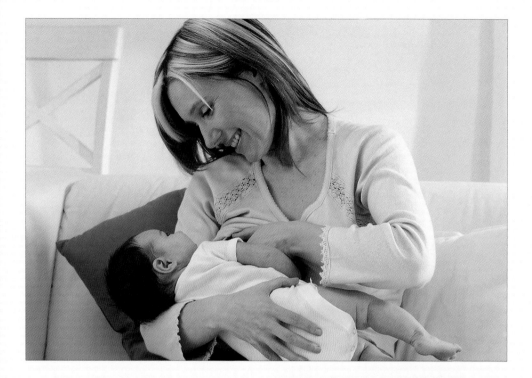

know this experience, and there will come a time when you can look back on the sleepless nights with a rueful smile.

It helps to remember that your child is a unique individual. No two babies, not even twins, are the same, and yours will have likes and dislikes right from the start. You will need to experiment to discover exactly how your baby likes to be held, and whether stroking or patting, for example, soothes him or her more easily. This is much easier if you take a flexible approach, rather than trying to follow a set routine from the outset. Spending these first weeks observing, listening to and cuddling the baby will help you to get to know your child and to understand his or her needs in a way that will store up benefits for the months and years to come.

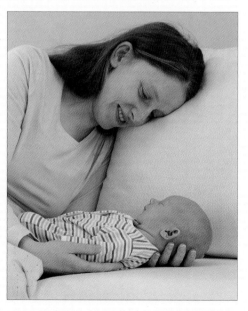

Top: Spend plenty of time getting to know your new baby. An alert baby will be just as curious about you and will gaze upon your face.

Some mothers fall in love with their babies at the first instant, but many women find that they take longer to form a really close attachment.

Bonding with your baby

A lot is said about the importance of bonding straight after the birth, and it is wonderful if the new family can be given the quiet and privacy they need to enjoy these first moments together. Your baby has been propelled from the dark, familiar cocoon of the mother's womb into a bright and noisy world, and is being bombarded with new sensations. In your arms is the most comforting and reassuring place to be.

The hour or so after delivery is also the ideal time to start breastfeeding. It not only encourages bonding but also stimulates digestion and ensures that the baby gets the protective benefits of the first milk (colostrum) straight away. Babies practise the sucking movement while in the womb, and if placed on the mother's stomach may find their own way to the nipple using their sense of smell.

At this time bright lights should be dimmed to create as relaxing and unobtrusive an environment as possible. Any weighing or non-urgent checks should wait, so that mother and baby can get to know each other. The room should be warm so that the baby can be placed naked on the mother's bare skin. If the father is there, he shouldn't feel that he has to immediately rush off to telephone relatives with the news. It is far more important that he stays to share the first few minutes of his baby's life. Everything else can wait.

All babies need loving touch. Research shows that premature babies who are stroked gain more weight, are more responsive and spend fewer days in hospital.

WHEN BONDING IS DELAYED

In the past, mothers and babies in hospital were separated soon after the birth to allow the mother to rest. Fathers' visiting rights were strictly limited. Bonding is now seen as so important that midwives and hospital staff do everything they can to facilitate a new family's need for time alone together. But the safety and health of the baby and mother come first, and if the delivery has been tricky or there are concerns about either, they may have to be separated for a while.

Even if the mother is physically close to her newborn, she may not feel the rush of love that she may have expected. She may be too exhausted from the labour and delivery to be able to feel anything other than relief that it is over; she may be in pain or shock or feeling woozy from the effect of drugs, or she may feel initial disappointment if the child is, say, a boy rather than a girl or has a physical defect such as a hare lip or a birthmark. If she had strong ideas about the type of birth she wanted and it turned out differently, she may be distracted by disappointment and less able to appreciate the beautiful baby in front of her.

Similarly, the father may have found the birth a much more distressing experience than he imagined, especially if there were complications. He may be too worried about his partner to feel much for his child. He may be disturbed

Many new mothers find that they cannot sleep the night after the birth, because they don't want to miss a minute of the child's first hours of life.

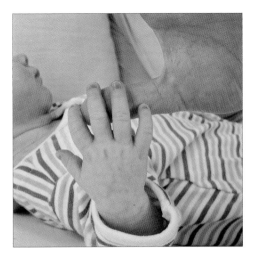

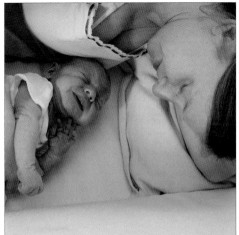

to find that the blood-streaked, blotchy newborn that he sees before him does not match the image of the angelic-looking baby he expected. And the realization that he is now responsible for this tiny being may feel overwhelming rather than exciting.

Some parents feel guilty if they do not feel instant love for their baby, and being separated from the child early on can be devastating. But it is a mistake to think that any delay in the bonding process will have a permanent effect on your relationship.

Bonding often starts slowly and grows over time. There is nothing special that you need to do to help this process along. It will unfold naturally as you get to know your baby, as you learn about his or her likes and dislikes, and – especially – as you tend to the baby's needs: changing, cleaning, bathing, comforting, rocking and feeding. Your baby will not remember those first hours of life, but over the months and years that follow will gradually become aware of being encompassed by your love and care.

SPECIAL CARE

Some babies need to be looked after in a special care unit. It can be very hard to see your baby in an incubator or covered in tubes. But even if you cannot yet bring the baby home, there is a lot you can do. Spend as much time as possible by your baby's side, talking softly so that he or she gets to know your voice. Hold the baby's hand and stroke him or her through the holes in the side of the incubator. Cuddle the baby as much you are able: skin-to-skin contact helps to regulate a baby's heartbeat, body temperature and breathing, and it is very calming.

Breastfeeding helps you to bond. It gives you the satisfaction of knowing that you are giving your baby the best possible nourishment and is also the one thing that you can do for your child that nobody else can. If the baby can't be taken out of the incubator, then you can express milk to be given through a tube. The hospital should help you to do this by lending you an efficient breast pump and giving you privacy to use it. It can be hard to establish a good milk supply by expressing alone, so ask for support from a breastfeeding counsellor.

Occasionally a baby needs to be taken to a different hospital for special care while the mother is too ill to travel. This is very distressing, and it will help if the father can become the main carer for a while. If you are a mother in this situation, it is important to remember that you will be able to start the bonding process later on. In the meantime, keep a photograph of your baby with you. Some hospitals use webcams so that parents can see their babies even when they cannot be with them.

Holding a young baby can feel daunting at first. It takes several weeks before new parents feel confident about handling their baby.

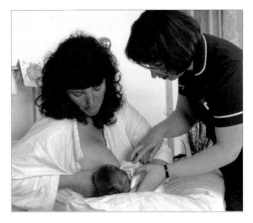

Nursing your baby soon after birth gets breastfeeding off to the best possible start. The antibodies in colostrum will help to protect your newborn from infection, and babies who are nursed early on may be less likely to develop sucking problems later.

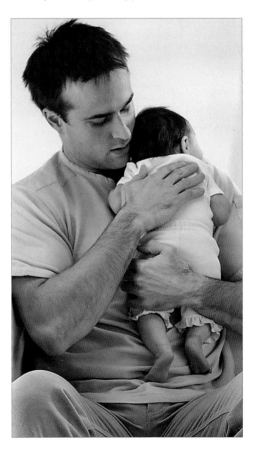

Your newborn baby

Not all newborn babies are cherubic visions of beauty. Their heads may be an odd shape after the birth (especially if the delivery was by ventouse or forceps) and their noses may look squashed. Their eyes may be puffy; their skin (especially if they were overdue) may be wrinkly and flaky, look greasy or be covered in downy hair, and it may have a bluish hue. Their genitals may be slightly swollen. All these strange features are normal and will start to disappear over the next few days and weeks.

WHAT YOUR BABY CAN SENSE

Babies enter the world fully equipped to apprehend and understand their environment. That is, they are in possession of all five senses – sight, hearing, smell, taste and touch – and begin to use them straight away.

Touch. Babies need touch in order to thrive. Your baby is most sensitive to touch around the mouth. Even tiny newborns respond well to gentle stroking, and older babies usually enjoy massage too.

Smell and taste. Research shows that babies have a natural preference for sweet tastes right from the start. They react to smells in the same way as adults: they recoil from bad odours and are drawn to sweet ones. They also quickly learn to differentiate their mother's smell from that of other people.

Hearing. Babies respond to sound in the womb, and may recognize music that they heard regularly before birth. But it is voices that they like best, and they show a preference for their mother's voice above all others. They also show dislike for certain sounds and will jump if they hear a sudden loud noise.

Seeing. Newborns find it easiest to focus on objects 20–30cm/8–12in away – roughly the distance of your face when you hold a baby in your arms or breastfeed. Babies show the most interest in faces, but are also fascinated by simple patterns.

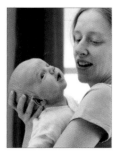

Babies don't have the muscle power to hold up their heavy heads, so you must keep a newborn's head well supported at all times. Gradually, the muscles in the neck grow stronger and they will be able to support the head, but watch out for sudden lapses as the head lolls.

YOUR BABY'S REFLEXES

A newborn baby is entirely dependent on your care, but is born with some instinctive reactions designed to help him or her survive.

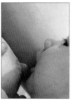

Rooting, sucking and swallowing: If stroked on the cheek, a baby will turn and search for the nipple (this is called rooting). Babies suck when they feel pressure on the hard palate in the mouth, and swallow automatically.

Gripping. If you put a finger in your baby's hand, he or she will grasp it. Your baby will also curl the feet if the soles are touched. These reflexes are left over from our primate ancestors, who needed to cling to their mothers' fur. They gradually develop into a deliberate holding action.

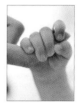

Crawling. When placed on their tummies, babies will curl their legs and arms beneath their bodies and may even produce a crawl-like movement. Gradually your baby's body uncurls from its foetal position and he or she will lie flat.

Stepping. If they are held so that their feet touch a firm surface, newborn babies will lift one foot after another in a stepping motion. This reflex disappears after a few days, and has to be re-learnt many months later when it is time to learn to walk.

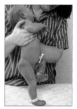

Startle reflex. If newborns are startled, they fling out their arms and legs as if to grab hold of something. Your baby finds this distressing, so see it as a reminder that he or she should be handled gently. The reflex disappears at about two months.

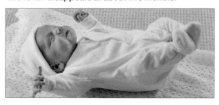

Lifting and putting down your baby

Babies need to be held securely and comfortably in the first few weeks, until their neck muscles have developed enough for them to support their own head. Always lift your baby slowly and gently to avoid startling him or her.

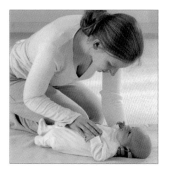 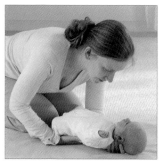 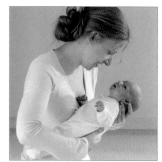

1 Alert the baby to your presence first by speaking softly, and putting your hand on their tummy. Lean over so that your body is close to the baby, and slide one hand under the head and neck.

2 Slide the other hand under the lower back and bottom. Take the baby's weight into your hands, and then bring him or her slowly towards you. When your baby is resting on your chest, begin to sit upright.

3 When putting the baby down, hold him or her close to you as you bend over. This means that the baby doesn't have to travel too far in mid-air. Keep your hands in position for a while before sliding them out.

HOW YOUR BABY COMMUNICATES

As helpless as newborns are, they can communicate in a way that almost guarantees they get their basic needs met: they cry. At first your baby's cries will all sound the same to you. But in time you may notice that he or she makes different sounds depending on what is wrong, and you may learn to distinguish between, say, a cry that means 'I'm hungry' and one that says 'I'm in pain'. After a few weeks, your baby will also start to communicate pleasure, by gurgling, cooing and making other repetitive little noises.

The person who looks after the baby most often – usually a parent – will probably see the first smile, which comes by about six weeks. At first babies will smile at any face – including a picture of one – by three months they smile more readily at the people they know best.

THE FONTANELLE

The bones of a newborn's skull have not yet fused together. The gaps between the bones, called fontanelles, are covered by a tough membrane and can't be damaged by normal handling. The largest one is on the crown of the baby's head, you may be able to see a pulse beating through it. This fontanelle can indicate a baby's state of health. If it is sunken, the baby is dehydrated and needs fluids urgently. A bulging fontanelle is another sign of illness, which also needs immediate medical attention.

Carrying your baby

When carrying your baby, both of you need to feel confident and secure. There are two safe ways to hold your newborn baby: the shoulder hold, which is good for winding and for general carrying around, and the cradle hold, which is a soothing way to nurse your baby.

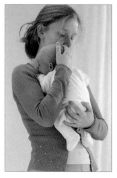 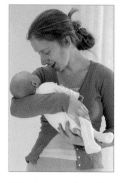

1 For the shoulder hold, support the baby against your chest, so that his or her head leans against your shoulder. Use one hand to support the bottom and back, and keep the other behind the back and head to stop the baby jerking backwards.

2 To use the cradle hold, hold the baby by resting his or her head and shoulders in the crook of your arm, and use your other hand to support the bottom and lower back. Newborn babies will feel most safe and secure held closely against your body.

The first weeks

In many cultures, it is traditional for the mother to stay indoors for 40 days after the birth – one for each week of pregnancy. During this time she is released from the burden of household chores, given special foods to restore her strength and encouraged to stay in bed to bond with her infant. Bedouin Arabs, Jews, Somalis and Latin Americans all observe 40 days of seclusion, while Chinese women 'do the month'.

Until very recently, western women were also encouraged to rest after giving birth – your grandmother probably spent a week or two 'lying-in', either in hospital or at home. But today new mothers are under immense pressure to get back to normal, regain their figures and show the baby off to all their relatives. This makes the first weeks after childbirth more exhausting and stressful than they need to be.

When you are caring for a small baby it is easy to forget to drink enough. Have a jug or bottle of water to hand.

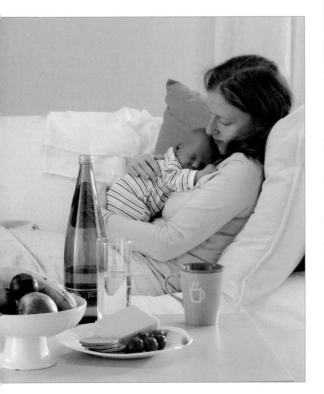

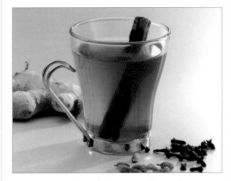

RESTORATIVE TEA

A spicy hot drink can invigorate and energize you. This mixture includes raspberry leaf tea, which encourages the healthy contraction of the womb, and nettle tea, which is a traditional tonic. Drink up to three cups a day.

3 cardamon pods
3 cloves
5cm/2in stick of cinnamon
2.5cm/1in chunk of ginger, sliced
3 tsp raspberry leaf tea
3 tsp nettle tea

Put 750ml/30fl oz water in a small, lidded pan and add the spices. Bring to the boil, cover and simmer for 10 minutes. Add the teas to the spice mixture, steep for 10 minutes then strain into a flask to keep warm. Drink when required.

A MODERN LYING-IN

It makes sense to withdraw from society for a while so that you can concentrate on your new baby. Everyone's idea of lying-in will be different, but it can be helpful to do the following, at least for a week or two.

Stay at home and don't get dressed. Pyjamas or a nightie are much more comfortable to wear than day clothes, and they help to remind you (and any visitors) that you are resting.

Make your bedroom the centre of your existence. Have everything you need close at hand – water, a bowl of fruit, healthy snacks, phone, books or magazines – to make this time pleasurable.

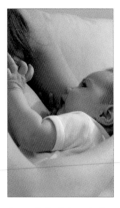
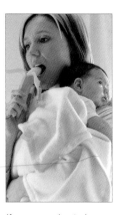
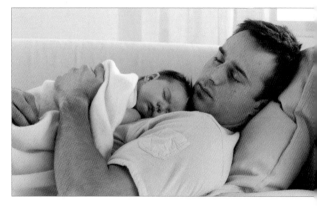

A new baby is happiest cuddled close against the breast. If the contact is skin to skin, even better, as your scent will add to the feeling of security.

If you are going to be on your own at home with a new baby, make sure you have plenty of healthy food that is quick to prepare and easy to eat.

Fathers will also need to get rest whenever they can. It is tempting to fall asleep together on the sofa, but don't, as the baby could become trapped between cushions.

Keep your baby with you all or most of the time. Follow his or her rhythms – feed the baby on demand, sleep when he or she sleeps.

Have another adult around. Ideally, the father will be at home to look after you and share the care of the baby. But if that isn't possible, ask your mother, best friend or another person close to you to stay.

Eat well. Have at least one hot meal a day (cooked by someone else) and lots of healthy, easy-to-prepare snacks at other times – fruit, cereal, yoghurt, oatcakes, smoked salmon, cold meats and so on. Make sure you drink lots of water.

Limit first visitors to close friends and family. For the first few weeks, arrange visits at times that are convenient to you, and keep them short. Ask your partner or supporter to encourage people gently to leave if you start to get tired.

If people offer help, accept it. Ask them to bring you a cooked meal or do some housework, so that you and your partner can concentrate on the baby.

Keep your first outings short and pleasurable. It is quite normal to feel a little strange at first. Many traditional cultures have a celebration at the end of the seclusion period, which serves not only to welcome the new baby but also to help reintegrate the mother into the world.

LOVING CARE FOR YOUR BABY

Looking after a newborn can feel daunting, not least because new parents are inundated with advice. Do ignore suggestions from well-meaning friends and relatives if they don't feel right for you at this moment.

What works for one baby doesn't necessarily work for another, and women who had their babies years ago – including your own mother and mother-in-law – may have ideas that are out of date.

The most important thing is to spend lots of relaxed time with your baby, concentrating completely on him or her, with no distractions, so that you get to know each other. Gradually, you will discover how to tell when the baby is hungry or tired, how he or she likes to be carried and what is most soothing, being rocked or shushed for example. This takes time, and it is important to trust your own instincts as you learn. In the meantime, the following pointers may help.

Babies thrive on physical contact. Cuddle your baby as much as you can, and limit the amount of time spent in a bouncy chair or pram.

Prioritize breastfeeding. As well as meeting your baby's basic needs for food and drink, it brings you physically close and helps with bonding.

Don't spend longer than an hour or two away from your baby. It's natural for mothers to want to be near their newborns, but other people can confuse you by telling you that you need time to yourself, and grandparents in particular may push to 'have a turn' at looking after the baby. Don't worry about other people's needs just now, and give in to this kind of pressure only if you really feel that you need a break.

The father is important, too. For the first year or so, the mother is usually at the centre of her baby's world, but the father will develop a much closer relationship with his child if he is involved in day-to-day care: changing nappies (diapers), cleaning, bathing and comforting. Fathers are often better than mothers at soothing babies who are distressed or windy, because the babies pick up on their mothers' anxiety.

Common problems for infants

Even the most beautiful and natural of births is physically gruelling for the baby, who is pushed and squeezed down the narrow birth canal. So it is not surprising that newborns are often bruised and marked and sometimes have bloodshot eyes. These little blemishes will fade in a few days and need no treatment.

If you have had a forceps or ventouse delivery, the baby's head may be misshapen for a while. This too will correct itself naturally. However, a baby who has had an assisted delivery may have a headache for a few days, which can make him or her cry more than normal. Lots of cuddling and nursing will help. If your baby continues to be very fractious, then gentle massage can help. It may also be worth taking the baby to a cranial osteopath, who can gently correct any distortions in the skull.

BIRTHMARKS
Some babies are born with a birthmark that is permanent. Three in every thousand have a pink or purple port-wine stain. This often occurs on the face, and is very occasionally linked to problems such as epilepsy. It can be upsetting when your child has a birthmark of this nature, and it may take time for their parents to come to terms with it. However, port-wine stains can be treated with lasers which can radically improve their appearance. Very occasionally, a baby is born with a raised brown mole. It's important to keep an eye on this and seek medical advice if it changes colour, shape or size: a mole can be surgically removed if there is cause for concern.

Breastmilk has natural antibacterial properties, so it is the perfect cleanser for a newborn's sticky eye.

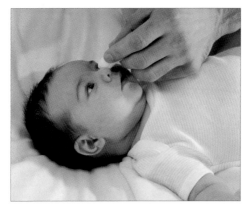

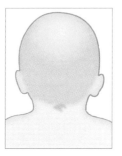 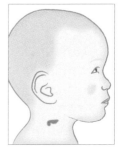

It is thought that stork marks may be the result of pressure on the head once the baby engages.

Strawberry marks can be quite prominent, but they usually fade and then disappear in a few years.

TEMPORARY BIRTHMARKS, SPOTS AND RASHES
Stork marks are so-called because it is fancifully said that they are caused by the beak of the mythical stork that delivers babies. They are pink or red marks on the brow, eyelids or back of the neck, which become more prominent when the baby cries. They gradually fade but can take up to two years to disappear completely.

Strawberry marks are red marks that start off flat and gradually become raised, increasing in size. They can be present at birth or develop a few days later. They have usually gone by the time the child is two or three. Mongolian spots are blue or grey patches that can appear on the buttocks or back. They affect black or Asian babies, and usually disappear by the end of the first year.

Most newborn babies develop minor skin problems in their first weeks. Heat rashes (tiny red spots) are very common because babies have immature sweat glands and are unable to control their temperature efficiently. If

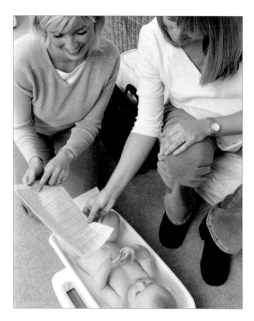

Babies may be weighed often in the early weeks to see that they are growing normally. Frequent checking can feel rather stressful for the parents, but so long as the overall weight gain is steady and your baby looks fit and healthy, there is nothing to worry about.

the sweat glands become blocked, tiny white spots (milia or milk spots) appear. They will disappear of their own accord in a few weeks. Do not pick at them or you may cause infection.

STICKY EYE

The eyes of newborns can produce a sticky, yellowish discharge. If this occurs in the first day or two it usually means they have picked up an infection in the birth canal. Use a cotton-wool pad (cotton ball) soaked in cooled, boiled water, or breast milk, to clean each eye, wiping from the nose outwards. See a doctor if it persists.

JAUNDICE

More than half of newborn babies develop jaundice two or three days after the birth. This is not a disease but a symptom: it means that bilirubin (a pigment produced by the body when red blood cells are broken down) has built up in their system. Usually the liver processes bilirubin, but a baby's immature liver is unable to cope with all the extra bilirubin produced when large amounts of red blood cells are broken down after the birth.

In most cases, the signs of jaundice are a yellowing of the whites of the eyes and the skin (which usually starts on the head and spreads down the chest and stomach).

Your midwife should check for jaundice but do point it out if you are concerned. Usually, no treatment is needed, and the jaundice clears up in a week or two. (In premature babies, who develop it five to seven days after the birth, it can take up to two months to disappear.)

If your baby's jaundice reaches the arms and legs, or there are other symptoms such as difficulty sucking, sleepiness, dark urine or pale stools, see your doctor promptly. Occasionally jaundice can have a serious cause, such as liver problems. The usual treatment is light therapy (phototherapy), which is done in hospital, but very occasionally a blood transfusion is needed.

INFECTED UMBILICAL CORD

It can take up to four weeks for the stump of the baby's umbilical cord to shrink and drop off, leaving a small wound that will heal in a few days. Doctors sometimes advise dabbing the stump with rubbing alcohol to prevent infection, but recent research suggests that it is best left to dry by itself. Clean the area around the stump daily with cooled, boiled water and pat dry with a clean towel. Fold down the top of the nappy so that air can reach the area. This will help it to heal faster. If the stump starts to ooze pus or smell, or the surrounding area becomes red, see a doctor, who will prescribe antibiotic cream.

THE SIX-WEEK CHECK

Babies are checked from head to toe soon after the birth and again six weeks later. At the six-week check, you'll be asked about your baby's feeding and sleeping patterns, as well as what you have noticed about his or her hearing and vision. The baby will be weighed (naked) and measured, and the results plotted on a centile chart to see how he or she compares with the national averages. The baby's vision, head control and muscle tone will be systematically checked and a hearing test may be done. The doctor will also look at your baby's eyes, heart, spine, hips and genitals to ensure all is well.

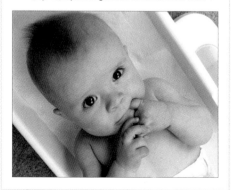

Common problems for new mothers

Every woman needs time to recover from giving birth. Even if you have had a natural vaginal delivery with no tearing, you are likely to feel bruised and tired. You may have aches and pains in odd places, especially if you had an active birth in which you moved around a lot. And, of course, your body is adjusting to the fact that you are no longer pregnant: your womb is shrinking back to its normal size, your hormone levels have dropped and your breasts are producing milk to sustain your new baby.

Much of the discomfort experienced by new mothers can be eased with the help of natural remedies. None of the remedies given will interfere with breastfeeding. However, it is important to see your doctor or midwife if you have severe pain or are worried about any symptom.

Afterpains are often at their most intense when you are breastfeeding, because this triggers the release of the hormone oxytocin, which encourages the womb to contract. Sit in a relaxed position and breathe slowly and deeply and relax your muscles to ease the cramp.

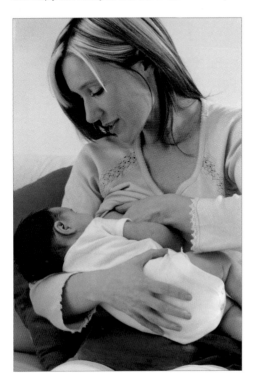

EXERCISING THE PELVIC FLOOR
You probably did pelvic floor exercises while you were pregnant, and it is important to continue after childbirth. Contract the muscles around your vagina and anus and imagine drawing them upwards (as if you were stopping yourself from urinating in mid-flow). Hold the squeeze for a few breaths then release slowly. Try to do this ten times or more, several times a day.

AFTERPAINS
Many women experience cramp-like pains in the abdomen when the womb starts to contract. These start within hours of the birth and usually last three days at most (often less). Afterpains can be intense, particularly during breastfeeding. They also tend to be stronger with second and subsequent children, as the womb becomes increasingly stretched.

There are simple things you can do to ease the discomfort: a warm bath or a warm hot-water bottle held against the abdomen help to relax the muscles. Sipping a soothing herbal tea such as chamomile, or an antispasmodic one such as ginger or crampbark, may also help. Raspberry leaf tea, so useful for strengthening the womb before childbirth, also helps it to readjust afterwards. Some women swear by the homeopathic remedy Mag phos, and Chamomilla can also be helpful.

SORE PERINEUM
If you have had a natural birth, your perineal area will have been stretched, so it will feel sore and bruised. Homeopathic Arnica tablets are excellent for treating the bruising, and will also help with any shock resulting from the birth. Doing your pelvic floor exercises will speed healing, since these encourage blood to flow to the area.

Take one or two warm baths a day to encourage healing and give you a few precious minutes to yourself; dilute a few drops each of tea tree and lavender oil in a carrier oil and add to the water. For immediate relief, apply a pad of cotton wool (cotton ball) soaked in witch hazel. Alternatively, use a home-made icepack (made by wrapping ice in a plastic bag then covering it in two layers of kitchen paper or a cotton cloth), but don't use this for longer than ten minutes at a time.

As you urinate, pour a jug of lukewarm water over the perineal area to prevent stinging. Pat rather than wipe it

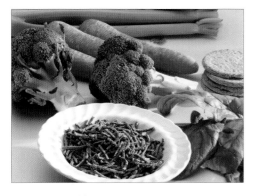

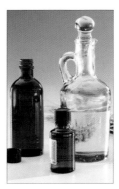

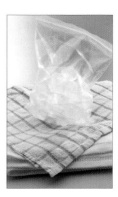

Include plenty of fresh vegetables and wholegrain cereals, including oats and bran, in your diet before and after childbirth to ensure that you get enough fibre and help prevent constipation.

Lavender and tea tree oils can help the healing of tears or cuts. Add 2–3 drops to a warm bath.

An ice pack – applied for up to ten minutes – can bring welcome relief to a bruised perineum.

dry. Many women worry about how it will feel when they move their bowels for the first time. You may be concerned that your stitches will tear, but be assured that they won't. However, the first bowel movements after childbirth will be more difficult if you are constipated, so drink plenty of fluids and eat lots of fruits and vegetables.

HAEMORRHOIDS

Even if you got through pregnancy without developing haemorrhoids, also called piles, they may well develop when you are pushing down in labour (about one-third of women get them after a vaginal delivery). If you don't have any itching or pain, you can leave them to heal naturally, but taking warm baths and doing pelvic floor exercises will be helpful.

The homeopathic remedy Hamamelis is often recommended for itchy or painful piles. You can apply a pad soaked in witch hazel to the area: this is cooling and

The homeopathic remedy Chamomilla can help with afterpains. You could also try sipping a cup of chamomile tea three times a day.

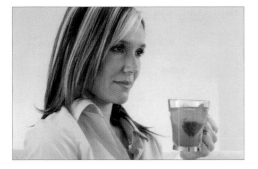

encourages shrinking. You can smooth Calendula cream on the piles between compresses. It's important to avoid becoming constipated (see above), since this will exacerbate the problem. Wash the area with water and pat dry after each bowel movement.

AFTER A CAESAREAN

If you had your baby by Caesarean section, recovery will take a little longer than with a natural birth – you have had major abdominal surgery, after all. You'll be encouraged to get moving as soon as possible in order to start the healing process, and you may be given gentle exercises to practise. But you will have to be careful about how you move and should avoid lifting anything heavier than your baby for at least six weeks. You should not drive for at least a month. Check this with your insurance company.

It is important to keep the Caesarean scar clean and dry. Frequent baths will help with healing; adding lavender and tea tree essential oils may prevent infection. Carefully pat the area dry afterwards, or use a hairdryer on a low setting. Arnica tablets are good for bruising and shock. Once the scar has healed, you can massage it daily with lavender oil and vitamin E oil diluted in a blend of almond and wheatgerm carrier oils.

THE POSTNATAL CHECK

All new mothers are invited to a check-up with their doctor about six weeks after the birth. This is usually done in tandem with the baby's six-week check. You'll be asked about how you are recovering and the doctor will examine you to see if any tears have healed. This is a good time to voice any concerns you have about any aspect of your recovery.

Handling your emotions

Giving birth is an incredible experience, often the most powerfully emotional event of a woman's life. But there is little time for you to reflect on it because there is a tiny, vulnerable baby needing round-the-clock care. Not surprisingly, the first few days after the birth can be a very emotional and bewildering time for both parents. You may feel exhilarated and joyous, exhausted and overwhelmed, proud and fearful, often in quick succession.

As a new mother, it is helpful to remember that your hormones are out of balance, and the physical opening of the body for childbirth has affected you on a deep emotional level. In a way, it would be odd if you felt utterly serene and completely in control as you adjust to the new person in your life.

BABY BLUES

About half of all new mothers get very tearful or anxious a few days after the baby is born, and it is common to experience mood swings. These 'baby blues' are probably due to the sharp drop in hormone levels, and they may also be connected with feelings of anticlimax after the intensity of the birth. The most helpful way of dealing with them is to relax, and allow yourself to feel the emotions. Cry if you need to, and be open about how you are feeling to your partner or to a good friend.

A healthy diet, with red meat for iron and oily fish for essential fatty acids, can help you to manage difficult emotions after the birth, and helps breastfeeding too.

EMOTIONAL STRENGTH PLAN

The baby blues are usually temporary, but can sometimes come and go over a few weeks. Prioritize your physical needs – eat healthily and often so that your blood-sugar levels don't drop, drink plenty of fluid and sleep whenever your baby does.

Good nutrition can help with depression. The fatty acids in oily fish help maintain a healthy nervous system; calcium (found in dairy products, green vegetables, nuts and seeds, beans and lentils) and magnesium (nuts and seeds, green leafy vegetables, wheatgerm, sprouted grains, soy beans and whole grains) are also helpful. Check your iron levels – anaemia makes you feel lethargic and one study found that low iron levels could hamper bonding. Liquid iron is more easily digested than tablets, while good nutritional sources are lean red meat, oily fish, pulses, nuts, dark green vegetables and dried fruit. Vitamin C helps your body to absorb iron: citrus fruits are a good source. In addition, doing the following will help keep you in good emotional health and will help you to get through any periods of unhappiness or low spirits.

- Be open about how you are feeling with your partner, close friends and health professionals.
- Talk to your midwife about the birth experience. This can be very useful if you have any ambivalent feelings about your labour or delivery.
- Treat yourself to a postnatal massage or acupuncture treatment. Some complementary therapists will come to your home.

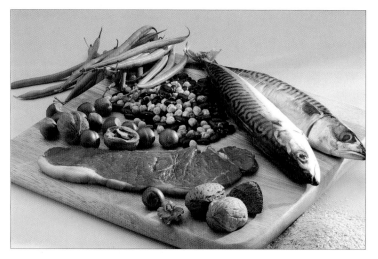

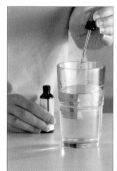

Rescue Remedy is a good instant remedy for any feelings of anxiety, panic or fearfulness.

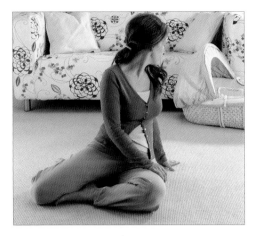

Yoga, or gentle stretching exercises, can have a calming effect and may help to counter feelings of depression.

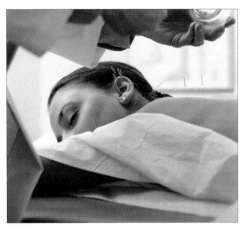

An acupuncture treatment can help you to feel more balanced after the exertion of giving birth.

- If you are on your own with the baby, make sure you see somebody every day. If you feel low, do some physical exercise every day, such as brisk walking and postnatal yoga. After six weeks – provided you get the all clear from your doctor – try a gentle postnatal circuit class or go swimming.

POSTNATAL DEPRESSION

Quite different to the baby blues, postnatal depression (PND) can start weeks or months after the birth, and can be long-lasting. It can make a woman feel so exhausted and lethargic that looking after the baby feels an impossible task, and it may cause anxiety and strong feelings of inadequacy. Fathers can also sometimes suffer from depression after the birth of a child.

Depression is hard to diagnose because it is normal to feel low and inadequate from time to time, but if feelings like this persist for more than a week or so you should seek medical help. There are various treatments for postnatal depression. Practical help, counselling, support groups and, if necessary, medication can all be helpful.

FIRST DAYS AS A DAD

It can be hard to be a new father. You are the parent of a tiny baby, which can feel overwhelming. Your relationship with your partner is likely to feel very different for a while and you may feel excluded by the bond between mother and child, especially if the baby is being breastfed. As new mothers tend to be tired and hormonal, your partner may seem irritable and unappreciative at first. The thrill of fatherhood is no less real or satisfying than the joy of

A new father may feel thrilled with his tiny child, but have moments of feeling overwhelmed or panicked too.

motherhood, however, and most fathers quickly carve out a role that is all their own, such as taking charge of bathtime or the first change of the day. Such things – however mundane they seem at the time – lay the foundation for the special and unique relationship between a man and his child.

Once the initial month or two are past, you will find that the presence of your child adds a whole new dimension to your relationship with your partner. Your baby is, after all, a tangible and constant sign of your love, a wonderful lifelong link between you.

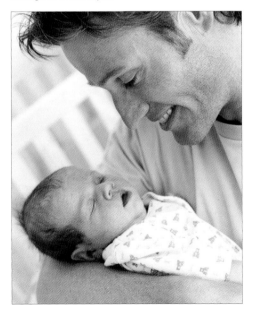

Basic baby care and feeding

" Breastfeeding naturally binds mother and baby together, making them inseparable for the first months of a child's life. "

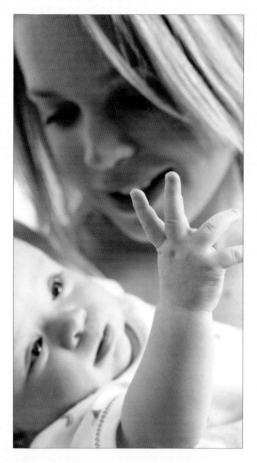

Lots of people talk about the hard work involved in looking after a baby. And it is true that a small baby requires almost constant care and attention. But there is also great pleasure to be had from lovingly attending to your child's needs.

These needs are, generally, pretty straightforward. Babies want feeding, probably more often and more erratically than you can imagine; they need changing when they are wet or dirty; they need to be kept warm; and they need to be held so that they feel safe. All these things are easily done, but the way you go about them can make all the difference between enjoying caring for your baby and finding it a burden or chore.

For instance, changing a nappy (certainly one of the less pleasant aspects of parenthood) is much more than a messy cleaning task. It is, in a strange way, a means of communicating your feelings towards your baby. When you put a towel on the cold changing mat to make it more comfortable, or speak soothingly as you touch and clean your baby, you are

A new arrival brings change and excitement to the wider family, as well as the parents. Siblings will want to be involved in caring for the new member of the family.

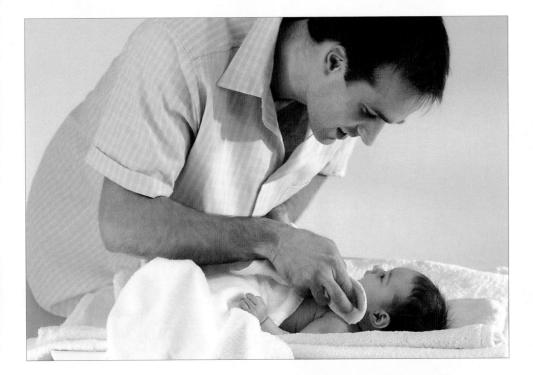

working to make the experience a positive one. Such attentiveness both requires and builds the loving tenderness a parent feels for his or her child.

Nature, through breastfeeding, has provided women with the perfect way to nurture their babies. Breastfeeding naturally binds mother and baby together, making them inseparable for the first months of a child's life. And while this might mean that as a new mother you cannot go out as you used to, it gives you the most wonderful opportunity to give yourself up to motherhood and to forge an unbreakable emotional connection with your child. If you decide to bottle-feed, you can make that connection in the same way, so long as you make a conscious decision to treat feeds as a special time to love and bond with, as well as nourish, your baby.

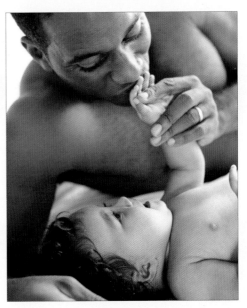

Top: Looking after a baby involves doing lots of small and repetitive tasks – but these can be incredibly fulfilling and enjoyable.

A baby's father will be able to find lots of ways to care for, and bond with, his child, even a breastfed one. Spend as much time as you can with each other.

Changing your baby

It's worth thinking about what type of nappy (diaper) you are going to use for your new baby before you give birth, so you can plan ahead. Parents spend a lot of time changing nappies. Your baby may need anything up to 12 a day at first, and could easily go through 4,000 nappies in the first two years. You should change your baby immediately a nappy is soiled, and at least every three hours otherwise. However, don't wake your baby up just for a nappy change.

WHICH NAPPY?

You can choose between disposable or cloth nappies, or you can use a combination of both. Disposables are convenient and quick to put on, but it's worth considering cloth nappies, especially if you are trying to reduce the amount of waste your family produces. Real nappies are better for babies' skin than disposables because they are

Smiles, eye contact and chat will help your baby to put up with having his or her nappy changed.

REUSEABLE NAPPIES

If you plan to use cloth nappies all the time, you'll need about 24 nappies and three covers. But if you plan to use some disposables, 10 cloth nappies and two waterproof covers should be sufficient. You'll also need two or three booster pads for nighttime, as well as liners. You can get flushable paper liners or reusable cloth or fleece ones.

Terry squares. These are the traditional option and the cheapest. They are good for newborns – a shaped nappy can look huge on a tiny baby. You can now buy plastic fasteners, which are safer than traditional pins.

Prefolds. These nappies are rectangular and have to be folded before use. They come in different sizes, so you will have to buy new ones as the baby grows, but prefolds are generally less expensive than shaped or all-in-one nappies.

Tie-up nappies. These come in one size and are folded in different ways depending on the size of your baby. They are secured using the attached ties.

Shaped nappies. These are probably the easiest to use, because they don't need folding. They come in a range of sizes, or in one size fastened differently depending on the size of the baby, and are secured by poppers or Velcro.

All-in-ones. These are shaped nappies that incorporate a waterproof cover. They are quick to put on, but they take longer to dry after washing and are also more expensive than other nappies. But they can be a good option for when you are out for the day, if you prefer never to use disposables.

shaped nappy

all-in-one

terry squares

plastic fasteners

prefold nappy

tie-up nappy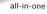

Nappy fold for a newborn

Even if you intend to use shaped nappies, it is worth investing in some terries for when your baby is very small.

As with other forms of real nappies, you'll need a waterproof liner to prevent leakage.

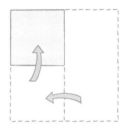 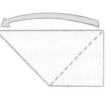 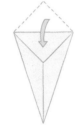 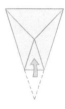

1 Fold the square in half lengthwise to make a rectangle, then again to make a small square.

2 With the four corners of the nappy at the top, pull the corner of the top layer across to make a triangle.

3 Turn the nappy over and fold the square edge over twice, so it forms a pad in the middle of the triangle.

4 Add a liner, put the baby on the nappy, fold up the base, bring one side over the other and secure.

Kite fold

The newborn fold is good for the first few weeks, but your baby will soon be too big for nappies folded in this way.

The kite fold is suitable for larger babies, and will extend the length of time you can use terry squares.

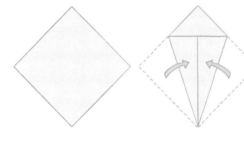

1 Place the square so that one corner is pointing towards you. Fold in the two side corners to make a basic kite shape.

2 Fold down the pointed top, then fold up the point at the bottom, as shown.

3 Place the baby on the nappy so that his or her waist is aligned with the top edge of the nappy.

4 Fold up the base, then fold one side over the other and secure with a nappy pin or plastic fastener.

---

made of natural fabrics and don't contain adhesives or superabsorbent chemicals, which can come into contact with the baby's skin. In the long term, real nappies work out cheaper than disposables, especially since you can re-use them for any other children you have. A local nappy laundering service, which delivers clean nappies and collects your dirty ones, is an alternative costing about the same in the end as using disposables.

If you prefer to use disposable nappies, consider using the eco-friendly brands that are now available from health stores, by mail order, on the internet and in some supermarkets. These have fewer chemicals and bleaching agents than most disposables, and contain more biodegradable materials. However, they tend to be more expensive – and bulkier – than ordinary disposables.

WASHING NAPPIES

You will need a large bucket with a tight-fitting lid to store used nappies, until you have enough to make up a wash that fills the machine. If you want to soak the nappies before washing (it isn't essential), add a few drops of tea tree oil – which has antiseptic qualities – or lavender oil to reduce smells, to the water.

To help keep the nappies free from stains, you can also add a tablespoon of bicarbonate of soda or two tablespoons of white vinegar. It is worth buying a mesh bag for the bucket to make it easier to get the nappies into the washing machine: when you are ready to wash, you simply transfer the whole bag to the machine. Use non-biological detergent, and close any Velcro fasteners to prevent snagging.

CHANGING YOUR BABY

During the day, make nappy changing fun. This is a great time for play – talk and sing to your baby, blow raspberries on his or her tummy, make silly expressions to make the baby laugh. Hang a mobile or mirror above your

Change your baby on a changing station or bed to ease your back and knees. Get everything to hand before you begin, and don't leave the baby alone for a second if the mat is above floor level.

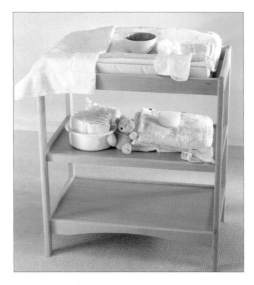

changing area as a distraction. At night, on the other hand, change your baby only if he or she is very wet or has soiled a nappy. Keep the room quiet and dim so that you don't disturb the baby any more than necessary.

CLEARING UP

Put disposable nappies in a nappy sack – you can get biodegradable ones that are made from starch rather than plastic. If you are using cloth nappies, flush soiled paper liners down the toilet and put wet ones in a nappy sack. Hold a soiled reusable liner in the toilet while you flush to rinse it, then place with the nappy in your nappy bucket. Wash your hands with soap and hot water.

PREVENTING AND TREATING NAPPY RASH

Most babies get nappy rash at some point. The best way to prevent it is by keeping your baby clean and dry: he or she is much less likely to get a rash if changed eight times a day or more, and if you leave the nappy off from time to time. It will also help if you use only damp cotton wool to clean the skin, and avoid wipes (especially those that contain alcohol), soap and strong detergents.

If your baby develops any redness, change him or her more often, and leave the nappy off for a few minutes at every change to let air circulate – give longer periods of

> **CAUTION**
> Don't use talcum powder on babies: they can inhale the tiny particles, which may be harmful to the lungs.

Cleaning and changing

Get everything ready before you start and have it close to hand. Cover the changing mat with a towel to make it more comfortable and to soak up any accidents. Keep talking to your baby to reassure him or her.

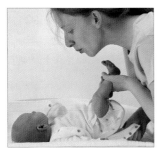

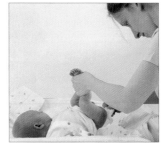

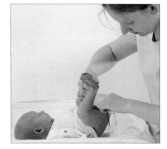

1 Remove lower clothing, and unfasten the nappy. If the stools are very liquid, use some tissue to clean off the worst of it, then clean the baby's bottom using wet cotton wool balls (cotton balls).

2 Lift up the baby's legs, fold the nappy in half and remove. Clean thoroughly, including creases in the legs. Wipe a girl from front to back. Clean under a boy's testicles but don't pull back the foreskin.

3 if there is any redness, apply a thin smear of barrier cream. Lift the baby by the ankles, then lay the clean nappy underneath, aligning the top of the back with the baby's waist. Lower the baby on to it and fasten it.

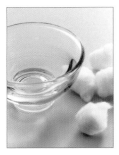

There are lots of nappy wipes on the market, but it is best to use cotton wool (cotton balls) and cooled, boiled water to clean your baby, especially in the first weeks. If you need to use wipes when away from home, use unbleached, chemical-free ones.

bare-bottom time if you can. Use a natural barrier cream, such as calendula nappy rash cream, at every change. See your doctor if the rash doesn't clear up within a few days or if blisters or pimples develop.

A GUIDE TO STOOLS

Babies' vary enormously in the number of soiled nappies they produce. Many will move their bowels at every feed, while some breastfed babies can go for up to a week without having a bowel movement. So long as the stools are normal and your baby is not in discomfort, this is nothing to worry about.

Normal stools. A baby's first bowel movement is black or green and very sticky: this is called meconium and it is passed in the first couple of days after the birth. Subsequent stools are usually yellowish in colour. In breastfed babies, they can be mustard yellow and runny

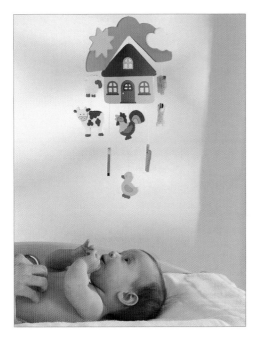

NATURAL SPRAY CLEANER

Bacteria can breed on a changing mat so make sure that you keep it clean. To make your own natural antibacterial cleaner, put two cups of cooled, boiled water in a new, washed, plant-spray bottle. Add 15 drops each of tea tree and mandarin essential oils and shake well before using.

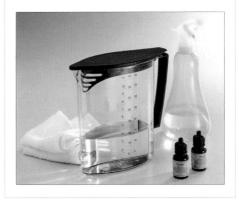

or dark yellow/light brown and grainy. The stools of bottle-fed babies tend to be dark yellow to light brown and firmer than those of breastfed babies.

Green stools. Some formulas can make a baby's stools green, but if they are also slimy, foul-smelling and frequent, then your baby probably has diarrhoea and should be checked by a doctor. A bottle-fed baby may need to drink cooled boiled water instead of formula for a short period; a breastfed baby can feed as normal. A breastfed baby may produce green, watery stools if he or she is getting too much foremilk and not enough of the rich hindmilk. To correct this, make sure the baby has emptied one breast before starting on the other.

Pellet-like brown stools. These suggest constipation. Breastfed babies almost never become constipated because breastmilk is easily digested, but bottle-fed babies may have this problem from time to time. Give cooled boiled water to drink as well as milk and make sure that you are using the correct amount of formula when making up the bottles.

Abnormal stools. Dark brown or black stools (other than meconium) in a young baby may indicate bleeding in the bowel: see your doctor for advice as soon as possible. Dark red or bloody stools may indicate an obstruction in the bowel, this must be checked urgently. Very pale stools may be a sign of jaundice and also must be checked with your doctor.

Hang a colourful mobile above your changing station so that your baby has something to look at.

Bathing your baby

Until a few years ago, mothers were taught how to bath their babies while still in hospital and a bath was seen as an essential part of the daily routine. However, frequent baths are not only unnecessary but also dry out a baby's skin. They can also be upsetting for young babies, who often don't like being naked, and stressful for parents. Handling a slippery infant with a floppy neck can be difficult, especially if he or she is screaming in protest. If your baby screams when you put him or her in the bath, wait a few days and then try again.

If you can, wait two to four weeks before giving the first bath. You can easily keep the baby clean in the meantime by washing his or her bottom at each nappy change, and topping and tailing at least once a day.

NAIL CARE

Most parents find the idea of cutting their baby's tiny nails daunting, but there is no avoiding it. Scratch mittens are useful for the first days, but you can't keep your baby's hands hidden away for long, not least because he or she needs to discover and use them. The easiest way to trim

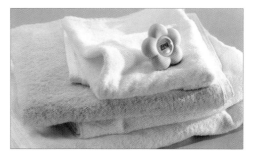

A bath thermometer takes the guesswork out of bathing your baby, but you should still double-check the temperature of the water with your elbow.

Topping and tailing

Clean your baby in a warm room, so that exposed skin doesn't get cold. You can use a changing table, a bed or sofa, or the floor, but cover the surface with a thick towel folded over a few times to keep the baby warm and comfortable. Either undress the baby completely and cover with a towel to keep warm, or remove clothing as you go along. Never leave your baby unattended on a raised surface, even if you think he or she can't yet roll over. Get everything ready before you start: you'll need a bowl of warm boiled water, cotton wool (cotton balls), a facecloth, a small, thin towel and a clean nappy (plus nappy rash cream, if necessary).

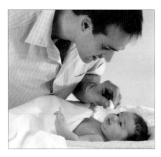

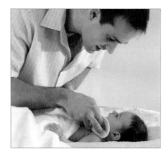

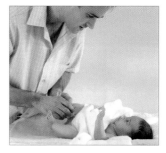

1 Cover the baby's lower half with a towel. Dip a small wad of cotton wool in the water, and wipe the baby's eye from the inner to the outer corner. Use a new piece of damp cotton wool to clean the other eye.

2 Use more wet cotton wool or a clean, damp facecloth to wipe the baby's face, including the nose and ears. Clean the folds of the neck (dried milk can collect here) and pat the baby dry with a clean towel.

3 Move the towel to cover the baby's top half. Now clean the nappy area, make sure you wipe all the folds in the legs and groin. Do not pull back a boy's foreskin or a girl's labia – these areas are self-cleaning. Pat dry.

Bathing

You can bath your baby in an ordinary bath, but using a baby bath is more convenient and uses less water. You can use a baby bath inside an ordinary bath, but it will be less strain on your back if you place it on the floor, or, better yet, on a stand. Make sure that the room is very warm before you undress the baby, and always check the temperature of the bathwater before immersing the baby in it. It's easier to get the right temperature if you fill the bath with warm water and then gradually add cold. Keep baths very short – a few minutes is all that is necessary – and hold the baby firmly to help him or her feel secure. It will be reassuring if you talk in a low, calm tone.

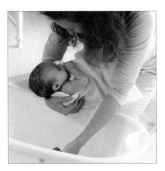 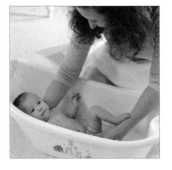 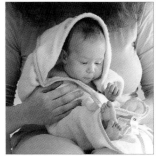

1 Undress your baby and wrap in a towel, leaving the head exposed. Hold the baby over the bath, supporting the back, neck and head with one arm and hand. Use the other hand to wash the baby's hair with water (there's no need for shampoo). Gently pat dry.

2 Remove the towel and lower your baby into the bath, holding under the arm with your hand and supporting the neck and head with your wrist. Support the bottom with your other hand. Continue to support the baby's back and neck while you use the other hand to rinse.

3 Lift the baby out and lay him or her on a towel, quickly wrapping it around him or her, covering the head as well as the body (a hooded towel works best). Dry well, all over, including the creases, and then put on a clean nappy and sleepsuit.

---

nails is to use baby clippers. Do it after a bath when the nails are softer, or when the baby is asleep. Hold the finger between your thumb and forefinger, and press the pad out of the way while you clip. You can also use a nail file, which doesn't leave sharp edges, or you can nibble your baby's nails short. Fingernails grow quickly, so check them every couple of days. Toenails should be trimmed in the same way, but they grow more slowly so won't need doing so often.

Trim your baby's nails when he or she is asleep, or is at least calm and still. Make sure there is enough light to see by – it is very easy to nick the skin by accident. Use baby nail clippers rather than scissors.

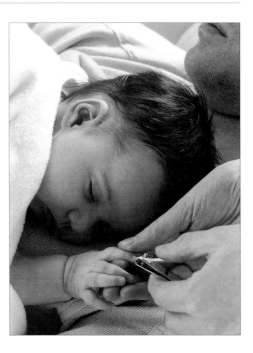

BATH SUPPORT

A framed towelling bath support makes bathing your baby much easier, since it leaves both your hands free and supports the baby's head. When your baby is a few weeks old, it will help to make bath time more enjoyable for you both. The towelling can become chilly when it is wet, so keep scooping water over it.

Caring for your baby's skin

Baby skin is very delicate and can easily become dry. The best way to protect it is to treat it as naturally as possible, and minimize any contact with chemicals. For example, use a soap-based washing powder rather than a detergent (biological ones are definitely to be avoided). Do not use fabric softeners, which can irritate a baby's skin. Always wash new clothing before putting it on your baby, since the fabric may contain chemicals left over from the manufacturing process. Where possible, choose clothes made from organic fabrics, such as cotton. Unbleached, undyed fabrics are the best choice for bedding and clothing that will be next to your baby's skin.

SKINCARE AT BATHTIME

It takes a few weeks for the oils in the skin of a newborn baby to form a natural protective barrier, so it is a good idea to avoid bathing your baby during this time: top and tail instead. Restrict baths to no more than two or three a week and don't use any baby bath products, especially those that contain petrochemicals, alcohol or perfume. Your baby is unlikely to get so dirty that he or she needs washing with soap, and you won't need baby shampoo for months – water will do the job all on its own.

It's fine to add the very gentle essential oils of Roman chamomile and lavender to a baby's bath so long as he or she is three months or more. Use one or two drops, diluted in oil or full fat milk before added to the water.

A baby's skin has a gorgeous natural scent. Perfumed bubble baths and other products aren't necessary.

Bathing in oatmeal

An oatmeal bath is an excellent way to soften and moisturize babies' delicate skin. It can also be used to help relieve the itching associated with eczema, chickenpox or insect bites.

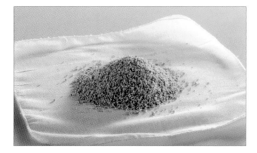

1 Grind two cups of oatmeal in a clean coffee grinder, blender or food processor until it is very fine. Combine the ground oatmeal with four cups of cold water, stirring well.

2 Add the oatmeal solution to a tepid bath – the water should look slightly milky and feel slimy to the touch (if the oatmeal drops to the bottom of the bathtub, it hasn't been ground finely enough).

3 Take care not to get any water in the baby's eyes during the bath since the oatmeal can irritate. You also need to be very careful when holding or lifting your baby because this bath makes skin extremely slippery.

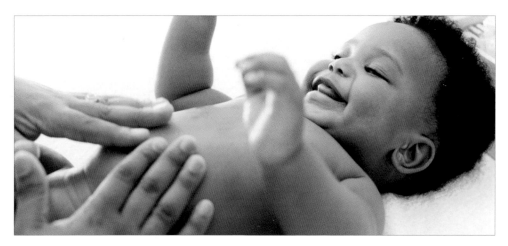

BABY MASSAGE OIL

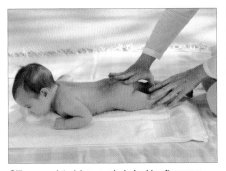

Oiling or moisturizing your baby's skin after every bath will help to keep it soft and hydrated. Using oil will also allow you to massage your baby without pulling the skin. But make sure that all the creases are completely dry before applying oil or you'll be creating the ideal conditions for fungal infection. You can use lavender and Roman chamomile essential oils on babies of three months or older. If your baby was born prematurely, wait until at least three months after your due date.

100ml (3½fl oz) sunflower oil
5 drops lavender essential oil
5 drops Roman chamomile essential oil

Pour the sunflower oil into a dark glass bottle then add the essential oils. Replace the cap and shake well to mix. When using for massage, pour a small amount on your hands and rub your palms together, then smooth over your baby's skin. Add more oil whenever you notice that the skin is starting to pull.

Plain water can be drying, so it is worth adding a little oil to the water to help keep your baby's skin soft and supple. Many parents like to use almond or jojoba oil in their babies' baths. But a few babies can react to nut-based oils such as these, so it may be safer to stick with vegetable oils like sunflower or olive at first. Alternatively, you can use oatmeal in the bath, which is a natural emollient.

CRADLE CAP

Lots of babies develop thick yellowish scales on their scalp. This happens when the sebaceous glands in the skin produce too much sebum, the oily substance that helps to keep skin lubricated. Cradle cap doesn't do any

Cradle cap can last for many months if you don't treat it. Smoothing olive oil into the scalp is a simple remedy.

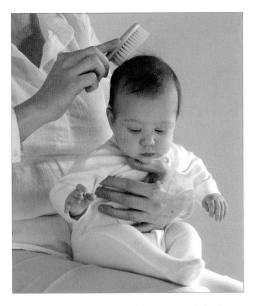

Use a baby brush, with very soft bristles, to help clear off the loose scales of cradle cap.

harm, but it can look unsightly and may persist for months if you don't treat it. To do so, gently rub some olive oil into the area and leave overnight, then wash off in the morning. To help cradle cap on its way, you can brush the scalp with a baby hairbrush to remove loose scales. Never pick off scales with your fingers or you may cause infection. If the cradle cap is very stubborn, try rubbing in calendula cream every night for a few days.

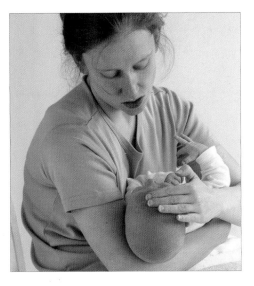

Clothes for your baby

Babies are not good at regulating their body temperature, so they must always be dressed appropriately for the weather. On a hot day, a nappy and perhaps a vest may be all your baby needs. On cold days, a vest, an all-in-one towelling sleepsuit and a light cardigan should be sufficient. Be ready to change your baby's clothing if the temperature changes or you go out.

You can tell if a baby is warm enough by feeling the back of the neck. If it is cold, you need to put on more clothing. But don't worry if the baby's hands and feet feel cooler than the rest of the body; this is quite normal. To check if a baby is getting too hot, feel the tummy or chest. Remove a layer of clothing if the skin is very warm.

Choose clothes made from fabric that is soft, stretchable and machine-washable – cotton is ideal. And make sure that everything is easy to put on and take off. You'll find all-in-ones with roomy necklines and snap fasteners a lot less restricting than denim jackets or party frocks. Shoes may look cute on a baby, but they can cramp the feet and restrict growth if they are too tight. It is much better to let your baby go barefoot so that he or she can wriggle his or her toes freely, or to put him or her in soft socks or tights to keep the feet warm. Make sure there is plenty of 'wriggle room' in the socks, and cut the feet off sleepsuits once they get snug in the feet.

BABY BASICS

Some of the most useful basic items of clothes for a young baby that will help you to have what you need whatever the weather are as follows.

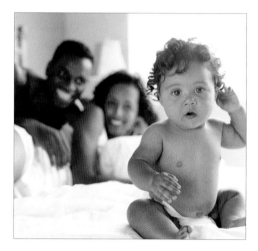

If it is hot, your baby may not need to wear any clothes at all. Some young babies feel insecure if they are naked and prefer to wear a vest, but most soon love the feeling of being bare.

Six short-sleeved bodysuits or vests. These may be all your baby needs to wear on summer days, and they make useful undergarments in winter. Long-sleeved bodysuits are good for winter but are harder to get on. **Six to eight long-sleeved sleepsuits with feet**. Great as pyjamas or daywear for young babies, but make sure they are roomy enough in the feet. You'll need fewer in

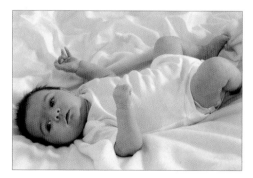

Lots of parents tend to overdress their babies. On a warm day, or in a centrally heated house, a bodysuit or vest on top of the nappy may be all he or she needs to stay comfortable.

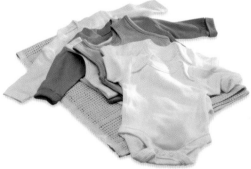

Baby clothes have to be simple and practical. Frills, fiddly buttons and fussy necklines all make dressing your baby hard work, and synthetic fabrics may irritate the skin and cause overheating.

Putting clothes on your baby

Many babies hate having their clothes changed, so do it only when their clothing is soiled or wet – there's no need to put a baby into a different sleepsuit for the night, say, if the one he or she has on is perfectly clean. Make sure the room is warm, especially in the early months, and place the baby on a comfortable surface. Work as gently and as quickly as possible, without getting flustered (it gets easier with practice). If the baby seems worried or distressed when naked, lay a small towel over him or her to give a greater feeling of security.

It will help if you maintain eye contact with your baby and sing or chat as you dress him or her. With an older baby, you can turn dressing into a game – play peek-a-boo as you pull a sleepsuit over your baby's face.

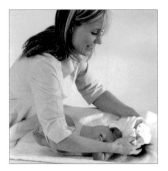 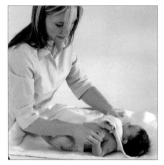 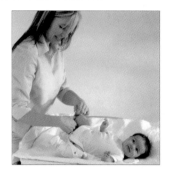

1 When putting on a vest or bodysuit, use your hands to stretch the neck as wide as possible. This will help you to ease it over the baby's head without scraping the nose or ears. Do this as quickly as possible since babies don't like having their faces covered.

2 If the garment has long sleeves, gather the sleeve fabric as close to the armhole as possible. Put your fingers through, gently hold your baby's hand and pull the sleeve over the arm rather than tugging a tiny arm through the sleeve. Repeat with the other arm.

3 To put on an all-in-one sleepsuit, open up all the fastenings and lay the suit on a flat changing surface. Place the baby on top. Gently ease the feet of the suit over your baby's feet. Pull the sleeves over the arms as before. Do up the fastenings from the feet upwards.

summer, when it may be too hot for the baby to wear them during the day.

Two to three cardigans. These are much easier to put on than garments that go over the head, but choose the kind that fasten with snaps rather than fiddly buttons.

Baby blanket. Good for wrapping the baby up when you need to go outside, or for use as a cover during naps.

Baby sleeping bag. A great alternative to blankets, which can be kicked off, a sleeping bag is a good way to make sure your baby stays warm. Combine a sleeping bag with a long-sleeved bodysuit, and add a cardigan if it is very cold. You can get bags with lighter tog ratings suitable for summer.

Three to six bibs. Useful if your baby spits up milk after feeds, or is dribbling a lot because of teething.

One or two hats. For summer, choose cotton hats with a wide, floppy brim (especially important if you are using a sling and need to protect the top of the baby's head). For winter, buy hats that are made of fleece or similar, with flaps that go over the ears.

Two to six pairs of socks. Get them all in the same colour, as you are bound to lose quite a few. You won't need many in summer.

Snowsuit with built-in mittens. This is great for keeping a baby cosy when you go out in winter. But you won't need one if you have a warm inner sleeve for the buggy or if you are carrying your baby in a sling; choose a cape or warm coat instead.

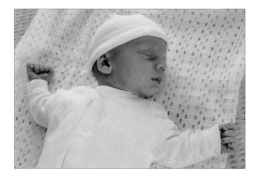

Babies should normally have their heads uncovered when they are indoors, but very small, or premature, babies may need to wear a hat in the first few days. Check with your midwife if you are unsure what is best.

Out and about

Going out with a young baby can feel quite stressful at first, so it is a good idea to keep trips short and relatively simple until you get used to the outside world again. Carrying your baby in a sling will help you both feel secure but can be hard on your back. Sooner or later you will need a buggy. Choose one that lies flat or use a pram for the first few months to avoid putting pressure on the baby's developing spine. A buggy with a seat that faces you will allow you to keep an eye on a young baby, and means he or she has your reassuring presence in view.

When you go out, your baby will need to wear extra layers and a hat (body heat can rapidly escape through the top of the head). To avoid overheating, you should take off any outer clothing and remove blankets and rain covers when you come back indoors or if you go into a warm shop or café, even if it means waking your baby up. Rain

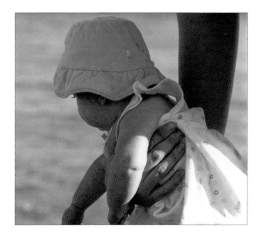

It is important to keep a young baby out of direct sunlight at all times. A wide-brimmed hat will help to shade his or her face.

Slings seem fiddly, with lots of straps and buckles to work out, but they are very comfortable and your baby will love being close to you.

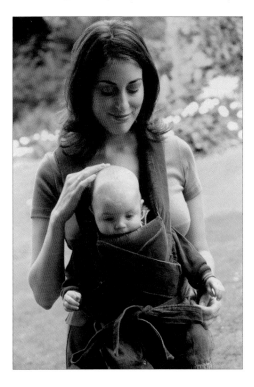

CHECKLIST: PACKING YOUR DAY BAG
It is worth investing in a proper changing bag, which is designed to carry everything you need for a day out. Write out your own list and keep it in the bag so that you can check you have everything whenever you go out.

- Nappies (diapers) and cotton wool (cotton balls)
- Flask of boiled water, or alcohol-free wipes
- Nappy sacks
- Nappy rash cream
- Complete change of clothes
- Muslins to protect your clothing and clean up baby
- Bottles of formula or expressed breastmilk, if using
- Bottle of cooled, boiled water, if using
- Snacks for breastfeeding mother
- Comforter or dummy (pacifier), if using
- One or two toys

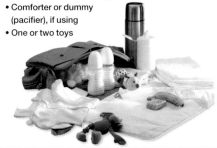

Take outdoor clothing off your baby when you enter a warm building. If the baby is asleep it is tempting not to do this, but he or she could become overheated.

covers and sunshades trap warm air around your baby, so be sure to open ventilation flaps whenever possible, and put covers and shades down when you go indoors. Using a UV-filter sunshade will keep your baby cooler than the buggy hood, and will give more protection from sunlight.

SUN PROTECTION

Babies under six months old should not be exposed to direct sunlight because their skin is too thin to protect them from harmful UV rays. Put a sunhat with a wide brim on a baby who is being carried in a sling, and cover arms and legs with a cool fabric such as cotton. If your baby is in a buggy, get an adjustable UV-filter sunshade so that your baby is kept in the shade.

CHOOSING A CAR SEAT

It is essential that you use the right type of car seat for your baby, even if you need it only for short trips. A car seat is one baby item that you should definitely buy new. Car seats that have been involved in an accident should not be reused, and you cannot be certain that a second hand seat has not been damaged, so it is risky to use one from an unknown source.

Each country has its own regulations for child seats, and in the US laws differ between states. Check online for specific rules, but most will state that for the first nine months or so, babies need a rear-facing car seat. This helps to protect their undeveloped neck muscles from a whiplash-type injury, which would be much more serious than in an adult. Check that the seat you buy conforms to United Nations or EU standards, and carries the appropriate quality mark, and choose one that has high sides to protect from side-impact blows. Once your baby weighs 9kg/20lb or more and can sit unsupported for at least 15 minutes, they can go in a forward-facing seat. For further information on different types of car seat, see page 456.

A travel cot provides your baby with a safe place to sleep wherever you are.

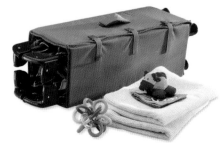

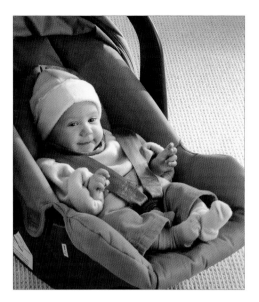

LEAVING HOME

Going away with your baby can be a daunting prospect, especially when you start to think about how much you need to take with you. But it's actually easier when a baby is very small, especially if you are breastfeeding. Here is a list of some of the things you may need.

SLEEPING
- Travel cot or Moses basket (unless your baby sleeps with you)
- Fitted sheet and flat sheet
- Blankets or baby sleeping bag
- Any sleep aids you may have been using (such as CDs or comforters)

CLOTHING
- Three complete changes for each day (fewer if you have washing facilities), and outdoor clothing
- Bibs, if using
- One or two baby towels

FEEDING
- Formula, bottles and teats, if using
- Sterilizer, if using (if you have access to a kitchen, you can boil bottles and teats in a large saucepan instead)

OTHER ITEMS
- Baby bouncer or play mat, if using
- Selection of toys (including any that your baby has grown attached to)
- Change of clothing for you
- Sling or buggy, if using, for going out and about

Why breastfeed?

Breastfeeding involves more than simply giving your baby milk. Snuggled at your breast, your baby enjoys your warmth, your scent and the familiar sound of your heartbeat. He or she can gaze upon your face, which is just the right distance away to focus on. Your baby is blissfully content. Before the birth, lots of women worry about whether they will be able to breastfeed their child. But almost everyone can, provided that they have a supportive environment in which to do it. And although you may experience some difficulties along the way, nursing can be as satisfying and loving an experience for you as it is for your baby.

SUCCESSFUL BREASTFEEDING

One of the keys to successful breastfeeding is simply trusting that you can do it. In societies where breastfeeding is the only safe way to nourish infants, new mothers assume that they can breastfeed – and they do. After all, our bodies are designed to nurture our babies both before and after birth.

Good support boosts your confidence and encourages you to continue through any initial problems. Studies have found that having a partner who is positive about breastfeeding can have a major effect. The support of friends and relatives, particularly women who have successfully breastfed themselves, can also make a big difference. It is well worth seeking out a breastfeeding counsellor or an organization such as La Leche League, who may run a drop-in support group in your area.

WHAT IS BREASTMILK?

Breastmilk is the perfect food for babies. It provides the nutrients they need in exactly the right quantities and it is packed with antibodies to help them fight off infection and illness. It is also completely sterile. Unlike formula milk, breastmilk is a living substance that adapts to your baby's needs. It varies from day to day, and from feed to feed. For example, it may contain specific antibodies to help your baby fight off any germs you encountered that day and it will have a higher water content on hot days. It is usually denser in the morning, after you have rested.

The first milk you produce is colostrum, rich in antibodies and nutrients, and with laxative properties that encourage your baby to pass the sticky first stools (meconium). True breastmilk comes in a few days after the birth. Each feed begins with thin foremilk to quench

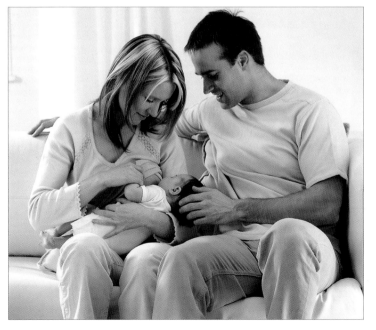

Fathers have a role in breastfeeding too: a supportive partner can be a key factor in successful breastfeeding, as can friends and relatives.

Nursing is an expression of love that only a mother can give. A baby who is upset or ill instinctively turns to you for the comfort of nursing.

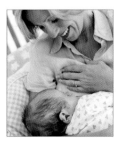

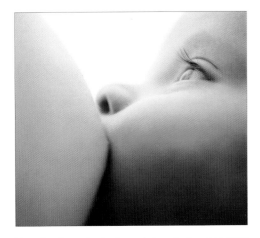

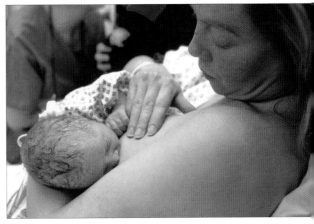

Breastfeeding not only gives a baby a feeling of security and comfort, it also has a soothing effect on the mother, and gives her a reason to relax and rest.

Even if you don't intend to breastfeed for long, nursing your baby for the first few days will give him or her some level of protection from infections.

the baby's thirst. As the baby continues sucking, denser hindmilk is produced. This is high in fat and proteins and gives your baby the energy he or she needs to grow.

THE ADVANTAGES OF BREASTFEEDING

It's more convenient. It is much easier to breastfeed than to prepare and warm a bottle, especially in the middle of the night.

It's better for your baby. Breastfed babies suffer from fewer tummy bugs than bottle-fed ones (one study found that American bottle-fed babies got diarrhoea more than 12 times more often). They also get half as many colds and are less likely to get respiratory diseases and ear and urine infections.

It sets the foundations for good health in adult life. Breastfeeding exclusively for six months helps protect your baby from allergies. Breastfed babies are less likely to be obese in later life, or to develop eczema, diabetes and high blood pressure. There is also evidence to suggest breastfeeding helps with brain development.

It encourages the development of the jaw and teeth. Breastfed babies may have fewer dental problems.

It exposes your baby to a wide range of tastes. The flavour of breastmilk varies depending on what you eat. This may help with weaning.

It is enjoyable. Babies nurse for comfort as well as food, and breastfeeding is the quickest way to calm a baby who is distressed.

It helps you to get back in shape. Breastfeeding stimulates the production of oxytocin, which helps your womb return to its normal size. And the fat stores you laid down in pregnancy are used in producing your milk.

It helps you to relax. You have to sit down to nurse your baby, which means you rest. Also, nursing mothers have higher levels of the hormone prolactin. This helps you to feel calm, so you can sleep quickly after a feed.

It has benefits for your health. Breastfeeding may reduce the chances of developing breast or ovarian cancer, and lower the risk of osteoporosis.

It delays the return of your periods. Breastfeeding has a contraceptive effect and you are unlikely to become pregnant if you are feeding on demand and do not go longer than four hours between any feeds. But if you need to be certain of avoiding pregnancy, you should use another method of contraception.

VITAMIN D

There is much debate about whether breastfed babies get enough vitamin D, which is important for bone health. It is present in breastmilk in low amounts and is manufactured in the skin when exposed to sunlight. Since we are now advised to protect babies from the sun, they are more reliant on breastmilk for their supply. The American Academy of Pediatrics recommends that all breastfed babies are given vitamin D drops as a precaution, while the UK Department of Health advises vitamin D (as well as C and A) for babies of six months who still have breastmilk as their main drink. They also now advise that all children continue to have vitamin drops containing A, C and D from six months to the age of five. This is to counteract poor diets in children who are then at risk of vitamin D deficiency. Talk to a health professional about what is best for your baby.

Feeding on demand

Your breasts will almost certainly produce as much milk as your baby needs, provided that you feed as often and for as long as the baby wants to. In the first weeks, this may mean you are feeding 10–12 times a day so that it feels like nursing is an almost permanent activity. You may find it hard to believe that your baby can be hungry so quickly after the last feed. But a baby's tiny stomach – about the size of a walnut – can take in only a small amount of milk at a time. Breastmilk is so easily digested that it doesn't remain there for long.

If babies get less than they need at a feed, whether it's because they go to sleep, or feed very slowly, they will want to nurse again sooner. By allowing your baby to nurse as soon as he or she is hungry, your breasts get the message that more milk is needed and will adjust their supply accordingly. It may take anything from a few days to a few weeks, but eventually your baby will start to go longer between feeds.

Every so often, you'll notice that your baby suddenly wants to feed more frequently again. These increases in demand often happen at around two weeks, six weeks

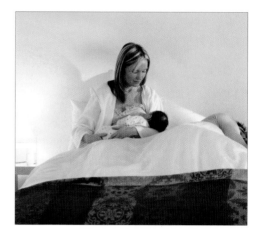

Feeding your baby on demand can be tough at first – most women find that they are nursing four or five times a night. But you get used to going back to sleep quickly, and eventually your baby will wake less often.

Lots of babies come off the breast when they are satisfied, but some like to go to sleep with their mother's nipple in their mouth. You may find that your baby wakes and cries when you remove it. If so, try letting the baby suckle once more and then taking him or her off again. You may have to do this several times before the baby will relinquish your nipple.

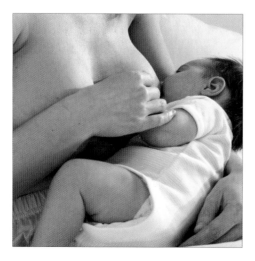

and 12 weeks, and indicate growth spurts. Again, if you let the baby nurse on demand, your milk supply will increase to meet his or her needs. Mothers often wonder how long a feed should last. The answer, annoyingly, is that it varies depending on how your baby feeds. Some babies keep sucking vigorously until they are satisfied, and they may get enough milk in 10–15 minutes. Others tend to feed in short bursts, resting in between. It may take an hour or more for them to feel sated. With slow feeders, it can sometimes feel as if one feed rolls into the next. There isn't a lot you can do about this: just accept that for now you will be spending most of the time nursing. Babies gradually become more efficient at feeding, so your feeds will get shorter.

EARLY BOTTLES

Don't give your baby any bottles of formula early on: if your baby is getting nourishment elsewhere, he or she will feed less often at the breast – and your milk supply won't increase in the way it needs to. Also, it requires less work for a baby to get milk from the teat of a bottle than the nipple, so if you give a bottle, the baby may refuse breastfeeds altogether. If you want to combine breast and bottle-feeding it is still best to breastfeed exclusively for six weeks to establish the milk supply. It is also best to avoid using a dummy (pacifier) during this time.

ONE SIDE OR TWO?

Mothers are sometimes advised to feed from each breast for a specific time. But if you do this, your baby may get only the thin foremilk, so you need to let the baby suckle at one breast for as long as he or she wants. If this empties the breast (which will then feel soft rather than full) but the baby still seems to be hungry, offer the other one. For the next feed, offer the second breast first, so the feeds start on alternate sides. To help you remember which side to start on, try attaching a safety pin or ribbon to your bra strap and moving it to the opposite side at each feed. Some women find that they can tell which breast to start on, because it is heavier.

IS IT WORKING?

The number of wet nappies produced can be the best indicator of whether your baby is getting enough milk: if there are fewer than six a day, you may need to check your latching-on technique or look at ways of boosting your milk supply. Make sure you are resting enough and drinking enough fluids. A baby mustn't be dehydrated, so talk to a health professional if you are worried.

If your baby is gaining weight slowly or in a different way to the development charts babies are measured against, don't assume you are not feeding successfully. It is normal for babies to lose up to 10 per cent of their birth weight in the first week, and to grow less in some weeks than in others. So long as they gain weight steadily over a number of weeks, they are probably feeding enough.

Like any new skill, breastfeeding takes practice and you may want to give yourself privacy at first. But once you and your baby get the hang of it, you can nurse discreetly without other people taking much notice.

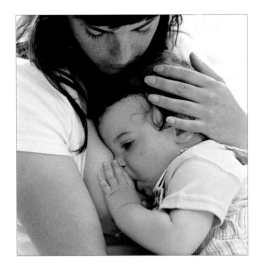

Breastmilk continues to have health benefits even after a baby is on solid food. Many women continue breastfeeding for two years or more.

HOW LONG TO BREASTFEED

Ideally, women would breastfeed their babies exclusively for six months and then continue to nurse for at least the first year, even after solids have been introduced.

Lots of women give up breastfeeding if they suffer from sore nipples or other problems early on. This is a shame, because breastfeeding usually gets much easier, quicker and more satisfying for the mother once the baby is a little older. You may find that you are able to go on longer than you expected, particularly if you get support and seek out other women who are breastfeeding for encouragement.

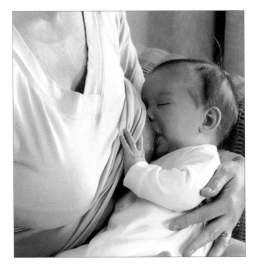

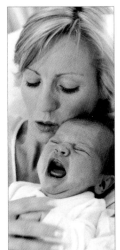

A hungry baby may cry, nuzzle against your breast or make rooting or sucking movements. Try to feed a hungry baby as soon as possible. Any period of breastfeeding will benefit your baby, so it is definitely worth starting, even if you don't think you will want to continue for very long.

Breastfeeding basics

Your baby will instinctively search for your nipple with an open mouth when placed on the breast (this is the rooting reflex that all babies are born with). But you need to give your baby some help to make sure he or she takes your breast in a way that enables him or her to get as much milk as is needed as efficiently as possible. It is also important that the feeding process doesn't make your nipples sore. This can be tricky at first, but with practice you and your baby will achieve the correct latch each time with ease. When a baby is latched on correctly, his or her gums press on the areola (the dark bit around the nipple) and stimulate the milk ducts inside the breast. As the baby sucks, the gums act in the same way as a pump, drawing milk into the nipple. The sucking also sets off the mother's 'let-down reflex' in the breast, which pushes milk from the production glands and into the milk glands.

WHAT NOT TO DO
- Don't put your hand behind the baby's head and pull it towards you. The baby will arch away.
- Don't position your nipple opposite the baby's mouth. Make sure that it is in line with the nose, or the baby won't be able to draw it deeply enough into the mouth.
- Don't press on your breast to make an airspace for the baby's nose – you could cause a blockage in a milk duct or move the nipple out of position. If the nose is squashed, try moving the baby's bottom closer to your body to create space.
- Don't continue if you feel pain that lasts more than a few seconds. Take the baby off and start again.

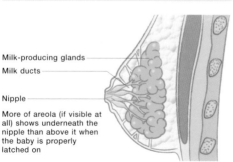

Milk-producing glands
Milk ducts

Nipple

More of areola (if visible at all) shows underneath the nipple than above it when the baby is properly latched on

A baby is properly latched on when the nipple is deeply inside the mouth. The tongue should be beneath the nipple, while the gums clamp down behind it.

LATCHING ON
As the baby sucks you should be able to see the jaw and ears moving and hear swallowing. If you can hear smacking sounds or the baby's cheeks are drawing in, he or she is not latched on properly.

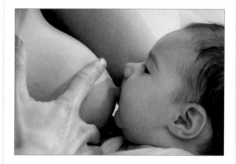

1 Hold the baby close to you, tummy against yours and nose opposite your nipple. Make sure the baby is completely on his or her side, with head, shoulders and back forming a straight line. Support your breast with your fingers, keeping them clear of the areola. Your baby may open his or her mouth and reach towards the nipple. If not, brush the baby's lower lip with your nipple.

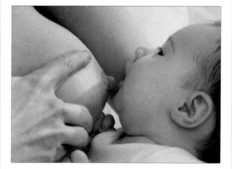

2 As the baby's mouth opens very wide, gently draw the shoulders towards you so that the baby can take the nipple and as much as possible of the areola into the mouth. The gums should close well clear of the nipple. If you feel discomfort for more than a few seconds, wet your little finger and slip it into the side of the baby's mouth to release the suction. Take the baby off the breast, then try again.

YOUR POSITION

You can breastfeed sitting down, leaning back, lying on your side or even standing up. All that matters is that the baby is in the right position for latching on and that you are comfortable and relaxed. You shouldn't have to lean or hunch over in order to get the breast in the baby's mouth – use pillows to support your back and the arm you are using to hold the baby, and put your feet up.

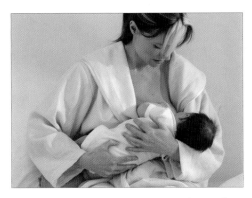

Cradle hold: The baby's head rests on your forearm, just below the crook of your arm, with his or her body supported along your forearm and bottom in your hand. Make sure you are tummy-to-tummy and place the baby's lower arm around your waist. This position is good for women comfortable with breastfeeding.

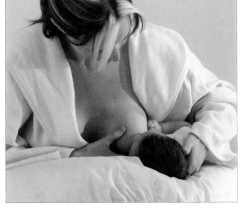

Clutch hold: Tuck the baby under your arm, facing you. The baby's head and shoulders are held in your hand, the back is supported by your forearm and the legs rest on a pillow behind you. This position allows you to guide the baby's head to your breast easily, so it is a good one to start with. It can be used if you've had a Caesarean, and also makes it possible to nurse twins simultaneously.

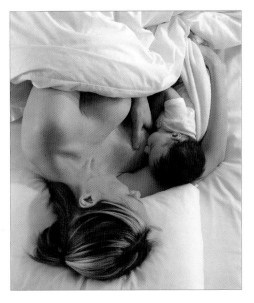

Lying-down position: You and the baby lie on your sides facing each other (put pillows under your head, behind your back and between your knees for extra support). Raise your lower arm above your head or use it to cradle the baby's shoulders and head. This position works well for night feeds but some women find it a bit tricky at first.

BURPING

Babies take in air when they feed and often need to burp afterwards. If your baby has fallen asleep feeding, you don't need to wake him or her to burp, but there may be one later. Some babies don't burp straight away so keep patting or change position, but if your baby doesn't burp after a while, then he or she probably doesn't need to.

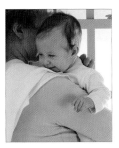

The simplest burping position involves holding the baby against your shoulder and gently rubbing or patting the back for a few minutes.

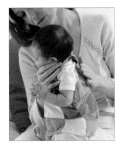

Alternatively, sit the baby on your knee, supporting the chin. Lean his or her chest on one hand and rub his or her back with the other.

Breast care and expressing

Even if you have breastfed a baby before, it can take your breasts some time to adapt to all the extra stimulation that they are getting. There is a lot you can do to prevent discomfort in the early weeks. Make sure you wear a proper nursing bra that fits properly. Most women find their breasts are a cup size bigger when their milk comes in, and a bra that is too small may cause your milk ducts to become blocked. You need three or four bras. Air your breasts often. If they are covered up whenever you are not feeding, warmth and moisture can build up, creating the ideal conditions for fungal infection. So expose your breasts to the air after every feed.

Don't wash your nipples with anything other than water – soap can be very drying and may encourage cracking. After each feed, rub a little breastmilk over the nipple and areola to keep them lubricated. Let them dry naturally. Eat

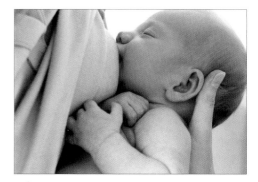

Wear loose, comfortable clothes that can be easily adjusted for feeding, especially in the first few weeks.

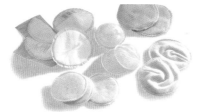

Breast pads protect your bra and clothing from leaking. You can get washable, reusable, unbleached ones, which are more environmentally friendly than the disposable sort. Plastic breast shells to collect the milk are helpful when expressing, or if your breast leaks a great deal when your baby is on the other nipple.

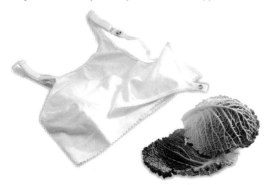

Your breasts may feel hard, hot and swollen when your milk first comes in. To relieve this, place a Savoy cabbage leaf, scored at the stem, inside each bra cup.

healthily and frequently. Breastfeeding women need an extra 500 calories a day, more if nursing twins. It is very important not to diet, since this will affect your milk supply and reduce your energy. Drink lots of water. Most women get very thirsty when they are nursing. Have a large bottle of water next to you when you feed, and drink regularly at other times too.

WHAT TO EAT
Both you and the baby will benefit if you have a healthy diet. Your daily requirements for vitamins and minerals go up when you are breastfeeding, but you can easily meet them by eating at least five portions of fruits and vegetables a day, plus whole grains, dairy foods or other calcium-rich foods, oily and white fish, lean meat, pulses and nuts. A balanced diet includes some fat, which you can get from healthy sources such as avocado, olive and vegetable oil, and oily fish.

EXPRESSING MILK
Before you had your baby, you may have assumed that you would express often so that your partner could feed while you rested. In reality you may find that you have neither the time nor the inclination to express. But if your

CAUTION
Do not take any prescription or over-the-counter drugs without checking that they are safe for nursing mothers. Check with your pharmacist or doctor.

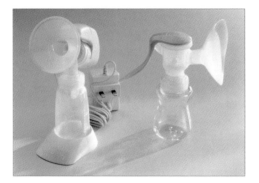

Electric breastpumps tend to be easier to use than hand ones. But expressing is a knack so don't worry if you get only a few drops at first.

baby is in special care, if you develop very sore or cracked nipples or if you have to go back to work, then expressing can be indispensable. There are three methods: by hand, by hand pump or by electric pump. Electric pumps tend to give the fastest results, but some women prefer a hand pump. Hand expressing is much slower, but it requires no equipment and can work very well for women who have a fast milk flow. If you know that you will need your baby to take a bottle, give expressed milk once a week from about six weeks.

STORING YOUR MILK

Expressed breastmilk can be stored in a completely clean, sterilized feeding bottle. Keep the bottle in the middle of the refrigerator (not in the door) for up to 24 hours. If you want to keep it longer, it is best to freeze it. When you are planning to use frozen milk, take it out of the freezer and place in the fridge to defrost for 12 hours. If you need it in a hurry, place the bottle in a bowl of hot water. Do not refreeze defrosted breastmilk.

One of the advantages of introducing a bottle feed is that fathers can take part in the profound bonding experience of feeding their baby.

Expressing by hand

Place warm flannels on your breasts or take a warm shower to encourage your milk to flow. Take a few moments to relax. Think about and look at your baby, or look at a photograph, to stimulate the let-down reflex.

1 Supporting your breast with one hand, use the other to stroke from the top of the breast to the nipple. Do this for 30 seconds or so, and be very gentle.

2 Cup the breast with your thumb and forefinger, placing them at the outer edge of the areola. Use a rhythmic squeeze and release motion, pushing your thumb and fingers slightly backwards (towards the chest wall) at the same time, until drops of milk appear.

3 Lean forward slightly so that you can collect the milk in a sterilized container as you continue to squeeze and release. Move your hand around the edge of the areola, so that you empty the breast. When the flow of milk slows, switch to the other breast. Repeat on both sides.

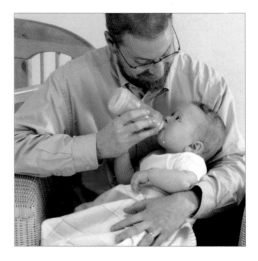

Common problems for nursing mothers

Breastfeeding problems often occur when a new mother is trying to do too much. So the best response is to take yourself off to bed for a couple of days with your baby. Ask someone else to take care of food and any chores so that you can concentrate on nursing. Frequent feeding and lots of rest can do a lot to help.

SORE NIPPLES

The problem new mothers complain about most – and with good reason – is sore nipples. Usually, soreness is due to incorrect positioning at the breast, so the best way to avoid it is to ensure that your baby is latched on properly every time. Rest assured that your nipples won't be sore all the time that you breastfeed – they will adjust and you will find latching on easier. In the meantime, you can help yourself in the following ways.

- Gently rub breastmilk over the nipple area after each feed and let it dry naturally. Airing the breasts regularly will also encourage healing – go topless when at home.
- Use lanolin cream to soften the nipples and heal any cracking. Calendula cream can also be used, but you need to wash off any residue before nursing your baby.
- Take the homeopathic remedy Castor equi.
- Do not restrict feeds, as this can cause the baby to grip the breast and suck harder.
- If all else fails, use nipple shields. These plastic caps cover the nipple while feeding. Some experts advise against using them because they can make it harder for your baby to suck, but they can be a good temporary

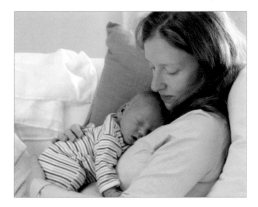

If you get a blocked duct, sore nipples or other breastfeeding problem, it may be a sign that you are doing too much. Spending one or two days in bed or on the sofa with your baby may be all you need to do.

measure if you are in pain, especially if the nipple is cracked. If milk collects behind the shield after your baby has been on the breast for a few minutes, then he or she is probably getting enough.

THRUSH

Occasionally, painful nipples may be due to the fungal infection thrush. If you have thrush, your nipples are likely to be red and itchy, and there may be white patches on them. In addition, you may be able to see white patches in the baby's mouth. You will both need to be treated, otherwise you will keep reinfecting each other.

The pain of thrush can make it hard to breastfeed, so it is important to treat it promptly. See your doctor for some antifungal gel: you spread it on your nipples and in the baby's mouth.

Occasionally, women get thrush in the milk ducts (which causes breast pain). This needs an oral antifungal treatment. It is also a good idea to take acidophilus supplements or eat bio-active yogurt to restore the 'good' bacteria in your system: this keeps the thrush fungus naturally under control. You can also get a probiotic suitable for young babies from good health food stores. Some women find it helps to cut out sugar and yeast for a while.

Arm swinging can help with blocked ducts or engorgement because it gets your milk flowing.

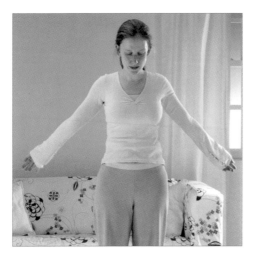

Thrush thrives in warm damp areas, so rinse your breasts after feeding (use plain water or a solution of one tablespoon vinegar in one cup of water) and expose to the air until dry. Be vigilant about hygiene: wash your hands with soap after using the toilet, before and after changing a nappy, and after feeding while treatment is ongoing. Use paper towels to dry your hands and discard; wash bath towels after each use in hot water (if possible, add a little white vinegar to the final rinse) Wash any toys or dummies in hot soapy water, then boil for 15 minutes.

BLOCKED DUCTS

If a milk duct becomes blocked, you'll notice a small hard lump in the breast. This may not hurt, but you need to clear it since an infection could develop, leading to mastitis. A blocked duct can be caused by a tight bra or by pressing your breast with a finger to make room for the baby's nose. It is often the result of the baby being latched on wrongly, so that some of the milk ducts are not being emptied. To treat a blocked duct:

- Change your bra or stop pressing on the breast.
- Apply warm flannels to the area before and between feeds. Some women find cold compresses (a packet of frozen peas wrapped in a small towel makes a good one) more helpful.
- Feed often (express if your baby is unwilling).
- Try an alternative feeding position so that your baby drains the breast from a different direction.
- While feeding, very gently stroke your fingers over the area and towards the nipple.
- Try arm circles before a feed, to help the milk flow.

MASTITIS

If a blockage is not cleared, then part of the breast can become inflamed. You will see a hot, red patch on the breast, which will feel hard. This is the early stage of mastitis. If it is left untreated, you will also get a high temperature and feel very ill (as if you have flu). If you

Mastitis starts with a hot, red patch on the breast. If you catch it early on, you may be able to avoid antibiotics.

react quickly enough, you may be able to treat mastitis by resting for a day or two (preferably in bed with your baby) and by following the advice for clearing a blocked duct. It is very important to keep feeding, and it is helpful to express any milk left in the breast after a feed to ensure that the breast is completely drained. A homeopath may recommend Belladonna or Hepar sulph, or you may want to take painkillers such as paracetamol (acetaminophen). See your doctor if you do not start to feel better after a day or so, or if you feel worse despite self-help measures.

If the mastitis is due to an infection in the breast, then it is best to take antibiotics to clear it. If it is left untreated, you may get a breast abscess. Many doctors recommend antibiotics at the first sign of mastitis. Most antibiotics are safe to take when you are breastfeeding, but they may cause your baby to become irritable or to produce stools that are looser than normal. To avoid another bout, be vigilant about positioning your baby correctly at the breast. If you get mastitis more than once you should discuss your technique with a breastfeeding counsellor.

ENGORGEMENT

If the baby goes a long time between feeds, milk can collect in your breasts, making them hard and swollen. Engorgement can also occur if the baby is incorrectly positioned, even for just one feed. To treat it:

- Have a warm bath or shower, or apply warm flannels to the area, then express a little milk before latching your baby on. Be gentle: engorged breasts bruise easily.
- Do some arm swinging before feeding.
- Use a cold compress on the breast to reduce swelling.
- Feed frequently, or express if your baby won't oblige.
- Try drinking fennel or marigold tea three times a day.

It is important that you keep feeding if you suffer from any breast problems. It is quite safe to do so: any bacteria will be destroyed by acids in your baby's stomach.

Herbal teas may ease breastfeeding problems. A fennel or fenugreek seed infusion is said to enhance milk supply, while marigold tea may help with blocked ducts.

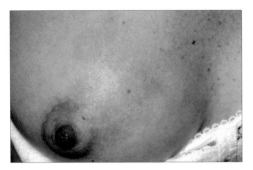

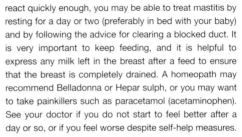

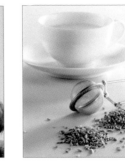

Common feeding problems

Most babies will quickly let you know if they have a problem with breastfeeding. They may cry during or after a feed, keep pulling off the breast or sometimes refuse point-blank to feed. This can be upsetting, but try not to take it as a personal rejection. Often there is a simple cause, which is commonly that the baby is not latching on properly. If it happens often and you can't work out why, a breastfeeding counsellor may be able to help. The following are all possible reasons for difficulty.

- If your breasts are engorged, your baby may find it hard to latch on. Express a little milk before the feed or hold a warm flannel against your breasts to help soften them a little.
- If your nipples are inverted or very flat, your baby may not be able to draw enough of the areola into his or her mouth (see box).
- Your milk flow may be so fast that it shocks the baby when he or she starts to suck. Try lying down or leaning well back (supported on lots of cushions) as you feed your baby. You can also try expressing a little milk just before the feed. Some women with a fast flow find that it helps to wear nipple shields while feeding.
- The baby may be frustrated when your milk flow slows down after the initial rush. Babies have to keep sucking in order to encourage more milk to be released from the production glands. If your baby stops feeding, it can help to switch to the other breast for a while before trying the first one again.
- Your milk supply may be low. There are several remedies you can try to enhance it (see below).

When breastfeeding goes well, it is deeply satisfying for mother and baby.

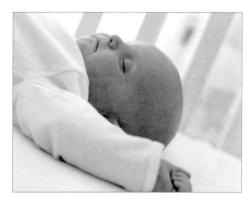

CORRECTING AN INVERTED NIPPLE
To help the baby grasp a flat or inverted nipple, take the areola between your thumb and first finger and gently press them together to push the nipple out. Then bring the baby towards you to latch on. Once the baby is attached, slowly release your fingers. Wearing breast shells between feeds can help to draw the nipples out.

- The baby may be windy. If your baby fusses halfway through a feed, he or she may need to be burped. Reflux, colic, teething or illness can also cause fussing.
- The baby may be distracted, particularly if he or she has just learned a new skill or if you are feeding in a noisy or unfamiliar place.
- You may have eaten or drunk something that the baby doesn't like.
- The baby may not be hungry. It's easy to get into the habit of nursing whenever your baby cries, but the problem may simply be that he or she is tired.

SLEEPY BABY
Some babies fall asleep after nursing for a few minutes, with the result that they need another feed very soon. This doesn't matter from time to time, but if it goes on you may want to encourage your baby to feed for longer.

- Make sure the baby is not too warm – feed in a cool room or remove a layer of clothing to help keep him or her awake.
- Rub the feet or walk your fingers up the back (either side of the spine) to keep the baby awake. Blow on his or her face, and stroke the cheek to stimulate the sucking reflex.
- Check that the baby's nose isn't squashed against your breast, since this can lead to sleepiness.
- Change the nappy halfway through a feed so that the baby is thoroughly awakened.

If your baby continues to be very sleepy and shows little interest in feeding, then he or she may be dehydrated or ill. See your doctor if you think this may be the case.

POOR WEIGHT GAIN
If your baby isn't gaining enough weight, don't be too quick to assume you can't make enough milk for his or her needs. A concerted effort to increase your milk flow can often solve the problem. Make sure you are getting

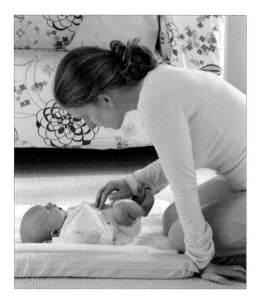

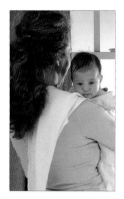

Left: It's hard to wake a sleepy baby. If you feel your baby has fallen asleep before they have enough, changing his or her nappy halfway through a feed will usually wake them up.

Right: There is not a lot you can do to prevent your baby from spitting up, but a cotton muslin will protect your clothes.

enough to drink and to eat – if you are dieting, it will be difficult for you to breastfeed. If you can, take your baby to bed with you for a couple of days; otherwise, spend as much time as possible together and feed frequently. Offer both breasts at each feed (starting on alternate ones each time). As with all breastfeeding problems, it is also worth checking your latching on, since if the baby is not attached to the breast in the right way he or she won't be able to empty it properly. Natural remedies for increasing milk supply include teas made from fennel, caraway or fenugreek seeds, nettle and blessed thistle. Certain foods such as oats and beans are also said to boost milk supply. In addition, it may be helpful to try to increase the fat content of your breastmilk by including more high-fat foods in your diet. Healthy options such as oily fish, nuts and avocados are best, but the odd bar of chocolate could help too.

SICKY BABY

Many breast- and bottle-fed babies bring up some milk after a feed, and some spit up quite a lot. This does not usually indicate a problem, so long as the baby is gaining weight normally, seems well and is producing wet nappies. But a baby who brings up part of a feed is likely to get hungry again quite soon. If the vomiting is frequent or forceful, the baby seems to be in pain or has watery stools, he or she needs to be seen by a doctor.

REFLUX

Some babies suffer from gastro-oesophageal reflux (heartburn). In this condition, the muscle at the entrance to the stomach doesn't close properly, which means that

stomach acid can travel back into the oesophagus. The baby often brings up large amounts of milk after feeding and may have poor weight gain. He or she may be distressed during and after every feed.

Try to keep your baby upright during and after feeds – use a sling and feed standing up, or try lying back against pillows and feeding so that the baby's tummy is against yours and he or she is facing the breast. Make sure you are both relaxed during feeds (breastfed babies tend to have less severe reflux at night when there is less distraction). Skin-to-skin contact, warmth and quiet will help. A homeopath may recommend the remedy Chamomilla or Nux vomica to ease discomfort. See your doctor if the symptoms persist.

Holding the baby so he or she is more vertical than horizontal can help babies with reflux or those who struggle with a fast milk flow. Leaning backwards may also help. Keep your baby's tummy against yours.

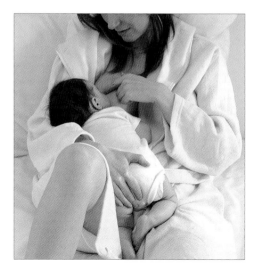

Deciding to bottle-feed

If you do not breastfeed, you will need to give your baby formula milk. Babies under the age of one can't have ordinary milk as their main drink because it contains too much salt and protein and not enough iron and other nutrients. Modern formula milks have been designed to resemble breastmilk as closely as possible. Most are based on cow's milk that has been modified to make it easier for babies to digest and to include the minerals and vitamins they need.

WHICH BABY MILK?

There is a range of baby milks on offer. There are not many differences between them, but some do not contain added iron, which is recommended. If you select organic formula there are fewer brands available.

There are two main types of formula: infant and follow-on. These have different ratios of the two main proteins in milk: whey and casein (curds). Infant milks are based on whey, which is more digestible. Follow-on milks are for babies of at least six months and contain more casein, which is denser and more satisfying. Many babies over six months are fine on infant formula and don't need to switch. Some manufacturers also offer a casein-based milk for younger babies – often marketed as being for "the hungrier baby". It is best to start with an infant milk and to switch to a denser formula only if your baby needs it.

Formula milk is available in powdered form or ready-made in cartons. Ready-made milks are convenient if you are out and about, but they are expensive, so most

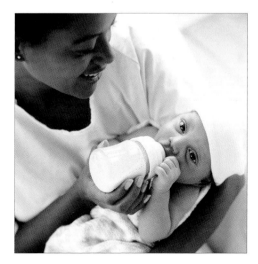

When possible, give your baby skin-to-skin contact during a feed and concentrate on your baby to replicate the nursing experience.

people use powdered milk, which needs to be mixed with boiled water. Most organic milks are available only in powdered form, though this may change as they become more popular.

ALTERNATIVE FORMULAS

If your baby proves to be allergic to baby milk (see box), he or she may be able to tolerate a special cow's milk formula called protein hydrolysate formula. In this milk, the proteins have been broken down into smaller particles to make them easier to digest. Health professionals can advise you on this.

Another alternative is soy-based formula, the only vegan option. Soy-based formulas contain high levels of the plant chemical phytoestrogen, which can have an adverse effect on thyroid function, so you should not use them before discussing the implications with your doctor.

If you are going to bottle-feed your baby, then you will need to sterilize the bottles to prevent tummy upsets. An electric sterilizer does the job quickly.

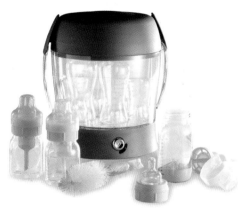

ALLERGIC TO FORMULA?
Signs of a true allergy include frequent diarrhoea, regular and forceful vomiting, excessive tiredness and skin rashes, but any of these symptoms should always be checked with a doctor since they may have other causes.

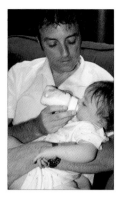

Left: Feeding time is a wonderful opportunity to sit quietly and cuddle your baby. Remember that sucking is a pleasure for the baby – concentrate on what you are doing together.

Right: Bottle-feeding allows the baby's father, or another person close to you to feed and bond with the baby.

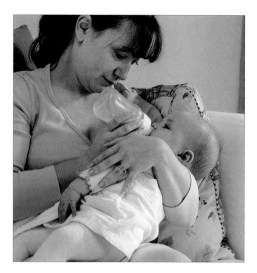

Some parents prefer to give their baby a formula based on goat's milk, which can be easier to digest than cow's milk. However, it contains some of the same proteins, so a baby who is allergic to cow's milk formula may also react to goat's milk formula.

BONDING OVER A BOTTLE

Drinking milk is not only nourishing for your baby, it is pleasurable too. So take your time with feeding, and make it a loving and relaxing experience. When possible, loosen your baby's clothing and place him or her on your chest so that you are skin-to-skin. Look at and talk softly to your baby during the feed. It will help mother and baby to bond if she is the one to give most of the bottles for the first few weeks, with the father or one other close person lending a hand.

Make sure you are comfortable and put a pillow under the arm you are using to hold the baby. You will need to hold the baby slightly upright (at a 45-degree angle), with

head well raised, so that the milk doesn't flow too fast. This will also help the baby to burp if necessary. To prevent the baby taking in too much air with the milk, hold the bottle up so that the teat is completely full. Never prop the bottle up and leave the baby to feed alone. Not only does this make feeding a rather lonely experience, it could lead to choking.

After the feed, help to release any air taken in with the milk by placing your baby against your shoulder and patting or rubbing the back until he or she burps. Sitting the baby on your lap, supporting the head with your hand or laying the baby on his or her tummy across your lap may also help. If any milk is left in the bottle you can keep it for up to an hour in case the baby wants more; after that it should be discarded.

HOW MUCH, HOW OFTEN?

Don't be in a hurry to put your baby on a feeding schedule. For the first few weeks, it is best to respond to the baby's needs and feed whenever he or she seems hungry. Babies' appetites vary and it will make both of you miserable if you restrict feeds or try to force the baby to accept more milk than he or she naturally takes. Offer the bottle whenever you think your baby wants it, and let him or her decide how much to drink – some babies will take a lot at one go and and then wait three to four hours before the next feed, others like to take less but feed more frequently. Over time, the gaps between feeds will get longer and you'll be able to plan your day around your baby's natural feeding pattern.

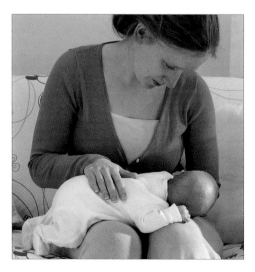

Experiment to find the best way of winding your baby. Try laying the baby across your lap, keeping the head slightly higher than his or her body.

Bottle-feeding basics

You will need at least six bottles and teats. You can reuse another baby's bottles, so long as they are not scratched, but you should always buy new teats, and there are lots of different ones on the market. Teats have different flow rates: slow, medium and fast. Generally, if your baby empties the bottle in just a few minutes, the flow rate may be too fast; if the feed takes half an hour or longer, the flow rate may be too slow.

If your bottles have wide necks, you can mix up the feed in them. If not, you will need a measuring jug and a plastic fork or knife (of a type that can be sterilized) for mixing the formula. You'll also need a bottlebrush and sterilizing equipment.

KEEPING CLEAN

Bacteria multiply quickly in milk, so it is vital that any bottles you use are scrupulously clean and sterilized to protect your baby from gastroenteritis and tummy upsets. Always wash bottles in hot water and washing-up liquid, and use a bottlebrush to clean around the rim of the bottle and the screw top. Squeeze washing-up liquid into the teat and use your fingers to clean it, turning it inside out to ensure that no residue remains. Rinse in hot water and then sterilize.

You should always wash your hands with soap and water before giving your baby a feed, and before making up the milk. Don't keep milk at room temperature for more than an hour or so, and always throw away any milk left over at the end of a feed.

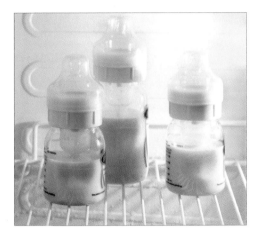

Always keep bottles of formula in the refrigerator once you have made them up. It is important to keep them cold to prevent bacteria from multiplying. If you haven't used the bottles within 24 hours, discard the milk.

WHICH STERILIZING METHOD?

Steam sterilizer units are the easiest and quickest way to sterilize feeding equipment, and don't use any chemicals. You simply add a little water, close the lid and switch on.

Boiling needs no special equipment except a large, lidded pan, which you should keep just for sterilizing. Fill with cold water, add the bottles and lids and submerge completely (making sure that no air is trapped in them), then boil for ten minutes with the lid on. Don't take the lid off until you need the equipment: once you remove the lid the water is no longer sterile, so you must take everything out (wash your hands before doing this).

Chemical sterilizing can be a useful method if you are away from home, but it is probably too time-consuming for general use. You can buy a cold-water sterilizing unit or use any large container, such as a bucket, with a lid. You will also need sterilizing solution or tablets. Make up the solution according to the manufacturer's instructions, and add to the bucket. Immerse the bottles, lids and teats

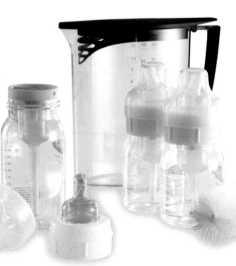

Before you embark on bottle-feeding, you need to have all the necessary equipment, including enough bottles to see you through 24 hours, a bottle brush, measuring jug, and plastic cutlery that can be sterilized.

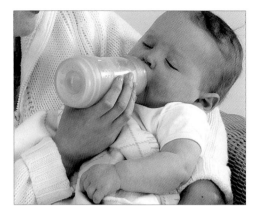

WHICH BOTTLE?
Many plastic baby bottles are made from polycarbonate plastic, which contains the hormone-disrupting chemical Bisphenol A. Minute amounts of this chemical may leak into the baby's milk, especially when the bottle is heated, or if the surface is scratched. Although the risks are very small, as a precaution you may want to buy bottles made from heat-resistant toughened glass (which can also be recycled) or from polypropylene plastic, which does not contain Bisphenol A. Check on the internet for manufacturers of suitable brands.

Some babies don't mind drinking milk cold, but most prefer it to be the same temperature as breastmilk.

completely (making sure that no air is trapped in them) and use a plate to weigh them down. Leave for at least two hours, or as specified by the chemical manufacturer. Wash your hands before taking out the bottles. If you want to rinse off the chemical solution, use boiled, cooled water, not tap water (which isn't sterile).

When your baby is ready for a feed, take the bottle from the fridge and heat in a bowl of hot water, keeping it out of children's reach. Shake the bottle, then test the temperature with a few drops on your wrist.

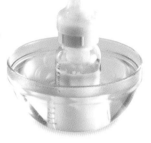

Making up a feed
You can make up each feed as you need it, but it will save time if you prepare all the bottles your baby will need for 24 hours in one go. It also means that if you've got a furiously hungry baby you have the vital feed ready at hand.

Put the caps on the bottles and store them in the fridge until required. Make sure everything you use for making up the feed – bottles, tops, teats, measuring jug, plastic knife and fork – is clean and sterile.

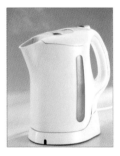

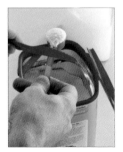

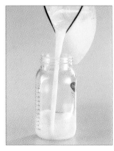

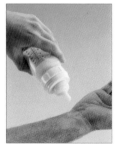

1 Always use freshly boiled water: empty the kettle, rinse it and fill with cold water. Boil, then leave it to cool. Wash your hands. Pour the correct amount of water into a measuring jug, or directly into bottles.

2 Add the exact number of scoops of formula recommended by the manufacturer (usually, one level scoop per 30ml/1fl oz water). Overfill the scoop and then level off the powder using the back of a sterile knife. Do not pack the powder down.

3 If you are using a jug, stir with a fork to mix, then pour the formula into the bottles. If you are mixing in the bottle, add the teat, the disc and the cap and shake well to mix. When all the bottles are full, put them in the centre of the fridge so they chill quickly.

4 Before a feed, warm the milk in a bowl of hot (not boiling) water. Don't use a microwave oven, which heats unevenly and can cause hot spots. Test it is at blood temperature by shaking a few drops on to your wrist; it should feel neither hot nor cold.

Crying, responding and sleeping

66 As babies get older they are more interested in noise, colour and movement, and will respond to your efforts to entertain them. 99

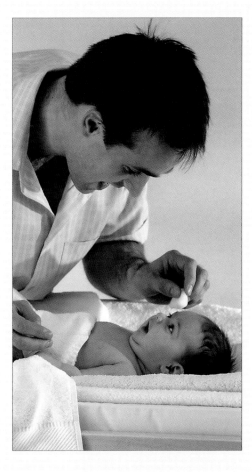

It's normal for babies to cry. It is the only way that they can communicate with us, to let us know when they are hungry, cold, uncomfortable or lonely. But some babies definitely cry more than others. A British study, conducted in Manchester, found that the amount young babies cried over the course of a day could be as little as a few minutes or as much as five hours.

Many babies are naturally easy-going. They cry only for obvious reasons, such as hunger or when they are startled. They may also be easy to soothe, once you have worked out what they like best: being rocked or sung to perhaps.

If your baby cries a lot, it is very easy to feel that you are doing something wrong. It is true that there is sometimes a clear cause for frequent crying, such as illness or persistent hunger, which obviously needs to be addressed. But often babies who cry a lot are highly sensitive, and simply find it hard to cope with all the stimuli that they are bombarded with in a normal day. If this is the case with your

There is no doubt that some babies are easier to care for than others. If you have a high-need baby, the calm moments can be all the more special.

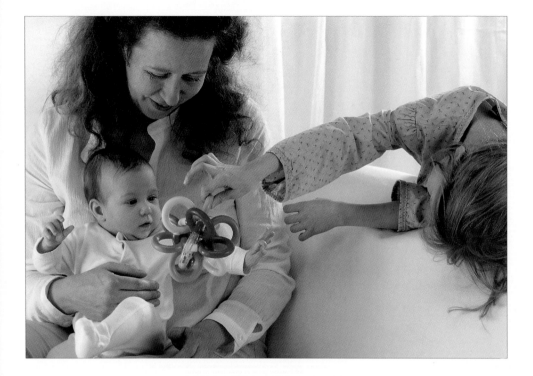

baby, you will have to call on all your reserves of compassion and patience to nurture him or her through this tricky stage. It can be very helpful to remember that it won't go on forever: sensitive babies often settle down after three or four months. This is also the time when you can expect your baby's sleep pattern to begin to coincide more with yours. Very young babies don't distinguish between night and day and, if anything, they tend to be more wakeful at night.

There is a lot you can do to help your baby sleep better right from the start. But, like so many aspects of parenting, having a relaxed attitude and realistic expectations is important and will help you to cope with the inevitable disturbances and disruptions to your painstakingly established routines.

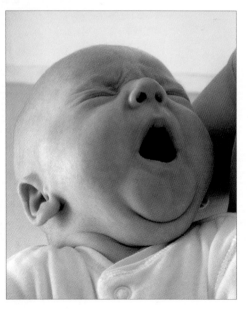

Top: As babies get older they become more interested in noise, colour and movement, and will start to respond to your efforts to entertain them.

Babies have all sorts of new things to look at and experience in a day. It's not surprising that they can become overwhelmed in these early months.

Why babies cry

Crying is the only way a very young baby can communicate. And it is a very effective method for the baby to get attention: when you rush to soothe your crying baby, you are doing what comes naturally to parents all over the world. Babies cry in different ways depending on what is wrong. In time you will learn to distinguish between cries, and recognize the different sounds your baby makes when hungry, uncomfortable or overtired. You may also start to pick up on certain gestures – for example, arching the back when windy – or you may become more aware of what triggers your baby's distress – such as too much handling by visitors.

CHECKLIST: WHY IS MY BABY CRYING?

In the early days, discovering why your baby is crying is a matter of trial and error. It's helpful to have a mental checklist of possible causes that you can run through to help you pinpoint the cause.

Is the baby hungry? Young babies can get hungry more quickly than you would think possible. They go through growth spurts, which means they suddenly need to feed more than usual. So even if you have fed your baby very recently, crying may mean he or she is hungry.

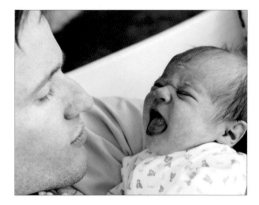

Don't worry that you are teaching your baby bad habits by attending to his or her cries. You are showing that you can be relied on to be there when needed.

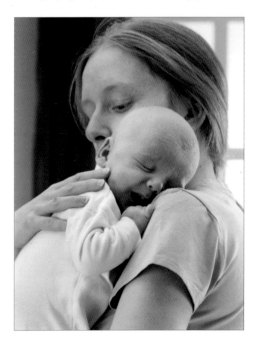

Is the baby wet? Some infants hate feeling wet, and will scream when their nappy is dirty or a cloth nappy is damp. Others don't mind it at all.

Is the baby uncomfortable? Babies cry if they are too hot or cold, if their clothing is tight or uncomfortable, and sometimes when they are having a bowel movement. Check that the room is warm enough and that your baby is dressed appropriately. Make sure that clothing isn't rubbing, scratching or pressing against the skin. Check fingers and toes, too – perhaps a hair is wound tightly around a tiny digit. Have a look at the nappy (diaper) area – the cause may be a painful rash.

Has the baby been startled? New babies often jerk around a lot, especially when they are dropping off to sleep. A baby who is frightened – by a loud noise, say – will cry. All the baby needs is to be held close until he or she calms down. Swaddling or holding close can help your baby to feel secure and prevent any sudden movements that will be disturbing.

Does the baby dislike being naked? Some babies cry whenever they are changed or washed. If this is the case with yours, be as quick and gentle as you can. Laying a small towel over a naked baby's chest and tummy may help him or her feel more secure. Making eye contact, talking and singing may also be reassuring.

At difficult moments, focus on calming yourself down – if you are tense, you will find it harder to soothe your baby. Relax your shoulders and breathe slowly.

Has the baby got wind? Babies cry during or after a feed if they need burping, and some may need burping again later on when the milk is being digested. Sometimes they need to pass wind: it can help your baby to do this if you pat his or her bottom rhythmically. Your breastfed baby may also cry if you have eaten a particular food that he or she is sensitive to.

Is the baby ill? Babies who are crying in a different way than usual may be unwell. Check the baby over: is there a rash, a temperature, a runny nose or other signs of illness? Call a doctor if your baby is crying strangely or persistently, or looks or behaves unusually.

Is the baby overstimulated? Babies can become irritable if they get too much stimulation; they cry as a way of shutting out external noise. If your baby is tired and overstimulated, he or she will find it hard to drop off.

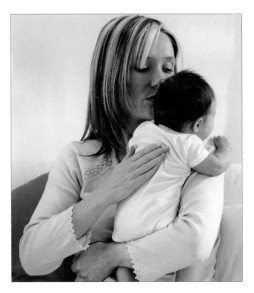

You will soon learn how to comfort your baby: some like to be held upright, others prefer being cradled.

Being held, rocked, or patted on the back is a good way to settle an overtired baby, but some seem to prefer being laid down in a quiet, dark place and allowed to cry for a minute or two, after which they will go to sleep.

Is the baby lonely? Babies need lots of physical contact, and will cry if they want to be picked up and cuddled. If you find it hard to hold your baby as much as he or she seems to want, take it in turns with a partner, enlist the help of a grandparent or friend, or use a sling to carry the baby while keeping your hands free.

You will often hear parents say that they are happy to leave their babies to cry so long as they know they are fed, burped and changed. But a baby may be crying simply because he or she feels fearful or lonely and needs your comforting presence.

AM I SPOILING MY BABY?

Young babies are not capable of crying in order to manipulate you – their brains don't work that way. They cry because they have a need that isn't being met; making a noise is the only way that they can signal that something is wrong. It's important that your baby learns he or she is safe and can rely on you. Don't hesitate to pick the baby up for a cuddle whenever he or she is upset. In this way, you help to establish a relationship based on trust and love.

Researchers have found that the more quickly their carers respond to their cries, the more quickly and easily babies are soothed. In other words, if you leave your baby to cry for ten minutes in the hope that he or she will settle, it may take you much longer to calm him or her down. Other studies show that babies whose cries are quickly and consistently responded to in the first months will develop into more independent toddlers than those who are often left to cry. So don't worry that you are teaching your baby bad habits by attending to his or her cries. You are letting the baby know that you can be relied on to be there when you are needed.

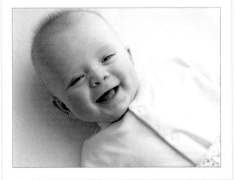

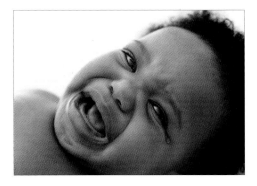

Soothing your baby

If your baby is crying, check the basics first: offer a feed and check for a wet or dirty nappy. Try burping to release any trapped air. If your baby is clean, fed and burped, but still crying, one or a combination of the following methods may be soothing.

GETTING PHYSICAL

Bear in mind that no one method works for all babies – finding out what calms your baby is a matter of experimentation, and nothing will work every time.

Hold the baby close. Physical contact has a calming effect, especially if you place your baby naked on your bare skin. Try shutting out any other stimuli by going into a dark, warm room. You may find that changing the way you hold the baby is also soothing – try an upright position or the colic hold (see Coping with Colic).

Try rocking. Most babies love to be swayed from side to side – it's the same movement they experienced in the womb. Researchers have found that parents automatically rock their children approximately in time with a heartbeat. If rocking doesn't seem to work for your baby, try upping the tempo a little – about 60 rocks a minute is good. Rocking your baby in a pram can also be very soothing, or you can use a sling and walk around.

Dance. If your baby is agitated, playing music or singing while you dance rhythmically with the baby in your arms

CAUTION

Even if you are at your wit's end from constant crying, you must never, ever shake your baby. A moment's frustration can have serious long-term, and possibly fatal, effects. If you feel that you may be in danger of shaking or otherwise hurting your baby, put him or her down in a safe place (such as the cot) and walk out of the room. Taking a few minutes to breathe deeply can help you to calm yourself. If possible, call someone else to come and look after the baby to give you a break.

may help to soothe him or her. You can gradually slow the pace as the crying subsides.

Let the baby suck on something. Some babies are very 'sucky' and like to nurse for comfort for long periods. If you are not breastfeeding – or if you are but your baby doesn't seem to want the breast – your clean little finger makes an excellent temporary pacifier. Dummies can also work well or you can try guiding your baby's own fingers to his or her mouth to suck on.

Keep the baby warm. A baby who feels warm and cosy may calm down more quickly. Heat the room to a comfortable temperature and wrap your baby in blankets or try swaddling (see Coping with Colic).

GOOD NOISE

Before birth, babies are exposed to constant noise from their mother's heartbeat, her muted voice and the low rumble of the womb. So similar kinds of noise can be comforting for distressed infants.

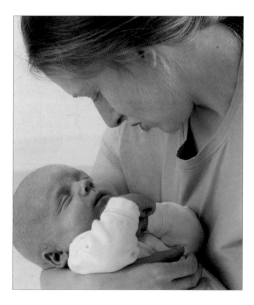

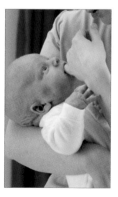

Left: Shushing helps to shut out extraneous noise and also relaxes the baby as it recalls the noise of the womb. This is why we instinctively use this sound to soothe babies.

Right: Holding your baby close for a while may be soothing, but you may also need to rock a crying baby, or offer your little finger to suck.

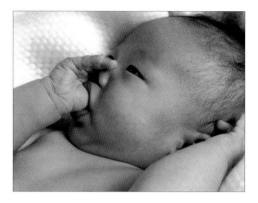

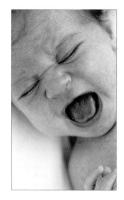

Left: Babies have been seen sucking a thumb in the womb – it is a great way of self-soothing.

Right: Long bouts of crying are rare in cultures where babies are carried all day, so it may just be that your crying baby wants to be held. Using a sling and more cuddling or nursing may reduce your baby's crying.

Shush. Shushing is a traditional and effective way to quieten a baby – simply place your mouth a little distance from your baby's ear and say 'sssssshhhhhh'. Do long shushes, increasing the volume if your baby doesn't seem to be responding.

Sing. The other sound traditionally used to soothe a baby is singing. It doesn't matter whether you have a good voice or not – your baby will appreciate your singing. It's worth learning a couple of lullabies for this purpose.

Use white noise. The roar of a vacuum cleaner, the hum of a washing machine or untuned radio static can all quieten a baby, sometimes in an instant. You can buy CDs of these sounds or record your own. It's not a good idea to operate a vacuum cleaner near your baby for long periods since this will affect the quality of the air that he or she is breathing.

Play music. Classical music has been shown to have a soothing effect on babies, and Mozart has been shown to be particularly good (no one knows why). But try light concertos rather than, say, operas.

CHANGE THE ENVIRONMENT

Consider your surroundings. If it is noisy and bright, with lots of activity, the baby may feel overwhelmed.

Take the baby somewhere quieter. Sometimes a change of place is all a baby needs to calm down.

Get some fresh air. Going outdoors will often stop a baby crying – and it can help you to relax too. Many babies fall asleep when driven around in a car for a while, even if they wake up the instant you stop the car.

Pass the baby to somebody else. If you haven't been able to soothe your baby, ask your partner or another close person to take a turn. Don't take it personally if the crying stops – it may just be that the change of company has distracted the baby.

A crying baby may be distracted from his or her distress by something new – an interesting toy, a funny noise or even a comical expression.

Try diversion. Offer a toy, walk in front of a mirror so that the baby can see his or her reflection, or walk around the house. Some babies find a warm bath very soothing; others don't.

AND FINALLY...

If all else fails, just stop trying to calm your baby down and accept the fact that for some reason he or she needs to cry. Continue to hold the baby close, but make a positive effort to release any tension that you might be feeling. Let your shoulders drop downward, take a long slow breath in and then out. Sit quietly for a few minutes, holding your crying child, controlling your breathing, and allowing yourself to accept the difficulty of the situation. If you can be relaxed about what is happening, you may well find that the baby stops crying in response.

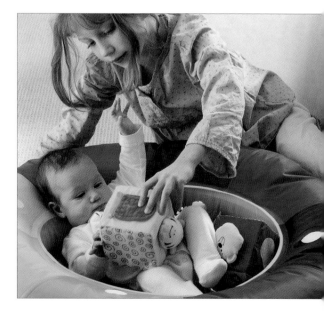

Baby massage routine

Massage is a wonderful way to build a loving bond of trust between parent and child, and can be a useful part of a bedtime routine. It has practical benefits, too: it can stimulate your baby's circulation and immature immune system, and it helps to improve the digestion. Massage is best done when your baby is already relaxed and calm, so aim to do it between feeds – a massage may be uncomfortable immediately after feeding, and if the baby is hungry he or she won't want to lie still. Don't try to do anything else, like watch TV, while you are

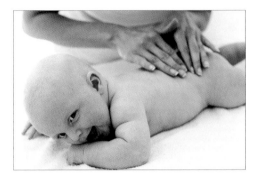

As your baby grows and becomes more robust, you can increase the pressure slightly, but never be firm or probing. Newborns should simply be gently stroked.

WHEN NOT TO MASSAGE

Check with your doctor or health adviser if your baby has health problems or if you have any doubts about the suitability of massage. Do not massage if your baby is ill or has a skin condition, and wait for 48 hours after immunization – longer if the baby has been adversely affected. Stop the massage if your baby doesn't enjoy it, and drop or adapt any movements that he or she does not seem to like.

massaging your baby – make this a quiet and precious time that you can both enjoy: go to a quiet place and switch off any bright overhead lights. As you massage, keep looking at your baby – smiling, chatting and singing will help to maintain his or her interest.

Massage techniques

You can massage your baby clothed or naked. A naked massage gives the skin-to-skin contact that babies enjoy, but use oil so your hands glide over the skin without pulling. An ordinary vegetable oil such as olive or sunflower is ideal. Make sure that the room is warm, and lay your baby on a thick towel so that he or she is comfortable (you can place a clean nappy under a naked baby). Take a few slow breaths to help you relax. Use light strokes that are just firm enough not to be ticklish – this routine is for babies of about one month or older. Do each stroke several times.

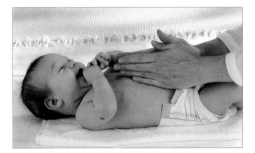

1 Lay your baby on his or her back and look into his or her eyes. Place your palms together and gently lay the sides of your little fingers on the centre of the baby's chest. Slowly open your hands, keeping the thumbs together and sliding the little fingers apart until your hands are flat on the baby's body. Stay like this for a few moments.

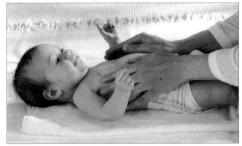

2 Tell your baby you are going to give him or her a massage. Slowly stroke down the baby's torso. Start by using both hands then turn your hand so that it covers the top of the baby's chest. Gently stroke down the torso. As you do so, place your other hand at the top of the baby's chest. Stroke one hand after the other in a smooth action.

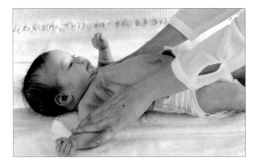

3 Rest your hands on the baby's chest and stroke upwards and outwards so that your hands pass down the baby's arms and hands.

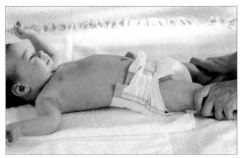

4 Now stroke both hands all the way down the torso, gradually lengthening the strokes to include the baby's legs. Take the left leg in one hand, using the other to support the ankle. Work your way down the leg using a gentle squeezing action.

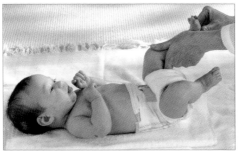

5 Take the left foot in your hand, supporting the heel with one hand. Use the thumb of your other hand to stroke over the sole, from the inner to the outer edge, and from the heel to the toe. Do the same on the right foot.

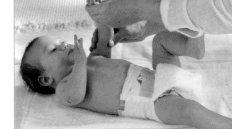

6 Now take the left arm in one hand, holding the baby's hand or wrist with your other hand. Work down the arm to the wrist, gently squeezing, then change hands so that you maintain a continuous action. Do the same on the right arm.

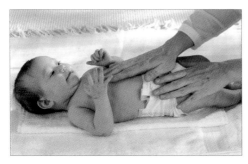

7 Gently rest your hand on the baby's abdomen and trace an arch from the bottom right of the trunk to the bottom left – this follows the digestive path. Take care not to press down.

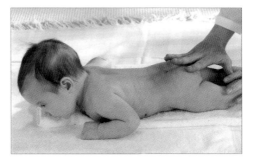

8 Turn your baby over, remove the nappy if you want to. Place your hands over the shoulder blades and draw your hands all the way down the spine and over the back of the legs. Using the flat of your hand, trace an arch from the right buttock to the left one, then stroke down the back of the body again.

Coping with colic

A young baby who has regular and long bouts of inconsolable crying with no apparent cause is said to have colic. About one in five babies are affected. Nobody knows exactly what colic is or what causes it, but there are many theories. In a few cases, it may be caused by a cow's milk intolerance or, in breastfed babies, by a reaction to something in the mother's diet. The crying could also be due to discomfort from reflux or wind. However, in many cases, colic may simply be a sensitive baby's reaction to all the stimulation received during the day. The immature nervous system becomes overloaded and the baby expresses this through crying.

Colic is hard for parents to cope with, but it is important to remember that it does stop in time. Try to arrange for help at the time of day when your baby is likely to cry. If you find the crying unbearable, don't hesitate to get support: your doctor or health visitor should be sympathetic, or you can call a voluntary organisation such as Cry-sis. Remember that you can place the baby in a safe place – such as the cot – and go into another room if you need a breather.

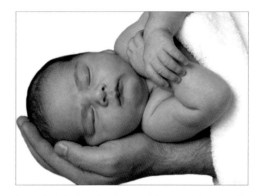

A small study of 28 babies found that cranial osteopathy reduced crying and improved sleep in colicky babies.

SOOTHING A COLICKY BABY

Reduce external stimuli – turn off overhead lights, music and the television. Then try doing all of the following, one after the other, or use the techniques separately.

- Swaddle your baby in a light blanket or shawl (see box)
- Hold the baby close so that you place gentle pressure on the abdomen: hold the baby along your forearm in the colic hold (see picture)
- Shush in the baby's ear or play white noise.
- Rock the baby in your arms.
- Give the baby something to suck on, such as your little finger or a dummy (pacifier).

IS IT COLIC?

Colic usually starts when a baby is two to four weeks old and lasts for up to four months. Babies are said to have colic when:

- they have lengthy bouts of crying on most days
- there is no obvious cause

Many colicky babies:

- have crying bouts at the same time each day, usually in the late afternoon or evening
- draw their knees up to their chest and clench their fists, as if they are in pain, and are red in the face
- may pass wind or have difficulty passing stools

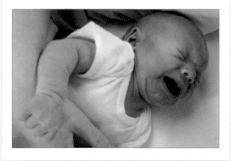

USING A DUMMY OR PACIFIER

Babies love to suck. You can sometimes encourage a baby to suck on his or her own fingers or thumb by guiding them to the mouth. Alternatively you can give the baby a dummy (pacifier), which, used wisely, is useful if your baby needs to suck a lot.

- Never dip a dummy in sugar or honey.
- Don't use a string or ribbon to tie a dummy around the baby's neck.
- Don't use a dummy in the first six weeks if you are breastfeeding.
- Don't give your baby a dummy whenever he or she is upset (it will become a hard-to-break habit).
- Ideally, restrict use to sleep times and colic.
- Wash and sterilize dummies between each use.
- Throw a dummy away if it shows signs of damage.

SWADDLING YOUR BABY

Some babies prefer to be wrapped so their arms and hands are free. You will need a stretchy, light blanket or cotton sheet about 90cm/3ft square.

1 Place the sheet diagonally on a flat surface and fold down the top corner by about 15cm/6in. Place the baby so that his or her neck rests on the folded edge.

2 Straighten the baby's arm at the side, then pull one side of the blanket over the arm and across the body. Tuck it under the back at the opposite side.

3 Fold the bottom of the sheet over the feet and the baby's body. Tuck it into the first fold to secure it. Straighten the free arm, then pull the other side of the sheet over it and across the baby's body, as in step 2. Tuck it under the back on the opposite side.

WORTH A TRY?

One common over-the-counter remedy is simethicone. However, studies have shown it to be no more effective than a placebo. The following are proven to help some infants with colic, so may be worth trying with your baby.

- If you are bottle-feeding and think your baby may be allergic to formula, ask your doctor about using a hypoallergenic formula.
- If you are breastfeeding, take note of what you eat and see if certain foods seem to make your baby's colic worse. Tea, coffee and colas, dairy products, alcohol, spicy foods, citrus fruits, onions, garlic, cabbage, broccoli and cauliflower may all have an effect. If you notice a correlation, cut out the offending food for a few days to see if your baby cries less. If you cut out dairy products, make sure you get enough calcium from other food sources or a supplement.
- Consider taking your baby to a cranial osteopath for treatment. Sometimes the pressure of the delivery can cause slight misalignments in the way the flat bones of the skull join together, causing headaches and distress. A cranial osteopath will very gently manipulate the bones to relieve any pressure, and this can sometimes have a miraculous effect on a previously colicky baby.

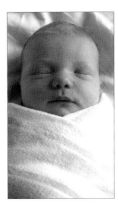

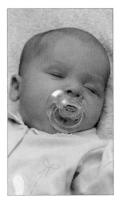

Many hospitals advise against swaddling at night because of the risk of overheating, but wrapping can be very soothing when you are awake and can keep an eye on your baby.

Some parents can't imagine life without dummies, others think they are an abomination. But, used wisely, they are useful if you have a baby who wants to comfort-suck a lot.

- To prevent wind and help with reflux, feed in an upright position and make sure you burp after every feed. If you are breastfeeding, get an expert to check your technique. If bottle-feeding, try using a teat with bigger holes; if they are too small, your baby may be swallowing lots of air with the milk.

For the colic hold, support the baby's crotch with your hand while the tummy rests on your forearm and the head is near your elbow. For the reverse colic hold, support the head with your hand; the baby's front rests on your forearm and the crotch on your elbow.

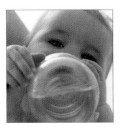

Cool, very dilute chamomile or fennel tea can help to soothe a gripy tummy. These teas are considered safe for children, but do let your doctor know you are using them in the unlikely event of allergy.

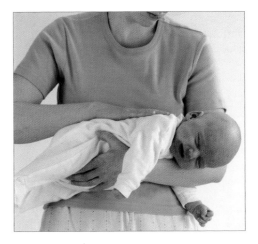

A place to sleep

Young babies sleep when they are tired, and they stay asleep as long as they need to. It doesn't matter to them whether they are in a cot or being carried through a crowded shopping centre. If your baby needs sleep, he or she will drop off without your help.

It is inevitable that your baby will fall asleep often when you are holding him or her, and cuddling a sleeping newborn is one of the silent joys of parenthood. But if this happens every time, your baby will associate sleeping with being held. As a rule, it is a good idea to put babies down when they are looking tired or yawning so that they learn to drop off in bed. It's impossible to do this all the time, especially if you are breastfeeding. But letting your baby fall asleep on his or her own sometimes will help establish good sleep patterns for the future.

If your baby protests at being put down, try stroking or patting him or her in the cot. Singing or playing soothing music can also help the baby to relax. A musical mobile can distract and lull the baby to sleep.

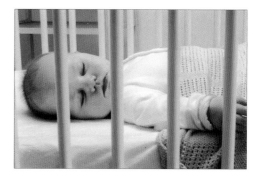

Putting your baby to sleep on his or her back is the best way to reduce the risk of SIDS. Some babies don't like this, but they will get used to it in time if you always put them on their backs. However, if you decide to let your baby sleep on one side, make sure the lower arm is to the front to prevent the baby from rolling forward.

CHECKLIST: SAFE SLEEP

All parents worry about their babies, and most find themselves checking on sleeping infants from time to time. The following steps reduce the risk of a baby suffering SIDS (sudden infant death syndrome).

- Always put your baby to sleep on his or her back.
- Put your baby to sleep on a firm mattress (not a sheepskin or pillow).
- Do not let anyone smoke near your baby (if possible, ban smoking from your home).
- Do not let your baby get too hot (or too cold) – keep the room temperature comfortable. Never put the cot next to a radiator or heater, or let your baby sleep with a hot-water bottle or electric blanket.
- Put the baby's feet at the base of the cot (the feet-to-foot position) so that he or she cannot wriggle down under the covers.
- Keep the baby's head uncovered. Make sure that covers reach no higher than the shoulders and are tucked in securely.
- Use sheets and thin blankets only (cellular blankets are ideal). Don't use duvets, pillows, wedges or bedding rolls.
- Don't use plastic sheets, cot bumpers or anything with strings or ribbons in your baby's bed. Keep toys out of the cot when your baby is sleeping.
- Seek medical advice promptly if your baby is ill.

A SNUG BED

Some babies happily sleep in a cot from birth, but most seem to prefer being in a cosier space (which is what, after all, they have been used to in the womb). A Moses basket, rocking crib or the carrycot from a pram are all suitable, and your baby can sleep in one until he or she gets too big for it, or is starting to roll over.

Your baby's mattress should be firm and clean – it is best to buy a new one for each baby. Choose one with a removable, washable waterproof covering or a complete PVC covering, and clean and air it regularly. Check that it fits well – there shouldn't be any gaps between the edges of the mattress and the sides of the cot.

A PLACE FOR NAPS

Opinions vary on whether it is best for your baby to be in the same place for every sleep, or whether it is helpful to differentiate between daytime naps and nighttime sleeping. Like many aspects of baby

You don't need a baby monitor unless your baby's room is out of earshot. If you do get a monitor, choose one that monitors sound only – a breathing monitor can just increase your anxiety levels, which is counterproductive.

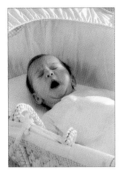
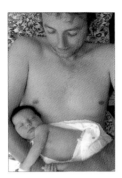
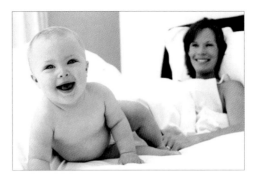

There is no need to keep quiet while your baby naps. Young babies can sleep through normal household noise, and it is a good idea to get them used to this.

Even though you are advised not to sleep with your baby, you'll certainly both enjoy spending time on your bed together.

care, it is down to what suits you and your baby best. You will probably find it easier to go out and about if your baby takes daytime naps in a pram. But some babies settle better when they are placed in their own cot in a darkened room. Experiment to see what works for you.

SLEEPING WITH YOUR BABY

It is recommended that your baby should share your room for at least six months. A baby who sleeps near his or her mother may be better able to regulate breathing. However, it is best for a young baby to sleep in a cot. An adult bed is not designed for a baby, who could become trapped between the mattress and headboard, or suffocate if a sleeping adult rolls on him or her.

In some countries, including the USA, parents are specifically advised not to sleep with their babies. Although a cot is the safest place for a baby to sleep, many mothers find that they do end up sharing their bed with their baby for part or all of the night, particularly if they breastfeed. Women who co-sleep tend to breastfeed for longer. A bedside cot with a side panel that seprates the baby's bed from your mattress can give you the best of both worlds. If you decide to bedshare, there are some extra safety precautions you need to take into account.

* Sleep on a firm, flat mattress – not a sofa, armchair, waterbed, beanbag or soft and sagging mattress.
* Do not place the baby between you and your partner – fathers are less aware of their babies and so may be more likely to roll on top of them.
* Make sure that your baby cannot fall out of bed or be wedged between the side of the mattress and the wall. A guard rail is useful.
* Dress your baby in no more clothing than you would wear in bed yourself. Use lightweight covers for your baby, not the duvet.
* Make sure that the covers cannot cover the baby's head and that he or she can't wriggle under a pillow.
* Don't leave the baby alone in the bed.

If you have twins, you may like to put them in the same cot. A study by the University of Durham showed that putting twins in the same sleeping space was safe, provided all the safe sleep guidelines were followed.

WHEN NOT TO SLEEP WITH YOUR BABY
Many experts believe that it is not safe to bedshare with a baby under three months. It is also not advisable to bedshare with a premature or small-at-birth baby or a baby with a fever. Never sleep with your baby:
* If you smoke.
* If you have drunk alcohol, or taken drugs, or are very tired or ill.
* On a sofa or armchair.

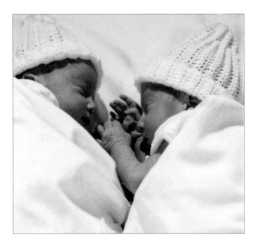

How babies sleep

Babies spend a lot of their time asleep, but they don't go about it in a way that is convenient for their parents. Small babies have lots of naps – an hour here, two or three there. This is because they have tiny stomachs and need feeding frequently. Bottle-fed babies tend to go longer than breastfed babies because formula milk takes longer to digest.

Unlike adults, young babies don't operate on a 24-hour cycle, and they don't distinguish between day and night. In the early weeks, there is very little you can do about this. So there is little point in trying to establish a sleep routine early on.

Gradually, your baby will adapt to the daily rhythm of light and dark. By the age of three or four months, most babies are sleeping about twice as much at night as during the day. Some babies may even sleep through the night at this stage, but most still wake up at least once a night to feed.

BABIES' SLEEP CYCLES

Like adults, babies sleep in cycles of active (dream) sleep and quiet sleep. A baby is more likely to wake at the end of one of these cycles, which usually last between 45 minutes and an hour. An adult cycle lasts up to two hours, but we usually don't remember waking up because we have learned ways of putting ourselves straight back to sleep.

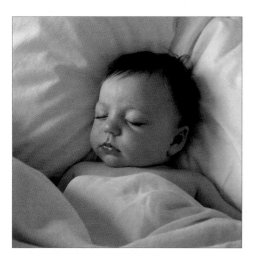

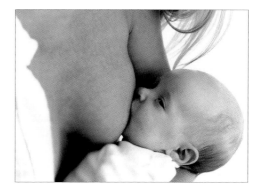

A good feed at bedtime will help to lull your baby into a long and restful sleep.

CREATING A GOOD SLEEPING ENVIRONMENT

You can encourage a young baby to get as much sleep as possible at night by providing a good sleeping environment for them.

- Keep the room warm (16–18°C/60–65°F). Make sure that your baby's cot isn't positioned in a draught.
- Darken the room. Use a low lamp to tend to your baby at night.
- Position the cot somewhere quiet. If it is near a window, outside noises may wake your baby up.
- Change your baby at night only when it's really necessary. Even then, keep activity to a minimum – speak as little as possible and only in a low voice.
- Similarly, make night feeds quiet and functional.

STRUCTURING THE DAY

Giving a baby a good daytime routine can help to improve nighttime sleep. If your baby tends to sleep late to make up for a restless night, try waking him or her up earlier to help the baby's body clock adjust to yours. Prioritize daytime sleep even if it means missing out on some activities or going for long walks in order to get your baby to drop off.

Young babies nap several times a day. Once they reach the age of three or four months, and start sleeping longer at night, they have longer periods of wakefulness during

The average newborn sleeps for about 16 hours a day – but yours may not need this much sleep, or may sleep much longer. Some babies get by on as little as eight hours a day.

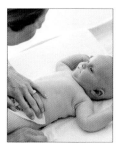
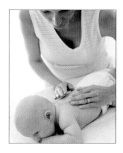

A set bedtime routine might be a warm bath, then being dressed before you do any final winding-down activities such as a feed.

A very gentle, soothing massage might be what your baby enjoys as part of the bedtime routine, but only if he or she finds it soothing.

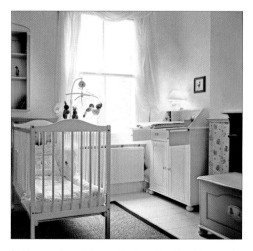

Babies need a quiet room to sleep in without too much stimulus. Keep toys hidden in cupboards and out of the cot, so that there is nothing to distract them from sleep.

the day. But they still need at least two naps. It is important to realize that babies get tired very quickly. Most need a nap about two hours after they wake up, and another longer nap in the early afternoon. So if they wake up at 7.00 am, they will need a sleep around 9.00 am and again at about midday. Young babies also need another sleep in the late afternoon (as may some older babies). It is best if this nap is kept short, though, or nighttime sleep will be affected. It's helpful to put your baby down for a sleep after a feed, which has a naturally soporific effect. Don't restrict daytime sleep in the hope that your baby will sleep better at night – it is likely to have the opposite effect. An overtired baby is likely to sleep fitfully at night.

Some babies take only short naps. If this is the case for yours, it may be worth noting the times when the baby wakes after first dropping off. Then try going to the cot a few minutes before the usual wake-up time and stroking or singing your baby back to sleep if there are signs of stirring. This may help the baby to sleep for longer, and eventually he or she should do this without you going in.

Schedule plenty of activity in the afternoon, then have extended calm-down time in the run up to bedtime. Most importantly, feed regularly. Some older babies are hard to feed during the day because they are distracted – and they then need to feed more at night. Feeding in a dark, quiet room can help them to concentrate.

A GOOD BEDTIME ROUTINE

Babies respond well to repetition, and an evening routine can help your baby to settle well at night. Three or four months is a good age to institute a bedtime routine, but you can start it earlier if you like. Try to stop boisterous play (such as tickling) at least an hour or so before the

Give your baby plenty of kick-around time. An active day can help a baby to sleep better at night.

baby's bedtime. Make this a quiet wind-down time, with gentle play. Your bedtime routine could include some of the following. It will help if you stick to the same elements in the same order each evening. But don't make a bedtime routine too complicated or it will take you ages to put your baby to bed.

• Warm bath
• Massage
• Being dressed in nightclothes
• Story or song
• Lights out
• Breastfeed or bottle
• Kiss and cuddle
• Time alone in the cot, perhaps with a musical mobile, a ticking clock, radio turned down low or a CD of lullabies to help lull the baby to sleep.

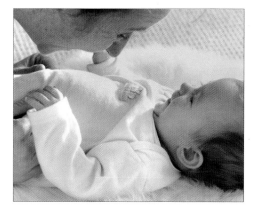

Helping a wakeful baby sleep

Most parents want their children to sleep through the night, but it is important to realize that in the early months most babies are unable to sleep for longer than five hours at a stretch. If your young baby goes from midnight to 5.00 am without waking, you can consider that to be sleeping through the night. By the end of the first year, your baby may sleep for 10–12 hours at a stretch. But many babies continue to wake up at least once at night. All babies will have wakeful periods from time to time, especially if they are teething or ill.

IMPROVING SLEEP

If your baby is still waking up several times a night after the age of three or four months, it may be that something is preventing him or her from sleeping longer. It is worth going through the following checklist to see if you can encourage a better sleeping pattern.

Is your baby getting enough fresh air? Research shows that babies who go out in daylight after 2.00 pm get a better night's sleep.

Is your baby having enough daytime naps? If a baby doesn't sleep much during the day, he or she may well have more disturbed sleep at night.

Is he or she sleeping too much during the day? Don't let your baby sleep for more than three hours at a time during the day, or night sleep may be affected. Keep naps in the late afternoon to no more than 30 minutes.

Is he or she getting enough stimulation? It is important to let your baby have a good kick-around on the floor and for you to provide new experiences to enjoy. Babies tend to be most alert in the afternoon and early evening, so this is a good time to take them out.

Make sure your baby has plenty of opportunity for stimulation and movement during the day.

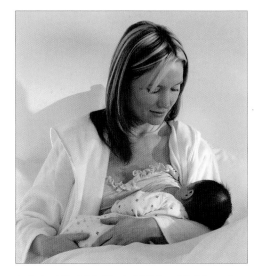

A study of English babies in 2003 found that fewer than a quarter of them were sleeping through the night by the age of ten months.

COMFORTERS

If your baby wakes in the night a comforter can help him or her get back to sleep. Provide the same soft toy or piece of cloth every time the baby goes to sleep. It will help if you imbue it with your scent – place it between you and the baby every time you breastfeed, or wear it next to your skin for a day or two. If your baby takes to the comforter, make sure you have at least one spare for when it is in the wash or in case it gets lost.

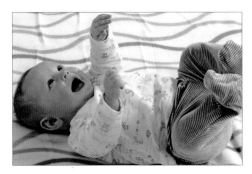

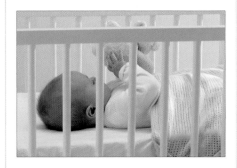

Is he or she getting too much stimulation? If your baby is being distracted when he or she is getting sleepy, it may be harder to drop off at night. Be alert to signs of tiredness: yawning, turning the head away, rubbing eyes.

Is he or she getting enough milk? A hungry baby may often be lulled back to sleep temporarily but will keep waking up until he or she is given milk. Both bottle-fed and breast-fed babies benefit from being given a feed at about 10.00 pm, or at the parents' bedtime, to help them sleep through the main part of the night.

Is bedtime early enough? Most babies like to go to sleep at 6.30–7.30 pm. If yours is getting to bed much later, try putting him or her to sleep 15 minutes earlier each evening until you reach this time.

Is the baby warm enough? If a baby is too cold, he or she will wake up. A baby sleeping bag is good if covers tend to be kicked off.

Is the room too light? Invest in blackout blinds if light from the street or the sun is waking your baby up.

Are your expectations too high? It is unrealistic to expect a young baby to sleep for many hours without a feed, especially if you are breastfeeding, because breastmilk is digested more quickly than formula.

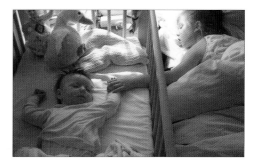

Your baby might settle more easily if he or she sleeps in the same room as an older sibling.

SHOULD YOU LEAVE A BABY TO CRY?

If you have a wakeful baby, then somebody may advise you to leave the baby to cry. But young babies are not old enough to assume that you are nearby. All they perceive is abandonment, so being left to cry may have a negative psychological effect. Even advocates of controlled crying say that sleep training shouldn't be tried with babies under the age of six months.

Gentle persuasion

If your baby tends to cry when put back down to sleep after a feed, he or she may want your company. If you want your baby to settle in the cot, try the following routine. You can also use this method to institute a regular bedtime. If the baby starts to cry at any point, revert to the previous action. You may find you have to run through the routine many, many times before your baby goes to sleep, but stay calm and persevere. Use the yoga exercise on the next page if you find yourself getting wound up, or let your partner take over. Don't feel you can't try again if you give up from time to time – if you repeat this routine regularly, your baby will eventually settle more easily.

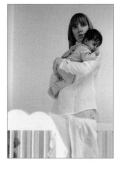

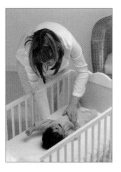

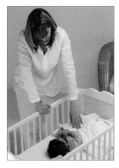

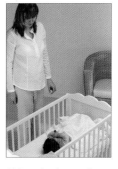

1 When your baby cries, go in to the room, don't put on the light. Pick the baby up and soothe him or her with quiet shushing noises. As soon as the baby is calm, lay him or her gently in the cot again.

2 Keep one arm under the baby. Stroke the baby's tummy with the other hand still shushing. If you use a dummy (pacifier), give it to the baby. Slowly slide the arm out from under the baby, with the other hand on the tummy.

3 Continue shushing. Gradually decrease the stroking, but leave your hand resting there for a few moments longer. Slowly take away your hand, and gradually reduce the volume of your shushing.

4 Move slowly away from the cot, still quietly shushing, until you are out of the room. If your baby protests, go back and put your hand on his or her tummy. Repeat the process if you need to stop the baby getting upset.

Coping with broken nights

Sleepless nights are probably the hardest aspect of parenthood. Every parent feels tired at some point, and some find the first weeks and months disappear in a blur of exhaustion. Accept that you will get less sleep than before you had your baby – disturbed nights can be easier to deal with if you are relaxed about them. Some breastfeeding mothers say that they come to enjoy night feeds as a quiet time to share with their babies. Many parents feel pleased to see their baby, whatever the time. The following techniques can all help you to deal with being woken at night and minimize sleep deprivation.

- Have everything you may need in the night to hand: nappies, cotton wool (cotton balls), warm water in a flask, a spare sleepsuit for the baby; a bottle of water for you. You'll get back to sleep more quickly if you haven't had to go hunting around the house for these.
- Wear nightclothes so that you don't get cold if you get up and you don't have to scrabble around for a T-shirt when the baby is crying.

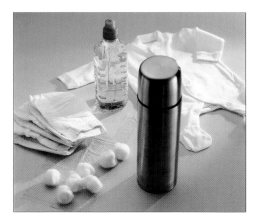

Being woken several times a night by your baby is hard. Keep fuss to the minimum by having everything you need to change the baby nearby.

Yoga relaxation exercise

This is a simple yoga pose that induces deep relaxation. You need at least ten minutes to relax fully. So it is best to do this exercise either when the baby has just gone down for a nap and is definitely asleep, or – better still – when there is somebody else in the house who can attend to the baby if he or she wakes.

Before you begin, make sure the room is warm and quiet – turn off any music, switch off the phone, close the curtains and ask anyone else in the house not to disturb you. Lie on a rug, yoga mat or large towel. You may like to cover yourself with a light blanket, and to put on some socks, to keep warm.

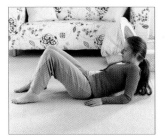

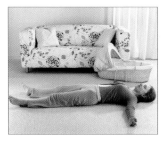

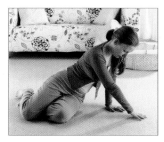

1 Sit on the floor, feet together and knees bent. Put your hands on either side of your buttocks. Slowly lie back, supporting your weight on your hands then elbows until you are lying flat, knees still bent. Lengthen the back of your neck as you put the back of your head on the floor. Stretch out your legs, feet apart.

2 If you feel discomfort in your lower back, place a cushion under your knees or leave them bent. Let your arms move comfortably out to your sides, palms upwards and fingers slightly curled. If your shoulders feel hunched, slide them down slightly. Close your eyes, relax and breathe for about ten minutes.

3 When you are ready to get up, bend your knees and roll over on to your left side. Come to a sitting position – taking your time – then get up slowly. Try to maintain slow steady breathing and a quiet frame of mind for a while. At the very least, don't instantly start to rush about.

- Make yourself go to bed earlier than you might otherwise, even if you don't feel sleepy. If you find it hard to drop off, institute a nightly routine for yourself as well as for the baby. Have a warm bath, with a few drops of lavender or chamomile essential oil added to the water. Have a milky drink. Don't watch television in bed or read for long before sleep.
- During the day, grab a nap whenever the baby sleeps. Don't use the time to catch up on chores or phone calls if you are really tired; go to bed and rest. Even if you don't sleep, lying quietly will help replenish your energy.
- Eat well and healthily. Tiredness is harder to cope with if you are hungry.
- Practise deep breathing to calm the nervous system. Whenever you get a minute or two to yourself simply sit up straight, relax your shoulders and breathe.
- Consider taking time out to go to a yoga or pilates class. Check that the class is suitable for new mothers – ideally, go to a specialist class (you may be able to take the baby along or you may prefer to ask a friend, relative or your partner to babysit so that you can concentrate on your practice).
- Get out of the house at least once a day, even if you are feeling really tired. Fresh air and some kind of physical activity will do both you and the baby good and you may find the baby sleeps better at night if you provide plenty of stimulation during the day.

DEVELOPING A NIGHTTIME STRATEGY

It's a good idea to have a strategy for dealing with broken nights. Discuss this with your partner in advance. It's much better to decide beforehand who is going to do what than to try and negotiate in the middle of the night when neither of you is likely to be feeling very reasonable.

Be realistic. Some partners may not be able or willing to do any nighttime parenting, especially if they have to get up early to go to work, and if you are breastfeeding, most of the night care will inevitably fall to you. Whatever strategy you have, there will be times when you need to be flexible. A father or helper can help at night in the following ways.

- If you are bottle-feeding, by giving a feed last thing at night. That way, you can go to bed earlier and get a few hours of unbroken sleep.
- By rocking or walking around with a baby who is ill or can't settle after being fed.

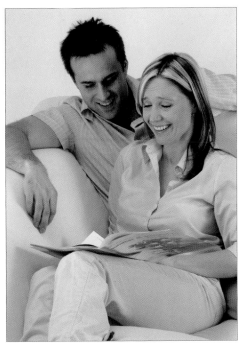

It is easy to get irritable when you are very tired, so take time to connect with your partner. Ask someone to take care of the baby to allow you to spend an hour or two alone together.

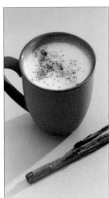

A drink of warm, cinnamon-spiced milk before you go to bed will help to relax you and encourage sleep.

- By getting the baby up in the morning so that you can get an extra hour's sleep.
- By taking care of the baby in the early evening, to give you a break.

Some new fathers opt to spend nights sleeping in the spare room or on the sofa. This can help both of you in the short term – your partner gets a full night's sleep (which may make him better able to help you at other times) and you may sleep better if you have the bed to yourself. But obviously it is not something either of you will want to do for long.

Development and play

> ❝ Every baby is an individual: each one develops at his or her own pace and in a different way from any other. ❞

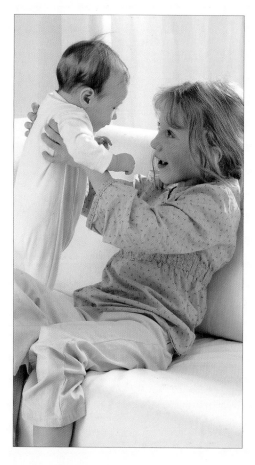

One of the real pleasures of parenthood is to watch your baby grow and develop. The tiny wriggling bundle you start with very soon becomes a fascinating child who sits up, laughs, babbles, and is curious about the world. Some changes happen suddenly – one day your baby is content to lie on a playmat, staring at a hanging toy; the next day he or she hits out at it. Other milestones, such as sitting up, take weeks of practice. And there are plateau periods, when your baby seems content simply to be. Doctors divide a baby's development into four key areas.

- Social development is about how your child interacts and responds to you and others, with smiles and little noises.
- Language development relates not only to how quickly and well a child learns to speak, but also to how much he or she understands what others say.
- Large motor development covers major physical actions such as sitting up, rolling over, crawling and walking.

The budding relationship between a baby and a sibling can be wonderful to watch. Babies often reward older children with the biggest smiles and belly laughs.

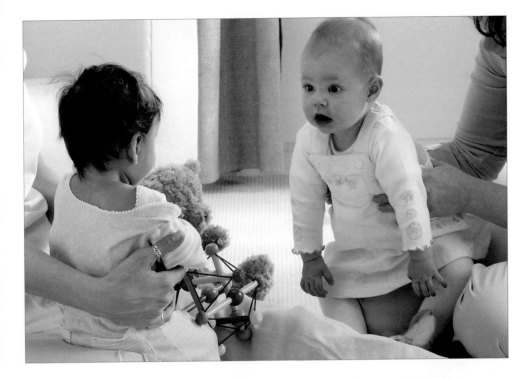

- Small motor development concerns more precise skills, including hand-to-eye coordination and the ability to hold and manipulate objects.

Health professionals will evaluate your baby's key achievements from time to time, to check that all is progressing normally. But if your child is late in developing certain skills, this doesn't necessarily mean there is something wrong. Every baby is an individual: each one develops at his or her own pace and in a different way. Some babies seem to learn new skills very easily, while others take longer to acquire them. Often a baby will be advanced in one area but late in others, and will forget about one skill for a while as he or she concentrates on learning something new.

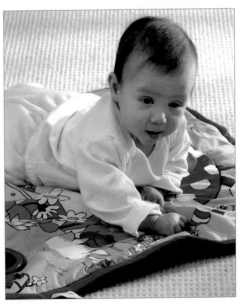

Top: Babies can be transfixed by other young children. At just a few months old, your baby may find another child much more fascinating than a new toy.

Your baby is preset to develop all the skills he or she needs. All you need to do is to provide him or her with a safe environment to explore.

Helping your baby to learn

Babies acquire new abilities when they are ready. As a parent, there isn't much that you can do to speed up this process. Pushing a child to learn a new skill before he or she is ready is at best pointless and at worst frustrating for you and potentially harmful for the child. However, you can make sure that your baby has a good environment for learning – one that is loving, stimulating and encouraging.

Babies are born with a drive to explore the world around them. The way they learn best is through human interaction, so lots of love and attention is what a baby needs most. Talk directly to your baby, sing to him or her, explain what is going on. Describe what you are doing as you, say, change a nappy, and point out interesting things when you are out together. Your baby won't understand the words you are using, of course, but will pick up on your interest and respond to it.

Until your baby can walk around and explore, you have to bring the world to the baby. Offer interesting things to look at and let the baby touch them. If you are looking at a plant in the garden, say, hold the baby close enough to reach out and grab it. Gently brush different materials – silk, cotton wool, corduroy – across the baby's skin to help him or her learn about texture.

Give your baby interesting things to smell, such as a citrus fruit or a lavender bag. Let the baby hold your watch or a sturdy necklace when sitting on your lap. From a few months old, your baby will start to put everything in his or her mouth: this is not an attempt to eat things, but an infant's primary mode of investigating physical objects.

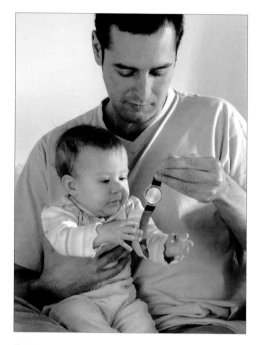

Babies need human company in order to develop well. A baby who spends hours each day in a cot or bouncy chair, without anything interesting to look at, will become bored and understimulated.

Sometimes a baby doesn't need a toy or other entertainment, he or she will be quite happy just watching you and following your movements.

While babies love to play with their parents, siblings and other close people, they don't need to be actively entertained all the time.

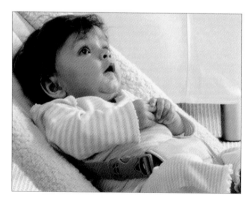

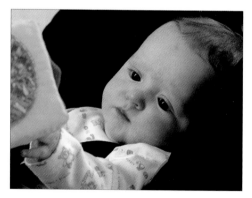

DEVELOPMENTAL MILESTONES

Keep a relaxed attitude to your baby's development. Most parents look at developmental charts at some time or other, and it is very easy to worry if your baby hasn't achieved a so-called 'milestone' at the usual time. If your baby seems to be very late, or has missed several milestones, then discuss this with a health professional. But don't get too hung up on whether your child is 'advanced' or 'behind'. The ages given for developmental milestones are simply statistical averages of certain easily observable behaviours. They are not an exam your baby has to pass. Reaching the stages early does not mean your child is phenomenally clever, and reaching them late does not imply anything about future academic achievement. Albert Einstein, one of the most incisive and original minds of the 20th century, was a 'slow' child who did not start to talk until he was three.

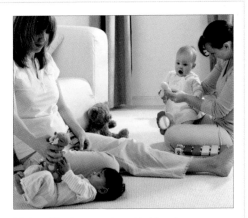

Mixing with other parents and babies gives you a good idea of how babies develop at different rates.

Lots of cuddles help babies to feel secure, and give a sense of a 'base' from which to explore their surroundings. But that doesn't mean they have to be held all the time. In fact, it is good to let your baby see things from different positions. Put the Moses basket or pram in a variety of places where there are interesting things to look at. Lay the baby on his or her front sometimes, so that he or she gets a new viewpoint and can practise different movements such as lifting the head.

FOLLOW THE BABY

Tailor playtime to your baby's temperament, likes and dislikes. Some babies are very active from a young age and enjoy being tickled, say, or bounced up and down. Others are more nervous and prefer gentler play. It is important to be sensitive to your baby and not to persist with games that make him or her unhappy or scared. Similarly, don't let anyone else play with your baby in this way – it is quite common for men, in particular, to play rough games with baby boys in the mistaken belief that this will toughen them up. If your baby doesn't seem to be enjoying a game, put a stop to it.

Always follow your baby's lead. If he or she is enjoying a particular toy, don't try to introduce another one. Let the baby explore this one fully, show him or her what it does, and join in the game.

Try to pitch activities at your baby's level, or just above it. This makes playtime stimulating but fun. If your baby is

Introduce your baby to different textures by stroking fabric over his or her tummy or palm. Try something soft such as a square of velvet or a furry soft toy, and see how the baby reacts.

taking an interest in a particular toy, say, you could play peek-a-boo with it. The baby will appreciate the surprise and will soon learn that things are still there even when they can't be seen – a key human attribute. If the baby likes to hold a particular rattle, next time try offering one that is a different shape, size or colour to explore.

Be aware of your baby's moods. If he or she is hungry it is time for a feed, not playtime. And even when happily enjoying a toy, a baby won't want to play with it for more than a few minutes. Starting to cry, turning away or getting a glazed look are signs that the baby has had enough: follow these cues.

Above all, mark your baby's tiny successes with enthusiasm. Babies, like the rest of us, like to be encouraged. Use exaggerated facial expressions and a joyous tone of voice. Your smiles, claps and exclamations of 'Clever baby!' will delight your child and make him or her want to try new things.

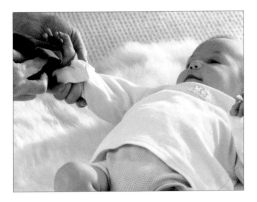

Seeing and hearing

People used to think that newborns were deaf and blind, but we now know that babies can see and hear from birth. Their vision is poor at first, but they can see almost as well as adults by the time they are eight months old. Hearing is the most developed sense in a newborn and is almost perfect by the time the baby is a month old.

SIGHT

The vision of newborn babies is limited and blurred, but they can focus on things that are 20–30cm/8–12in away. Faces are what interest babies most at this stage, but they will also be transfixed by simple patterns that have good contrast – try showing your baby simple black and white geometrical designs.

By two months, babies are able to track a moving object with both eyes. They are just starting to be able to distinguish colours at this point – they may show an interest in bright primary colours as well as more complicated patterns. This can be a good time to begin to show a baby colourful board books.

Babies start to get a sense of perspective by about four months, and this helps them with their new-found grasping skills. They are now able to focus on small

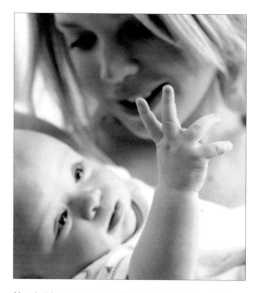

New babies are unaware of their hands, but suddenly they discover these fascinating things belong to them.

Check it out

Your baby's vision and hearing will be checked at routine developmental reviews, but it is important to see a doctor if you think your baby is not responding to sound or that there may be a problem with his or her sight. Many problems are easier to correct if they are picked up early on. You can check your child's hearing in the following ways, but don't panic if your baby doesn't respond: he or she may just be absorbed in something else, or be tired and distracted. Don't keep going; just give up and try again another time.

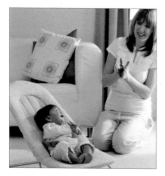

0–3 months: Clap your hands behind a baby's head (not by an ear). If the baby reacts, hearing is normal.

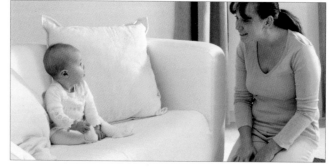

4–6 months: Call your baby's name to see if he or she turns to you. Babies of this age should also turn towards the source of an unusual sound – try tapping on a glass with a fork or making a squeaking noise.

Babies are born with perfect pitch and enjoy listening to all manner of soothing sounds – such as a ticking clock or a set of wind chimes.

Babies are fascinated by shiny objects that catch the light. Try holding up a length of foil and watching your baby react.

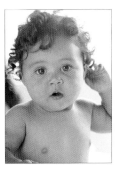

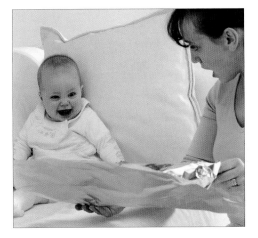

objects as well as large ones. Over the next month or so, they begin to spot small items from farther away, and get better at tracking moving objects. They also find it easier to distinguish between different colours.

HEARING

The sense of hearing develops in the womb, and there is evidence to suggest that babies can hear sounds outside the womb as early as 25 weeks. One study found that newborns could recognize the theme tune of the Australian soap opera *Neighbours* if their mothers had watched it regularly while pregnant.

From birth, babies are interested in human voices: they show a preference for their native language and they prefer their mother's voice to anyone else's. They also respond more keenly to high-pitched tones than low ones – most people sense this and automatically assume a higher pitch when they talk to babies. But even though your baby is listening intently to you, he or she may not turn towards you when you speak until the age of about three months. Babies also show an innate appreciation of music; they enjoy soothing music from birth, and they seem to prefer songs to purely instrumental music.

FIVE GOOD TOYS FOR YOUNG BABIES

Newborns babies don't need toys, but by three or four weeks old your baby will be able to appreciate some of the following.

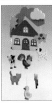

Mobile. A mobile makes a wonderful amusement. Hang it within easy focusing distance – ideally, about 25cm/10in away – and to the baby's right or left (babies usually lie with their head pointing to one side rather than upwards). Babies can't distinguish between colours until they are three months old, so choose one that has sharp contrasts – either black and white or bold colours.

Mirror. Babies are fascinated by their own reflection – although they don't understand that they are looking at themselves until they are well over a year old. Choose soft toys or books that have a special unbreakable mirror attached.

Black-and-white patterns. A new baby will be fascinated by geometric black-and-white patterns, and you should be able to find cloth books or soft toys that use these designs. Alternatively, draw some simple designs on paper and stick these to the wall next to the Moses basket.

Rattle. Babies are interested in noises so they like playing with rattles. Moving a rattle around helps to make the connection between cause and effect, as the baby learns that shaking the rattle makes a noise.

Baby gym. A baby gym can give your child months of pleasure. When lying on his or her front there are different textures, colours and sometimes sounds to enjoy. Lying on his or her back, the baby has space to kick around and toys to look at, swipe and grasp. Hang the toys in different places so that there are different ones to reach for.

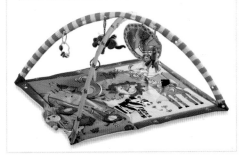

How movement develops

Newborns aren't able to control their movements, and any seemingly purposeful movements they make – such as sucking or grasping – are due to survival reflexes. However, both before and after birth babies will kick, fling out their arms and twist their bodies. These simple random movements strengthen the muscles and stimulate the nervous system. Gradually, your baby learns how to lift and move different parts of his or her body.

The development of motor control follows a set pattern in all babies: it moves from the top downwards and from the centre outwards. So, babies will learn to hold up their head long before they can move their legs. And they will use their arms to hit out at an object before they can close their hand in order to hold it.

HEAD CONTROL

In very young babies, the neck muscles are too weak to hold up the heavy head, so you need to support it whenever you hold your baby. By six weeks, there is some degree of head control: when held, babies start to lift their head up for a few seconds at a time, and may move it from side to side. They can keep their head steady when sitting in an infant carrier or a bouncy chair.

When they lie on their tummy, three-month-old babies will lift their head off the floor and turn it so that they can look around – a few babies are strong enough to do this when they are just a few weeks old. They won't do it for long at first, but as their strength grows, they'll start lifting up on their hands so that their shoulders come up too. This is an important precursor to crawling.

By four months, your baby will be able to keep his or her head up as you carry him or her around (though you may still need to support the head if you are performing an awkward manoeuvre, such as getting the baby into a

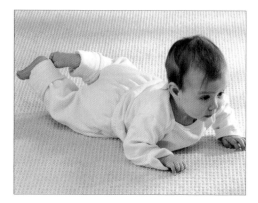

Head control develops very slowly, so you need to support your baby's head for several months. But he or she will try to lift the head from an early age.

car seat). And by six months most babies have developed neck muscles strong enough to keep themselves upright if their lower bodies are supported. Soon they will be able to sit up by themselves; some already can at this age.

ROCKING AND ROLLING

The first independent movement babies make is rolling (usually from their front on to their back). Instead of lying wherever you have placed your baby, he or she discovers how to get a toy that is just out of reach or change his or her viewpoint. It's hugely exciting for both of you, and once your baby has mastered the skill, he or she will roll at every opportunity. Babies sometimes roll from front to back as early as two months, but rolling from back to front takes greater control of the head and arms. It usually happens between five and seven months.

Because rolling sometimes happens without warning, it is essential that you never leave a baby unattended on a high surface (such as a bed or changing table). Don't turn away for a second.

TRYING TO SIT

Babies start trying to sit up from three or four months, once they have some head control. If you lay babies of this age on their back, they may lift up their head so that

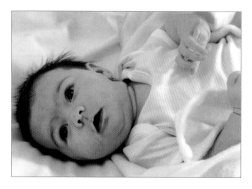

The first step towards rolling over is when a baby starts to crane the head while lying on the back. It takes many practice goes before he or she manages to flip over.

Encouraging rolling

Like all physical skills, rolling happens when your baby is ready. But you can encourage back to front rolling with a toy that they reach for. Make sure he or she is lying on a flat surface – a crumpled blanket will impede movement.

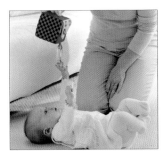 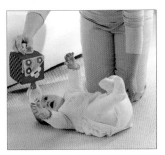 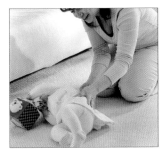

1 Lie your baby on his or her back. Attract your baby's attention by holidng a favourite toy above him or her, just out of reach.

2 Hold the toy away to one side to encourage the baby to stretch towards it, and begin to rock on to his or her side.

3 Gently hold the baby on his or her side for a few moments. Then slowly turn the baby on to his or her front, making sure he or she is happy.

Encouraging Sitting

Babies start trying to sit up from an early age. But they have to develop neck muscles strong enough to support the head. When this happens, your baby will enjoy being pulled to a sitting position.

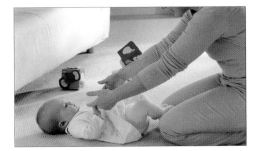 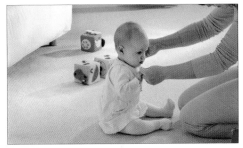

1 Wait until your baby is lying on his or her back. Offer the baby your hands and see if he or she tries to rise up. If so, you can gently help him or her come to a sitting position. Make sure that the neck stays in line with the body.

2 From a sitting position, you can slowly lower your baby back onto their back. Again, make sure that the neck is in line with the body. A few well-judged sound-effects – 'dooooown', 'uuuuuuup' – will make it more fun.

---

they can look around. If you give them your hands, they'll try to pull themselves up to a sitting position.

Babies enjoy being propped up so that they can see what is going on around them. A bouncy chair is ideal for this, especially one that can be adjusted from an almost reclining position to a more upright one as the baby's head control improves. When the neck and back muscles have strengthened to the extent that your baby is nearly sitting up (usually at about five or six months), you can use an L-shaped breastfeeding cushion or ordinary pillows to support him or her. Make sure that there are cushions all around so that the baby isn't hurt if he or she falls forward or sideways.

As soon as they master some head control, babies love to sit up and watch what is going on around them. Prop your baby up on some cushions for brief periods, but as he or she will inevitably slip gradually downwards, you'll have to be there to make sure he or she stays upright and doesn't topple over.

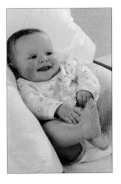

Fun with movement

All babies really need for the development of large motor control is a safe space to move about in. If they are always in a bouncy chair, sling or pushchair, they won't be able to learn how their body moves. So, give your baby plenty of time on the floor where he or she can enjoy a good wriggle around.

You can help your baby to practise his or her new-found muscle control by playing physical games. Always

From about six weeks, put your baby on his or her tummy often to practise lifting his or her head, which will strengthen the neck muscles. A few minutes a day is all that is needed. Sit on the floor close by and chat to encourage your baby to look up at you.

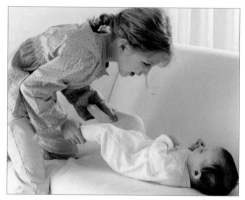

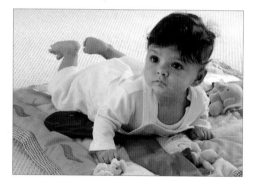

Babies love using their bodies. 'Bicycling' is a great way to help them experience a different movement.

be gentle and do what your baby seems to enjoy. When your baby is lying on his or her back, try bicycling: move the legs alternately towards the body, bending them into their chest and then stretching them out towards you. Lift the baby up into the air and move him or her around before bringing him or her back to the safety of your lap.

Give your baby lots of tummy time so that he or she can practise lifting up the head and upper body. Some babies don't like going on their tummies, but there are lots of ways you can make this fun. Get down there too,

Ball play

This little game of catch will keep your baby amused during his or her tummy time. It is also good exercise for the neck, arm and leg muscles, making it a good preparation for crawling. Stop as soon as your baby seems uncomfortable.

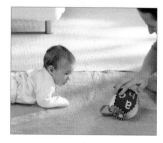

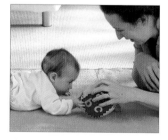

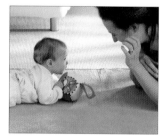

1 When your baby lifts his or her head, roll a ball about 60cm/2 ft in front of him or her. At first the baby will be content just to watch it move.

2 As he or she gets stronger, the baby will reach out to grab the ball as it rolls. Give lots of praise whenever this happens.

3 Always end the game by giving your baby the ball to play with. He or she is more likely to stay interested in a game than ends in success.

Baby yoga: wind-relieving posture

This aptly named yoga pose works on the digestive system and helps a baby to release any trapped wind. If your baby is windy or colicky, it is a good one to include in a massage routine, or you can just do it by itself.

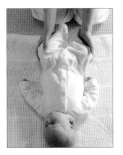

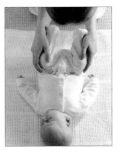

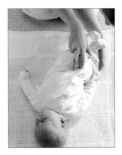

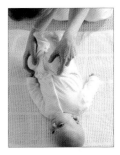

1 Place your baby on a blanket on the floor. Holding the baby's knees, open his or her legs out so that the knees are wider than the hips.

2 Slowly bring the knees to touch the body. Make the movement smooth and relaxed. Release the pressure, and then repeat twice more.

3 Keeping the baby's knees bent, bring the legs over to the left. Hold for a moment, pressing the knees gently into the side of the abdomen.

4 Release the pressure and slowly return the legs to the centre. Move them to the right and hold against the side of the abdomen. Repeat twice.

so that your baby doesn't feel scared: make eye contact, talk or sing, and make silly expressions to keep him or her amused. Use a playmat that has different textures and colours to explore. Place a mirror in front of the baby so that pushing up is rewarded by his or her own face.

Hold your baby under the arms so that he or she can 'stand' on your lap; the baby will push down to straighten his or her legs and may enjoy bouncing up and down. Once he or she has good head control (at about five or six months) the baby will probably appreciate being in a baby bouncer for short periods. Some babies who can raise themselves up on their arms when lying on their front enjoy the 'wheelbarrow' position: try lifting your baby's legs, then lowering them back down and repeating. Show the baby you are excited by these achievements by exclaiming, smiling and making plenty of eye contact.

BABY YOGA

Yoga helps babies to learn about and enjoy their bodies. If you are interested in baby yoga it is worth going to classes, but you can also do some simple movements at home. Babies are naturally flexible, so the postures are more like massage techniques than exercise, and you can easily incorporate them into a baby massage routine. But it is very important to be gentle; never force a movement or persist with the poses if your baby seems unhappy.

Baby yoga; butterfly pose

This is an adaptation of another favourite yoga pose, which works on the hips and pelvis.

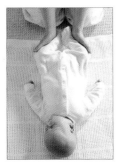

Babies have very flexible hip joints so they love this movement. Hold both your baby's ankles with your hands. Move the feet together so that the soles are touching. Gently push the feet into the abdomen, hold for a moment and then release. Then try pushing the legs slowly in and out in a rhythmic way.

Handling and chewing

Newborn babies are born with the grasping reflex but it takes months before they can reach for an object and pick it up. During the first weeks of life, babies' hands are curled into fists. They may hold a small toy if they are given it, but won't really explore it for some weeks to come. At about eight weeks, your baby may start to hit out at objects, such as the items hanging on a play gym, or toys attached to the bouncy chair or pram. It is a good idea to make sure they are within arm's length, so that the baby doesn't become frustrated. At this stage, babies play with their own hands from time to time, but they don't yet realize that they actually belong to them – they won't look at their hands unless they happen to be in their line of vision.

From about eight weeks, babies start to open their hands. If given a small toy to play with, they will instinctively grasp it and may finger it for a little while. A noisy toy, such as a rattle, is ideal because the sound it makes will draw a baby's attention to his or her hands. By three months, babies' hands are their favourite playthings. They examine them intently, put them in their mouth, bring them together and apart again. They also enjoy batting toys within reach, and occasionally manage to grab hold of one.

All this activity helps to develop hand-to-eye coordination. By three or four months, babies can pick up large objects they see and will deliberately grasp a toy

A small wooden toy with moving parts like this one is perfect for fingering, and will keep your baby entertained for several minutes at a time.

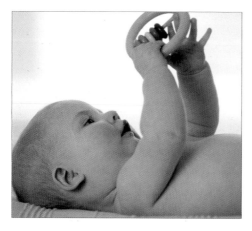

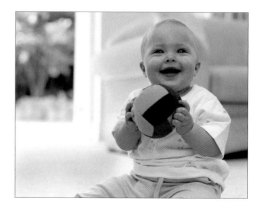

A soft ball can be grabbed easily and provides an interesting texture to explore. If it has a bell inside, then the amusement factor is even greater.

that is held out to them. Make sure that you give your baby the time he or she needs to reach out, though, as it can take a baby a little while to respond. Try using a squeaky toy to add to the fun.

Once babies can hold objects, they will put them in their mouth. The mouth has more nerve endings than the fingertips, so it is the best tool for exploration. This means that everything within reach of your baby should be safe for sucking. Don't give a baby anything that could be toxic or allow him or her to handle anything small enough to choke on (such as a string of beads).

By six months, babies can pass a toy from one hand to the other and reach for an object without looking at their hands as they do so. And they can work out whether a toy is within reach or not – they won't try to grab it if it is too far away.

GOOD TOYS FOR GRASPING
When your baby is at the swiping stage, hang an interesting mobile so that the items are within batting distance. A play gym is excellent for this, especially if you can move the toys around to keep up the baby's interest. Your baby can play with other things besides toys, of course. Household objects that have no sharp edges – such as a whisk, a set of measuring spoons or some plastic pots – are ideal for your tiny explorer. Once your baby can take hold of things, provide a range of toys to explore, including different sizes, textures, sounds and shapes, such as the following.

- Toys that have small protrusions for easy grabbing.
- Toys with two handles for passing from hand to hand.
- Toys that a baby can safely put in his or her mouth – this is good for teething.
- Toys that are brightly coloured with sharp contrasts.
- Toys that are interesting to feel – squishy fabric blocks, smooth plastic objects, soft toys, toys that have contrasting textures.
- Toys that make any kind of a noise, such as rattles and squeaky toys.

GRASPING GAME

A good game you can play to encourage grasping is to attach a brightly coloured soft toy to a piece of string or ribbon. Prop your baby up in a sitting position and then dangle it in front of him of her. When the baby reaches for it, say 'Well done,' with lots of smiles. Always end the game by giving the toy to the baby to play with, but detach the string or ribbon first.

TOYS AND SAFETY

Make sure that anything your baby plays with is safe. In particular make sure you follow these guidelines:
- A toy should not be small enough to fit completely into the baby's mouth.
- There should no detachable parts that are small enough to choke on.
- It should be lightweight, so that it will not hurt if your baby drops it on to his or her face when lying down.
- It should be made of non-toxic materials.
- A soft toy should be machine- or surface-washable. Check that the seams are securely sewn and make sure there are no trimmings, such as eyes, noses, buttons or ribbons that can be pulled or bitten off.
- All toys should meet the recognized safety standards.
- Don't give a toy that is intended for an older child to

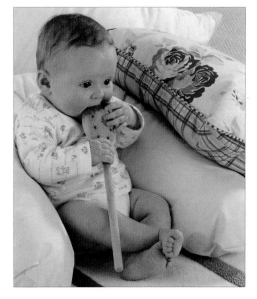

From two or three months, babies can hold objects and will lift them up to their mouths to suck. Small items of kitchen equipment hold as much fascination as any toy – try giving your baby a set of plastic measuring spoons, or a wooden spoon to explore.

your baby. Toys are labelled with recommended ages for safety reasons.
- Don't give a balloon to a baby. It may burst, which will be frightening, and if a small part of the balloon is swallowed it may cause choking.
- Don't attach a toy to a cot or pram with string or ribbon.
- Remove mobiles and other hanging objects once a baby begins to push up on hands or knees.

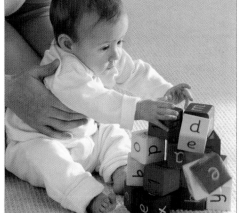

Once your baby can sit, he or she will enjoy knocking down a tower of bricks that you have built.

Encourage your baby to grasp by holding out a toy. If he or she reaches for it, give it to them.

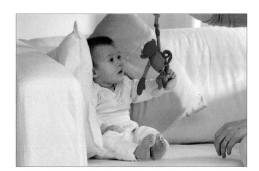

Sociability and language

Babies are social beings. Right from the start they need company, and are happiest when they are getting plenty of cuddles. Young babies don't have a sense of being a separate person – they don't know their hands are their own, for example, and they can't tell where their mother's body ends and theirs begins. They just instinctively know that it is good to be around people.

Young babies like to look at faces more than anything else, but they can't at first tell the difference between a real face and a picture, and they cannot recognize expression: a scary face is just as interesting and enjoyable to a tiny baby as a smiling one.

By about three months babies can recognize individuals, and will smile more readily at those they know well – their mother, father, siblings and so on. Over the next weeks and months, they become increasingly attached to their main carer. This is usually the mother, but if both parents share the care – or if a grandparent or childminder is very involved in the child's life – then the baby will naturally develop strong attachments to those people too.

But babies are also interested in new people. It's a good idea to give your baby plenty of opportunities to meet people, and to let him or her engage with relatives, friends and people that you come into contact with when you are out. This helps to foster the notion that the world is a friendly place – which is good for socialization skills.

First smiles are a response to a familiar voice. It's not until about eight or nine weeks that a baby will smile when you smile. When he or she realizes that smiling gets attention and cuddles, the baby does it a lot more.

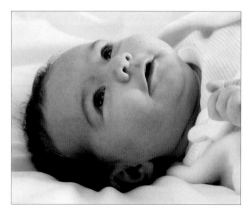

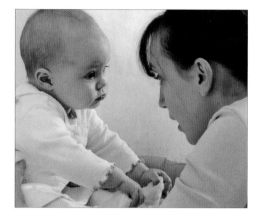

Your baby will learn to speak by listening to your voice and copying you. It will help if you make eye contact, and give him or her a chance to respond.

BABY TALK

At first your baby communicates only through crying, but after the first weeks, he or she will start to coo and gurgle. The first sounds – 'aah', 'eeeh' and other vowel sounds – will be random at first. But soon you will notice that the baby coos at you or at a particular object that has captured his or her attention.

Your baby will also start making easily articulated consonant sounds – 'ma', 'da' and 'ba'. Some babies do this as early as three months, some not until six months. Whatever age they start, they enjoy practising their new sounds. They also love it if you make the same sounds to them – try it and see how your baby reacts. Gradually babies start babbling: practising strings of consonant sounds such as 'babababa', 'dadadada', 'mamama', over and over. Six months is an average age to do this – but many babies will do it considerably later.

By now, you'll be waiting for your baby to say 'Mama' or 'Dada'. Lots of babies can do this at about eight months, and 'Dada usually comes first. But they won't use these words to mean their parents for another few months to come.

As well as practising sounds, babies start to laugh at about three and a half months. They also learn to screech to attract your attention. Don't worry that you are teaching bad habits when you respond to a deliberate scream – your baby will adopt different ways of calling you as soon as he or she is able.

GOOD WAYS TO TALK TO YOUR BABY

- Read to your baby from a young age. Look at a brightly coloured picture book together and make up your own words. Read the same story again and again. Give your baby cloth and tough board books that can safely be chewed.

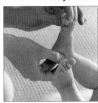

- Play games – count your baby's toes and play 'This little piggy' on them, play "Round and round the garden" on his or her palm and 'Incy-wincy spider' on the baby's tummy.

- Recite nursery rhymes. If you have forgotten the words, buy or borrow a children's book.
- Sing to your baby often. Play lots of music too – classical music helps to stimulate areas of the brain that deal with literacy and numeracy.

- Have 'conversations'. Even very young babies move their mouths, as if trying to speak. Respond to this with 'How interesting', 'That's a good story' and so on.

- When your baby starts to makes sounds, copy them – you'll get a smile when you do. Remember to pause so that the baby can 'answer' you.
- Point out things of interest when you are out and

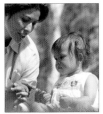

about. Name common objects – 'cow', 'car', 'flower' – as the more often your baby hears words in context the more quickly he or she will learn them. Talk about whatever you are doing – changing or bathing your baby, say.

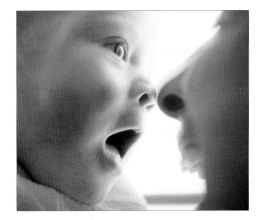

A baby will observe your face closely, so make exaggerated expressions when you talk to him or her. Try opening your mouth and sticking out your tongue – even a very new baby may copy you.

are helpful: they serve to reiterate the main sounds of the words, giving babies a second chance to hear them and commit them to memory. Diminutive endings – 'teethies', 'doggies' – are another universal element of baby talk: this way of speaking is also helpful, as 'framing' the consonant sound between vowels makes it easier to hear and learn. So don't feel embarrassed about lapsing into baby talk when you chat to your child – you are just doing what comes naturally.

BILINGUAL BABIES

Learning to speak is a fantastic intellectual achievement – one that all babies accomplish by the age of three. Strange as it may seem, it is no harder for a baby to learn two languages than one. So, if you and your partner speak different languages, each of you should stick to your own. Your baby will assume that there is a mummy language and a daddy language and will rise magnificently to the challenge of acquiring both.

HOW TO TALK TO YOUR CHILD

Some people find it very easy to chat to their babies; others think it is pointless talking to a baby who cannot understand them. But talking gives babies emotional stability, and it helps with language development and learning. Children learn their native language because they hear other people using it, so you have to give them the "raw data" to work with.

Most people naturally adopt a pitch higher than normal when talking to babies, as they are more responsive to this. 'Baby talk' also includes lots of rhymes – such as 'milky-wilky' and 'itty-bitty' – and repetitive elements – 'night-night', 'bye-bye'. Both rhyme and simple repetition

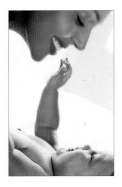

It's great if your baby is happy to go to other people for a cuddle, but he or she will always want to come back to you. You may also notice that your baby grabs at your face and pokes his or her fingers in your mouth with great gusto, but is a lot more restrained when held by someone less familiar.

section five

your older baby

six months to one year

The experience of caring for a baby is a mixture of anxiety and joy. But as you become seasoned parents, the joy starts to predominate and everything seems easier to accomplish. You will be astonished by the rate at which your baby changes during the second six months. You can almost see him or her develop before your eyes, as an individual personality begins to emerge.

General care and feeding

❝ It is immensely satisfying to know that you are training your baby's palate, laying the foundations for a lifetime of healthy eating. **❞**

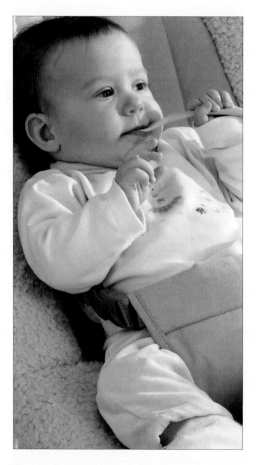

By now you will be better accustomed to caring for your baby and will be able to meet his or her basic needs with a more practised ease: long gone are the days when you struggled to get that sleepsuit over tiny arms and legs.

But babies grow fast and parenthood brings with it an ever-changing set of challenges. Around the six-month mark, your baby will start to cut his or her first teeth. Some babies do this without seeming to notice it; others feel a lot of pain and require lots of gentle aid to help them through the teething process.

The advent of teeth is a sign that your baby is getting ready for real food. Don't be surprised if you find it hard to give up the deep connection that comes with breastfeeding: this is a normal feeling. It is one of the many acts of letting go that are integral to parenthood. If you are committed to providing your baby with natural food, you will find that the changeover to solids involves a great deal of work at first: there are all those fruits and vegetables to cook, purée and pour into ice-cube trays for freezing. But it

Your baby may find a first experience of solid food strange, but he or she will soon get the taste for it and may grab the spoon out of your hand.

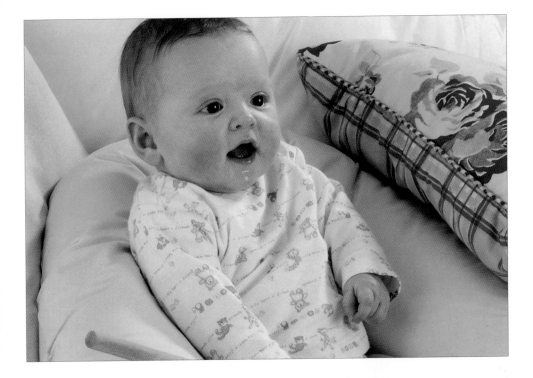

is also immensely satisfying to know that you are helping to train your baby's palate, laying the foundations for a lifetime of healthy eating. And, like all aspects of childcare, feeding your baby gets much easier with practice.

Many women return to work in their baby's first year, for perfectly good reasons, but if you find that you cannot bear to leave your baby after all, you are not alone. It's worth considering whether you can extend the time you spend together by negotiating more flexible working hours, for example. But if you do need to go back to work, for whatever reason, you will naturally want to choose your childcare carefully. Leaving your baby is much easier once you are confident that he or she is being looked after lovingly by someone you trust.

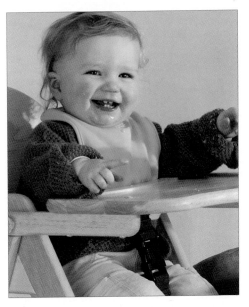

Top: Your baby will be much more aware of, and entertained by, his or her surroundings, and will watch your face and activities with absorbed interest.

Weaning is fun. There is huge pleasure to be had in introducing a baby to new flavours and seeing his or her growing enjoyment of good food.

Teething and tooth care

Spotting that tiny white line on your baby's gum is an exciting event – the first tooth is on its way. This can happen at any time in the first year, but teeth usually start coming through when a baby is around six months old.

WHEN THE TEETH COME THROUGH
Baby teeth tend to come through in pairs in a set sequence. But your baby's teeth may emerge in a slightly different order to the one described here, and they may appear earlier or later than the average ages given. They will look crooked when they are coming through, but will soon straighten out. Eventually your baby will have 20 milk teeth (compared to an adult's 32 permanent teeth).

TEETHING PAIN
The first teeth are sharp, thin incisors, so they usually cut through the gum quite easily. But if your baby is cutting more than one tooth at once, or if one of the large flat molars is emerging, this can cause a lot of discomfort.

To help your baby cope with the teething process, try rubbing the gums with a clean finger or a finger-toothbrush. You may be able to feel a bump on the gum before a tooth comes through. Something cool to bite on can help: a smooth hard toy or a clean facecloth dipped in cold water both work well, or you can use a teething ring that's been cooled in the fridge (not the freezer). Some people find that a stick of peeled carrot, a breadstick or a sugar-free teething biscuit helps; stay close by in case your baby manages to bite off a bit. You

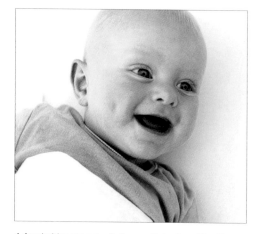

A few babies are actually born with teeth, while others don't develop any until after they are a year old.

can also breastfeed for comfort. Teething babies often want to nurse more frequently and need lots of fluid.

Many babies find homeopathic teething granules (Chamomilla) very soothing. But if natural methods don't seem to work, try rubbing teething gel on the gum. This numbs the area and can help a baby get off to sleep, but it is suitable only for babies over the age of about four months. You can also give your baby infant paracetamol (acetaminophen) to help with pain and reduce any fever.

This is a general guide to when you can expect which of your baby's teeth to appear.

Get your baby a toothbrush as soon as the first tooth comes through.

Front incisors, top – 7 months
Neighbouring incisors, top – 9 months
Top canines – 18 months
First two molars, top – 14 months
Back two molars, top – 2 years

Back two molars, bottom – 20 months
First two molars, bottom – 12 months
Bottom canines – 16 months
Neighbouring incisors, bottom – 7–8 months
Front incisors, bottom – 6 months

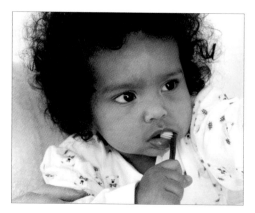

PROTECTING YOUR BABY'S TEETH

- Don't give your baby any sugary foods.
- Limit dried fruit to an occasional treat.
- Limit drinks to water and milk only.
- Always use sugar-free medicines.
- Take your baby with you when you go to the dentist for your own check-ups, so that the surgery becomes familiar. Always talk about going to the dentist in a positive and enthusiastic way.

TOOTH CARE

Start cleaning your baby's teeth as soon as the first ones come through. You'll find this easier if you lay the baby on your lap so that you are looking down at his or her mouth. If your baby doesn't like you using a baby toothbrush, try using a piece of damp gauze wrapped around your finger. Put a tiny smear of toothpaste on the gauze and clean the teeth very gently using circular movements, twice a day.

Don't worry if your baby won't let you brush his or her teeth at all; just give the brush to the baby to chew on. So long as you are using a fluoride toothpaste, this will help to strengthen the teeth and protect them from decay. It is important not to let tooth cleaning become stressful. At this stage it should be enjoyable and fun; but once several teeth are through they will need to be cleaned.

THE RIGHT TOOTHPASTE

Most dentists recommend that you use a specially formulated children's fluoride toothpaste for your baby. Adult toothpaste contains higher levels of fluoride, so it is not suitable: too much fluoride can cause discoloration of

Babies are fascinated by toothbrushing. Try giving your baby his or her own brush at the same time as you use yours, to copy you. Let your baby have a go at "brushing" your teeth while you are cleaning his or hers.

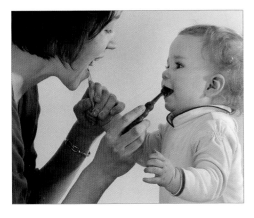

CHECKLIST: IS YOUR BABY TEETHING?

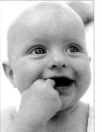

Be careful not to confuse real illness with signs of teething. If your baby seems to be in real pain, has a high temperature, a rash, diarrhoea or other symptoms, see a doctor. The following are the classic signs of teething.

Dribbling: More saliva is produced, so your baby is likely to dribble a lot more than usual. Many babies get a runny nose as well.

Distress and irritability. Pain will make your baby fractious and possibly more clingy than usual.

Biting and gnawing. Pressure on the gum relieves the pain so your baby may want to chew on everything (including you). The baby may bite his or her bottom lip before the first teeth come through.

Swelling on the gum. The gum may look red, bumpy or sore.

Flushed cheek. One or both cheeks may be red.

Fever. A slightly raised temperature is common with teething, especially at night.

Nappy rash. Many babies produce runny stools and are prone to nappy rash when teething.

Wakefulness. The baby may wake up more than usual at night.

the teeth. Fluoride is a mineral found in water. Additional fluoride is added to the water supply of some British regions and almost all US states to improve dental health. If there are only low levels of fluoride in your water, you may consider giving your baby a fluoride supplement, but you must take advice on this from a dentist: you could damage your child's teeth if you give too much fluoride.

Bikkie pegs are natural, rock hard, teething chews that some babies enjoy gnawing on.

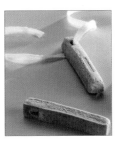

Homeopathic teething granules don't ease pain, but have a soothing effect on any fretfulness.

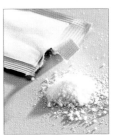

Bathing and dressing an older baby

Bathtime is a lot more fun once your baby is old enough to enjoy toys, games and lots of splashing in the big bath. Most older babies love having a bath, and a soak in warm water can be an excellent way of calming them down before bedtime. But having a bath straight after a meal can make a baby sick so leave a gap.

Make sure the bathroom is very warm and have a towel ready so that you can wrap your baby up as soon as you lift him or her out of the water. Until your baby is a confident sitter, you will have to lean over to support him or her throughout bathtime. This is hard on your back: make sure you are facing the bath squarely so that you are not twisting it.

BATHTIME GAMES

The best way to get your baby enjoying water is by playing in the bathtub.

- Lay your baby down on his or her back in the water, supporting the head and bottom, and swoosh him or her up and down the bath. Then turn the baby over and do the same, this time with your hands under the chin and tummy.
- Scoop water up in a beaker and pour it gently over the baby's tummy. Hold the beaker high and pour water into the bath in front of the baby so that it makes a glistening stream. He or she will reach out and touch it.

If your baby stops wanting to go in the bath, try getting in too. Take extra care when you are getting in and out, or have someone else there to lift the baby out for you.

BABY BATH OIL

To give your baby a beautifully aromatic and calming bath before bedtime, add a few drops of oil scented with mandarin orange to the water. Combine ten drops of mandarin essential oil with 100ml/3½fl oz sunflower oil, and store in a dark glass bottle out of direct sunlight. This oil will keep for 12 months.

- Gently trickle water on the baby's face using a facecloth or a scoop toy. This should help your baby to cope with any splashing in the pool if you go swimming together.
- Get some bath toys to play with. A natural sponge is great fun, and your baby will enjoy filling and emptying stacking cups or plastic bowls and beakers.
- If you have an older child, let them take a bath together – your baby will love playing in the water with a big brother or sister.

WASHING YOUR BABY

It is best to avoid baby bath products that contain chemicals, since these strip the natural oils from your baby's skin. You don't usually need to 'wash' your baby at this age anyway: you can do without shampoo, soap and bubble bath. If your baby has some grubby patches, you can use an oatmeal 'sponge': simply put a handful of oats in a muslin square, and twist to make a pouch. Water dries out the skin, so add a little oil to the bath. And of course, you don't have to bath your baby every day; a daily sponge bath of face, neck, underarms, hands, nappy area and feet is enough to keep a baby clean.

Babies love water games, and a natural sponge and a few simple toys add to the fun of bathtime.

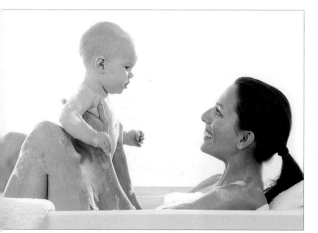

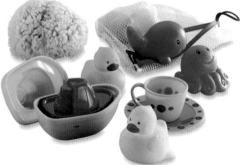

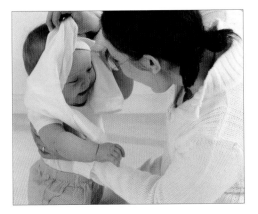

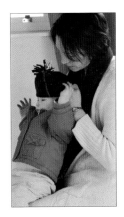

Left: Your baby will enjoy your cry of "Where's baby?" as his or her face disappears inside a top, and your start of surprise when a face is revealed. Play peek-a-boo with baby's hands and feet as you slip them into clothes.

Right: It may take lots of perseverance and patience to convince your baby to wear a hat.

CLOTHING YOUR BABY

Some older babies take an active role in getting dressed, pushing their hand through a sleeve opening or 'helping' you pull a jumper off. But if they are not in the mood, dressing can be a challenge. Try to make it as much fun as possible – smile, make eye contact, chat, sing and play games. Clothes that are easy to get on and off make the whole process easier: look for wide necks and sleeves, stretchy fabrics and popper fastenings. If your baby is crawling, choose clothes that keep the knees covered.

A hat is important for warmth in cold weather and to give protection from the sun. But getting a baby to wear one is tricky. If your baby pulls it off as a matter of course, wait until he or she is distracted and then put it back on. Alternatively try saying 'No' firmly and replacing it. You may have to do this many times, but once the baby realizes you mean business the hat may stay in place – for a while at least. It will help if the baby has a coat with a hood that you can pull over the hat, or if you choose a hat with straps that fasten under the chin.

Babies don't need shoes until they are walking. Keep the feet bare whenever you are in the warm. If your baby is wearing socks, make sure they are the non-slip variety in the right size: the tiny bones in a baby's feet are very soft, and tight socks can cause damage. Outdoors, a baby's feet may need some extra protection: soft pram shoes are best. Once your child learns to walk, buy proper shoes with lightweight, flexible soles from a specialist shop with trained fitters.

SAFETY IN THE BATH
- The water should be warm but not hot. Always check the temperature before putting the baby in the bath.
- Keep the room warm; babies lose body heat very quickly when they are wet.
- Keep the bath shallow – no more than waist-deep when your baby is sitting down.
- Never leave a baby alone in the bath, or under the care of another child.
- Don't let your baby pull himself or herself up in the bath unless you are holding on. It's best to discourage standing in the bath altogether.
- Wrap a wet facecloth around the hot tap as soon as your baby is old enough to reach for it.
- Put a non-slip mat in the bottom of the bath.

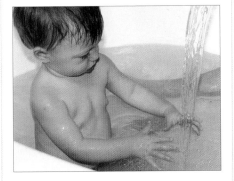

SAFETY IN THE SUN
- Keep your baby out of the sun as much as possible.
- When using a buggy, attach a parasol or, better still, a UV-filter sunshade.
- Dress your baby in lightweight fabric with a tight weave to protect the skin.
- Make your baby wear a wide-brimmed hat.
- Use a sunscreen of factor 20 or above, and re-apply frequently. Choose a natural sun cream specially formulated for children.
- Take precautions on warm cloudy days as well as on sunny ones.

When to wean

By the age of six months, your baby will almost certainly be ready to start eating solid food. The iron stored at birth will have begun to run out, and the baby may need more calories than he or she can get from milk alone. At this age, most babies are interested in new experiences and are more likely to take to eating than if you wait until much later in the first year. Ideally you will start giving solids at six months, but some parents start earlier, and so long as the baby is not at risk of developing allergies and you give only recommended foods, this shouldn't be a problem. However it is important not to start giving your baby food any earlier than four months, because a young baby's intestines are immature. Starting solids early or giving certain foods may encourage long-term digestive problems or allergies.

Young babies also find it quite difficult to eat – which suggests that they are not ready for the experience. They can't sit up properly, so swallowing is difficult, and they tend to poke their tongue out when they sense something alien in their mouths. This tongue-thrust reflex protects them from choking. It disappears between four and six

If your baby shows an interest in food, a bouncy chair is a convenient place to have his or her first meals.

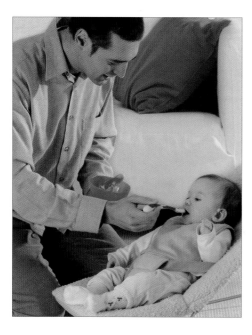

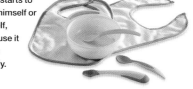

ESSENTIAL EQUIPMENT
You don't need a lot of special equipment when introducing solid food to your baby, but the following are useful.
Baby chair. It is much easier to feed with a spoon when you are facing your baby. If he or she can sit up well, use a highchair. If not, a bouncy chair set at the most upright level makes a good substitute for the first weeks.
Spoons. Shallow weaning spoons are easy to get into a baby's mouth and make it easy for him or her to lick the food off. Plastic spoons are easy to clean and sterilize, and they won't hurt your baby when he or she starts waving them around.
Bibs. Feeding is a messy business so you will need three or more bibs. Cloth ones are the most comfortable, and Velcro fasteners are much easier to use than ties.
Bowls. You can use ordinary bowls, but it is easier to serve tiny amounts in a small, shallow bowl, which also allows the baby to see the food. A bowl with a sucker on the base is good for when a baby starts to feed himself or herself, because it stays steady.

months, when they learn to use the tongue to manoeuvre food to the back of the mouth and swallow it. An older baby can also let you know that he or she wants more food by leaning towards the spoon with an open mouth or has had enough by turning away with a mouth firmly shut.

IS MY BABY READY FOR SOLIDS?
Wait until your baby is showing signs of being interested in food before you think about introducing solids. These are some of the typical signs to look for.
- Your baby still seems hungry after a feed.
- Your baby wants feeding more often.
- Your baby watches you with interest when you eat.
- Your baby begins waking up more frequently in the night after a period of sleeping through.
- Your baby is putting things in his or her mouth.
- Your baby can hold his or her head up well.

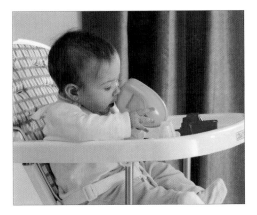

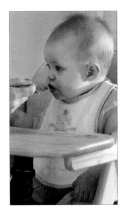

Left: Before you use the highchair for feeding, get your baby used to it. Put some toys on the table for them to play with. If they start putting a toy in their mouth, give them something they can eat.

Right: Starting your baby on solids is quite an event. At first it can feel like hard work, but you – and the baby – will soon get the hang of it.

Talk to your health visitor if you are not sure whether to start solids or not. A premature baby won't be ready to start on solids until at least four to six months from his or her expected, rather than actual, birth date.

WHICH HIGHCHAIR?

The most natural option for a highchair is one that is made from wood from a sustainable source. Make sure the design is simple and that it doesn't have any awkward crevices that will be difficult to clean.

A chair with an adjustable seat or footrest will be more comfortable for the baby, but will probably take up more space than one that folds up. The chair should have a fixed five-point harness for absolute safety. You will need some cushioning to protect the baby's head from banging on the back of the chair.

Some highchairs are designed to be drawn up to the table so that the baby can join in family meals from the beginning. This is a great idea in theory, but you may prefer to choose one with a tray to contain the mess. A highchair with a detachable tray can be used either way.

ALLERGIES

If a baby's father, mother or any siblings suffer from allergies or allergy-related conditions such as asthma, eczema or hay fever (allergic rhinitis), the baby may inherit the allergy. The best way to protect him or her is to breastfeed exclusively for six months, and to continue breastfeeding for the rest of the first year.

Introduce solids very slowly and do not give any foods that you or your partner are allergic to until your baby is at least a year old. Dairy foods, wheat, citrus fruits, eggs, fish, shellfish and nuts are the most common food allergens, so they should be introduced with caution. Sesame seeds and peanuts, and any foods containing them (such as peanut butter, groundnut oil and sesame oil) should not be given until your child is at least three; you may wish to exclude all nuts from your child's diet.

Even if there is no family history of allergy, it is still important to take weaning slowly. Introduce one new food at a time and be on the lookout for any allergic reactions. These usually occur within minutes of eating and can include the following: facial rash (especially around the mouth), sneezing, runny nose, coughing, wheezing. Very occasionally, a baby may develop breathing difficulties or swelling of the lips: this needs urgent medical attention and you need to call an ambulance.

If a baby is intolerant of a certain food – meaning it is difficult to digest – he or she may experience bloating or passing wind, diarrhoea or vomiting within a few hours or sometimes over a couple of days after eating it. If your baby seems to have a reaction of this kind to a certain food, try introducing it again a few weeks later to see if the reaction recurs. If it does, you probably need to eliminate the food from your baby's diet. Children often grow out of allergies and intolerances, so you may be able to re-introduce the offending food later, but get individual advice on this from a health professional.

When a baby is ready for weaning, he or she should take food from a spoon or your finger with just a little encouragement.

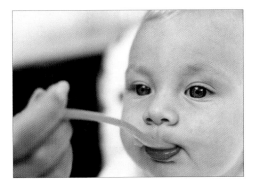

First foods: 4–6 months

Your aim when introducing solids is to get your baby used to different tastes and textures, not to replace milk. Start with just one 'meal' a day, offering just a teaspoonful of food to start with. If your baby seems eager for more, you can offer a couple of teaspoonfuls the next time and gradually build up to a couple of tablespoons or so. Don't worry if your baby seems to eat more one day and then less the next; this is quite normal.

A good time to introduce solid food is mid-morning, ideally between milk feeds. That way, your baby won't be so hungry that he or she will be wanting milk, nor so full that he or she won't be interested in trying something new. Once the baby is used to the idea, you can combine solid food with the lunchtime feed. Give milk before the solids, so that you don't cut down on milk feeds too quickly. Or try giving a little milk first, then the solids, then the rest of the milk.

If your baby rejects the food repeatedly, he or she probably isn't ready for solids yet and you should wait a week or two before trying again. Don't try to force the baby to eat more than he or she wants – babies have a good sense of when to stop and it is important to be led by what your baby wants.

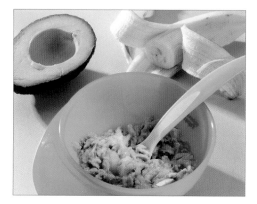

Avocado and banana, mashed together, are healthy raw foods that you can feed to young babies.

INTRODUCING NEW TASTES

Give baby rice for at least a week or two before introducing another new food. Take the weaning process very slowly, introducing new foods one a time. Leave about a week between the first three or four new foods

Starting solid

A good first food is baby rice, which is gluten-free and unlikely to cause any reaction. Commercial baby rice comes in dried flakes and usually has added nutrients such as iron. Mix it with your baby's usual milk (expressed breastmilk or formula) so that this first 'meal' has a familiar taste. It should have a soupy consistency.

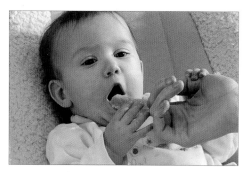

1 Put a little of the milky baby rice on the tip of your finger so that your baby can suck it off. If he or she doesn't seem interested, try dabbing a little on his or her lips or tongue. You may find that the rice is poked straight back out until your baby gets the hang of moving it to the back of the mouth for swallowing.

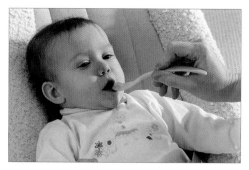

2 If your baby takes well to sucking food off your finger, offer a little rice on a shallow spoon. Give a few more spoonfuls if the baby shows interest by leaning forwards, opening his or her mouth when you offer the food, or grabbing your finger or the spoon. If the baby turns away or pushes your hand away, he or she has had enough.

and wait three to five days before introducing subsequent ones. This will allow your baby's digestive system to get used to each new food, and will also make it easier for you to pinpoint the problem food if your baby develops an allergic reaction.

The following fruits and vegetables make excellent first foods because they are bland and can be mashed or puréed to a smooth consistency. Add a little milk or milky baby rice so that the consistency is fairly runny. To make food more interesting, combine different purées that you have already introduced – try carrot and apple, parsnip and sweet potato, papaya and banana.

Root vegetables. These have a naturally sweet taste and are easy to digest. Try carrots, sweet potato, butternut squash, yams, parsnips and swede (rutabaga). Peel and cut into pieces (remove the seeds in squash), steam until very soft and then purée or mash. Your baby may also like puréed potato.

The best way to cook fruits and vegetables for babies is to steam them – it preserves more nutrients than any other cooking method.

Pears and apples. These fruits are gentle on the stomach and most babies love them. Peel, core and cut into pieces. Steam or cook in a little water until very soft, then purée or mash. An older baby can eat mashed, uncooked pear if it is very ripe.

Bananas, papayas and avocados. These are very digestible fruits that don't need cooking. Simply mash and mix with a little milk to give a suitably runny texture.

COOKING FOR A BABY
The best cooking method is steaming, which preserves most nutrients. Boiling and baking (without oil) are also healthy, but don't boil foods for too long. Avoid frying and roasting, which makes food more difficult to digest. Microwaving not only destroys some of the nutrients in food, but also heats it unevenly, so it is best avoided.

To save time, you can cook and purée a batch of vegetables or fruit, take what you need for one meal, cool the rest and freeze straight away in ice-cube trays. When the cubes are frozen, transfer them to a freezer bag. Don't forget to date and label the bag. Cooked frozen foods cannot be refrozen once defrosted, and if your baby does not eat much of a meal you must throw the rest away, however wasteful that seems. It is fine to defrost frozen food cubes in a saucepan, but make sure that you heat the food through thoroughly, then cool before feeding.

THREE MEALS A DAY
A few weeks after you start giving your baby solids mid-morning, you can introduce breakfast, too. Most babies are very hungry when they wake up, so give a milk feed first and then a teaspoon or two of solids. After another few weeks, start giving the baby some solids in the early evening, too. You can gradually increase the amount at each meal to suit his or her appetite – follow your baby's lead and give what he or she seems to want. Older babies will also need healthy snacks between meals, such as fruit, rice cakes and oatcakes.

Preparing a batch of tiny meals in advance takes the stress out of feeding.

Baby rice is quick and easy to prepare, and most babies like it.

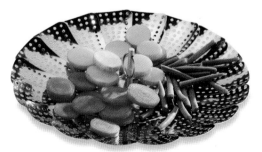

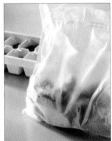

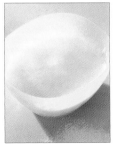

Second foods: after 6 months

Once you have introduced the idea of eating solid food, the next step is to extend your baby's palate. Don't assume that your baby won't like strong flavours such as, say, courgette (zucchini) or natural yoghurt; he or she may well surprise you. It will help if you introduce each new food in a relaxed and confident way – if your expression says 'Beware', then your child will. Often a baby will be more willing to accept a new food that has a distinctive flavour – spinach, say – if it is mixed with the carrot or parsnip that he or she already knows and loves. Start by adding a tiny amount and then gradually increase the ratio of spinach to carrot as the baby gets used to it.

NEW FOODS TO TRY

The following foods are good ones to introduce after first foods. Remember to introduce them one at a time, and to leave three to five days between each new food.

FOODS THAT NEED TO WAIT

Some foods are more likely to cause an allergic reaction than others, so they should not be among the first foods that you introduce to your baby.

After six months, you can try:
- Cow's milk dairy products – yoghurts, butter, cheese and fromage frais, but don't give unpasteurized cheeses to a young child.

After eight months, if no history of allergies, try the following (wait until twelve months if there is a history of allergy:
- Foods containing gluten – wheat, rye, barley or oats
- Egg (make sure it is well cooked)
- Nuts and seeds that have been ground (excluding peanuts and sesame seeds)
- Fish (but children should not have shark, marlin or swordfish because they contain levels of mercury that could affect their developing nervous systems)
- Citrus fruits and juices

After twelve months, you can try:
- Honey (avoid for the first year because it may contain a bacterium that causes infant botulism)
- Peanuts (crushed) and sesame seeds (avoid until three years if there is a family history of nut allergy)
- Finely chopped nuts (do not give whole nuts to under-fives because of the choking risk).

CAUTION
Never leave your baby alone when eating: stay nearby in case he or she chokes on a piece of food.

Vegetables. Try purées of steamed courgette, spinach or green beans, broccoli and cauliflower, as well as puréed boiled frozen peas. Home-cooked beetroot (beet) is a good food to combine with mashed potato.

Fruits. Lightly cooked mangoes, peaches and nectarines make good purées, or try mashed ripe melon (cantaloupe is one of the sweetest) from about seven months. Dried fruits such as apricots, dates or prunes can be cooked in water and then puréed, but give them sparingly as they are very sweet. Some babies are allergic to kiwi fruit and strawberries, so wait until at least nine months before introducing these fruits and watch for any reaction.

Grains. Introduce millet or oats (which can be made into a smooth porridge) before wheat-based cereals, which are more likely to cause a reaction. Once your baby is taking textured food, couscous, quinoa and barley are good grain foods and you can also introduce tiny pasta shapes (buy the ones intended for soup).

Dairy products. Give plain unsweetened yoghurt, plain

Babies have a natural instinct to do things for themselves, and most really enjoy feeding themselves with finger foods. Rice cakes are ideal to start off with because they disintegrate when sucked.

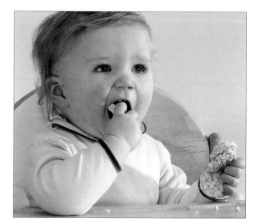

fromage frais, cream cheese, cottage cheese, Cheddar and other hard cheeses. Always use full-fat dairy products – growing babies need lots of calories so you don't want them to fill up on low-fat foods.

Lentils and beans. Try a purée of red lentils – you can add a sliver each of garlic and ginger to the cooking water to add flavour (remove the ginger before puréeing). From about nine months you can try butterbeans, haricots, split peas and soya.

Chicken and meat. Chicken and turkey usually go down well. They can be puréed or mashed with root or green vegetables or dairy products. Once your baby is happy with white meat try lean red meat such as lamb.

Fish. Introduce white fish from about eight months: poach it in milk, flake it and check very carefully for bones before feeding to your baby. Once your baby is happily eating these foods, you can try introducing oily fish such as salmon.

EXTRA FLAVOURS

You can make your baby's food more tasty by adding flavourings such as sautéed onion or leek, garlic and ginger, and finely chopped parsley and other soft-leaved herbs. It is also a good idea to introduce mild spices from about eight months – try sprinkling a little cinnamon on porridge, or adding cumin or paprika to savoury dishes.

Don't add any salt to food for a baby less than a year old, and avoid processed foods such as baked beans, which contain added salt. Similarly, don't sweeten food with sugar or give sugary 'treats'. There can be a lot of

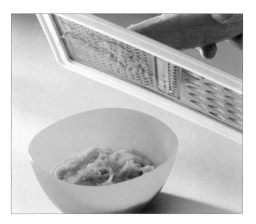

Adding grated food to purées is a good way of getting your baby used to a new texture.

sugar in fruity yoghurts and fromage frais, baby rusks and processed foods, and all are best avoided.

TEXTURE, TOO

At first your baby can manage only smooth and runny purées. But if you go on giving these for a long time, he or she may reject lumpier food. So it is a good idea to start mashing rather than puréeing food from about seven months, and to gradually increase the lumpiness of the food you serve. Once your baby is eating lumpier food, try stirring in some finely grated or chopped foods to introduce different textures. You can also give your baby finger foods from about seven months.

Don't limit your baby to bland foods. Babies are much more receptive to new flavours than older children, so it is a good idea to expose them to flavours such as ginger, cumin, garlic and fresh herbs.

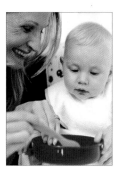

Introduce your baby to different textures and tastes. Try a whole banana, oatcakes, a few raisins or dried apricots, a handful of whole butter (lima) beans, chunks of hard cheese, thin slices of apple or pear and tiny sandwich squares spread with cream cheese.

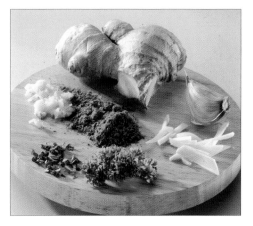

Healthy eating for babies

As your baby's appetite for solid food increases over the first year, he or she will start to take less milk. Once solids become a more substantial part of the diet, you need to start providing a good mix of different foods to ensure that your baby is getting all the right nutrients. A balanced daily diet for a nine- to twelve-month-old baby would include the following.

One or two servings of protein foods. Protein is made up of amino acids, which are needed for the growth and repair of all the body's cells and tissues. Lean meat, chicken and turkey, fish, eggs, cheese, yoghurt and tofu (soya bean curd) are complete sources of protein. Pulses and beans are healthy protein foods but contain only some of the essential amino acids. Your baby also needs to eat some grain foods (rice, oats, bread or pasta) or nuts and seeds over the course of the day to get a good balance of amino acids.

Three or four servings of starchy foods. Carbohydrates are the body's main fuel. The best sources are starchy foods such as oats, rice, bread, barley, rye and potatoes; lentils, pulses, fruits and vegetables also contain carbohydrates. It is best not to feed babies high-fibre foods as this will fill their tiny stomachs without providing the necessary nutrients. Refined grains such as white rice and ordinary pasta are much easier to digest.

Four or five servings of fruits and vegetables. These contain the vitamins and minerals that are essential to good health, and they are the best source of fibre for babies and young children. The best way to make sure that your baby is getting enough is to offer as wide a range as possible.

Grains and starchy vegetables give your baby the carbohydrates he or she needs for energy.

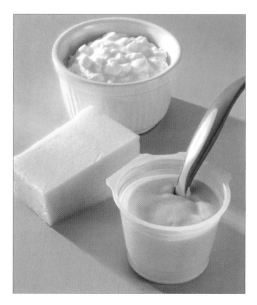

Cheese, yoghurt and other dairy foods are a good source of calcium, but be sure to give full-fat versions.

Calcium. Babies get calcium from their milk, which is still their most important food. If your baby is not drinking quite enough milk, other good dietary sources include dairy products (cheese, yoghurt, fromage frais), almonds, brazil nuts, green leafy vegetables and tofu.

Some healthy fats. Fats are a concentrated source of calories, which growing babies need – both breastmilk and formula have high fat contents. Always give your baby full-fat versions of any milk, cheese, yoghurt or other dairy products you offer. Include healthy

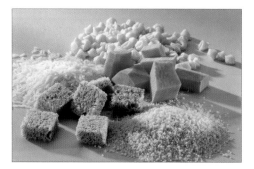

GOING ORGANIC
Buying organic food is an easy way to reduce the chemicals your baby is exposed to: organic fruits and vegetables are produced with fewer pesticides and fertilizers, and the animals used for organic meat are not routinely given antibiotics. Organic farming methods may also produce some food with higher levels of nutrients: one study found that organic milk had higher levels of essential fatty acids, vitamin E and antioxidants, which help fight infection.

Vitamin	Needed for	Good sources
Vitamin A	Growth, healthy skin, good eyesight	Green leafy vegetables, carrots, squash, sweet potatoes, apricots, mangoes, liver, oily fish, egg yolks, butter, margarine and cheese
Vitamin B group	Growth, healthy nervous and immune systems, healthy skin, nails and hair, good digestion	Green leafy vegetables, broccoli, oats, lean meat and liver, tofu, fish, fortified breakfast cereals, bananas, avocados, milk and yoghurt
Vitamin C	Strong gums, teeth, bones and skin, healthy immune system, helps with iron absorption	Citrus and berry fruits, mangoes, papaya, nectarines, blackcurrants, potatoes, green leafy vegetables, peppers, tomatoes
Vitamin D	Strong bones and teeth	Salmon, sardines, tuna, milk, fortified margarine, eggs, fortified breakfast cereals
Vitamin E	Maintaining the body's cell structure	Vegetable oils, nuts, seeds, avocado

unsaturated fats in the baby's diet, from vegetable oils, avocados, nuts and seeds, and oily fish. Foods such as processed cakes and crisps contain unhealthy trans-fats and have no nutritional value so they should be avoided altogether.

Some iron-rich foods. Iron is important both for physical and for mental growth, but babies can easily become anaemic (iron-deficient). Use a formula milk with extra iron if you are bottle-feeding. Good dietary sources of iron include red meat and liver, oily fish, pulses, green leafy vegetables, dried fruits such as apricots, and fortified breakfast cereals. Iron from animal sources is easily absorbed by the body. Iron from plant-based sources is absorbed more easily if they are accompanied by a food that is rich in vitamin C (red (bell) peppers, tomatoes and all citrus fruits are particularly good).

Protein foods such as meat, fish, lentils and eggs are an important part of a baby's diet.

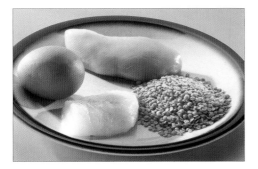

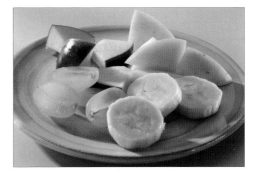

Try to get your baby to try different kinds of fresh fruits, to provide a good range of vitamins.

VEGETARIAN BABIES

A vegetarian diet is perfectly healthy for babies so long as they get enough protein: offer two servings a day. An easy way to increase the protein content of a vegetarian meal is to add cheese, chopped egg yolk or a smooth cashew or almond nut butter (from about eight months). You'll also need to ensure that a vegetarian baby gets sufficient iron, especially if still being breastfed (formula has added iron), and vitamin B12, found in dairy products, breakfast cereals and yeast extract (suitable after one year).

A vegan diet is very restrictive, so it is harder to make sure your baby is getting all the necessary nutrients. You'll have to plan meals carefully in order to provide the baby with enough protein, vitamin B12 and vitamin D, and you may need to give vitamin supplements. It is worth getting advice from a paediatric dietician or doctor before starting to wean your baby if you intend to follow a vegan diet.

Milk and the older baby

Babies need to continue drinking plenty of milk, even after solids are introduced. They need about 600ml/1 pint a day up to the age of twelve months. Give your baby milk first thing in the morning and at bedtime, and at other times if necessary.

Breastmilk is the best milk for your baby for the first year. If you are breastfeeding, it is impossible to tell how much milk your baby is getting. But if you are giving four or more full feeds a day, your baby is almost certainly getting enough.

Bottle-fed babies over the age of six months can continue to drink infant formula or can switch to a follow-on milk if the infant formula doesn't seem to be satisfying them. Cow's milk and goat's milk are not suitable as a main drink until your baby is at least twelve months old, because they don't have enough iron and other nutrients.

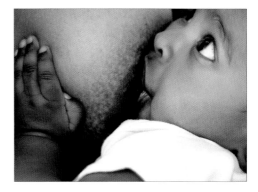

Mother's milk is still the best nutrition a baby can have – it has a high fat content to give energy and plenty of calcium for growing bones.

OTHER DRINKS

Other than milk, the best drink to give is water. There's no need to give other drinks, which fill your baby up without providing vital calories. It is a good idea to get your child used to drinking water from an early age. Give him or her sips from a cup at mealtimes.

Babies over the age of six months can drink water straight from the tap, but you may want to filter it first to remove impurities. Don't give bottled mineral water – some have high levels of salt and are unsuitable for babies, and the water may have been sitting in the bottle for months.

A spouted cup is useful when you are out and about, and there is a wide range on the market – you may need to experiment to find one your baby likes to use. Remember it is still important to sterilize your baby's cups, bottles and teats.

Fruit juice, even if it is well diluted, is too acidic for young babies. Even after six months, it is best not to give your baby fruit juice to drink because it contains sugars, which can cause tooth decay. Sometimes parents are advised to give babies diluted juice at mealtimes to help

Weaning your baby off a bottle and on to a cup can be a long process. Try cuddling your baby in the same way you would when they were taking a bottle, and maintaining the close association milk has with you.

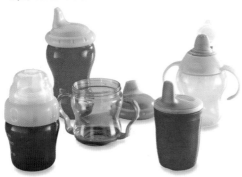

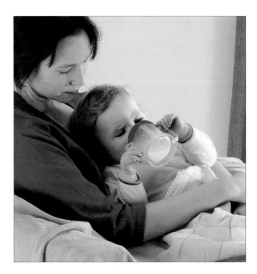

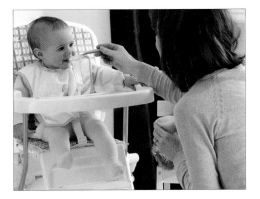

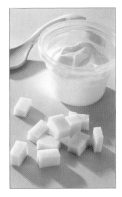

Left: There's no need to give your baby sweet fruity yoghurts. Try him or her on plain bio-active yoghurt, which is better for the teeth and can help the digestion.

Right: Dairy foods, such as milk, cheese and yoghurt, are a good way of ensuring that babies get enough calcium in their diet.

them absorb the iron in food. But fruit or vegetables rich in vitamin C will do the job just as well. If you do decide to give juice at mealtimes, dilute it with water – ten parts water to one part juice – to help protect your baby's emerging teeth, and to stop them getting full on liquid. Other drinks, such as squashes, teas or fizzy drinks, should never be given to a baby.

MOVING TO A CUP

It's a good idea to start getting your baby used to a cup from six or seven months. With a bottle, liquid tends to collect in the mouth and over a prolonged period this can lead to tooth decay, particularly if the baby tends to comfort suck. Frequent sucking on a teat can also interfere with the correct development of a baby's teeth.

The best kind of cup to use is an open one; you can get slanted 'Doidy' cups, which are easier for a baby to drink from than the usual baby cup with a spout. You are bound to have accidents when using an open cup, so you may want to restrict it to times when your baby is sitting on your lap or in a highchair and use a beaker with a spout (a sippy cup) for water at other times.

It can take a long time to get a bottle-fed baby used to drinking from a cup. Take your time – and don't be surprised if it takes six months or more to completely wean the baby from a bottle. The bedtime bottle is usually the last one to go, but don't worry, just enjoy the warmth and closeness it brings. Here are some ways to help.

- Let the baby play with an empty cup.
- Introduce a cup at mealtimes first, and help your baby to hold it.
- When you think your baby is ready, give one milk feed from a cup. Choose a feed when the baby doesn't drink as much – usually the mid-afternoon one.
- Keep your baby cuddled on your lap while he or she is drinking the milk – some babies are reluctant to give up the bottle because they associate it with being held.
- Once your baby is taking the cup at one feed, substitute it for the bottle at other feeds, one at a time.

WEANING FROM THE BREAST

The decision to wean your baby from the breast is a complicated and emotive one. Babies benefit from having breastmilk as their main drink throughout the first year, but many nursing women decide that they want to stop or reduce breastfeeds earlier for a variety of good reasons.

- Don't stop breastfeeding abruptly, since this can be traumatic for your baby and uncomfortable for you.
- Accept that weaning takes time. Leave at least a week or two between each dropping of a feed.
- Substitute a bottle or cup of milk for each feed you drop so that your baby doesn't go short of milk.
- If the baby is reluctant, try giving expressed breastmilk until he or she gets used to the idea of taking milk from a source other than the breast.
- If your baby won't take a bottle or cup from you, then try getting his or her father to give it. Stay out of the room so that you don't distract the baby.
- Give your baby lots of cuddles. It is important that he or she doesn't feel rejected and continues to get the closeness you both enjoy when you breastfeed.
- Make the bedtime feed the last one you drop. You may decide that you are happy to continue with this, and a morning feed, say, for a few months longer if your baby is drinking formula at other times.
- Wear a well-fitting bra. Express a little milk to prevent engorgement if necessary.

SUPPLEMENTS FOR BREASTFED BABIES

While breastmilk is generally healthier than formula milk, formula does have iron and vitamins added to it. Breast-fed babies may not get enough vitamin A, C and D from milk alone, so vitamin drops are generally advised. However, once they start eating solids, babies can get these vitamins from other foods. Despite this, current UK advice is for all children from six months to five years receive vitams A, C and D.

Helping your baby enjoy food

Eating is one of life's great joys. It's common for parents to worry about how much and what their baby is eating, but such anxiety can introduce an element of tension into mealtimes that is counterproductive. Having a relaxed, positive attitude towards your baby's food will go a long way to helping him or her enjoy it.

MAKING FOOD FUN

Let your baby eat with his or her fingers. Food will go all over the place, but it will show that eating is fun and that the baby can feed himself or herself rather than having to rely on you to spoon food into his or her mouth. Once old enough, your baby will love to pick up peas or other small morsels and pop them into his or her mouth. Serve easy finger foods alongside mashed or minced food – try steamed strips of vegetables, thin strips of chicken, strips of rolled-up pancakes, butter (lima) beans, small pasta shapes and squares of toast.

Give your baby a spoon as soon as he or she wants to hold one. Let the baby try to use it, while you use a second spoon to get food into his or her mouth, and accept the fact that babies make a mess at mealtimes. Don't hover around wiping your baby's face or hands after

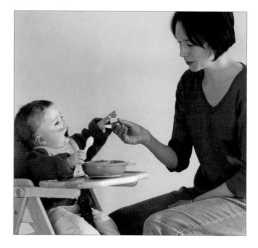

Your baby may assert a fierce sense of independence at mealtimes. Feeding will probably work best at this stage if you both have a spoon.

every mouthful – you'll be sending out the message that food is dirty or bad. Use a bib and put newspaper or a plastic sheet under the highchair to contain the mess. Wait until mealtime is over to clean the baby up.

RELAXED MEALTIMES

Always sit with your baby when he or she eats: mealtimes should be sociable events, and you need to stay close by in case of choking. Include the baby in family meals from as young an age as possible. Offer suitable bits and pieces off your plate, feed the baby a minced or mashed version of what you are eating or provide some finger foods to play with.

Always be positive about your baby's food. Be careful if you are offering something that you personally don't like – your baby may pick up on your distaste and refuse it. And get into good habits yourself. Your child is more likely to eat fruit at breakfast, say, if he or she sees you doing the same.

Let your baby decide how much to eat. His or her appetite will vary from day to day, and from meal to meal. Don't force food into the baby's mouth or spend ages trying to encourage him or her to eat one last spoonful. Your baby will quickly realize that it's possible to get your focused attention by refusing food, and mealtimes could become a battleground.

Setting a good example

Eating food from the same plate as your baby is a good way of encouraging him or her to eat.

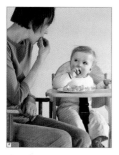

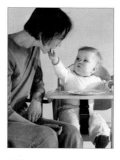

1 If your baby seems uncertain about trying a new food, try popping a bit in your own mouth. Look as though you are enjoying it, and your baby will love to copy you.

2 The next stage will be them wanting to feed you. Accept their offering, however sucked and squishy it might be. They will automatically pick up this positive attitude.

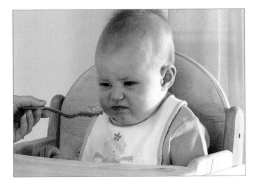

If your baby refuses food, don't keep pushing him or her to accept it – it's more important that the baby sees food as pleasurable than that he or she eats up that last bit of carrot.

EXCITING FLAVOURS

Give homemade food most or all of the time. Most commercial baby foods have a similar taste and they are all processed to the same smoothness. So a baby fed mostly from jars won't experience the distinct flavours and different textures of homemade foods. If you limit your baby to just a few dishes, he or she may be less willing to accept new foods later on, so provide lots of variety. Now is the time to get the baby enjoying as many of the wonderful flavours of food as possible.

REFUSING SOLIDS

Some babies do not take to solids well. If your baby doesn't seem interested when you first offer them, he or she may not be ready for food. Trying waiting at least a week or two before offering it again.

Even babies who take well to solid food will refuse it from time to time, especially if they are ill or teething. The best way to handle this is to stay calm. Continue to offer meals, but leave it up to your baby whether or not he or she eats. Most babies will start eating again when they feel ready, though it can take a few weeks before their appetite returns fully. Similarly, babies will often eat only a few foods – fruit and toast, say – or suddenly refuse foods that they have previously enjoyed. Again, this is normal. Keep offering other foods alongside the ones your baby is eating; let the baby see you eating them. It may also help if you give the baby meals with the rest of the family. Eventually curiousity about new foods will grow again.

WHEN BABIES DON'T EAT

A few babies don't take to eating until much later in the first year. So long as your baby is gaining weight and is healthy, starting solids later is unlikely to be a problem. Talk to a health professional if you are worried. If your

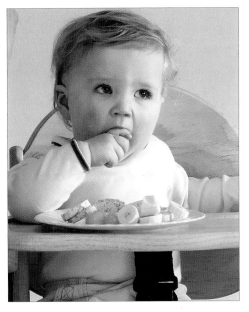

Giving your child a selection of fruit such as grapes and sliced banana after a meal is just as nice – and a lot healthier – than a sugary pudding.

baby is older than eight months and still showing no interest, try cutting down on milk feeds – babies don't need more than 600ml/1 pint per day.

It is worth bearing in mind that a baby who is prone to allergies may be better off feeding only on breastmilk for most of the first year. Nutritionally, babies can get almost everything they need from breastmilk, with the possible exception of iron. Breastmilk contains small amounts of iron, but it is more easily absorbed than that in infant formula, so a breastfed baby may be getting enough.

Your baby will enjoy mealtimes more if he or she is allowed to touch, squash and smear food around. This helps babies to get familiar with food and appreciate it.

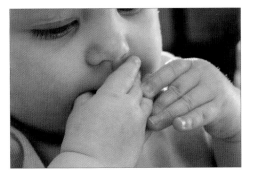

What childcare?

Knowing that your baby is happy and well cared for will make it easier for you to leave him or her if you go back to work. It's important for both of you that you choose the right childcare and that you feel confident about whatever arrangement you make.

DECIDING WHEN TO GO BACK TO WORK

Some mothers are keen to return to work as their baby gets older, while others prefer to take as long a period off work as they can manage. If you are feeling happy with the original arrangements you made about returning, the next step is to decide on the right carer or nursery, but if not you could consider extending your maternity leave. Don't stick with the decision to return to work on a certain date because it seems easier than re-negotiating. Have the courage to follow your instincts about what is right for you and your baby, even if that means admitting you have made a mistake.

Be open and honest with the baby's father (if you are together) about how you are feeling, and listen to how he feels too: he may be unable or unwilling to take on the burden of being the sole breadwinner, he may prefer it if you stay at home to care for your baby or he may want to give up work to do this himself. Often parents have more options than might be immediately apparent; for example, one of you might be able to afford to stay at home if you forego holidays, meals out and so on. It is important that you decide together what is right for your family.

If you want to go back to work but are worried about leaving your baby for long working days, you could consider reducing the number of hours you work. Many women decide to work part-time after they have a baby, and a growing number of fathers are doing the same.

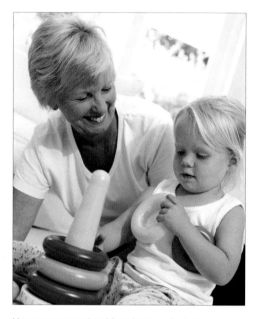

Your parents may be able to help you look after your baby. This form of childcare can work very well, but make sure everyone agrees on who does what.

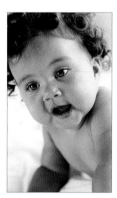

Your baby will prefer to be at home and looked after by you than anyone else. Delaying going back to full-time work for at least the first year is a good option if you can manage it.

WHAT'S BEST?

A long-term study led by the respected childcare expert Penelope Leach, which began in 1998, looked at the emotional and social development of 1200 children in Britain, aged three months to four years. It rated childcare options for babies under 18 months old in the following order of preference:

1 Full-time care by parent
2 Nanny in child's own home
3 Childminder (home day care)
4 Grandparent or other informal carer
5 Nursery (commercial day care).

It is important to keep this and other research in perspective. Remember that any study of day care looks at a wide range of children; what is right for your child may be very different. And of course everything depends on the individual carers: for example, a fantastic nursery with attentive, loving staff is better than a lazy and uncaring childminder.

If this is not possible, see if you can change your hours to fit in with your childcare arrangements. It may be that you and your partner can work at different times, to increase the length of time your baby spends at home.

CHILDCARE OPTIONS

These are the main childcare options.

Nanny. A nanny looks after your baby in your own home, so the baby stays in familiar surroundings and has the full attention of a carer. This is the most flexible option, because the nanny can fit around your hours and follow your routine. Most nannies have studied first aid and childcare, but this is not compulsory so it is important to check qualifications. Nannies may live in or out, and it is possible to share one with another family.

A nanny needs a living wage so this is a costly childcare option. If she (most nannies are women) works in your home, you will be her employer. This means that you will need to draw up a contract detailing the job description, hours, sick and holiday pay and so on. You will also need to take out public liability insurance in case of accidents and will have to pay the nanny's tax and insurance contributions.

Childminder (home day care). There are male and female childminders, but most tend to be mothers with children of their own. They usually work in their own homes, caring for a fixed number of children. Hours can be flexible, but some childminders work only in the school holidays or on particular days.

If both parents work flexible or part-time hours, you will be able to reduce the time your child spends in care.

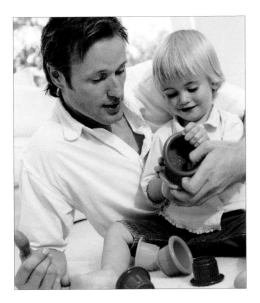

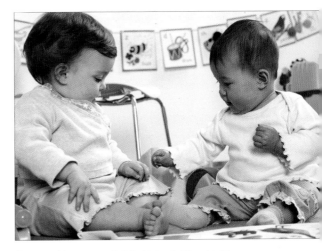

A nursery (day care centre) that takes babies should have a special room where the babies can be cared for away from toddlers and older children.

The legal requirements vary from country to country. In the UK, for example, childminders have to be registered with the local authority and are allowed to look after no more than six children (of whom no more than three may be under five years old). They are also required to complete a basic training course, including first aid. Always ask to see a childminder's registration, insurance and first aid certificates, and sign a written contract covering hours, pay, sick and holiday pay.

Grandparents. Many parents see a grandparent as the ideal carer for their baby. The arrangement is usually unpaid, and can work very well if the grandparent is willing to follow your routine and respect your views on eating and sleeping. However, anyone who cares for your baby must be fit and agile, and aware of health and safety issues. If a grandparent is looking after your baby in his or her own home, make sure it is safe.

Day nursery (commercial day care). Nurseries (day care centres) are often favoured by working parents because they offer reliable and professional care. However, babies cannot go if they are ill, and hours are usually restricted. Some employers offer a workplace crèche, which means that your baby is near you while you are at work. Children are usually looked after in groups, and babies are separated from toddlers and young children.

The main disadvantage of this kind of care is that your baby is likely to be looked after by a series of different people in a day, though many nurseries assign each child to a key worker to provide a sense of continuity. Choose a registered nursery, and ask about staff turnover: if staff tend to come and go, your baby won't get a chance to develop a relationship with the carers.

Arranging your childcare

Start looking for childcare a few months before you need it. This gives you time to evaluate the options properly; you don't want to have to make a decision about where to leave your baby when you are under pressure and in a hurry. Looking for good childcare can feel daunting, and it will help if you work out exactly what you need beforehand. For example, if you work long and unsociable hours, say, then you will need a nanny or childminder who will do the same. If your child is disabled or has special needs, you will need a nursery or carer who is able and willing to care for him or her sensitively.

Spread your search wide. Ask as many people as possible whether they can recommend someone. In particular, the following can be useful.

Your local authority. They should have a list of registered childminders and nurseries in your area.

Other parents. Those with older children may have a trusted childminder they are no longer using.

Nursery workers. If you are looking for home-based care, it is worth asking the staff at your local nursery. Trained staff may be available to look after your baby part-time, or they may know of an experienced childcarer who is looking for a new charge.

Young babies generally do better with a single carer than in a nursery. But if a nursery is well staffed and the carers are warm and loving, it can be a good option.

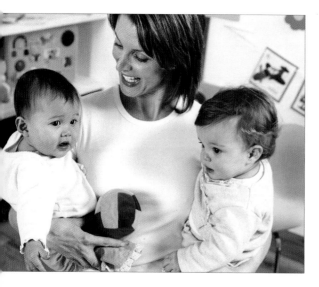

CHECKLIST: CHOOSING A NURSERY

A good nursery should be spacious, clean and light, with some safe outdoor space. It is important that there is be a good ratio of staff to children: for the under-twos this means no more than three children to every member of staff.

- Ask for a tour of the nursery during a normal day. Observe whether the children look happy and well cared for.
- Look at the areas for eating and sleeping – will your child be comfortable?
- Check that your baby will be cared for in a separate area, away from older children.
- Find out if your child will remain on the premises all the time. If not, ask where else they will go and how such outings are organized.
- Chat to as many members of staff as possible: do they seem loving, kind, friendly and interested in the children?
- Take your baby with you and observe how staff interact with him or her.
- Go back at least once; take your partner or another close person with you for a second opinion.

Health professionals. Your healthcare providers are in contact with parents and babies every day, so they may be able to recommend a good childminder or nursery.

Parents' groups. The co-ordinator of your local playgroup or breastfeeding group may have some useful contacts.

Childcare training college. Ask the principal if there is anyone he or she can recommend.

CHOOSING A CHILDMINDER OR NANNY

It is important to meet any potential carer at least twice. Take your child with you: the way the carer interacts with the baby is a good indication of whether she is suitable for the task of looking after him or her.

Ask the carer why she looks after children as a job, and what she enjoys about it. Discuss the practicalities of the daily routine: when and what your child will eat, when and where he or she will sleep, and what he or she will do during the day, including any trips he or she may be taken on. You will have more say about this if you are using a nanny, but a good childminder should be able to facilitate your wishes to a large extent. Don't forget to ask to see any relevant certificates: childminder's registration, first-

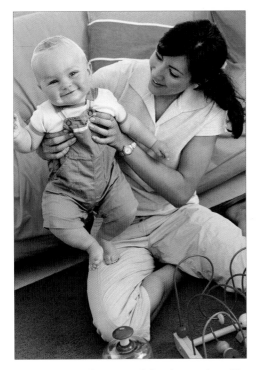

Say a proper goodbye to your baby when you leave him or her with a carer; don't just sneak off and disappear when the baby isn't looking.

aid certificate and so on. Check that the carer knows how to fit a car seat properly if your child will be driven around.

Always see a childminder in her own home. Check that all the relevant rooms are clean, tidy and safe, and that your baby will be comfortable there. Check the ages of any other children who will be present, and time at least one of your visits so that you can meet them.

It is vital that you feel good about the person who is going to care for your baby. Ask yourself if you feel that this carer will look after your baby in the way that you want. Are you happy and relaxed about leaving your child in this person's care? If the answer is yes, follow up the carer's references and ask your partner or another close person to meet her for a second opinion. If the answer is no, even if you can't pinpoint the reason, keep looking.

SETTLING IN

Agree a trial period of two to four weeks for any childcare arrangement, so that you can call a halt without penalty if it doesn't work out.

Arrange for your baby to spend some time with a new carer while you are present before leaving them alone together. A nanny can spend a day with you and your

baby, following your usual routine. If you are hiring a childminder, start by spending half an hour at her home with your baby. The next time, leave your baby with the childminder for half an hour or so while you wait outside or walk around the block. Then try leaving your baby for a couple of hours. If all goes well, try a half session and then a full one. Nurseries usually operate a similar settling-in scheme.

Always say goodbye to your baby when you leave. Be cheery and use the same form of words each time, such as 'See you later'. Your baby may not want you to go, but most children quickly adjust once you are out of sight. Ring to check: if your baby continues to cry after you have gone, this arrangement may not be the right one.

IS IT WORKING?

Your baby is the best barometer of whether childcare arrangements are working. Does he or she seem happy and alert when you return, or fretful or withdrawn? Does your baby seem well cared for? For example, is he or she clean, with a recently changed nappy?

Think about the carer's demeanour and attitude. Is she cheerful and relaxed? Is she happy to tell you about your baby's day? Or does she seem irritable and glad to hand your baby back? Does the carer seem to like and understand your baby?

There are bound to be times when your baby is fractious after a day away from you, but if he or she consistently seems unhappy or the carer is unhelpful, you may need to start looking for a new arrangement. If you are unsure, try arriving early one day just to see what is happening when you are not expected.

Your relationship with your baby's carer should be respectful and warm. It is important that you are both punctual and that you keep each other informed of any developments in your baby's life.

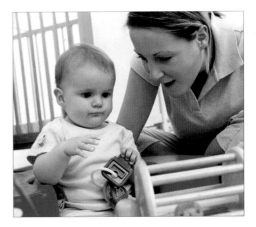

Crying, comfort and sleeping

  ❝ Of course, some broken nights are inevitable. They are an inalienable facet of parenthood, well into the toddler years. **❞**

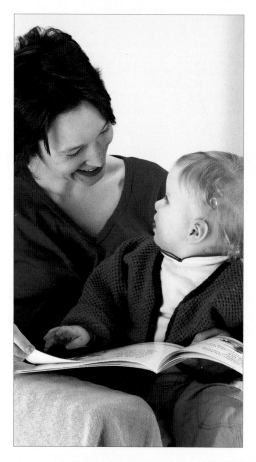

As your baby grows older, you will probably find that he or she cries less frequently. Some of the things that used to be upsetting might now be amusing instead. And while the discomfort of, say, a wet nappy will still trouble a baby, crying will often cease as soon as he or she knows you are attending to the problem. Sometimes your child will just whimper to let you know that something is wrong. In short, your baby has understood that crying is a form of communication, but you still need to respond quickly and compassionately. This can get harder from about eight months, when your baby's intense attachment to you means that he or she may wail in despair if you leave the room. This fear of abandonment, known as separation anxiety, can be very trying for you. When your baby demands to be with you every second, even a simple household task such as boiling the kettle becomes difficult. But the more gently and lovingly you respond to your baby's feelings, the better: he or she needs reassurance to get through this tricky stage.

The bond between parent and child grows stronger in the second six months – and your baby may not want to let you out of his or her sight for a while.

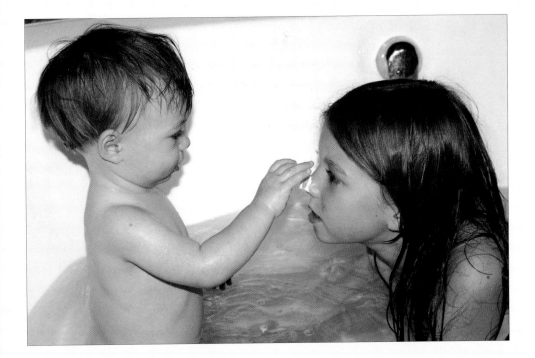

Dealing with nighttime crying is a tougher problem to solve, because you need your baby to spend the nights without your presence. Even babies who have been sleeping well begin to object to going to bed at this age, and no baby likes to wake up in the small hours and find that he or she is alone in the room.

Most babies need guidance to help them sleep well by themselves. This chapter suggests some ways to help your baby to wind down at the end of the day, and how to set clear and consistent rules about bedtime. These techniques will improve a wakeful baby's nights, but to make them work you need to make a clear decision about how you want your baby to sleep, and you must plan to achieve it. Of course, some broken nights are inevitable. They are an inalienable facet of parenthood, well into the toddler years.

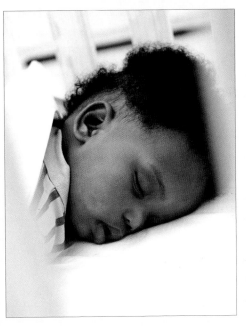

Top: Adopt a bedtime routine that stays the same each evening and gives time for your baby to settle down and relax. This will help him or her to fall happily asleep.

With a little forethought and determination, you and your baby can look forward to a refreshing night's sleep more often than not.

Why your baby cries

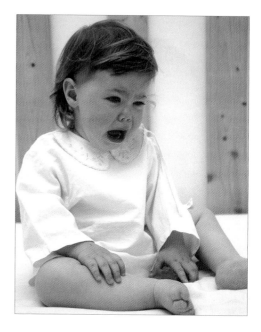

Older babies cry for many of the same reasons as younger ones: hunger, fear, teething and so on. Older babies cry when they are tired, but don't realize what they need is to go to sleep: unlike young babies they can, and do, keep themselves awake. Good daytime and nighttime sleep routines will help to avoid this problem.

There are also a few new causes for tears, arising from babies' increasing activity and growing perceptions of their world. As your baby learns to crawl, pull up to standing and cruise around the furniture, there are bound to be a few bumps. Crying is more likely to be caused by the shock than any pain, but he or she needs your reassuring hug fast. Older babies also need more stimulation and may cry from boredom: gone are the days when you could walk around shops with the pram for hours at a time. Your baby may quickly get fed up with being confined, and probably has a new moan or whining cry to signal displeasure.

Older babies may scream with fury when things don't happen the way they want. They hate it when they cannot quite make a toy work or find that they are propelling themselves backwards when they are trying to crawl forwards. This sense of frustration isn't necessarily a bad

Babies have intense emotions, but unhappiness doesn't last long if they are given comfort or distraction. Older babies are quite capable of crying simply from boredom and lack of stimulation.

Don't leave a baby crying in their cot unless you are following a controlled crying routine. If a baby is crying they are calling for your care and attention, they are not being 'naughty'.

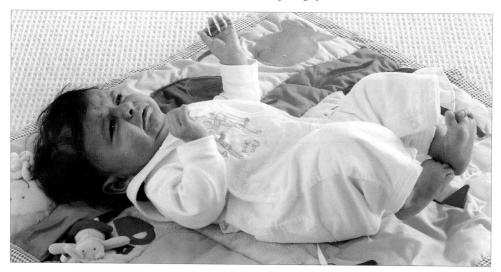

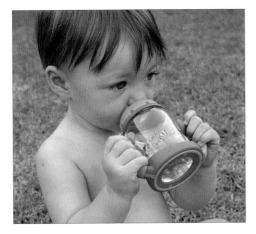

Try not to get into the habit of offering your baby something to eat to stop him or her crying – a few sips of water or an interesting toy will do just as well, and will avoid creating a link between comfort and eating.

thing. It eggs babies on to new achievements, and the screams that accompany their attempts are sometimes a way of expressing the effort they are putting in, but you will obviously want to reduce and minimize any distress.

Help your baby out by showing how to make that troublesome toy work or by removing an obstacle in his or her path. But don't take over – encourage the baby to have another go if the task is within his or her capability. Distraction is the subtlest tool that a parent can deploy. If your baby is getting very frustrated, divert his or her attention by doing something unusual, like making a funny face or a new noise. Remain calm yourself. Cries of frustration are a normal and inevitable part of your baby's development, and patience and reassurance are sometimes all a parent can offer.

THE START OF DISCIPLINE

Lots of people talk about babies being manipulative when they cry. It is true that once a baby learns that you will come running when you hear crying, he or she may do it simply to get your company. But this doesn't make the baby 'naughty' or 'cunning' – it simply means that he or she wants you to be there. The fact that the crying stops as soon as you arrive shows how delighted your child is to see you.

The next few months, though, are the time to lay the foundations of discipline. As the baby learns to assert himself or herself, you are bound to find that your wishes conflict. For example, your child may scream and resist whenever you try to put him or her in a car seat, or howl in protest when you take that sharp pencil away. Try not to forbid your baby to do things if there is no need. Going

CAUTION
Remember that unexplained crying can be a sign of illness; do see your doctor if you feel worried or if your baby has any unusual symptoms.

into the car seat is obviously non-negotiable, but perhaps it doesn't matter if the baby pulls all the food containers out of the cupboard: this is only exploring after all, and your baby doesn't know that they are not toys. So choose your battles wisely: it will make life easier for you both.

Be firm. If you have decided that your baby cannot do something – such as playing with your mobile phone – don't suddenly give in.

Be consistent. Don't stop your baby pulling books off a shelf one day and then ignore this same behaviour the very next day.

Be inventive. If your baby is resisting going into the highchair, say, put an exciting object on the tray to encourage him or her to go willingly.

Think prevention. You can avoid a lot of tears by ensuring your baby's environment is safe to explore.

Reinforce words with action. Don't expect your baby to stop doing something because you call 'No' from the other side of the room without moving towards them; it is good to say 'No' in a firm way but you should also go and gently take the troublesome object away to reinforce the message. Add some easily understood words of explanation as well – for example, 'Hot!' as you move the baby away from the oven.

If a child is crying from anger or frustration try to keep calm yourself, and keep giving love and cuddles.

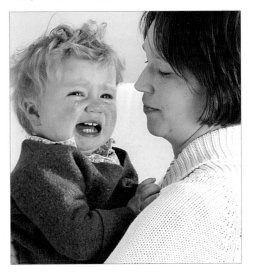

Fear and anxiety

There is a whole category of things that can make your baby cry that are nothing to do with the physical world but are psychological in nature. By now your baby has built up an expectation of how things happen in his or her world. If something out of the ordinary happens – even if it is not a bad thing in itself – the baby may cry because it is unsettling. For example, if you take your child to a swimming pool for the first time, he or she may cry even before you go into the water, because the smell, look and sound of the pool environment are very unfamiliar. Similarly, if a babysitter appears when the baby wakes in the night, instead of you or your partner, he or she may become very distressed – even if the babysitter is somebody your baby loves.

The best way to help your baby through these difficulties is to try to let him or her know whenever something new is about to happen. The babysitter could call to your baby while approaching the room, so that the baby knows someone different is coming in before he or

Fathers need not be upset if their baby cries when handed over. Babies naturally feel closest to their mother at first: the uniquely wonderful and complex bond with the father takes longer to develop.

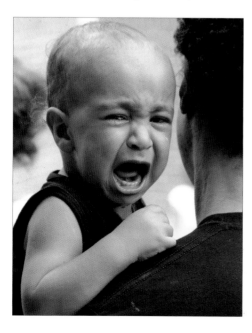

she is picked up and comforted. And, of course, your baby will be much easier to soothe if left in the care of someone he or she knows well. At the swimming pool, cuddle the baby for a while and point out other children playing in the water before you even attempt to get in there too. Babies are very adaptable and usually enjoy new experiences, so long as they are introduced gradually and from a home base of safety.

FEARS

Older babies may develop very specific fears of everyday things. A classic one is the vacuum cleaner. Even if you used the sound of a vacuum cleaner to lull your newborn to sleep, you may find that an older baby develops a real fear of it. This may be so great that the baby whimpers on catching a glimpse and cries at a similar sound – such as the blender, say, or a hedge trimmer being used outside.

Although your baby's fears may seem irrational, don't dismiss them as 'silly' or try to force him or her to confront them – you will only increase the fear. Babies need to feel safe in the world and to know that they can trust their carers to look after them. So if your baby is scared of the vacuum cleaner, keep it out of sight and use it only when he or she is sleeping or in another room. If the baby seems to be scared of the dark, get a nightlight or leave the hall light on and the bedroom door open.

As your baby is reassured about being protected from frightening things, his or her confidence will grow. Eventually the baby may start to get curious about the very thing that was scary – he or she may want to look at that vacuum cleaner and even touch it. Don't rush this – let the baby conquer such fears one step at a time, when he or she is ready.

SEPARATION ANXIETY

Young babies think of themselves and their main carers as one: they have no sense of themselves as individuals and are completely unaware that those tiny fists waving in the air belong to them. As they learn to control their movements and make things happen, they gradually become aware that they are independent beings. One clue is the realization that they can make the carer come by crying out, which happens at about four months.

By about seven months, they have worked out that they and their carers are separate entities. This marks a huge leap in understanding, but it also makes babies anxious: for if they are separate, that means they can be left alone. Separation anxiety, as it is known, manifests as

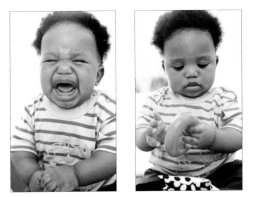

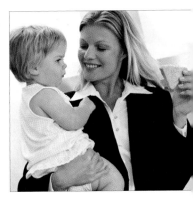

Left: It is amazing how the most heartbreaking tears can be soothed and then forgotten by a live-in-the-moment toddler.

Right: If you are leaving your child, be sure to say a proper goodbye that isn't rushed or stressful. Sneaking off may avoid some tears at the time but it will make him or her feel insecure.

a tendency to cling. It usually starts between eight and twelve months; but it can be later and some babies are not affected at all.

Your baby may start to cry if you try to give him or her to other people, especially if they are not very familiar. The baby may also protest or burst into tears if you leave the room for a moment, even when being cuddled by the grandfather he or she loves. At this stage, your baby cannot understand that you will return – all he or she feels is abandonment.

All the effort you put into your baby's feelings of security and confidence in the early years helps them, as they get older, to spend more time without you.

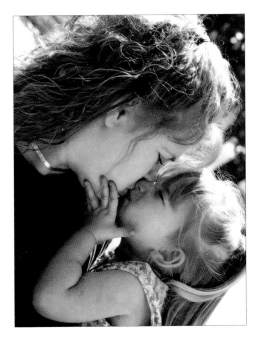

HANDLING SEPARATION ANXIETY

Your baby needs to be secure in his or her attachment to you. Only through love and reassurance do babies gain the confidence to explore the world.

Keep your baby with you as much as possible. It is often easier to take the baby with you into the bathroom, say, than to cause unnecessary distress. If your baby becomes nervous of strangers, which is very common during the second half-year, don't pass him or her over for a cuddle. Ignore anyone who says he or she is spoiled or clingy; your child will go to other people when he or she is good and ready. If possible, however, get your baby used to being with at least one other trusted person beside you and your partner. This means that there is someone else to care for him or her in an emergency, or if you really need a break.

When you are leaving, always say goodbye – sneaking off when your baby's attention is distracted for a moment will undermine his or her trust in you. But keep goodbyes short, cheery and calm – if you show that you are upset or anxious, you will be reaffirming and increasing the baby's sense of unease. It's a good idea to use the same form of words (perhaps with an accompanying gesture) each time. For example, say 'One minute' (and hold up one finger) if you are just popping into another room to get something; say 'See you later' (and blow a kiss) if you will be away for longer. And if you have said you will be 'one minute', don't be gone for ages – always stick to your promises. Your baby doesn't understand the concept of time yet, but will come to realize that 'one minute' means a short separation.

Give your full attention to your baby when you get back. Have a loving cuddle straight away if the baby wants one; if he or she is happily absorbed in doing something, watch and perhaps join in until your baby is ready to come to you. Be cheerful but calm so that the baby learns your return is quite normal and not something to make a big fuss about. Gradually your baby will learn that you always come back.

Changing sleep patterns

By now your baby will almost certainly be sleeping a lot more at night than in the day. Babies over six months commonly sleep for ten to twelve hours at night, as well as having daytime naps. But your nights are still unlikely to be the long unbroken stretch you may be craving. Even though your baby may be sleeping for as much as six to eight hours at a time, the longest sleep will probably coincide with your evening and the early part of your night. Most babies wake up at least once a night until they are twelve months old.

It is still important to put older babies on their back to sleep. If you find that your baby rolls over, gently move him or her back again. However, if this happens repeatedly or if the baby wakes up when turned, it is probably better to leave him or her be.

DAYTIME NAPS

Most babies need at least two naps a day – one in the morning and one in the early afternoon – until the end of the first year. Ideally, the afternoon nap should be the long one, as it will help keep your baby going until bedtime.

Some babies drop a nap even before they get to twelve months. You might find that they just enjoy a quiet period at that time for a couple of weeks.

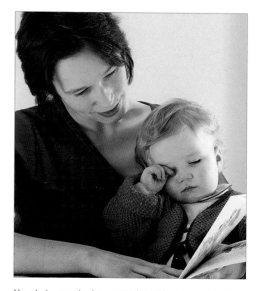

Your baby may be happy to play with some toys in the cot even if he or she doesn't want a nap. If not, schedule in some quiet time – look at a book or do a simple jigsaw – as a break in an action-packed day.

Now that your baby is more aware of what is going on, he or she may resist going to sleep during the day, because who wants to nap when there is all that exploring to do? But rest is important, otherwise the baby will become irritable during the day and, paradoxically, will find it harder to sleep at night.

Do what you can to facilitate naps, whether this means putting the baby down in a darkened room or rocking him or her to sleep in a buggy. If possible, put your baby down soon after lunch, even if there is no sign of tiredness. Without a sleep in the early afternoon, he or she is likely to be exhausted by late afternoon, the worst time for a nap because bedtime is not far away.

Don't worry too much about how long your baby sleeps. Although the average baby naps for about three hours a day, yours may need a lot less sleep than this. Be guided by your baby's humour and habits – if he or she is in a good mood during the day and sleeps well at night, then it doesn't matter if the naps are very short.

Some babies drop a nap before they reach twelve months. Usually the morning nap is the first to go, but some drop their afternoon nap, which means they have a

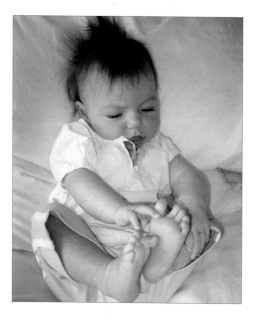

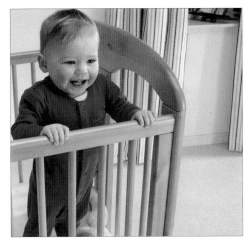

Moving your baby to his or her own room may improve the nights for all of you. The baby may be more inclined to settle him or herself after waking at night.

long time awake before bedtime. One solution might be to give your baby an early lunch – 11 am, say – and to put him or her down for a nap after that.

BABY'S OWN ROOM

Six months is a good age for a baby to move out of your bedroom and into his or her own space. Your baby is now more likely to wake up when you go to bed or if you turn over in the night. But if you don't have a lot of space, are still breastfeeding or feel that your baby benefits from sleeping near you, you may prefer to go on sharing a room for longer.

Avoid changing your baby's sleeping arrangements when in the throes of separation anxiety, during teething

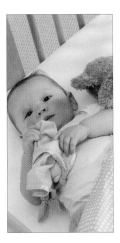

Left: If your baby whimpers in the night, don't pick him or her up too quickly: make sure that the baby really is awake. Try to settle the baby without picking him or her up if you can.

Right: A quiet cuddle before bedtime will help to get your baby into a relaxed state conducive to sleep. Make this the final thing you do, after toothbrushing or a nappy change.

or illness, or if the baby is experiencing change of another kind – for example, a new carer – and make sure that the baby is happy in the new room before you move the cot there. Buy or borrow a few new toys and place some favourite books there to make it fun. Spend as much time as possible in the room during the day for at least a week before moving the baby in. If your baby is easy to settle, you can use the new bedroom for daytime naps – in the buggy or a travel cot if you have one.

Move the cot in the morning. Put a couple of interesting activity toys in it plus one or two old favourites, including your baby's comforter if he or she has one. Give the baby two or three play sessions in the cot during the day. Stay nearby for these; if possible, busy yourself in the room so that the baby plays independently. Take the baby out as soon as he or she starts to get fed up. Follow your usual bedtime routine, and then put your baby to bed at the usual time in the cot. If he or she wakes up, make sure you get there quickly to help him or her settle back to sleep. You could consider putting a spare bed or mattress in the baby's room, so that you can sleep there if the baby becomes distressed rather than taking him or her back to your room.

Don't forget to give your baby plenty of attention and cuddles during the day to help him or her feel secure. Avoid any unusual absences or making any other changes to your baby's routine for a few weeks.

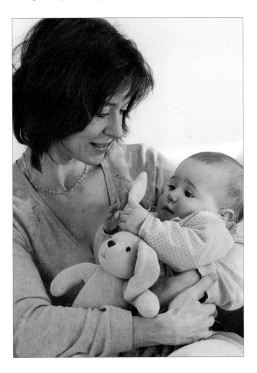

Improving sleep in an older baby

How you deal with broken nights depends very much on whether you think a baby should learn to fit in with your routine or feel that it is your job as a parent to tend to the baby's needs, even when it causes you a lot of inconvenience. Both attitudes have their supporters, but whatever you do, some sleepless nights are inevitable. Here are some simple ways to minimize them.

The baby may be getting hungry. Try to ensure that he or she gets enough food during the day by prioritizing mealtimes and by giving a full breastfeed or a bottle at bedtime. If the baby falls asleep during this feed, give it a little earlier – before a bath or story.

Check that your baby's bedroom is conducive to sleep. Some babies are more sensitive than others and need a carefully controlled environment in order to get through the night. Is it dark and warm enough? If your baby pulls the covers off and then wakes up because it is cold,

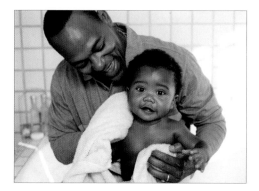

A warm bath is the ideal way for many babies to wind down before bedtime. You can encourage sleepiness by adding a couple of drops of lavender or chamomile essential oils, well diluted in a carrier oil or in milk.

LIGHT MORNINGS

Early-morning waking is very common, especially in summer, and it is hard to handle. Generally speaking it doesn't work to start putting your baby to bed later – he or she will almost certainly wake up at the same time. The most helpful thing that you can do is to ensure your baby's room is really dark – put up blackout blinds or curtain lining to eliminate the first chinks of light. It is also a good idea to treat all feeds before, say, 6 am as quiet night feeds. You can also try putting a couple of toys in the baby's cot so that he or she discovers them on awakening. You may find that he or she will then play happily in the cot for 20 minutes or so while you enjoy a few precious minutes' extra sleep.

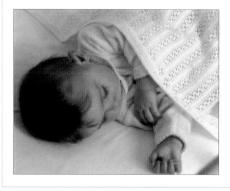

consider using a baby sleeping bag instead of blankets. Your baby may need quiet to sleep, but some find it easier to drop off if there is some noise – try leaving the door open so that the baby can hear the household sounds, or leave a ticking clock, a soothing musical mobile or a radio turned down low. A nightlight can also help some babies to sleep better.

Have a consistent bedtime routine that allows your baby to wind down properly – say, a warm bath, a story or song on your lap and then a feed. If you can, get your baby into bed while sleepy but still awake, to learn to drop off on his or her own (this is hard if you are breastfeeding and have a baby who falls asleep at the breast). Introduce a comforter if your baby doesn't already use one. This can be particularly useful if you are trying to move your baby into a cot from your family bed. And if you are breastfeeding and want to stop night feeds, get your partner or a supportive helper to attend to the baby during the night for a while.

ADOPTING A COMFORTER

You can encourage your baby to adopt a comforter if you think it will make settling at night easier. Over time your baby will associate it with love and sleep, but remember that once this association is made, the comforter will be extremely important to your child – you won't be able to go away for a night without it.

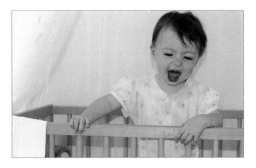

Children do tend to wake up earlier than their parents, and protest vigorously if they don't get a response.

Make sure that you are allowing your baby the opportunity to settle him or herself. It's easy to get into the habit of picking up your baby as soon as he or she makes a sound, especially if the baby is sharing your room. But babies often whimper, cry out or cough in their sleep without actually waking up properly. Wait for a few moments and listen – your baby may continue sleeping if you do not disturb him or her unnecessarily.

CHECKLIST: WHY IS MY BABY WAKING UP?
Here are some of the reasons why an unbroken night's sleep might be eluding you and your baby.
Hunger. If your baby wakes up and won't settle, he or she may need a feed. Keep the room dark as you feed and put the baby back to bed straight away.
Comfort feeding. Lots of breastfed babies wake up several times a night to nurse. Sometimes this is hunger but it can also be because they enjoy having their relaxed mother to themselves.
Anxiety. Babies may become more restless if they are unsettled by a major change – starting at nursery, for example. If your baby is experiencing separation anxiety, he or she may start to resist going to bed.
Developmental leaps. Your baby may be more wakeful at night when acquiring a new skill.
External disturbances. An older baby may be disturbed by noises or by your movements. This doesn't mean your home has to be kept silent – normal household noises can be comforting.
Physical needs. Teething pain – and any accompanying fever – can make for very disturbed nights. Your baby may also wake if too hot or cold, with a soiled or very full nappy, or if he or she is ill. If you think your baby's wakefulness may be due to illness, see your doctor.
Habit. Babies who are used to being nursed to sleep, for example, may find it hard to drop off on their own when they wake up at night.

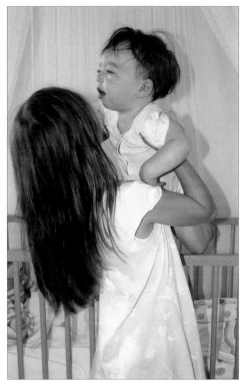

A responsible older sibling may be willing to amuse the baby for a short period so that you can get more sleep.

If your baby doesn't seem to like being in the cot, let him or her have a few play sessions there during the day while you potter about in the room. However, take most of the toys out of the cot at bedtime: one stuffed animal or a comforter is enough.

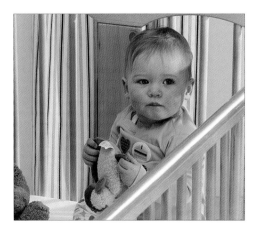

Sleep training

All babies wake up from time to time throughout the night. But if your baby is used to being fed or stroked to sleep at bedtime, he or she will need the same help to drop off during the night. The point of sleep training is to teach a baby to get back to sleep on his or her own.

If your baby is continuing to wake up several times a night, you may decide that now is the time to take action. Unless there is a medical reason for the crying – and it is important to check this with your doctor before embarking on sleep training – you should be able to teach your baby to sleep better using one of the methods described below. Set aside at least a week to do it, and don't choose a time when any major change is going on in your child's life, when your partner will be away or you will be going out in the evening.

Don't forget that your baby's sleep, or lack of it, is only really a problem if it is affecting his or her mood and ability to function, or making daily life difficult for you. If you are both happy, it doesn't matter if your child continues to wake up at night – some mothers are happy to give night feeds for the first year and beyond.

If you can, continue with the method throughout the night. But it is also fine to do the sleep plan until a certain time – 1 am, say – and then to revert to your usual methods if you find that easier. Stick with your sleep plan for at least a week if you can, to instil the idea that once your baby goes into the cot, he or she stays there. It is important that you and your partner agree your approach to sleep training if you are both going to be involved.

Sleep training aims to teach a baby to get to sleep without your help, so that he or she doesn't need to disturb you during the night unless something is wrong.

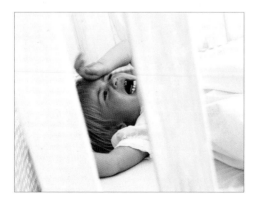

Make a decision about what you want, and work out what steps you are going to take to get there. Be clear about who is going to do what – it is difficult to make sensible decisions when you are faced with a crying child at 3am.

CONTROLLED CRYING

This is the sleep-training method recommended by many health professionals. It doesn't involve leaving your baby to scream unattended for a long time; instead you keep checking so that your baby knows you are there. This can make the baby furious – if you are coming in, why aren't you picking him or her up? – and the process can take longer than if you simply leave the child to scream it out. But it won't leave your baby feeling abandoned and it will mean you can check that nothing else is wrong – such as wind, or a lost dummy (pacifier) or comforter.

Controlled crying is stressful for everyone concerned, so try gentler methods first. If you do decide to do it, be certain that it is the right choice for both parent(s) and child. Be clear with your partner about who is going to do what before you begin. Stick to the method for at least four days – crying often peaks on the third. Remember that you can adapt the method to suit yourself. For example, you may decide that ten minutes is your limit for crying or that you will stroke your baby when you go in.

1 Follow a bedtime routine and put the baby to bed when sleepy and relaxed. Kiss goodnight and leave the room.
2 If the baby cries, wait one minute then return. You can shush, but don't linger or pick up. Gradually increase the time that you leave the baby to cry – to two minutes, then three, then five, then eight, ten and finally 15. Don't leave the baby crying any longer than 15 minutes at a time.
3 Be resolute – if you give in, your baby will hold out for longer the next time you try the method. Continue checking every 15 minutes until your baby falls asleep.
4 If your baby wakes up later in the night, go through the same process of checking and leaving for increasing periods of time, up to 15 minutes. Never just leave your baby crying without checking.

> **CAUTION**
> Any form of sleep training is stressful. Be clear about what you want to achieve and stay calm. It works best if one person tackles each night, but it is a good idea to have your partner or a supportive helper on hand to take over if you become overwhelmed.

Settling a reluctant baby

Some babies do not want to go to bed on their own because it means being away from you. They may be in the habit of falling asleep while breastfeeding, or coming into bed with you to get to sleep. Unless you want to sleep with your baby and go to bed very early every night, this is something you do need to tackle. Here is a gentle way to settle a reluctant baby. It involves gradually reducing the amount of soothing you do. Once you are down to the bare minimum, you should find that your baby finds it easier to drop off on his or her own.

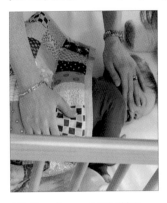 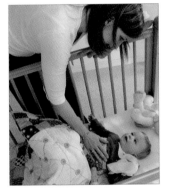 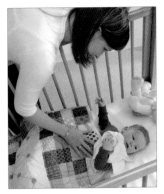

1 Go through your usual bedtime routine. Cuddle or feed until your baby is sleepy, and then put him or her in the cot. Stay in contact – leave one hand underneath the baby's back and stroke his or her head or tummy with the other. Soothe the baby verbally at the same time – try shushing, repeating a key phrase such as 'Sleepy time', or singing the same song.

2 If your baby gets very distressed, you may want to pick him or her up. Once comforted, put the baby back in the cot straight away – you may have to do this many times before he or she becomes calmer. If your baby is standing up, lie him or her down. Often a baby will scramble up again immediately. Just keep lying them down again until he or she gets the message and gives in.

3 Once your baby is lying down, keep reassuring them. Combine physical comfort with verbal soothing, reducing the volume as your baby calms down. Stay calm yourself – do some deep breathing if you need to. You should find that the baby's protests gradually become less vocal and insistent, but it can take a lot of patient perseverance before this happens.

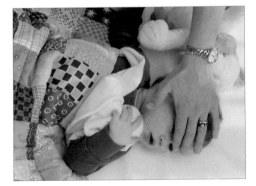 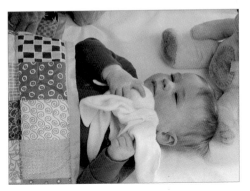

4 Once the baby is calm and sleepy, try stroking your hand from the forehead downwards. As your hand passes over the baby's eyes, they automatically shut and this can help lull him or her into sleep. Continue the verbal soothing, becoming quieter and quieter as the baby drifts off. Slowly remove your hand as you continue to shush or sing. Stand by the cot for a few minutes before retreating.

5 After a few days, your baby should be quietened more easily. Once he or she starts to go into the cot calmly, try simply sitting beside the cot and comforting him or her from a distance – but still go and offer physical comfort if he or she cries. Eventually, when you judge the time is right, you may be able to leave the room and let the baby drift off alone.

Development and play

❝ This new ability to get around will make your baby more physically independent, but emotionally his or her attachment to you will grow. **❞**

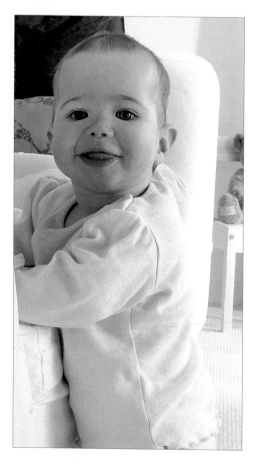

The second half-year of your baby's life is a most eventful time. In the space of a few short months he or she will learn to sit up, and then to get about – by crawling, bottom-shuffling or simply wriggling across the floor. No longer does your baby have to wait to be moved or given interesting things to examine – now he or she can just go and get them.

At some point during these months, your baby will discover how to pull up to a standing position, and will figure out how to edge around a room by holding on to the furniture. This new ability to get around will make your baby more physically independent, but emotionally his or her attachment to you will grow, and a strong bond will also develop with other important people in the baby's life.

Excitingly, your baby will also have some new ways to interact with you. Older babies understand the word 'no', although they may not always obey it, and they know their own names and turn round when you call them. By the end of the first year, many

Cruising gives your baby a degree of independence, which he or she will exercise to the full. Standing and moving about will become a favourite activity.

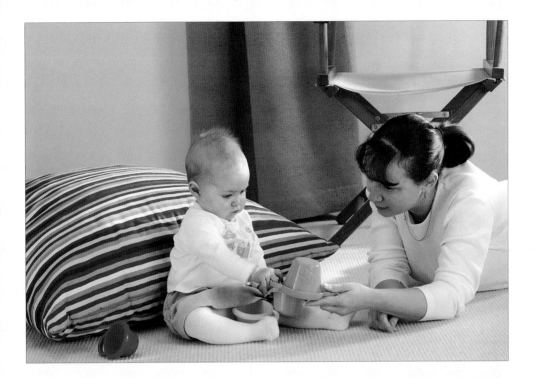

babies can use a few hand signals to communicate: they may wave goodbye, point at something they want and clap hands. Most babies love showing off these new skills, especially when they meet with approval and delight in those around them.

All these new developments mean that outings become more fun. Your increasingly curious and sociable baby will really enjoy music classes now he or she can see what is going on, and will love to shake a percussion instrument or clap with the music. Baby gyms provide your baby with the opportunity for a bit of rough and tumble.

At a developmental review (well-child visit), during this time you will be asked about your baby's eating and sleeping and new achievements. This is a good opportunity to raise any concerns you may have.

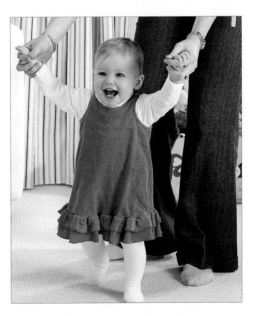

Top: The time when your baby sits up but cannot yet move about is probably the easiest stage of parenthood. He or she will be contented to sit and explore toys.

Babies who are beginning to stand will love being walked round. Some babies start walking independently, though most won't do this until well after one year.

Sitting and crawling

Babies love to sit, but it usually takes six months before they can stay upright by themselves. Before then, you can help your baby practise by sitting him or her in a circle of cushions or rolled-up blankets; the baby will rock from side to side as he or she tries to balance.

Sitting is great fun for babies because it gives a much more comprehensive view of what is going on. It also allows them to stretch further to grab interesting objects, and of course their hands are now free for exploring any item within reach. Expect your sitting baby to topple over a lot. Even after mastering the skill, it takes time to learn exactly how far he or she can reach out without tipping over. Until then, continue to use cushions or rolled-up blankets to give a soft landing. Stay close by: if your baby falls head-down into a pile of cushions in an awkward position, he or she could get stuck.

Most babies are at least nine months old before they can move from a lying-down position to sitting up, without help. Before this they will use any means available to haul themselves up, whether this is your hands, a tablecloth or the sides of a buggy. Be vigilant about strapping your baby into the buggy and highchair, so that he or she can't fall out. If you are still sitting your baby on a sofa or bed, it is definitely time to stop: he or she could easily tip on to the floor.

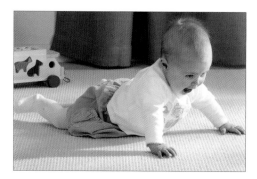

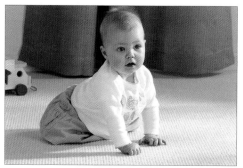

Babies who are just learning to sit haven't yet worked out how far they can lean forwards without falling over. They need a helping hand to explore safely.

Because motor control develops from the head down, babies' arms are much stronger than their legs at first. So they may use their arms to pull themselves along, commando-style, before they start to crawl properly.

CRAWLING

Not all babies crawl. Some get about by shuffling on their bottoms, using one hand to push themselves forward. Others travel on their hands and feet with their bottoms

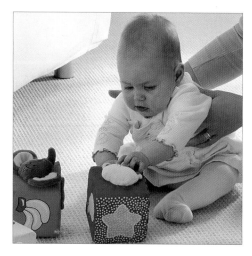

CHECKLIST: SAFETY FOR MOBILE BABIES
- Dress your baby in clothes that cover the knees to protect them from hard surfaces or carpet.
- Check wooden floors for splinters, gaps and any protruding nails.
- Put up stair gates.
- Check your child proofing.
- Remember that babies can learn a new skill quite suddenly. If your baby is getting ready to crawl, take precautions straight away.

MOBILITY

Babies vary so much in when and how they start to get mobile that crawling isn't included as one of the developmental milestones. It doesn't matter if your baby doesn't crawl, just so long as he or she finds some way of moving around. But if your baby isn't mobile by the age of one, or doesn't seem to use all his or her arms and legs when moving, you should consult a health professional. Remember that premature babies often do things later than other babies born at the same time.

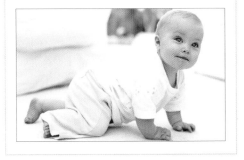

Once your baby becomes mobile, you will need to make sure that your home is safe and be on the lookout for hazards when you are out. Keep one step ahead of your baby's development, since he or she may progress quite suddenly.

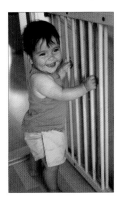

anything on the floor, so check for dropped coins and stray objects under sofas and so on. Put up stair gates, but once your baby is confidently mobile, let him or her practise crawling up stairs while you follow. You can also let your baby come down the stairs feet-first on his or her tummy, so long as you are there in case of a fall. Consider investing in a playpen or travel cot so that you can keep your baby safe if you need to cook, say, when he or she is awake. But don't use it for long periods.

high in the air – the 'bear-walk'. And some cut out this middle stage altogether, going straight from sitting to cruising and walking. Babies who do crawl usually start between eight and ten months, but they start to practise well before this. Often they start by pushing themselves up on their hands and knees when they are lying on their stomachs. It can take them many weeks to figure out how to move forwards from this position: they tend to rock backwards and forwards without going anywhere.

When they do start to move, it is often backwards. This is because their arms are stronger than their legs, but they soon learn how to push with their knees to move forwards. And once they work out how to use opposite arms and legs together, they can go much faster.

You can't help a baby to crawl, but you can provide the opportunities to practise and a safe space to play in, and put the baby down on his or her front often. Placing an interesting toy just out of reach can encourage a baby to try to move forwards. Once crawling starts, it is fun to make a mini obstacle course using cushions, which your baby then has to go around or climb over in order to get to you or to a favourite toy. This can help build confidence and improve balance and coordination, but do help out if your baby gets stuck or frustrated.

CHILDPROOFING YOUR HOME

It is a good idea to crawl around your living spaces to look for hazards such as trailing cords, sharp corners and uncovered plug sockets. A mobile baby will investigate

You can buy childproofing safety packs from DIY stores and pharmacies. They include plug guards to prevent your baby poking things in a socket, and corner protectors to cover sharp corners of coffee tables.

Loop up trailing wires of appliances and secure with an elastic band.

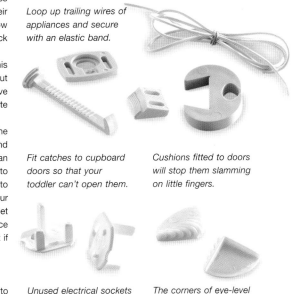

Fit catches to cupboard doors so that your toddler can't open them.

Cushions fitted to doors will stop them slamming on little fingers.

Unused electrical sockets can be made safe with these plugs.

The corners of eye-level tables can be cushioned with covers.

Standing and cruising

Babies long to stand on their own two feet in every sense. Moving independently is a great step towards other kinds of independence: they can entertain themselves, reach toys, and set off to find the people that have moved out of view. Babies seem to sense these possibilities for extending their experience: you need only look at the delight on a child's face after negotiating the route from sofa to table leg, from table leg to chair to see this. But learning to walk, like learning to sit, doesn't happen suddenly, it will develop in stages.

From the time they are a few months old, babies love to stand when being held on a lap. They quickly discover that they can bounce up and down if they bend and straighten their knees, and this will probably be one of their first games. At about seven months, they may start to alternate their feet as if they were walking. But most babies haven't yet developed the strength to take their own weight, and they feel insecure if they are 'walked' along the ground before they are ready.

Early walkers may take their first steps at eight or nine months, but most babies don't walk unassisted until they are between 12 and 15 months old. A few are older than 18 months when they start.

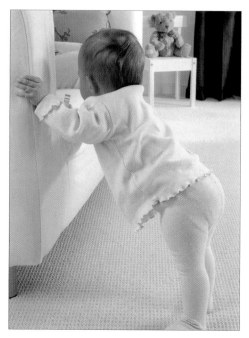

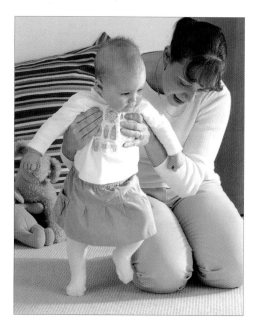

Once your baby starts to cruise, you will probably be astonished by some of the clever ways he or she finds to navigate a room. He or she will use this new skill whenever and wherever possible, so look out for unsafe items on furniture that they will be able to reach.

Most babies have developed enough strength in their legs to stand properly by the time they are about eight or nine months old. But apart from a few early developers, they can't usually maintain the necessary balance to stand independently or to walk. However, they quickly learn to pull themselves up with the help of a chair or the bars of their cots and playpens. They will also enjoy 'walking' with your help.

This is a tricky stage for both parent and baby – your baby will repeatedly pull himself or herself up and stand holding on to something at every opportunity. However, the baby hasn't yet worked out how to sit down again. So he or she will shout for you to help – and then promptly stand up again – or will fall on his or her bottom and be shocked by the impact. Be patient: it will take only a few weeks for the baby to figure out how to get back down to the safety of the floor.

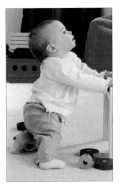
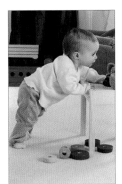

Babies start pulling themselves up from about eight months. But they won't work out how to get down for another month or two.

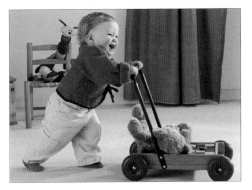

A toddle truck is the perfect toy for a cruising baby. Look for one that has a stable base and won't tip over. Wooden trucks are often sturdier than plastic ones.

CRUISING

Once your baby can pull up, he or she will soon start to 'cruise' – that is, walk while holding on to something. Cruising is likely to become your baby's favourite activity, and he or she will spend many happy minutes walking from one end of the cot to the other, or shuffling along the edge of the sofa.

As he or she gains in confidence, your baby may surprise you with ingenious ways of getting around a room: leaning with the flat of a hand on a wall, stretching up to grab the edge of a table or even pushing a chair along like a walking aid. The baby may navigate to the corner of the refrigerator, say, and then pause to consider how to get to the next piece of furniture. He or she will eventually take the odd unsupported step – like a leap into the unknown – without being aware of it. Your baby is ready to walk, but doesn't quite know it yet.

Don't get shoes until your baby is walking (and even then put them on only when he or she is outside). It is

It's best for babies to learn to walk in bare feet, since this helps with balance and coordination. So hold off putting your baby in shoes indoors.

much better for babies to learn to walk barefoot, which allows them to feel the ground and make the tiny adjustments they need to balance. If socks are necessary to keep a baby's feet warm, make sure they are the right size and the non-slip variety.

STANDING AND CRUISING SAFELY

You can't help a baby to stand or cruise; all you can do is provide a safe environment in which to practise. When ready, your baby will pull himself or herself up by any means possible: it is up to you to ensure it is a safe one.

Move flimsy pieces of furniture out of your living space or put them somewhere out of reach. Your baby can easily pull a light table over, which will not only hurt but will damage his or her confidence.

Remember that once your baby can stand up, he or she will be able to reach for things overhead. So, don't put coffee cups or anything else that can be pulled over on the edge of a table, and take any breakables off low shelves. Abolish tablecloths.

If you haven't been using a baby sleeping bag, don't start now. If your baby isn't used to one, he or she will try to stand up in it and fall over.

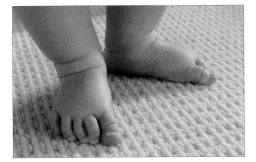

CAUTION

Never put your baby in a baby walker. These toys are dangerous: in 1991, almost 28,000 American children were admitted to hospital following accidents with baby walkers. They are not even a good development aid because they tend to reduce a baby's interest in getting around under his or her own steam. They may also even affect the proper development of the leg muscles if used a lot. Reputable baby stores no longer sell them.

Aqua baby

Swimming is a wonderful activity for you and your baby to enjoy. Water provides a whole new environment for babies to explore and in which to enjoy their bodies. In water they don't need strength or balance: they can experience what it is like to move freely. Swimming can help with muscle development and coordination, and it may also improve sleeping and eating patterns.

If you want your baby to be able to dive underwater and swim at an early age, it is worth joining a specialist swimming class. Most baby swimming classes are held in private or hydrotherapy pools, which are heated to a higher temperature than ordinary swimming baths. Swimming teachers recommend starting classes early, because young babies have no fear of water and have a natural dive reflex that enables them to hold their breath underwater. Babies are most likely to enjoy swimming if they go for the first time before the age of nine months. It's fine to take a baby who is older, but be prepared to proceed very slowly and gently since he or she is now more likely to be frightened of the water. Visit the pool when it is quiet or during a parent-and-baby session. Your baby may feel nervous if the pool is crowded and noisy.

GETTING STARTED

Remember that the point is to get your baby comfortable in the water. Hold the baby close to you at first, and gradually lower yourself into the water until the baby is immersed up to the shoulders. Don't rush this first stage.

Babies love playing games in the water, so it's a good idea to make swimming a group activity with a few parent-and-baby friends. Try making a circle with your babies, and then swooshing them out of the water and into the middle of the ring.

CHECKLIST: POOL KIT
- Swimming nappy (usually optional)
- Baby swimming pants (usually compulsory)
- A hooded towel
- A couple of pool toys (such as a ball)
- Milk and a snack for afterwards
- Your usual nappy bag
- Swimming costume and towel for yourself
- Toy or book for while you are dressing

If your baby is nervous, start by bobbing up and down so that only the tips of his or her toes hit the water. Then, as the baby relaxes, go a little further.

When your baby seems happy and confident in the water, slowly move him or her away from you and then back again, holding securely under the baby's arms. Have a big smile on your face, talk to your baby and keep eye contact. If he or she is happy doing this, swish him or her from side to side while you keep them at arm's length. Keep your face on a level with your baby's to help him or her feel safe. If the baby's face goes underwater, give him or her a cuddle and reassurance if necessary.

A good teacher can show you how to get your baby so comfortable underwater that he or she will dive with you. Choose a small class that offers plenty of individual attention. Your baby will be in the water for a while so it must be very warm.

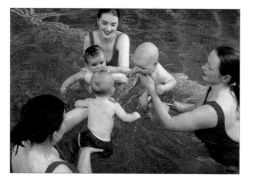

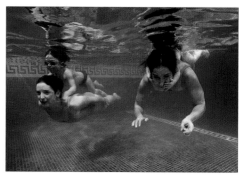

One-arm hold

Once your baby is comfortable in the water, and you are feeling confident too, try this more relaxed hold. It gets babies used to having less support without making them feel insecure. Eventually you can try using a foam woggle instead of your arm.

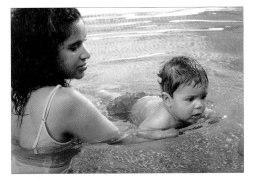

Rest your baby's chest on your forearm, so that his or her arms are in front of it. Place a reassuring hand on the baby's back. At first, keep your baby close to your body. Then slowly extend your arm outwards in an arc-like movement. Gently take your hand off the baby's back. Turn so that your arm traces a circle through the water. Put a ball in front of your baby to keep him or her amused and encourage use of the arms. Keep your arm relaxed.

Next, try turning the baby around to face outwards; keep your hands on either side of his or her ribcage below the armpits. Dip the baby in and out of the water, matching your words to the actions: for example, 'Up we go' and 'Splaaaash'. Hold the baby at arm's length and swish from side to side. Put a ball or interesting bath toy a little distance in front and move the baby forwards as he or she reaches towards it. Young babies naturally kick in the water, but older ones may not. If your baby doesn't

Practising back floating

This is a good exercise to encourage your baby to float on his or her back. Start with the baby in the water in a sitting position, using one hand to support the bottom and the other to support the neck, back of the head and top of the shoulders.

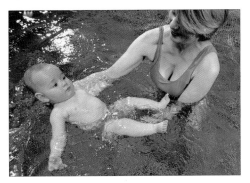

Gently lower the baby backwards into the water, then sit him or her up again. Do this several times in a rhythmic movement – try saying or singing 'Baaack, uuuup' as you do so. In time, the baby will be able to spend longer lying on his or her back and you'll be able to remove the hand under the bottom. Once the baby finds his or her buoyancy, you can lessen the support under the neck.

kick spontaneously, wait until you can support him or her one-handed (see below) before trying to help. Then use your other hand to move the baby's leg in a kicking action. Say 'Kick-kick-kick' whenever your baby is kicking, and eventually he or she will learn to kick in response to the words. Don't worry about the kicking style – babies have different ways of kicking, and there is no point in trying to refine their technique until they are swimming without assistance.

SWIMMING WITH A BABY: KEY POINTS

- Don't take a baby swimming if he or she is unwell or has a cold.
- If your baby has eczema, the condition may be exacerbated by chlorinated water. Keep a close eye on the baby's skin, and stop if it gets worse.
- If possible, choose a pool that has steps rather than a ladder. If yours has a ladder, get someone to go with you so that you don't have to negotiate the rungs while holding your wet, slippery baby.
- Keep swimming sessions short – start with ten-minute sessions and build up slowly to 30 minutes.
- Always take your baby out of the water as soon as you

think he or she is getting tired or chilly. Wrap the baby in a towel (with his or her head covered) as soon as you leave the water.
- Don't give your baby solid food just before swimming (it is fine to give a milk feed).
- Don't use armbands or rubber rings, which stop your baby from discovering his or her natural buoyancy.
- Always respect your baby's feelings. Even babies who have been swimming since they were very young may suddenly develop anxiety about being in the water. Never force a baby to do anything that he or she is unhappy with.

Dexterity, doing and thinking

By the age of six months, babies have already learned to grasp an object, put it in the mouth and to pass it from hand to hand. Now, although they still like to put objects in their mouths, they start to use their hands more: watch your baby stroke and pat an object before picking it up, and then shake, roll or bang it on the ground. Try laying your baby on different surfaces – grass, rough carpet, a soft rug, a silky cushion – so he or she can explore the feel. Offer textured books – the baby will quickly work out which part of the page to stroke – as well as toys with interesting textures and shapes.

Over the next few months, your baby's dexterity will improve dramatically. Babies learn to hold objects in their palms by wrapping their fingers and thumb around them, the thumb working like an extra finger rather than a separate unit. This clumsy hold doesn't allow them to manipulate the object very well. At about seven months, they learn to use the four fingers and the thumb as different units, making it much easier for them to pick up and handle things.

The next stage is to control individual fingers. The first sign that your baby can do this is when he or she starts to point, at about eight months. Some time around nine months, babies learn how to hold an item between index finger and thumb, using the pincer grip that is unique to

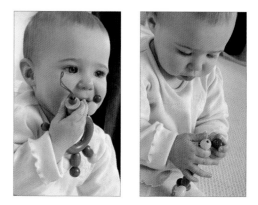

Young babies predominantly use their mouths to explore things. But as they become more dextrous, they start to use their hands a lot more.

humans. This enables them to pick up even very tiny objects and to perform sophisticated movements such as turning the pages of a book. You can help your baby to practise the pincer grip by putting a few cooked peas or grains of rice on the highchair's feeding tray at mealtimes: he or she will enjoy the task of picking them up one by

OBJECT PERMANENCE

Very young babies are unaware that anything they cannot see continues to exist. So if they have dropped a toy, say, they won't look for it because in their mind it is no more. Experts differ on when babies start to understand that objects are permanent, but most put it between four and seven months. At some point around this age you will notice that your baby will pull a cloth aside to find a toy that is partially visible. By nine months, a baby will look for a toy even if it is completely hidden. This leap in understanding means that an older baby will be much harder to distract when you take something away. You can help your baby to learn about object permanence by playing variations of the game 'peek-a-boo'. Cover your face with your hands and then reappear. Hide a squeaky toy under a cloth and make it sound before the baby can see it. Your baby will also enjoy surprising you by playing peek-a-boo back – covering his or her face and then slowly uncovering it. He or she will love it if you respond with surprise.

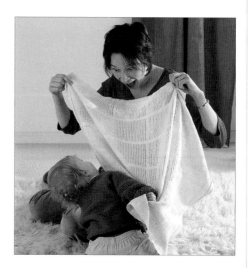

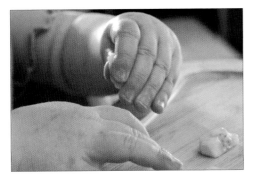

The pincer movement shows that your baby has control over individual digits. A key sign that it is about to happen is when he or she starts to point.

one. Unfortunately this also goes for any other small item, which will also go in the mouth. This means that you have to be vigilant about what is on the floor: a dropped button or pin could be a real danger.

Your baby will be able to hold only one thing at a time at first and will hold on until he or she loses interest and drops it without noticing. If you try to offer a second toy, he or she will automatically drop the first one in reaching for it. But by seven or eight months, a baby is able to hold two things at once, one in each hand.

Your baby will love to hand things to you. Say 'thank you' when he or she puts a toy into your hand – this is the very start of learning to share.

DROPPING AND THROWING

Babies have to learn how to let go of things. At first, they simply hold on until you take an object from them, or they drop it accidentally when their attention is caught by something else. But at about the same time as they learn the pincer grip, they discover how to open their fingers and deliberately drop something that they are holding. This quickly becomes a fun activity they will want to practise again and again. Your baby will love it if you give him or her a small toy and then ask for it back – put your hand under it so you can catch it as it drops.

Be prepared for a few weeks of picking things up whenever your baby is in the highchair – it will add to the baby's fun if you exclaim in mock protest every time you have to do this. You could put a metal tray on the floor where the objects fall so that your baby can hear that different items make different sounds when they hit it: try a metal spoon, a soft toy, a wet flannel and a bouncy ball. To stop your baby's new game becoming a real annoyance, restrict toys for the buggy to those that can be attached to it: the baby can then enjoy throwing them over the side and hauling them back in.

Your baby will also enjoy batting a ball back to you after you throw it. This is a good way to practise hand eye coordination. At first he or she will swipe at the ball and probably miss, but will quickly learn to how to hit it back in your direction.

Once your baby has discovered how to drop things, he or she will enjoy your reaction as they repeatedly hurl toys or dishes down from the high chair.

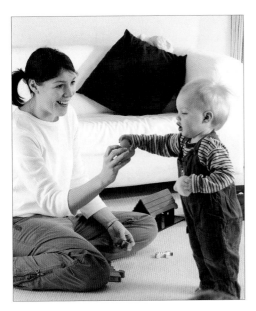

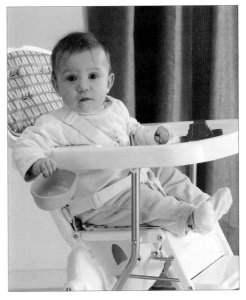

Sociability and language

Now that your baby can sit up and look around, he or she will get a lot more from going out and meeting people. You'll notice that your child starts to become more interested in other babies and children, and may stretch out to touch another baby's hand or face.

Babies love to socialize, and from the age of six months it is important to give them plenty of opportunities to interact with others. This can be as simple as taking your baby with you to the supermarket – it is good to experience positive interactions with strangers, who may smile and play little games while you are in the checkout queue. Your baby will also enjoy classes and parent-and-baby groups, as well as visits to the park to see other children playing.

As the first birthday approaches, you'll notice that your baby becomes more aware of the distinction between familiar people and strangers. For a while, new acquaintances will be scary. One moment the baby may be happy to be cuddled by another adult or to play in front of another baby; the next he or she may be crying for you. This is an aspect of separation anxiety and a normal stage of baby development. Your baby's budding

Your baby won't yet have any understanding of social skills, but you can certainly introduce the concept of being gentle when touching you or another baby. This is the root of empathy, the important notion that you should treat other people kindly.

LANGUAGE SKILLS AT 12 MONTHS
A few babies say their first word by 12 months, but most take longer. Your baby is likely to recognize the following words at one year old.
- His or her own name – the baby may turn towards you when you call it.
- 'Hello' and 'bye bye' – the baby may start to wave on hearing them.
- 'No' – though babies take real delight in ignoring it.
- A few naming words for familiar items – such as 'ball', 'duck' and 'teddy'.
- Some basic commands, such as 'Give it to mummy.'
- Simple questions such as 'Where is your nose?' – which the baby may then point to.

awareness of whom he or she belongs to and who belongs to him or her is the beginning of a sense of community, of being part of a family, a friendship group, a nation and a wider world.

LANGUAGE AND THE OLDER BABY
Most babies have started to manifest the rudiments of language by the end of their first year. At this time, you will probably find that your baby babbles more often and in a conversational tone that sounds like real language, as if

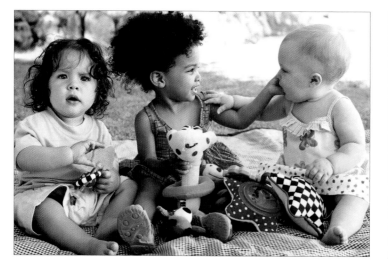

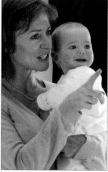

Pointing out things of interest and telling your baby about them is something that most parents do instinctively.

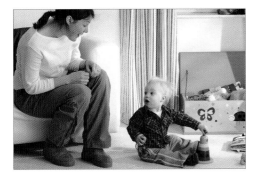

One of the first words that babies learn to recognize is their own name. If they hear it often, they will quickly learn that this particular sound means them.

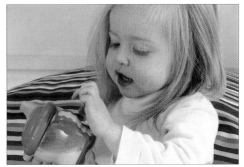

Talking to your child about things that are in front of him of her is the best way to encourage him or her to learn useful everyday words such as 'cup'.

telling a little story. He or she may even say a few words, though these are unlikely to be perfectly enunciated – for example, 'duh' for 'duck' or 'ook' for 'look'.

We tend to judge language development by when a baby says the first word, but your child's understanding is racing ahead of his or her ability to articulate. A one-year-old knows a lot more than he or she says, and when a baby chooses to speak the first word is not an indicator of developmental level.

Before your baby speaks, you will see the first green shoots of verbal communication in his or her behaviour. You may notice that the baby listens with greater attention when you talk, and seems to understand words that crop up often. He or she seems to know when you are asking a question – a quizzical expression shows this. And your baby may even know the answer to some frequently asked questions – pointing to a photograph when you say 'Where's granny?'; shaking his or her head when you offer another piece of banana (though sometimes this will be for fun, and the baby will take the banana from your hand straight afterwards).

Your baby will also begin to associate certain words with particular situations, which is a stepping-stone towards linking a fixed sound with a definite concept. The baby may, for example, routinely say 'Peep-oh' when playing the hiding game or invent words that seem to bear no relation to his or her native language. All this is thrilling for you as a parent. The time when your little baby can tell you what is on his or her mind is just around the corner. Some fascinating and sometimes hilarious conversations lie ahead.

HELPING YOUR BABY TO TALK

Your baby will pick up the meaning of words naturally, but here are some ways you can help.

Talk about things your baby can see. At dinner time, talk about the baby's food, cup, spoon; if you are in the park, talk about the swings, the children and so on.

Use simple sentences that include key labelling words such as 'Here is your teddy', 'Pass the teddy to daddy', 'Where is teddy?' Your baby has to hear a word in context many times to understand what it signifies.

Get down to your baby's level. Make eye contact when you speak, use big hand gestures, exaggerated facial expressions and a sing-song tone to help your baby grasp the gist of what you are saying.

Spend time talking to your baby each day. Find some time when there are no other distractions (such as older children wanting your attention) or background noise (such as the TV or radio).

Be on the lookout for first words and respond to them, even if they are made up. Your baby will be delighted to see that you know what he or she means.

Second children may spend less one to one time with their parents, but they will benefit from having a sibling to talk to, play with and learn from.

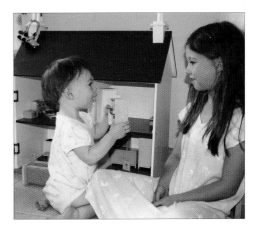

Signing with your baby

There is nothing out of the ordinary about babies using signs to communicate. This is something that they do quite spontaneously and without conscious prompting. From about eight or nine months, your baby may start to clap, wave 'Bye-bye', point to things, shake his or her head, lift his or her arms to be picked up and so on. Babies learn to signal before they can speak because hand signals are more visible and easy to copy than the complicated mouth movements that constitute speech.

Teaching your child baby sign language takes this natural process one step further. All it requires is for you to match an action to a word that crops up regularly, and to perform the gesture whenever appropriate.

WHY LEARN BABY SIGNING?

Baby signing can have real benefits for both baby and parent, because it allows a baby to communicate beyond his or her ability to articulate speech. It is fun for both of you – you get to find out more about what your baby is thinking, and the baby enjoys telling you.

Baby signing can facilitate language development, one study found that signing babies recognized more words and had larger vocabularies than non-signing ones. Baby

Signing isn't necessary for language development, which happens quite naturally as a result of interaction, but it can be a fun extra activity to do with your baby.

signing teachers claim that signing babies often learn to speak earlier as well. Baby signing may also help with brain development. Advocates say that signing, because it involves visual awareness as well as language skills, uses more parts of the brain than normal speech, and therefore creates more synapses (conceptual pathways) in the brain.

Another possible benefit is that signing can reduce frustration and possibly tantrums. If your baby can make signs that you both understand, it may be easier to tell you what he or she wants (a sleep, a drink, a favourite toy) rather than having to wait while you work it out.

WHEN CAN YOU START?

You can start signing with your baby any time from about six months, but the baby probably won't start to sign back until between eight and ten months. Toddlers can also benefit from signing, and since they have more advanced motor skills may reward you by signing back much more quickly – an 18-month old could pick up some simple signs within a few days.

HOW DOES IT WORK?

You can use a sign language developed for the deaf – American sign language (ASL) or British sign language (BSL) – to sign with your baby. Some of the signs are too difficult for a baby to reproduce, so you may need to

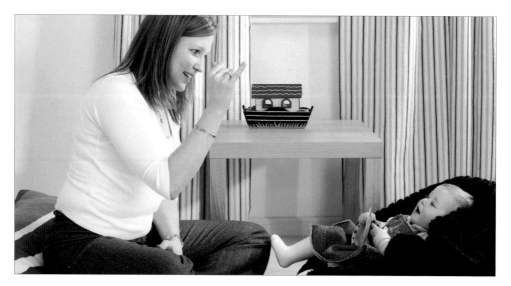

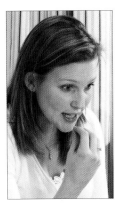

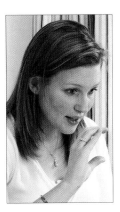

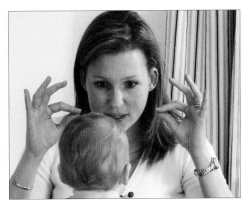

Eat: Bring your fingers together and then move your hand towards your mouth several times.

Drink: Hold your fingers and thumb apart to make a C-shape. Bring your fingers up to your face as if drinking from a cup.

Cat: Pinch the index finger and thumb of each hand together under your nose and then draw them out to the sides, as if preening a cat's whiskers. For "dog" slap your right hand against your leg a couple of times, then click your fingers as if attracting a dog's attention.

teach a simplified version. Alternatively, you can use your own invented signs – such as a few pats on the head for 'hat' or your hands cupped together for 'ball'.

Unless you want your baby to be able to sign to a deaf person, it doesn't really matter what system you use – your baby will adapt to any signs and is unlikely to continue signing once he or she can speak fluently. It can be easier to use an established system like ASL or BSL than to think up a host of new signs yourself, but you'll need to go to classes or buy a signing dictionary.

SIGNING AT HOME
Start with a manageable number of signs – six is enough – and make sure you have your baby's attention before you sign. Get close up, make eye contact and then do the gesture. Make sure that you always say out loud the word for the sign you are using. Remember that the point of the exercise is not to teach your baby perfect sign language,

but to provide a temporarily useful way of communicating until the baby is able to speak well. Try to sign in exactly the same way each time – your baby will learn by repetition. It is important to sign in different contexts – for example, sign 'cat' when you see one in the garden, when you come across one in a storybook, and as you draw one. Sign one thing at a time at first – don't sign two words in succession, or your baby may be confused.

Be on the lookout for your baby's first attempts to sign back. It doesn't matter if this sign ends up being different from the 'real' one; the baby may refine it as his or her motor skills improve, and you can then perhaps adapt yours. Make sure that you respond to your baby's signs, and give lots of praise. If possible, let other carers know what signs you are teaching, so that they can use them too. And be very, very patient. It may take many weeks for your baby to use a sign that you teach, or for you to recognize it as such.

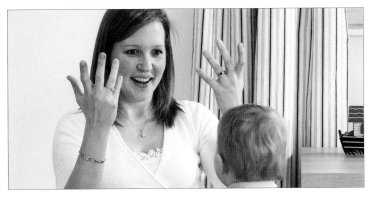

Right: To signal 'finished' open your hands, palms facing your chest, then turn them outwards in a flicking movement.

Fun for older babies

New manual dexterity means that your baby can explore toys more thoroughly, and you'll notice that he or she starts to have more interest in what they can do. So the baby may push a toy car along the ground, but place one building brick on top of another.

The best way to encourage your child's learning is to tailor play to abilities. Babies tend to be most interested in skills that they are just about to master or have recently learned. It is up to you to provide activities that are just hard enough to be fun and stimulating: if they are too easy or familiar, the baby will get bored; if they are too difficult, he or she may become upset. You will have to be the judge of when your baby is ready to give them a go.

ROLLING TOYS

A mobile baby will love to chase after toys that roll: a wheeled car or truck, a soft, slow-moving ball or even a toilet roll. Make sure that any rolling toys are too large to fit in the baby's mouth and that they are suitable for this age (don't let your baby play with an older child's car, say, which may have lots of small parts). The baby will also like pulling or pushing toys.

Babies are equally interested in 'boy' and 'girl' toys, so don't try to limit them. Your little girl may enjoy playing with planes or cars, which she can push along the floor; a little boy may love cuddling a baby doll, which, after all, looks just like him.

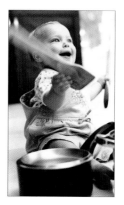
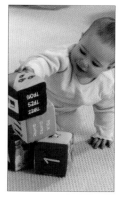

In the hands of a baby, a couple of saucepans and a wooden spoon can be magically transformed into a drum kit.

Babies love to knock down towers of bricks, and will eventually start to try building them up for themselves.

TOYS THAT DO THINGS

As your baby gets more dextrous, he or she will enjoy playing with toys that do something, especially if they offer the thrill of surprise. A truck that takes off when you push a button or a jack-in-the-box that pops up when you turn a dial will be a source of real fascination. Let the baby practise setting the toy off: this will help develop dexterity and strength. Toy telephones (and real ones) that ring or buzz are universally popular.

EMPTYING GAMES

Older babies love to empty things out of containers, drawers, cupboards, bags and boxes. To make a game out of this you can fill a fabric shopping bag or a box with a selection of small objects that the baby can take out one by one. Change some of the items every so often to keep the game interesting. As well as toys, you could include things like a wooden spoon, a baby hairbrush, an old notebook, a set of clean, unwanted keys on a ring, an old purse, a plastic pot or an orange. It is a good idea to let the baby help you put them all back in the right place – showing that 'tidying up' can be a fun part of playtime.

DISCOVERING WATER

Water is a source of wonder to all babies: it changes shape, cannot be held and glistens in the light. Your baby will love to play pouring games in the bath. Provide a

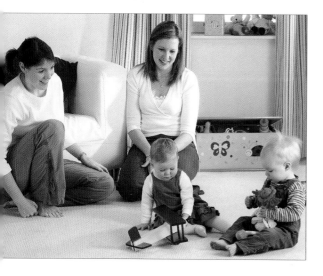

variety of containers of different sizes, and show how to pour water from one to the other. Natural sponges make great bath toys: fill one up and then show your baby how to squeeze the water out of it.

STACKING TOYS

A set of stacking cups will provide months of amusement. At first your baby will simply enjoy exploring similar objects of different sizes. Then he or she will have endless fun putting one of the small cups inside a larger one. This is one way that he or she starts to work out how things are different, and learn important concepts such as big and small. The baby will love to knock down a tower when you build it, and will want to do it over and over again: it is an early way of showing that he or she can change what is happening, giving an enjoyable sense of power and achievement. Eventually, the baby will have a go at putting one cup on top of another, or threading a set of stacking rings on a pole.

MUSICAL TOYS

Babies love things that make noises. Wooden maracas, a tamourine and various shakers will be popular with babies of this age and older, but you don't have to buy musical toys; you can also make your own. An upturned saucepan make a good drum to bang with a wooden spoon, while a few cotton reels in a well-sealed plastic container make a great shaker.

HELPING YOUR BABY ENJOY PLAY

Keep giving your baby new things to play with: babies need lots of variety and get bored if they play with the same toys all the time. But they don't need lots of expensive playthings – your baby really will be as happy exploring a cereal box and other household items as an expensive toy. Reignite your baby's interest in toys he or she has enjoyed by hiding them away for a while and then letting the baby discover them afresh. Allow your baby to make a mess. Babies scatter toys everywhere, and they

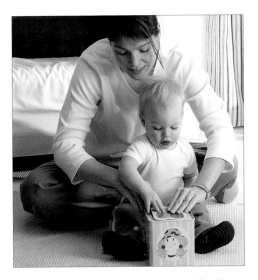

Babies learn by watching other people as well as by exploring things for themselves. So get down on the floor and show your baby how each toy works. He or she may not succeed in copying you, but will have a go – and will remember what to do with that toy next time.

love to empty out a cupboard or a bag of shopping. Be prepared for a less-than-spotless house for a while; you can always tidy up when the baby has gone to bed.

It will help to contain the mess if you restrict emptying games to a special cupboard filled with non-breakable things that can be flung on the floor. Whenever the baby tries to do the same to other cupboards, gently say 'No' and lead him or her back to the special cupboard. If you do this consistently, your child will eventually get the message. Be reasonable about what your baby can and cannot do. Move things that you don't want played with, rather than constantly saying 'No' every time the baby goes near them.

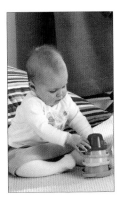

Left: Stacking cups or rings will give good value for months as a baby's manual skills develop.

Right: As your baby explores objects by handling, he or she starts to work out how things relate to each other. A baby will become totally absorbed in the task of putting a small beaker into a larger one.

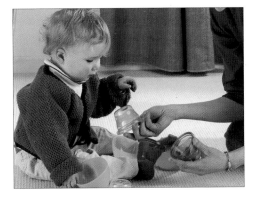

section six

toddlers and older chidren

Toddlers are amazing creatures: they are curious, strong-willed, unselfconscious, as changeable as the weather, and always ready to share love and laughter. You will find that it is a real education to go for a walk with your child and to get a privileged glimpse of the world through his or her eyes. Once your child learns to talk, you will have some of the most engaging conversations you will ever have.

General care and feeding

> 66 It is delightful to watch your little child wash his or her own face with a flannel or to put their wellingtons on the wrong feet. 99

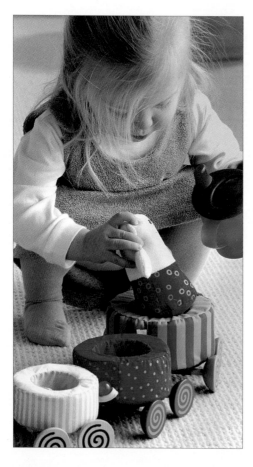

One of the real delights of being a parent to a toddler is seeing how their determination to do things for themselves gradually grows into true independence. But toddlers can have very strong opinions, so simple daily tasks such as getting dressed and washed or eating breakfast can turn into a battleground. Mealtimes are a flashpoint in many families. Your toddler may start to eat more messily, spread his or her dinner everywhere or hurl his bowl on the floor.

It is essential to keep your perspective. After all, it doesn't really matter if your child wants to wear, say, odd socks, or a fairy costume. Don't make a confrontation out of things that don't matter.

The key developmental goal at this age is bladder and bowel control. Toilet training is bound to involve a few accidents, but your child will get there more easily and quickly if he or she is keen to use the potty and if he or she is completely ready for the challenge when you start. In this chapter there's information on the key signs to look out for, as well as advice on

It's good to hand over control of small things to your toddler. Even something as simple as letting a toddler manage his or her own drinks can instil independence.

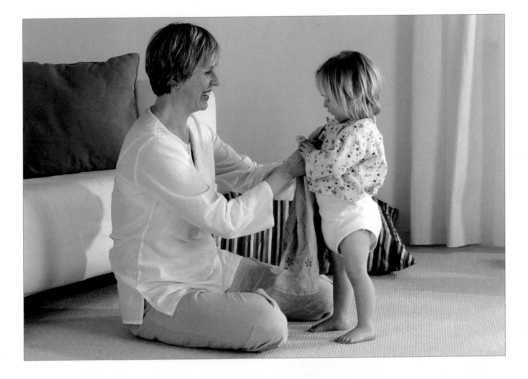

how to introduce the potty and encourage your child to use it. Another common life change in the third year, one over which your toddler has absolutely no control, is the arrival of a younger brother or sister. This is something that has to be carefully managed, but with a little tact and forethought the growth of your family can be as joyful a time for your older child as it is for you.

Always remember that your toddler's growing independence is a positive thing, even if it might make life trying from time to time. It is delightful to watch your little child wash his or her own face with a flannel or to put their wellingtons on the wrong feet, and it gives him or her great pleasure too. So as far as possible, try to nurture your child's natural enjoyment in doing things for themselves.

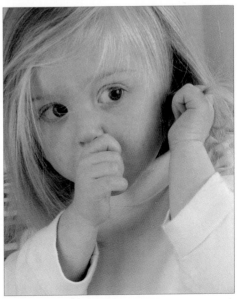

Top: It's fun to see your child gradually working out how to do things for him or herself. Most children want to help get themselves dressed from an early age.

However independent toddlers may seem at times, they are still babies emotionally. Your child may become more needy if a new baby arrives on the scene.

Washing and keeping clean

As your toddler gets older, you begin the process of teaching him or her to become more independent, starting to feed, wash and take care of themselves, or at least becoming aware of what is involved. Your toddler may embrace these new activities with enthusiasm – little children take great delight in doing things for themselves, especially if they perceive a task as a grown-up one. They are also inveterate copiers, and will enjoy performing tasks and jobs with you rather than only under instruction.

CLEAN HANDS

Toddlers inevitably get grubby, and an evening bath is the easiest way to get them clean after a busy day in the sandpit and the garden. In between times, though, it is important that young children wash their hands before meals and after using the potty or helping to take off a used nappy (diaper), so it is a good idea to instil regular handwashing habits early on. Your child will still need your help until about the age of three.

Get a step so that your toddler can reach the washbasin, and teach him or her the difference between the hot and cold taps. Demonstrate how to turn on the cold tap. Teach your child not to touch the hot one – and consider reducing the temperature of your hot-water supply to less than 55°C/130°F to prevent accidental scalding. Begin by lathering your own hands and then gently rub the soap bubbles all over your toddler's. Make it fun by blowing the bubbles into the air, or by having hand-washing races.

A toddler may positively enjoy washing his or her hands just like mummy and daddy. Choose a natural soap without harsh chemicals.

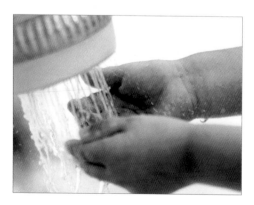

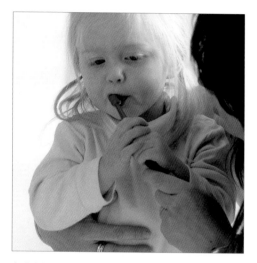

As babies get older, they often enjoy the twice-daily ritual of cleaning their teeth. But they can't brush them properly on their own until they are much older.

GETTING CLEAN

Your toddler's skin is very delicate so it is important to avoid harsh soaps or bath products. A handful of oats gathered in a piece of muslin makes a good alternative to soap, and you can avoid using shampoo altogether if you wish and simply rinse your child's hair with water: the natural oils in the hair will keep it clean. If you want to use products, choose natural ones free from chemicals, and limit hair washing to once or twice a week.

Many toddlers dislike having their hair washed. If you have this problem, you can sponge the hair to get rid of clumps of food. But from time to time, you will have to wash it. If you use shampoo, choose a gentle one that won't sting if it gets in your child's eyes.

NAIL CARE

It's easier to keep fingernails and toenails clean if they are short – long nails can harbour dirt and germs. But most toddlers hate having their nails cut and it is almost impossible to do this safely if your child keeps wrenching his or her hand or foot away. The best solution is to cut the nails when your child is asleep, but you could also try doing it as part of a game such as 'This little piggy'. Child-sized nail clippers are usually the best way to cut small nails, but some children prefer to have them filed.

TOOTHBRUSHING

If your toddler is reluctant to let you clean his or her teeth, try letting him or her do yours first or brush a favourite toy's 'teeth'. Tooth cleaning is important, so persevere even if it is difficult. Try doing it after supper rather than just before bedtime if it becomes a flashpoint. Take your toddler with you when you visit the dentist. Children don't need a check-up until they are about two, but it is good to make the dentist's surgery and the "special chair" a familiar environment long before that.

BATH TIME

You don't have to hold your toddler in the bath like a baby, but you do still need to be vigilant. Remember that small children can drown in just a few centimetres of water and in a few moments, so don't ever leave a toddler in the bath unattended or in the care of an older child, however sensible he or she may seem. Encourage your toddler to remain seated in the bath – to prevent slipping – and teach him or her to avoid touching the hot tap (wrap a wet flannel around it as an additional safety precaution).

FEAR OF THE BATH

Most children love baths, but some toddlers become frightened of the water or develop a dislike of the sound and sight of water disappearing down the plug hole. It is as if they fear they will go down with it. Treat these fears seriously – forcing a reluctant child to get in the bath will do more harm than good, and it's not a problem to give your toddler sponge baths for a few weeks. After a while, though, you will want to encourage your child back into the bath. Be sure to go slowly.

Start by getting in the bath together (if possible, have someone else on hand to lift the child in and out). Invest in a few new and exciting bath toys – wind-up toys are particularly good for this – to encourage play in the water. Once your toddler is feeling more relaxed about getting into the bath with you, try putting him or her in alone. But let the child stand up if this is easier (with you holding on as he or she could easily slip). Try scooping water over the child's ankles, then legs, bottom, tummy and back while he or she continues to stand.

Have plenty of toys in the bathwater: empty, cleaned shampoo or bubble-bath bottles, natural sponges, a flannel and plastic pots and beakers are good. Let your toddler bend down to pick a toy up. When you think he or she is ready, put the child in a sitting or kneeling position and then quickly provide a distraction by setting off a moving toy or pouring water from one pot into another. Keep the bath short, let your child hold on to you and have lots of physical contact during the bath, and cuddles afterwards. Don't pull the plug out until your child is out of the water (or out of the room if necessary) if it makes him or her feel scared.

MILK BATH

Here is a fragrant mixture to add to a toddler's bath. Milk is gentle on the skin, and an ideal medium for diluting essential oils. Mix the bath milk just before you need it because it won't keep.

100ml/3½fl oz full-fat milk
3 drops lavender essential oil
3 drops neroli essential oil
5ml/1 tsp blue or red food colouring (optional)

Pour the milk into a bowl or jug and add the essential oils, then the food colouring if you are using it. Stir to mix and pour the mixture into a warm bath.

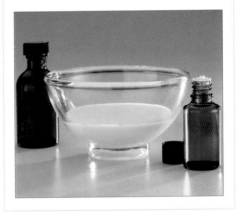

Children usually love baths, and if your child shows some reluctance it is more than likely to be a short-lived phase. He or she will soon be enjoying them again.

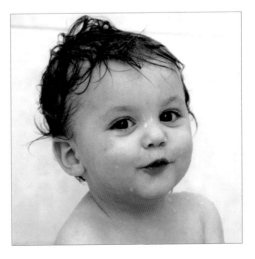

A healthy diet for toddlers

Toddlers have busy lives and small stomachs, so they need to eat little and often. Three meals a day – breakfast, lunch and dinner – is a convenient routine to aim for, but you will also need to offer a mid-morning and mid-afternoon snack to keep your child going between meals. Don't expect your toddler to eat the same amount every day – his or her appetite will vary hugely. It's completely normal for a young child to refuse food on some days and to eat extra helpings on others.

A VARIED DIET

You probably won't be able to get your child to eat perfectly balanced meals every day, but if you offer a wide variety of healthy food, this should add up to a reasonably good mixed diet over a week or so. It is very normal for children to refuse all but a few chosen items from time to time, but so long as your toddler is eating one or more foods from each group, you don't need to worry. Ideally your child will eat a good mixed diet consisting of the following foods each day.

Five or more servings of fruits and vegetables. Try to include as many types as possible.

Four or five helpings of starchy foods such as rice, potatoes, pasta, couscous or quinoa. Don't be tempted to put a young child on a high-fibre diet: wholegrains are bulky and they fill young children up without providing the necessary nutrients.

One or two servings of protein foods such as lean meat, fish, pulses, eggs or nuts. If your child doesn't eat meat or fish, give two servings of other protein a day.

Milk 500ml/17fl oz up to the age of two years; 350ml/12fl oz after two, or the equivalent in cheese, fromage frais, yoghurt and so on. Use plain, full-fat dairy products: fruit yoghurts often contain lots of sugar and small children shouldn't eat low-fat dairy products.

Some iron-rich foods the best sources are red meat, chicken or fish, but tofu, beans and lentils, leafy green vegetables, dried fruit, fortified breakfast cereals and bread also contain some iron. Eating vitamin C-rich foods such as brightly coloured fruits and vegetables at the same time helps the body to absorb the iron.

Some healthy fat – olive oil and avocados are good sources. Give oily fish at least once a week.

DRINKS

Drinking lots of water with snacks and at mealtimes will help to keep your toddler's digestion healthy. Juice isn't necessary, but if you want to give it to increase your child's vitamin intake, make sure that it is well diluted (one part juice to ten parts water for young toddlers, slightly stronger for older ones). Fizzy and sweetened fruit drinks and even fruit juice will coat the teeth in sugary liquid, so, ideally limit drinks to milk and water.

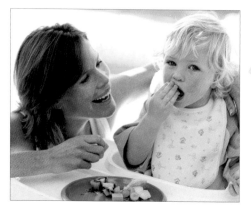

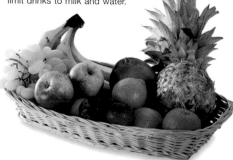

Left and above: It's important to encourage healthy eating habits from an early age. Fortunately most children love fruit – try to give them as wide a variety as possible and keep trying new types.

SWEETS AND CRISPS

It is much easier to ensure that your child eats healthily if you limit the intake of empty calories. All children love crisps and sweets, but they have no nutritional value, and they tend to ruin a child's appetite for more wholesome foods. That is not to say that such foods should be banned altogether (although it is a good idea to hold off introducing them for as long as you can), only that you and your child should see them as occasional treats. Set an example yourself by eating healthy foods: if you enjoy chocolate and biscuits after lunch, then your child will want some too.

If you do give sweets, choose kinds that dissolve quickly in the mouth rather than sticking to the teeth – chocolate instead of chewy sweets, for example. And get your child to eat them in one go: a lot of sweets eaten in a few minutes will actually do less harm to the teeth than eating a few at staggered intervals through the day. If possible, get your child to drink a glass of water afterwards, or to eat a piece of cheese, which helps to neutralize the effect of sugar on teeth.

DAIRY PRODUCTS

Milk is a good source of calcium (which is needed to build strong bones and teeth), vitamin A (for healthy skin, eyes and immune system) and fat (needed for energy), as well as protein. If you have stopped breastfeeding, you can now give full-fat cow's or goat's milk as your baby's main drink, or you can stick to follow-on formula milk if you prefer. Choose organic milk and dairy products whenever possible. Don't give skimmed milk or low-fat dairy products to children under five, because they need plenty of calories. You can start giving semi-skimmed milk to children over two, so long as they are eating and growing well. If your toddler stops drinking milk, give three servings of cheese, yoghurt, fromage frais or milk-based dishes a day. Here are some suggestions.

- Porridge or pancakes made with full-fat milk.
- Homemade fruit milkshakes or yoghurt smoothies.
- Dhal or soup with yoghurt stirred in.
- Quick 'rice pudding' made with cooked rice and plain yoghurt (it doesn't need sugar).
- Mini sandwiches made with Cheddar or cream cheese as a mid-morning snack.
- Cooked vegetables made with cheese sauce.
- Mashed potatoes made with lots of milk and butter.
- Chunks of Cheddar, hard goat's cheese or edam, served with slices of fruit.
- Greek or plain yoghurt.

NON-DAIRY ALTERNATIVES

There is a lot of debate about the health benefits of eating dairy foods, and it is clear that some children (such as those with milk-allergy-related eczema) are better off

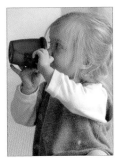

Leave a cup of water close by when your child plays so he or she can help him or herself.

avoiding them altogether. If you want to restrict the amount of dairy products you give your child because of intolerance or for other reasons, here are some good alternative sources of calcium. A paediatric dietician can advise you about planning your child's diet to ensure that it is not deficient.

- Unsweetened rice milk or soya milk with added calcium (don't give sweetened soya milk, which is bad for the teeth). But be aware that some children who are intolerant of dairy products are also intolerant of soya.
- Tofu (made with soya beans) or beans.
- Ground nuts and seeds.
- Canned salmon and sardines (with bones), mashed well.
- Leafy green vegetables: spinach, kale, greens.
- Dried apricots and figs.

Offer your child only healthy food choices for as long as you can. This is much easier if you eat healthily too – your child is much more likely to eat a piece of fruit if he or she sees you eating one.

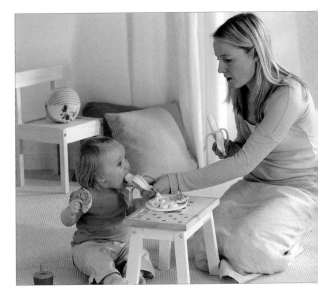

Helping your toddler to enjoy food

Toddlers are often picky eaters and a child's eating habits can cause parents a great deal of stress. But there are many ways you can help to give your child a positive attitude to food. As a general rule, it is best to let your toddler's appetite be your guide. You will naturally find yourself gently coaxing your child to eat vegetables, but it is pointless to try to force a child to eat more than he or she wants. If your toddler is a healthy weight and has plenty of energy, then he or she is almost certainly getting enough. Check with a health professional if you are not sure.

HAPPY EATING

Your child can eat pretty much everything you eat (with the exception of very salty or spicy foods) provided it is chopped small enough to manage easily. It is a great idea to include your toddler in family mealtimes as soon as possible, and make eating a sociable activity. Push the highchair up to the table, and later get a booster seat so that he or she can sit comfortably at the table.

It's best if your child sits down for snacks and there is less chance of choking that way. He or she will love food to be served on a toddler-size table or low stool.

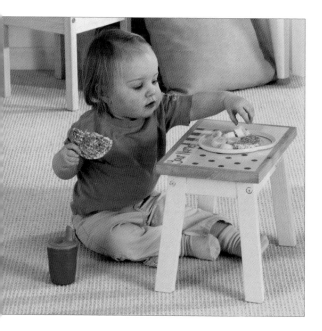

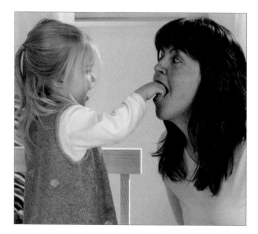

Children like to copy their parents and to try what you eat. Eating together and sharing food is a good way to make food an enjoyable part of life.

If you like to eat a little later than a young child's blood-sugar levels will allow, treat your child as an extra snacktime for him or her. Don't wait until your child is so tired or hungry that he or she is cranky before eating. Having regular meals and snacktimes will help to regulate his or her energy levels.

Let your child have a spoon and feed himself or herself as soon as he or she seems willing. Having control over how much and what is eaten helps to foster a positive attitude towards food. You can get forks with rounded tines for older toddlers. Your toddler will be more willing to eat an amount that looks manageable than a huge pile of food, so serve small portions. You can always give your child a second helping if he or she wants one.

LIKES AND DISLIKES

Be tolerant about food fads. Most children go through stages when they reject foods they have previously enjoyed, or when they have certain rules about how food must be presented. It is common, for example, for children to dislike 'mixed-up' food and to insist that each element of a meal be served in a separate pile that doesn't touch the others. It's often good to humour these fads, but talk to a health professional if you think your child's attitude to food is extreme.

Young children like to copy grown-ups (or older children) and studies show that children whose parents eat lots of fruits and vegetables tend to eat them too. So chop a raw pepper at snacktime and share it with your toddler, or offer some green vegetables off your plate. But children should never be forced to eat foods they dislike or to finish a meal if they are no longer hungry. Remember your own childhood meals. If you were made to eat a food you disliked, or told to sit at the table until you had scraped the plate clean, you may recall how it didn't make you eat any better. Worse still, the child will realize that refusing to eat is a good way of getting your attention and may use this as a way of exercising independence.

Don't assume that your child doesn't like a new food if it's initially rejected. Children may need to be offered a food ten times or more before it becomes familiar enough for them to eat it. So keep serving that portion of red pepper or spinach alongside other foods that your child will eat. It's very tempting to get out, say, bread and cheese if your toddler rejects the meal you have prepared. This doesn't do any harm from time to time, but if you do it often you may be storing up problems for the future.

If your toddler picks at meals, consider whether he or she is having too much milk or snacks at other times. Limit milk to the recommended daily amount, and don't give a snack within an hour of a meal – if a toddler is really hungry, it is better to bring the mealtime forward.

FRUIT AND VEGETABLES

Here are some ways to get your toddler eating plenty of fruits and vegetables.

• Serve fruit at all or most mealtimes. For example, chopped banana or pear in morning porridge; slices of apple after lunch; and peaches and yoghurt after supper.

Make mealtimes calm, happy times. Avoid discussing difficult issues or commenting on your child's eating habits in a negative way.

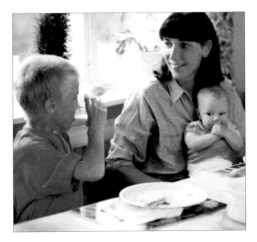

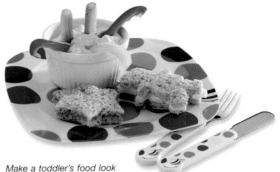

Make a toddler's food look appetising. Offer brightly coloured vegetables with every meal – red and yellow peppers alongside breadsticks with a dip, say. Sometimes you may like to use biscuit cutters to make little sandwiches in the shape of teddies or stars.

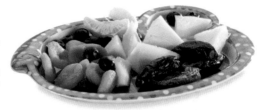

Serving fruit at every snack time will help to up your child's vitamin intake. Encourage them to try exotic fruits as well as the standard apples and bananas.

• Make sure you always have two or three different kinds of fresh fruit in the house. Keep homemade fruit purées in the freezer and serve them alone or stirred into yoghurt or plain fromage frais.
• Give your child raw vegetable sticks as snacks or to keep him or her amused while waiting for a meal – sticks of carrot and cucumber are good served with a dip: hummus or guacamole are good healthy options.
• Include vegetables in every savoury meal. Ideally have one green vegetable and one other vegetable to get a good range of vitamins.
• Keep vegetables in the freezer so you don't run out. If you can't find ready-frozen organic vegetables, make your own: chopped and lightly steamed carrots, green beans, baby sweetcorn and broccoli all freeze well.
• Stir chopped, puréed or grated vegetables into rice, mashed potato, dhal or tomato sauce for pasta. Grated carrot or courgette (zucchini) go well in pancakes.
• Remember that children don't have preconceptions about which foods should be served together. It is fine to use vegetable soup as a pasta sauce or to stir chopped dried fruit into a lamb casserole. And if you are resorting to a tin of (low-salt, low-sugar) baked beans, stir in some peas or spinach to increase the vitamin content.

general care and feeding   **369**

Preparing for toilet training

Learning to use a potty is an important part of growing up. Teaching your child to do it can be an easy process – provided that you wait until he or she is ready. If you start too early, it will take longer and there will be more accidents along the way. Most children are potty trained somewhere between the ages of two and a half and three years, but some take longer or are ready earlier. Most children master control over the bowel before the bladder, and will be dry during the day long before they can stay dry all night long. Remember, however long the journey, they all get there in the end.

IS MY CHILD READY?

Children start to become aware that they are doing a wee or poo at around 18 months. At this stage, they may clutch themselves and look down at a puddle of wee if they are naked – a sign that they understand they have produced it. It usually takes another year or more before they know in advance that they need to go to the toilet and have the necessary control to wait for a few minutes. When this happens, your child is ready to start potty training, provided there are no other major changes going on – for example, you are about to move house, a new baby is expected or your child is starting nursery. Here are the signs to look out for.

- Your child tells you that he or she is about to do a wee or poo – whether it is communicated in words, by facial expression or by actions.
- Your child remains dry after a nap or for more than two hours at a time.
- Your child makes it clear he or she objects to having a dirty or wet nappy (diaper).
- Your child is able to understand simple instructions, and knows what toilet-based words such as 'wee' and 'poo' (or whatever words you decide to use) mean.
- Your child is happy to try sitting on the potty and understands what it is for. Some children may ask to use the potty if they see their friends doing it.
- Your child has mastered all the physical skills needed to use a potty successfully – that is, walking well, sitting down and standing up unaided, and pulling his or her underwear on and off.

WHAT YOU NEED FOR TOILET TRAINING

A potty. Choose a sturdy one that won't tip over when your child sits on it and is easy to clean. If your child already knows about potties, he or she might like to choose one – narrow the choice down to two or three different types.

Proper cotton pants. Choose pants that your toddler will enjoy wearing, perhaps with a favourite character or motif on. You'll need at least ten pairs to begin with.

Training pants. Some parents find towelling training pants useful because they retain wee or poo, but can still be pulled up and down like proper pants. You can use them as a halfway stage, or as a safeguard when out and about. That way, your child will feel wet after an accident – which can help with potty training – but you won't have to deal with a public puddle. Change them quickly and emphasize how nice it is to be clean and dry. It is better not to use disposable trainer pants as they wick away the wetness too efficiently. This results in your child getting the treat of wearing pull-down pants without having to stay dry for the privilege.

Steps and a child seat for the toilet. Some children don't like the idea of a potty, but are keen to use the big toilet. If this is the case, you will need to buy a set of child's steps, so that your child can get on to the toilet on his or her own. A child's toilet seat is vital, so that the toddler feels secure when sitting on the toilet.

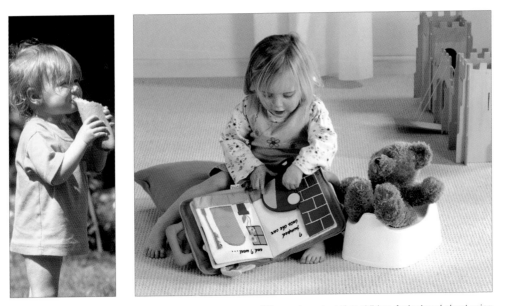

Bare-bottom time helps your toddler to notice how weeing feels. Your child may view the puddle with great interest months before he or she is ready for the potty.

It is very important that children feel relaxed about using the potty. Keep it in the living room before beginning to use it and watch how your child includes it in play.

PREPARING YOUR CHILD

It is important that your toddler feels good about going to the toilet. He or she probably gives some telltale signs that mean a poo or wee is coming: going red in the face, squeezing the legs together, standing on tiptoes, clutching the crotch and so on. Tell your child what is happening in a calm but interested way, and don't look disgusted when you are changing a nasty nappy.

If you feel able to, it is a good idea to let your child see you use the toilet – take the opportunity to explain what you are doing. If you have older children, ask them if your toddler can watch them go to the toilet, too, but don't put them under pressure – they have a right to privacy if they want it. It's particularly helpful if a girl sees mummy use the toilet, and a boy sees what daddy does.

GETTING READY

The first step is to get your child used to having a potty around. Keep it in the bathroom near the toilet, but bring it out to the play area from time to time too.
• Get a colourful book about a child learning to use the potty, so that your child starts to understand what it is for.
• Play at putting teddy or dolly on the potty. Later on, your child may like to have teddy sitting on the travel potty while he or she sits on the real one.
• Put a few toys or books around the potty to encourage the child to sit on it while fully clothed. Don't press or, worse still, force your child to sit on it. It is vital that he or she feels comfortable at every stage of potty training and that you are relaxed about it.
• Once your child is happily sitting on the potty, put it back in the bathroom and keep it there. He or she may like to sit on it while you use the toilet. You can also try casually suggesting that your child sits on it when naked before a bath – but don't push this.

As your child gets accustomed to the potty as part of their play, you can start to encourage them to sit on it themselves as part of the game.

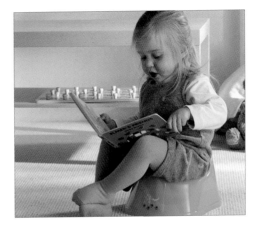

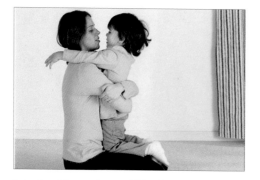

Lots of cuddles can help a child to feel better about accidents or difficulties during potty training.

TOILET TRAINING YOUR CHILD

Once you have embarked on potty training, there are some key things to remember.

Praise. Congratulate your toddler whenever he or she manages to wee or poo in the potty.

Reminders. Your toddler can't wait for long, so keep asking if he or she needs to do a wee.

Make it easy. Keep the potty where your child can find it. If your home has bathrooms on different floors, you may want to put a potty in each one. Dress your child in clothes that are quick to pull off – such as trousers instead of dungarees.

Give privacy. If your toddler wants to turn his or her back or take the potty into a corner, that's fine.

Take it slowly. Wait until your child is dry during the day before you tackle the nights. Back off if the child becomes anxious, and go back to nappies for a few weeks.

Be consistent. Once you've started potty training, keep going unless your child becomes distressed. Don't let the child use nappies one day and the potty the next, or go back to nappies because you are going to stay with friends or going out for the day.

Be patient. Clean up the inevitable accidents without much comment – 'Never mind, next time you can do it in the potty' is enough.

BOWEL CONTROL

Children usually learn to control their bowels before their bladder. If your toddler tends to poo at the same time each day (many children go within half an hour of eating a meal), try leaving the nappy (diaper) off just beforehand. Wait until you can tell that the child is about to do a bowel movement, then suggest trying to do a poo in the potty. If your child says no, put a nappy on. If he or she looks interested or doesn't respond, produce the potty quickly. Help with undressing and stay with your child. Remember that he or she may need to concentrate, so don't chat too much. Let the child get up if he or she has tried for a few

USING THE TOILET

It's better for a boy to sit down to pee at first when he starts to use the big toilet, but if he insists on standing up, try putting something he can use for target practice in the bowl: shaving foam, confetti or even coloured ice cubes (if you use blue food colouring his wee will turn the water green – a pleasing 'reward'). Make sure the seat won't fall down while he is using the toilet. Show him how to put it up properly and teach him to put it down when he has finished.

minutes and not produced anything and give lots of praise if he or she does poo in the potty.

Clean your child up. You can show older toddlers how to wipe themselves (tell a girl to wipe from front to back), but they still need your help. Wiping is easier with a wet wipe, but choose the flushable variety and don't flush more than two or three wipes at once. Empty the contents of the potty into the toilet and both wash your hands.

Some children love to flush their poo away – especially if they are not usually allowed to touch the toilet at other times. But others find flushing a terrifying prospect. The poo is their own creation, after all, and in their eyes it is something to be proud of. If this is how your child seems to feel, then it is best to flush after he or she leaves the bathroom. Some children are fascinated by their faeces

Some children are fascinated by the process of flushing the toilet and will watch things disappear eagerly. But others find this frightening.

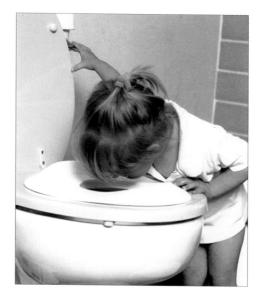

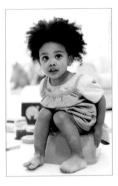

Don't feel that you can't get out and about when you are potty or toilet training. Get in the habit of taking at least one change of clothes with you when you go out, as well as a plastic bag to put the wet ones in.

and want to play with them. It is important not to allow this, of course, but take care not to use words such as 'dirty' about the faeces or your child may think that you are referring to him or her.

Make sure your child is eating enough fibre by giving him or her lots of fruit and vegetables during this time – if passing a hard stool causes any pain while on the potty, this may put the child off using it.

BLADDER CONTROL

Urine control can take longer than bowel control, because there isn't much gap between a child recognizing the feeling of a full bladder and the urge to go. It can be a good idea to have a few practice runs before starting potty training for real. Choose a morning or afternoon when you and your child are at home together. Leave the nappy off (perhaps after the first change of the day, or after the afternoon nap) and tell the child that he or she can use the potty for wees as well as poos. Don't make a big deal out of it: be as low-key as you can.

While playing, ask the child from time to time if he or she needs to use the potty – it is also helpful to sit your child on the potty before and after naps, after meals and if he or she hasn't had a wee for a couple of hours. If there is an accident – as there almost certainly will be – be sure not to criticise or tell your child off. If he or she was

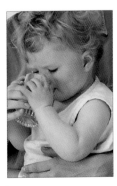

Left: Giving your child plenty of water to drink will give more opportunity to practise bladder-control and potty training. If you are trying to achieve night-time dryness, however, limit their liquid intake after tea time or supper time.

heading for the potty, give your child credit for trying – say, 'Well done for trying; next time you'll get to the potty in time.' Once you are having more successes than accidents, set aside a few days when there isn't much happening. Take your child to choose some new cotton pants for themselves (or trainer pants if you prefer). If he or she is excited about wearing these special pants, this will help to make potty training fun.

Most parents find it helpful to limit outside activities during potty training, but you can't stay home for days on end with an active toddler. Instead, make outings short, manageable and at child-friendly places; go to the local park or a good friend's house: get your child to use the potty before you go and take a travel potty with you, or use trainer pants.

NIGHT-TIME DRYNESS

Staying dry through the night nearly always takes longer to achieve than day-time dryness. Wait until you notice that your child's nappy has stayed dry for a few nights in a row before you begin (it's a good idea to give praise for waking up dry, even if the child is wearing nappies). Then try washable trainer pants or just go straight to pyjamas. Use a mattress protector on the bed and expect a few accidents. It will help to limit them if you encourage your child to use the potty just before bedtime and restrict drinks after suppertime.

Teach about hygiene at the same time as you potty train and get the child to wash his or her hands properly after using the potty.

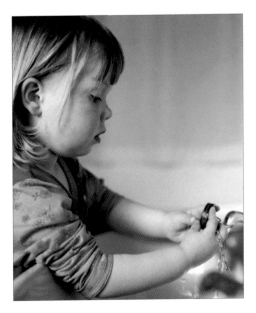

Toilet training problems and special circumstances

The process of toilet training can sometimes create a lot of tension. Parents may feel bad if their child is the last in a group to be toilet trained, or they may be under pressure from family members who insist that their children were trained before the age of two. It is important to know that some children (particularly boys) are not ready for potty training until they are over three. If in doubt, it is better to wait than to force the pace.

If you feel anxious about toilet training, it is worth seeking reassurance and advice on how to proceed. Remember that lots of children have problems with potty training, and an experienced health professional will almost certainly have already encountered any problem that your child has.

SETBACKS

Even children who have been successfully potty trained can start having accidents again, or suddenly refuse to use the potty. This can sometimes be due to a physical problem, such as a urinary infection, so see a doctor to check if this is the case.

If your child is in daycare, take several changes of pants and clothes when you are potty training. Discuss your method with nursery staff to avoid giving conflicting messages or using different terminology.

More often, setbacks are the result of emotional upset, such as the child being unsettled by an event such as a house move. Deal with the mess as calmly as you can and consider whether you need to offer some extra help for a while. Your child may want you to stay with him or her while using the potty, or something may be needed to refocus the child's attention – new pants, for example, or some stickers for the potty, and probably lots of extra loving attention too. If the problem persists for longer than a week or two, you may want to consider going back to nappies for a while and starting potty training afresh in a few weeks. Seek advice from your health visitor.

Children sometimes have a sudden increase in accidents simply because the activity they are involved with is more interesting than going to use the potty. If you think this is what is behind an apparent step backwards, say that it is not right to wait; your child must use the potty when he or she needs to go. Revert to asking often whether the child needs a wee, and put him or her on the potty at regular intervals for a while. But don't get angry.

SOILING

Some children may hold back from doing a bowel movement because they are frightened of doing it in the potty. Eventually they will soil themselves, because they can't hold on forever, and this adds to their distress. Be

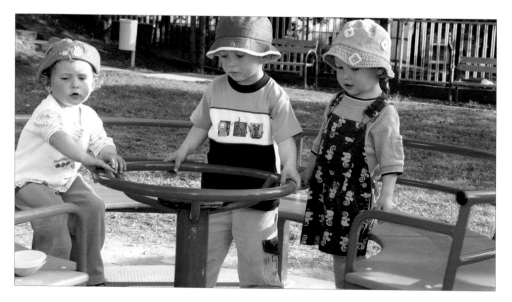

TRAINING TWINS

If you have twins, you may find it easier to train one before the other, or to train them simultaneously. Both methods can work well, so long as the children are ready for potty training when you start, are treated as individuals and their progress is not compared. You will need two potties, and it may be a good idea to get them in different colours and to let each twin personalize their own. However, some twins will want potties that are exactly the same.

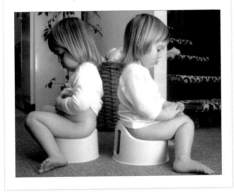

calmly sympathetic as you clean the child up and explain briefly that this happened because he or she held on. This may be enough to prevent it happening again. Children are more likely to do it if they are unsettled, so give extra attention and cuddles. Again, it can help if you stay with a child who is using the potty, and if you let the child leave the room to play before you flush the faeces away.

Sometimes soiling is the result of constipation, as liquid stools may leak past the hard ones. The child may not even realize that a bowel movement is happening until it is too late. If your child soils regularly and you think constipation may be the cause, seek professional help. Your child may need a laxative, but this should only be given under medical advice. Once the initial problem has been sorted, you'll also need to take steps to prevent your child from becoming constipated again.

CONSTIPATION

If your child is reluctant to do a bowel movement in the potty and is passing hard pellets, adding more fibre to the diet can help. Increase the amount of vegetables and fruits, and get the child eating some prunes and dried fruits. It is also helpful to increase the amount of wholegrain cereals and bread. Avoid bananas for a while and give the child plenty of water to drink. Excess intake of milk can sometimes be a factor in constipation, so keep an eye on how much your child drinks. See a health professional if the problem persists.

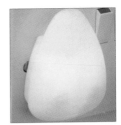

Using a plug-in light in the hallway may encourage your child to use the toilet in the night. It gives a very gentle glow and can provide reassurance as well as enough light to guide the child to the toilet.

BEDWETTING

Many young children wet the bed occasionally. Most grow out of this by the age of five, but if your child is wetting the bed often, you may want to try the following.

- Consider if you have started night-time training too early – talk to a health professional if you are not sure.
- If your child has been dry but has now started wetting the bed, he or she may be upset about something. It's also possible that a urinary infection or threadworms are to blame, so see a doctor if the cause is unclear.
- Try not to be cross. Remember that your child is not doing this on purpose, and the more calmly you deal with the problem the easier it will be to solve. Shaming or telling off a child will only make things worse. Don't accidentally encourage your child either by, say, bringing him or her into your bed whenever it happens.
- Restrict drinks after 5.00pm – but make sure the child has enough fluid earlier in the day.
- Put a cover on the mattress to minimize the damage, and have fresh sheets and pyjamas on hand so you can clean everything up quickly.
- Wake your child up for a wee when you go to bed. Most children will go back to sleep quite easily.
- Make sure the way to the bathroom is well lit during the night or have a potty in the child's room if he or she is afraid to go to the bathroom in the night.

If your child won't do a bowel movement in the potty, but is happy to wee in it, try some extra inducement. Fill a special 'potty box' with small gifts – crayons, stickers, balloons and little toys – and let the child pick one every time he or she manages to do a poo in the potty.

Crying, behaviour and sleeping

> ❝ A good bedtime and sleep routine is one of the key factors that will help your child to behave reasonably. ❞

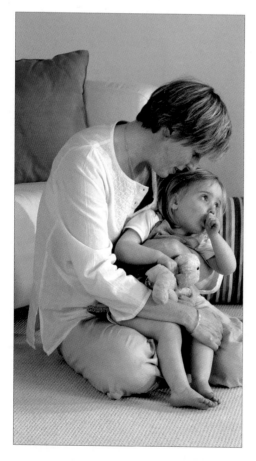

The years between the ages of one and three are probably the most emotionally tumultuous in a child's life. This is a time when your toddler may zig-zag between tearful neediness and fierce insistence on doing things his or her own way. Your child wants to be independent, but lacks the physical skills to manage without help. He or she wants to have you near all the time, but is furious if you try to show the way. This contrariness is what makes hard work of the job of parenting a toddler, but it is also what makes it such an absorbing experience. There are few things more fulfilling than sharing in your child's glee in attainments that bring him or her ever closer to the world of bigger children and adults: walking to the shop, repeating 'Woof' whenever a dog appears, wielding a fork or successfully negotiating the stairs.

Your toddler will be testing all kinds of boundaries, so this is the time to start laying down some basic rules. There are simple ways to help your child to behave well when wilfulness spills over into conflict

Tantrums can abate as suddenly and rapidly as they arise, leaving that furious struggling child sobbing, frightened and in need of a loving cuddle.

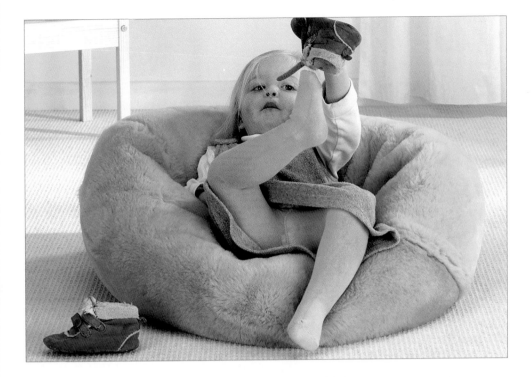

or tantrums. Some children have personalities that are more intense than others, and a very determined, creative or sensitive child is more likely to have tantrums than one who is naturally laid-back or timid. But the way you respond to crying may also play a part in determining how tantrum-prone your child becomes. A good bedtime and sleep routine is one of the key factors that will help your child to behave reasonably. A regular sleep pattern is the foundation of a daily schedule: get this right, and your toddler is more likely to be happy and equable during the day.

In this chapter there are ideas and techniques to help your child manage his or her moods and sleep well at night. Not all the suggestions will work for every child – it is up to you to choose the ones that suit you and your family.

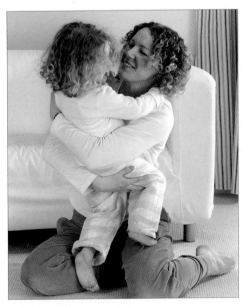

Top: That drive towards independence is ever-present, but toddlers don't understand the easiest way to go about things and need lots of tactful help.

Although parenting a toddler can be hard work, it is fantastically rewarding too. Nothing beats the affection you get from your child.

crying, behaviour and sleeping   377

Why toddlers cry

Toddlers may cry several times a day, and their upset may seem out of all proportion to the cause. But it is important to remember that your toddler simply isn't equipped to deal with difficulties yet. Young children don't have the experience to know that what they are feeling is rage, still less that it will soon pass. Crying is the only way they have of coping with unpleasant emotions. It is also still a key mode of communication, since they can't express their needs or feelings accurately with their limited vocabulary.

FRUSTRATION
There is a huge gap between the things your toddler wants to do and what he or she can manage. Frustration can be positive because it helps to spur a child on to new developmental achievements. But it isn't a comfortable feeling and it can quickly lead to tears of rage. Your toddler will also feel frustrated when prevented from doing something that is enjoyable – a small child doesn't understand, after all, why drawing on walls is bad or why he or she should have to get out of the bath.

FEAR, ANXIETY AND LACK OF ATTENTION
The world can seem a strange and overwhelming place to a young child. Toddlers often develop a fear of, say, the bath, dogs, the dark or certain noises, and will cry when they encounter them. Separation anxiety is normal in toddlers, who want to stay close to their carers and resist being left with other people. Your toddler may no longer cry when you leave a room, but may become distraught if you go out or leave him or her at nursery.

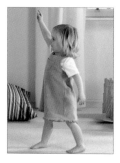

It's important to give growing children lots of ways to release physical energy, it can help to reduce tantrums too. You don't have to go outside for this, try putting on some lively music and having a dance around the house. It will probably improve your mood too.

Most children will cry when they are told off, because they fear the withdrawal of love from you. To an extent, this is a necessary part of socialization, but it is important to reassure children that you still love them even when they are naughty. Young children have an insatiable need for attention. If you are absorbed in another task, chatting on the phone or – worst of all – cuddling a friend's baby, your child may start to cry or behave badly simply because he or she wants you to play.

HOW YOU CAN HELP
Some crying is inevitable, and part of your child's way of expressing themselves, but you can minimize mood swings, and perhaps avoid a tantrum, as follows.
Rest. Your toddler will cry much more readily when tired. Make sure he or she is getting enough sleep and do all you can to help your child relax: a walk in the buggy or some quiet play on your lap can be almost as good as a sleep in restoring a toddler's spirits.

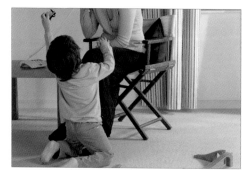

However happily absorbed in a game, your toddler is bound to want your attention the minute he or she notices that you are otherwise occupied.

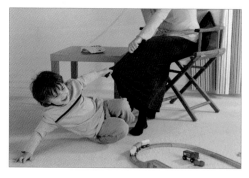

Not getting his or her own way can lead to an increasing sense of frustration and may easily end in an explosive tantrum.

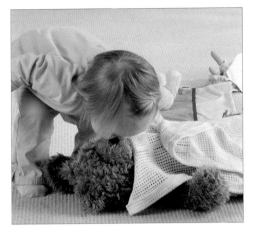

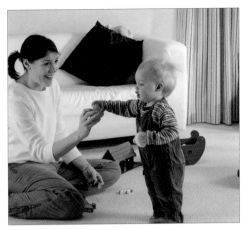

Toddlers have no sense of time and no conception of anyone else's needs. So don't expect them to stop playing just because you need to move on. Give a child time to adjust by saying you will be leaving in a while.

One of the most charming things about toddlers is their desire to be helpful. Your child may wipe the highchair tray or pass you something when you ask for it. This is a good behaviour trait to encourage.

Fuel. Low blood-sugar levels or dehydration make children (and adults) irritable and fretful. So give regular meals and snacks, with plenty of water to drink. Avoid sugary snacks, which give an initial boost but soon lead to a dip in energy and mood.

Physical release. Toddlers have lots of energy that they need to expend. Go on at least one outing a day, more if your child is very active or has regular tantrums. Toddler gym classes are great, but simple outings or indoor activities such as dancing can work just as well.

Sympathy. Be swift to reassure your child if he or she has a bump or is frustrated when playing with a toy. Be sympathetic about any fears – don't dismiss them as 'silly' or, worse, try to force your child to confront the thing that is frightening. Your child will almost certainly get over any fear more quickly if you are reassuring.

Independence. Toddlers are determined to do things for themselves, but don't always have the skills necessary to carry it out. Lend a hand where possible, but be tactful – your child will resent being 'babied'. Offering a few simple choices – does he or she want an apple or a banana, say, or to wear trousers or shorts, can help a child feel that he or she has some small mastery of the daily routine, and will boost self-confidence.

Preparation. Don't demand a sudden change of activity. If your child is involved in a game but it's time to leave, give five minutes' warning, and then a one-minute warning, too, so he or she is prepared for the change.

Distraction. If your toddler starts to get upset, try starting a new game or activity, exclaiming at something you see out of the window, singing a song and pulling faces, or taking the child out for a change of scene.

DELIBERATE CRYING

Toddlers gradually become aware of what crying can achieve and its effect on adults, and realize they can use it to get something that they want – think of young children whining for sweets in the supermarket. At first, this is not so much devious as experimental: your child is naturally going to test all the methods available to see what works and once he or she discovers crying can get results, a toddler is bound to try it on from time to time. It is up to you to differentiate between genuine upset and deliberate whining, so you don't reward bad behaviour.

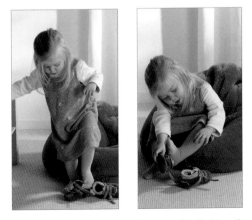

Help your toddler to do as much as possible for himself or herself, even though it is bound to take longer. If a child wants to try putting on his or her own clothes, leave plenty of time to get ready.

Dealing with tantrums

All children have to learn what is and what isn't acceptable behaviour, and this learning process starts early. Toddlers are driven by their own desires and have little sense of other people's feelings, so you can't expect them to know how to behave by themselves. Your child needs clear guidance from you.

Be reasonable. Have as few rules as possible, but put your foot down when it is important.

Be consistent. Make sure you, your partner and any other carers stick to the same basic rules.

Set a good example. If you shout at your child or your partner, your child is likely to copy you.

Encourage your child to ask nicely rather than to whinge or shout for what he or she wants.

REINFORCING GOOD BEHAVIOUR

Acknowledge pleasant behaviour with praise and extra attention and ignore bad behaviour when you can. It is easy to get into the habit of telling a child off for being naughty but ignoring all the good things. If your child gets most attention from you for being 'naughty', then that is what he or she will be. So stop your child from doing naughty or dangerous things, but don't tell him or her off unless it is really necessary.

Avoid confrontation when you can. If your child doesn't want to walk up the hill, say, suggest you have a walking race. If he or she wants to play with a sibling's favourite

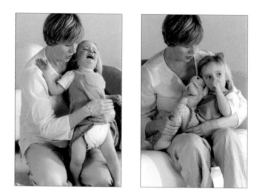

Young children may do best being held during a tantrum; they are then in the best place for a kindly cuddle and calming words once the temper abates.

toy, take it away but give the toddler something as a substitute. If you do need to tell a child off, get down to the child's level and make eye contact. Use a firm, low voice (don't shout) and tell the child the behaviour was unacceptable. Say: 'Hitting people is wrong. We do not hit people.' Don't say 'You are naughty.'

TEMPER TANTRUMS

Almost all young children will have temper tantrums from time to time and some intense toddlers have several a day. Tantrums often start at around 18 months, coinciding with a surge in independence. They may continue until

Older children may throw a fake tantrum. This is usually because they have discovered tantrums are a successful tactic.

If your child has lots of tantrums, try keeping a diary to help you pinpoint what the triggers are and then try to avoid them.

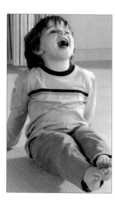

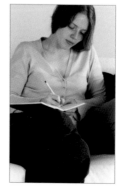

> **TACTICS FOR DEALING WITH A TANTRUM**
> When a tantrum starts, do the following.
> - Make the environment safe so your child cannot get hurt or hurt other people.
> - Some toddlers are helped by being held firmly, but this can make others even angrier.
> - Do not engage: do not talk or argue with your child. Either stay nearby but avoid eye contact (read a book) or remove yourself altogether, if it is safe to do so. Deprived of an audience, your child may call a halt to the tantrum more quickly.
> - If you are out, pick your child up and go somewhere quieter – your car, a quiet part of the park, a different room in grandma's house.
> - Never, under any circumstances, give in.

the age of three or older, when children develop the language skills they need to express themselves. Adults have their own strategies for dealing with anger and fear, some healthy, some not. But all that young children feel is the overwhelming physical sensations that these emotions bring with them – tense body, tingling in the fingers and a head that feels it is about to explode.

A tantrum is usually the result of frustration, or sometimes of fear. It is more likely to happen if a child is also feeling overwhelmed, fatigued, hungry or thirsty. You may be able to prevent tantrums by avoiding key triggers or by diverting your child's attention once you see them building up, but once a tantrum has started there is usually nothing that you can do to stop it: a child in the midst of an explosion of rage is out of control, beyond reason, punishment or reward.

Waiting until the storm blows over is difficult, even for the most laid-back of parents. Most tantrums are awful to watch: children may fling themselves around the room, throw themselves down and drum their heels on the floor, hit out at you and scream. Some children yell so hard and for so long that they make themselves vomit, and others hold their breath until they turn blue in the face or even faint. Rest assured that it is impossible for children to stop themselves breathing for long; the body's natural reflexes step in well before any harm is done.

COPING WITH A TANTRUM

Remember that however hard it is to witness your child in the throes of a tantrum, the experience is worse for the child, who may be genuinely terrified by the maelstrom of emotion that has welled up inside, and who will need your comfort and reassurance as soon as it is over. Calm is the best weapon you have. If you get angry, or show amusement, you will simply add fuel to the fire. And if you

A temper tantrum can erupt in a moment, and is sometimes the only way young children know to release the pent-up rage inside them.

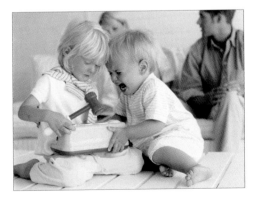

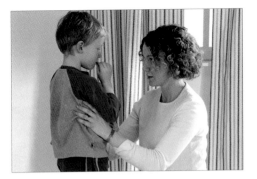

The underlying cause of tantrums is often the child's inarticulacy. As the child grows older, he or she will be able to talk more easily about his or her frustration.

try to draw a screaming toddler into a discussion, you are wasting your time. Your basic aim is to show your child that the tantrums do not frighten you (as they frighten the child), they do not push you into doing what your child wants and they do not stop you loving him or her.

Above all, do not give in. If the tantrum was precipitated by your refusing your child a treat, say, do not suddenly offer it, even if you now think your refusal was unwarranted. If your child learns that tantrums are a good way of getting what he or she wants, there are bound to be more of them. For the same reason, don't 'reward' a toddler for a tantrum by producing a treat afterwards.

Don't punish your child, either. When the tantrum stops, be ready to have a cuddle if he or she will allow it, and say that you are glad the tantrum has stopped. Reassure your child that you love him or her but you don't like that behaviour. Then continue with your day as planned; don't cancel arrangements because your child has been naughty.

With an older child, consider talking about the behaviour afterwards. Your child may benefit from discussing the anger, how the tantrum felt and ways he or she could alert you to the onset of this feeling next time. You will help your child to become emotionally literate if you put a name to the uncomfortable sensations of frustration or anger he or she has experienced.

Think about triggers for tantrums and consider ways to avoid them. For example, if the tantrums occur in the supermarket, make sure your child is well rested and has had a snack and a drink before you go shopping. Keep the child occupied: for example, pass him or her the groceries to put in the trolley. And keep the trip as short as possible. If your child has lots of tantrums, give him or her oily fish at least once a week. It may also be worth trying a fish-oil supplement specially formulated for children: a large UK study found that taking fish oils reduced tantrums and difficult behaviour.

Toddlers and sleep

Most young children need 10–12 hours sleep a night, but this won't necessarily be in one long stretch. If your child isn't sleeping through the night, take heart from the fact that you are not alone: around one in three toddlers has difficulty settling at bedtime or wakes frequently through the night.

DAYTIME NAPS

Most toddlers continue with day-time naps until they are at least two and a half. A one year old will probably still need two naps a day: one in the morning and one in the early afternoon. Over the next few months, he or she will probably drop one of these and the second will probably go a year or so later.

Making these transitions can be difficult. Two naps may leave your one year old wide awake at bedtime, but one may leave a child overtired and cranky by the end of the day. When your child drops the last nap, you may want to try having an early supper and then putting him or her to bed at, say, 6.00 instead of 7.00 pm. Be patient at this time, it won't last long. Arrange a quiet interlude at the time when the nap used to be. Your toddler may be happy to lie on the bed for a while, or sit down for a story.

HOW MUCH SLEEP?

Children vary in how much sleep they need, but this is how long an average toddler will sleep over a 24-hour period:

At one year – 13.5 hours
At two years – 13 hours
At three years – 12 hours

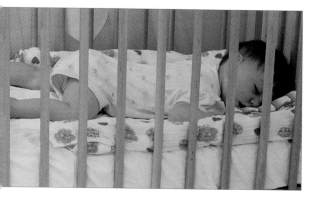

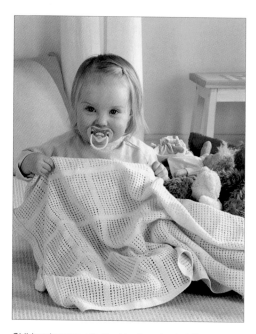

Children become attached to dummies but they can interfere with speech development. Using them at nap times only will make it easier to get rid of them later on.

MOVING INTO A BIG BED

A toddler can move from a cot to a proper bed any time between the ages of 18 months and three and a half years. There is no rush – it's better to wait until your child is keen to try a big bed rather than to push him or her into it too soon. If your child has learned to climb out of the cot, but isn't ready for a bed, make sure the mattress is on the lowest level and check that he or she is not using toys as steps. Put a duvet on the floor to provide a soft landing and move any furniture away. Consider keeping the side down so the child can climb out safely. But if your child can easily climb out of the cot, or is too big to sleep comfortably in it, it is probably time to make the move. It is also a good idea to move your child into a bed before you start night-time potty training, since he or she may need to get up in the night.

Most toddlers will carry on needing a sleep during the day, to ensure that in 24 hours they are getting around 12 hours sleep in total.

Here are some ways to help your child make the move from the cot happily.

- Don't do it when your child is undergoing any other big change, such as getting used to a new carer.
- If a new baby is due, either make the move to a bed two or three months before the birth, or wait until a few months after it.
- Let your child choose some exciting new bedding for his or her 'big bed'. It might be easier to pick this from a catalogue rather than going to a store, which could feel intimidating.
- Put the bed where the cot used to be for familiarity.
- Get your child to help you make the bed for the first time, and ask which toys he or she wants to sleep with. Let the child keep his or her cot blanket for comfort.
- Put a guardrail on the bed to stop the child falling out.
- Praise your child for staying in a grown-up bed at night.

LOSING THE DUMMY

Lots of young children like to suck on a dummy (pacifier) for comfort. This can help to get them to sleep, but prolonged use can cause the front teeth to push forwards in some children and it may also interfere with speech development if it is used during the day. Be clear that dummies are for sleep times only. Don't let your child play or talk while sucking on a dummy.

Experts differ on when you should get rid of a dummy – some say by the child's first birthday, others by the age of three. You will have to judge when your child can lose a dummy without causing undue distress. Most children become less interested in their dummies as they grow up,

Moving into a big bed is an important transition that you want your toddler to feel good about. Don't move a child because you are having another baby and need the cot. Borrow or buy a second cot (get a new mattress) rather than oust your toddler too soon.

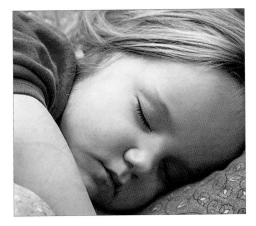

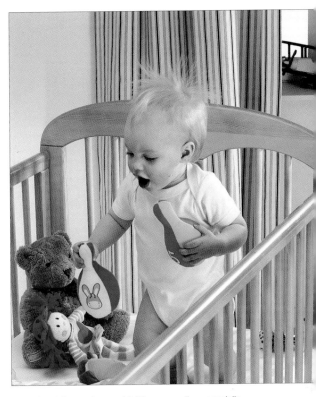

Lots of toddlers wake up at 6.00am or earlier, especially if they sleep through the night. The best solution is probably to go to bed earlier yourself. But your toddler may be happy to play for a while if you leave a different interesting toy in the cot each night.

so your child's dependence on the dummy may be lessening naturally. Try putting him or her down to sleep without it from time to time. If this works, simply offer the dummy less and less frequently.

If your child is old enough, talk about using the dummy. Say that you think he or she is now grown-up enough to stop using it. Ask your child's opinion about this. If the child is clear that he or she still wants it, let the subject drop for a while before bringing it up again. If your child is willing to consider giving up the dummy, suggest that a favourite toy can be used for comfort at night instead. A reward chart – with a sticker every time the child goes to sleep without the dummy – may help. Give lots of praise too. Don't use shame or ridicule to encourage your child to give up a dummy.

Some children benefit from ritual: a dummy fairy may come in the night and take the dummies away, leaving a gift in exchange, or your child could deposit the dummy at the dentist's in exchange for a new toothbrush.

Problems at bedtime

Some children who have slept through the night from a young age start to wake up again or resist going to bed. This is sometimes due to separation anxiety, but often it is simply down to excitement: now that your child can do so much, why would he or she want to go to bed?

BEDTIME ROUTINE

You'll find it much easier to get your child to sleep at night if you have a consistent bedtime routine. This helps a toddler to relax and get ready for sleep. Keep activities after tea gentle and quiet to help your child wind down from the day's events. It is also important to have a set bedtime – somewhere between 6.30 and 7.30 pm works well for most children, but some won't settle until later. If your child is used to a very late bedtime, bring it forwards by ten minutes a day until he or she is going to sleep at a time that works for you both.

Keep your bedtime routine short and simple – it shouldn't take longer than about half an hour. A good routine could be: playtime in the bath, getting into pyjamas, a drink of milk from a cup, toothbrushing, cuddle and storytime, then bed and lights out. Avoid doing anything upsetting at this time: if washing your

Story time is a good part of the bedtime routine, because it gives children focused time with their parent. It often becomes a treasured childhood memory.

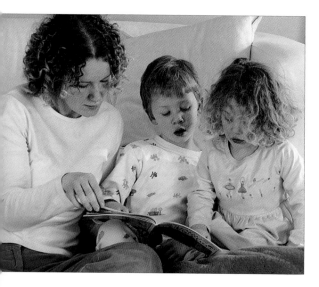

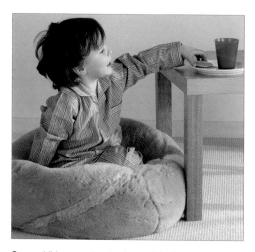

Some children need a simple snack before they go to bed. Avoid giving them anything, such as cheese or chocolate, that may affect their sleep.

child's hair makes him or her scream, do it in the morning. Resist an older toddler's attempts to extend the routine: he or she may ask you to read more stories, say, to delay bedtime. Be firm. Giving some notice of what will happen next – 'After your story, it is bedtime' – will help your child to accept the inevitable.

Make sure that your child has any comforters or favourite stuffed animals that he or she needs to help get to sleep. Get a nightlight or leave a light on in the hallway if the child doesn't like to be in the dark. Some children find it comforting if you say goodnight in exactly the same way each night – for example, 'Night night, darling, see you in the morning.'

GETTING YOUR TODDLER TO DROP OFF ALONE

If you always stayed with your baby until he or she was asleep, your toddler is unlikely to drop off alone now. You may still be happy to stay, but you may find that going to sleep takes longer and longer. If you want your evenings to yourself – or if you have older children who need your attention as well – you will have to make a firm decision to teach your child to go to sleep without you.

Most parents find that they can improve their child's sleep within a week. But you do need to give your child a clear, consistent message about bedtime throughout this time. For this reason, you should start a sleep training programme in a week when you will be around for every bedtime and when your child is not having to deal with any other disruptions to the normal routine, or other challenges in their life. Younger toddlers can benefit from the routines suggested for older babies, but older ones also respond very well to the kiss method.

THE KISS ROUTINE

This works best if your child is in a bed, so that you can easily bend down to kiss him or her when lying down. It could take a couple of hours and several hundred kisses if your child is very persistent. Kiss your child only when he or she is lying down, and don't be drawn into any discussion or play. Say again that you will be back in a minute to give your child another kiss, and do it as often as seems necessary.

1 Do your usual bedtime routine. Put your child to bed and give him or her a kiss goodnight.

2 Say you will be back in a minute with another kiss.

3 Turn away and then turn back and give your child a kiss straight away.

4 Move away a little further this time, then turn back and give another kiss.

5 Now do something in the room such as putting toys away or folding an item of clothing. Then turn back to your child and give another kiss.

6 Leave the room as if you are going to do something, come straight back and kiss your child again.

7 If your child gets up to follow you, act surprised and lead him or her gently back to bed. Give another kiss and then leave the room again.

8 Continue in this way for as long as it takes for your child to fall asleep. Gradually extend the period you leave between kisses.

9 Do the same on subsequent nights. You should find that it takes less time to get your child to sleep as the week draws on. But don't be surprised if you have a few setbacks: the third and fifth nights are often the worst.

THE MOVING CHAIR METHOD

An alternative method to use is the moving chair method. It can be good if your child cannot bear you to leave the room before he or she is asleep.

After your usual bedtime routine, sit on a chair beside the child's bed and turn the child so that he or she is facing away from you. Switch off the light and tell your child it is 'sleepytime' (or whatever phrase you prefer to use) and to close his or her eyes. Then every time he or she tries to chat, simply say 'ssshhhh, sleepytime'. You will probably have to do this many times, but persevere however long it takes for your child to drop off. Over the next few nights, do exactly the same, but move the chair a little further away from the bed and towards the (open)

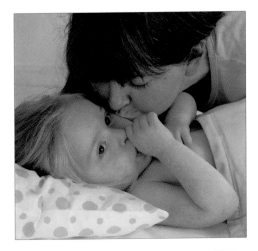

The kiss routine is a gentle way of getting your child to drop off alone, often without even realizing that that is what is happening.

door each night. Eventually you should be sitting outside the door. By this time your child should be able to drop off alone and you can leave the bedroom after you've said goodnight. Go back to sitting outside the door if he or she seems to need that reassurance for a while longer.

Help your child to see his or her bedroom as a pleasant place to be. Encourage the child to play in his or her bedroom and feel happy and relaxed in there. Don't make the bedroom a negative place by using it as a place to send older toddlers as punishment.

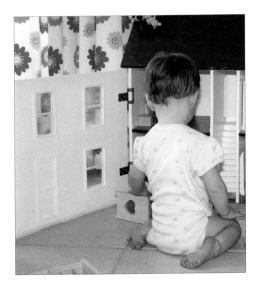

Night waking

It's hard to deal with children waking up during the night. Most of us will do anything to soothe our children so that we can get back to sleep ourselves. If your child is continually waking up and it is affecting your sleep, you probably need to steel yourself to use a sleep training technique to help him or her fall asleep without you.

It's best to start by establishing a bedtime routine first, which may resolve the problem. Give your child as few reasons as possible to get up in the night: leave a glass of water by the bedside if he or she wakes up thirsty, give the child a snack at bedtime and make sure he or she uses the toilet. If your toddler is happy to go to sleep at bedtime, but continues to wake you during the night, try to address any obvious causes first. But if your toddler simply wants your attention at night, you can do the kiss routine, controlled crying or the back-to-your-own-bed method as appropriate. As with any sleep training, you need to make a clear decision that this is what you want to do and to stick with it for a week.

WHY IS MY CHILD WAKING UP?

Night waking can have a straightforward cause and be simple to solve. Before trying any sleep training methods, consider whether your child does any of the following.

Sleeps too much during the day. Try shortening the daytime nap to one and a half hours. Don't let your child nap later than about 2.30 pm.

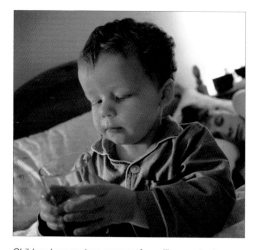

Children have various reasons for calling you in the night. Doing something as simple as leaving a glass of water in their reach can help them settle themselves.

Doesn't sleep enough during the day. Prioritize naptime. If your child won't nap, arrange some quiet time or go out for a restful journey in the buggy.

Is disturbed by outside noises. Consider moving the cot or getting thicker curtains to blot out noise. Leaving a radio set on low in the child's room helps to make outside noises less intrusive.

Is disturbed by you. Don't rush in to soothe your child; wait for a minute or two to see if he or she settles.

Gets too cold or too hot. Modify the bedding as necessary. If your child is waking from the cold when your heating goes off, add another blanket at your bedtime.

Is anxious when alone. Give lots of attention during the day and put your baby in a room with a sibling if you have other children. Consider moving your child's cot into your room, or put another bed in the child's room. When he or she wakes up, soothe your child briefly and then lie down until he or she goes back to sleep. You can then either go back to your own room or stay where you are. You can teach your toddler to sleep alone when the time is right.

Is ill or teething or has nappy (diaper) rash. Accept some broken nights as inevitable, but return to your usual routine as soon as possible.

Has night terrors or nightmares. Comfort your child immediately – don't leave him or her to cry. Put the child back to bed to sleep, but consider leaving a nightlight on.

NIGHT WAKING IN NURSING TODDLERS

Breastfeeding toddlers may continue to wake up at night to feed. If your child wakes often and you are finding it hard to function, the following may help.

- Feed more during the day. Try feeding your child in a quiet, darkened room where there are few distractions.
- Tell an older toddler that you are no longer going to feed at night – sometimes children just need to be given clear parameters.
- Ask your partner to go to your toddler at night. Your toddler is likely to protest at first, and your partner may need to be lovingly persistent in order to settle him or her. This will be easier if your partner first takes over bedtime for a few nights.
- If you are sharing a room, consider moving your child into a different room, or sleep elsewhere yourself for a few nights.

CONTROLLED CRYING FOR NIGHT WAKING

When your child cries in the night, listen to the cries. Go in straight away if you think the child is frightened or in pain. If you are sure he or she is just calling out for you, you can try this method. Remember that you can adapt it: your limit could be five minutes of crying.

1 Wait for a minute or so before you go in. Briefly check that the child's clothing isn't wet or tangled and that his or her comforter hasn't got lost. Soothe the child with a few shushes or by stroking his or her back. Don't pick your child up or linger longer than 30 seconds or so.

2 Let the child cry but go back at increasing intervals to repeat the soothing. Start with two minutes, then three, then five, then eight, then ten, then 15.

3 Keep returning at intervals of 15 minutes until the child falls asleep. If he or she wakes up again, repeat the process over again.

YOUR TODDLER AND YOUR BED

Lots of children get up in the night and come into their parents' bed. This is fine if you are happy with it, and it doesn't affect your sleep, your partner's or your child's. But you will probably find it does disturb you, and that either you or your partner ends up sleeping elsewhere while your child lies horizontally across your pillows.

If you are happy for your child to come in with you:

- Consider setting a limit to give you and your partner some privacy – for example, no toddlers in your bed before 2.00 am.
- Get a large bed that accommodates everyone.
- Put a small mattress next to your bed, and get your child to sleep there. Tell him or her to come in quietly "like a little mouse" so as not to disturb you.

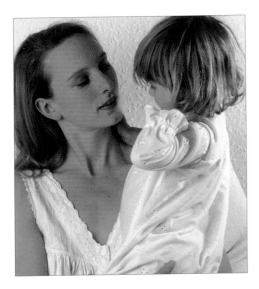

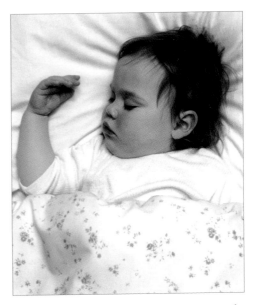

How your child naps during the day can be a cause of poor sleep at night. Think about whether he or she gets too little naptime – or too much.

The back to your own bed method:

1 When your child appears at your bedside, take him or her back to bed. Say it is bedtime, give the child a cuddle and then go back to your own bed.

2 The next time the child appears in your room, do the same thing.

3 If the child continues to appear, then gently lead him or her back to bed in silence. Do this as often as it takes until he or she stays there, even if you have to do it 30 times or more.

4 Don't get annoyed, and don't engage in any chat or explanations. Make sure your partner has the same approach: it is essential to be consistent.

After a nightmare, soothe and reassure your toddler before helping him or her get back to a peaceful sleep in his or her own bed.

NIGHT TERRORS

Some children have night terrors, in which they may scream, thrash about, sit up and look terrified for several minutes. Stay with your child while this is going on, but don't wake him or her. If the terrors tend to happen at the same time each night, try waking your child up 15 minutes beforehand and keeping him or her awake for a few minutes.

Toddler development and play

❝ You will be constantly surprised and delighted by your toddler's skills and attainments and you will bask in the reflected glory. ❞

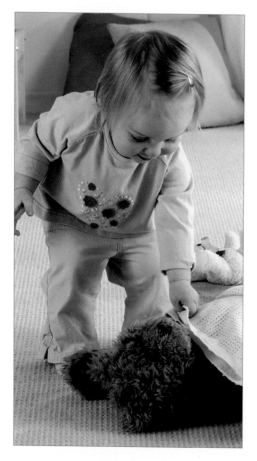

uriosity is the defining characteristic of young toddlers. From the age of about 16 months, your child will acquire an insatiable appetite for new sights and experiences, novel words and situations, and will want to share this new knowledge with you. He or she may exclaim 'Car!' every time one goes past (even if that's every two seconds as you go down the street), or may cry 'Woof!' at every four-legged beast in the park, on the television screen or in the pages of a book.

The world is full of interest for toddlers and it is fascinating to watch them explore as their daring and confidence grow. You will be constantly surprised and delighted by your toddler's skills and attainments and you will bask in the reflected glory when your child succeeds in coming all the way down the stairs, sliding on his or her bottom. This is the time of walk and talk. Your child can now get out of the buggy and walk down the street with you and his or her capacity for language will suddenly race ahead at an exponential rate.

A growing emotional maturity may show itself in caring behaviour. Your child may like looking after a teddy or dolly, putting it to bed, "feeding" it and so on.

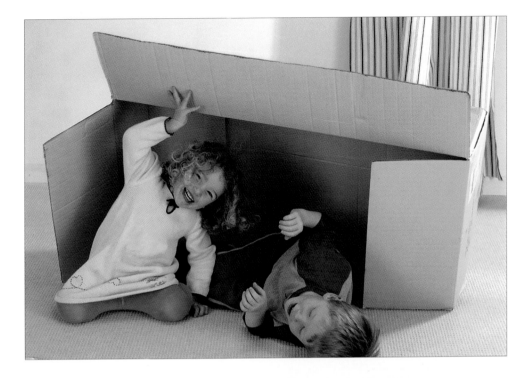

But at the start of their third year, children are in many ways still babies. Toddlers are totally concerned with themselves and do not yet understand about other people and their needs. Yet they already have views of their own about what they should be doing, and will protest loudly if adults try to make them do something they disagree with. This can be frustrating – lots of people dub this time the 'terrible twos' – but it is very natural. Your toddler is learning how to be a separate, self-sufficient person. As a parent, you have the tricky job of policing and keeping your child safe, while encouraging this new-found independence and individuality. Your toddler will frustrate and exasperate you at times. But this age is also fun. Your child's emerging personality will make you proud and keep you constantly amused.

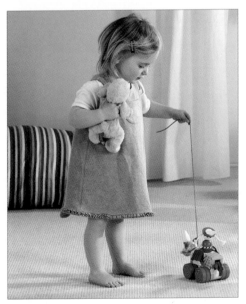

Top: Toddlers enjoy playing alongside other children from the age of about 18 months. An older child will keep your toddler happily engaged for long periods.

A treasured favourite toy may accompany a toddler everywhere for a while, even if he or she is actively playing with another toy.

First steps

Babies officially become toddlers when they learn to walk by themselves. Most children learn to walk when they are between 11 and 14 months, but some children walk as early as nine months and some can wait until 18 months. A child who isn't walking by then is probably just taking his or her time, but it is worth checking with a doctor to be on the safe side.

Your toddler will start walking as an extension of cruising. A gap between two pieces of furniture provides the impetus to take the first step: you can deliberately move them apart when you think he or she is ready to do this. Having been brave enough to take the first independent steps, your child will love to launch himself or herself from a piece of furniture towards you, or, better still, from one person to another – kneel on the floor, hold your arms out and call to him or her as encouragement. It can take several weeks before your baby gains the confidence to go further and walk across a room.

When they first start walking, toddlers rock from one foot to another, keeping their feet wide apart to help them balance. They also hold their arms away from the body for the same reason. As they gradually get steadier on their feet, they walk with the feet closer together. Your toddler will learn to bend and pick something up from the floor without losing his or her balance and will enjoy carrying

Learning walking skills starts early: a baby will enjoy supported standing from a few months old, and, once they learn to step, they will love to walk with your help.

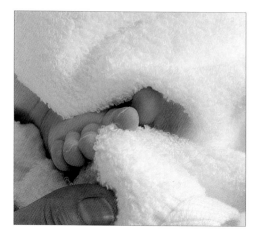

Wash your child's feet every day and dry between the toes – toddlers' feet can sweat a lot. Keep toenails trimmed, or they will press against the shoes and may become ingrowing.

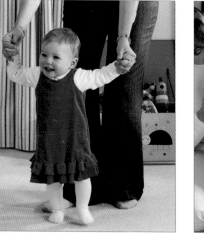 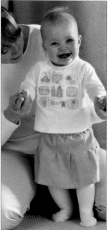

something from one part of the room to another. A sturdy toddle truck will be a favourite toy, but almost anything will be pushed along the ground: a cardboard box, a chair, the buggy. As your child will now be moving more quickly than when crawling, you'll need to watch him or her closely all the time.

Once your child is good at walking, let him or her walk outside. Think of short walks you could do together rather than always using the buggy or car seat. Many parents frown on reins because they think they are restrictive, but they are a good way of giving active toddlers more freedom while keeping them safe.

WHAT SHOES?

Walking barefoot helps to strengthen the muscles in the feet, so don't put your child in shoes until he or she is ready to walk outside. Even then, let your child go barefoot indoors or just put on socks for warmth.

When you shop for shoes, it is very important that you go to a store that measures children's feet properly and offers shoes in different widths as well as lengths. The bones of a young child's foot are very soft so they can easily be damaged if they are constricted by a badly fitting shoe. Never buy shoes off the peg, and don't put your child in second-hand shoes – they will have slightly distorted to the shape of the previous wearer's feet, and

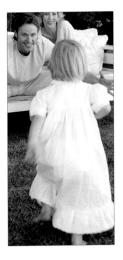

Left: The first steps are short and wobbly. But your baby will be incredibly pleased with himself or herself for managing such an awesome feat, and will be thrilled by your delight in this accomplishment.

Right: Push-along toys can help to give a new walker extra confidence. Later on, your child may pretend it is, say, a vacuum cleaner in imaginative play.

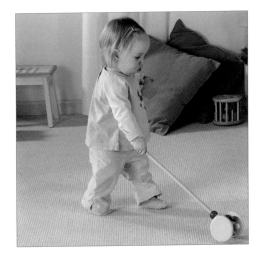

won't give proper support to your child's feet. A properly fitted shoe should have lots of 'growing room' in the toe area, and the sole should be flexible, so that it moves with your child's foot. The shoe should fasten securely with a buckle, Velcro or laces. The heel of the shoe should fit securely: it shouldn't come off the heel when your child stands on tiptoes. Choose shoes made of natural materials (such as leather or canvas), which allow the foot to 'breathe'.

Have your child's feet measured every six to eight weeks, a good shoe shop should do this – and check that your child's shoes are still fitting properly – without putting you under any pressure to buy.

SAFETY CHECK
Your toddler will be able to stretch for things when standing up – which means he or she can get to objects that were previously out of reach. Assess your living space afresh and take steps to make it as safe as possible.
- Don't leave cutlery, cups or glasses near the edges of tables.
- Make sure that carpets and rugs are smooth: a rucked-up rug is a hazard for your uncertain walker.
- If you have a hard floor surface, don't put your child in slippy socks: he or she needs to be barefoot or should wear non-slip socks.
- If older children are playing a game nearby, move a toddler out of their way or he or she is likely to get knocked over.
- Don't allow play with lightweight toy buggies until your toddler's balance has improved to the point where he or she doesn't tip them over.

IS SOMETHING WRONG?

Toddlers walk in a different way to adults – they tend to keep their feet apart, and they 'waddle' because they walk with flat feet. Normally these little oddities resolve themselves in time, but do seek medical advice if you are concerned about your child's feet or the way that he or she walks, or if any of the following conditions are severe or affect one leg only.

Pigeon toes (toeing in). Some children walk with their toes turned in. This usually corrects itself in time, but see your doctor if your child turns only one foot in or out, or if there is no improvement by the age of seven or eight.

Dancer toes (toeing out). Other children keep their toes turned outwards when they first start to walk. This usually improves within a year or so.

Flat feet. All children are flat footed when they start to walk; this gives them more stability. The arch of the foot doesn't start to develop until a child is about two, and your child won't walk with a heel-to-toe step for another year after that. If flat feet persist after age three, ask your doctor to refer your child to a podiatrist (foot specialist).

Bow legs. You'll see a gap between your child's ankles and knees until the age of about two. But if the gap is very pronounced or persists, ask a health professional to take a look – very occasionally this is a sign of rickets.

Knock knees. Lots of children hold their knees together when they walk: a gap of up to 6cm/2¾in in between the ankles is normal. Knock knees usually go by age six.

SOCKS
Only buy cotton socks for your toddler and make sure that they fit properly. Tight socks can be as damaging as tight shoes.

Your young toddler's development

Six months or so after learning to walk, your toddler will start to run, but he or she will find it hard to stop or slow down to turn corners. Chasing a child towards a sofa that he or she can land on safely is great fun and helps to strengthen the leg muscles and improve control. Outdoor games, such as football, will help with balance – your toddler won't be able to kick a ball accurately for a while, but he or she will have a lot of fun trying.

A toddler is hardwired to practise all the movements needed to improve his or her coordination and control. A child who has balance will instinctively squat to pick something up. This builds flexibility in the hips and knees and strengthens the leg muscles. He or she will also practise walking backwards and sideways. Most young children love dancing, which gives an ideal opportunity to practise a whole range of different movements: dance together and incorporate knee bends, swaying, arm movements and different steps into your routine.

The stairs will continue to be a source of fascination. Young toddlers learn to walk up them instead of crawling, but have to bring both feet on to one step at a time, at first holding on to the step above. The next stage is to walk up without holding on, but they can't do this using alternate feet until they are about three. It's good to let

As your child's thinking ability develops, you may notice that he or she pauses before tackling a task to consider how to go about it. Shape sorters teach children about shapes and sizes and give a sense of accomplishment.

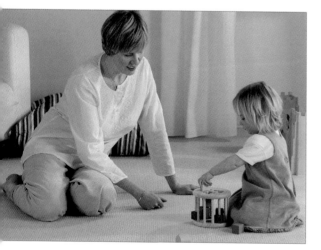

your child practise going up and down stairs, but you'll need to be close behind. A toddler is very likely to pause halfway up and, forgetting where he or she is, may lean backwards with inevitable results. Coming down is harder than going up; teach your child to do it backwards, on his or her tummy. Continue to use stair gates to prevent your child from shimmying up or down unaccompanied.

USING THE HANDS

During the second year, children learn to rotate the wrist, which allows them to be much more controlled in their hand movements. They can build a tower, placing one brick on another: by about 18 months they can manage a tower of three or four bricks, and will be able to add a couple more by the age of two. They can bring a spoon to their mouth without spilling too much food and can learn to drink from an open cup, provided they are given the opportunity.

At the same time, the small motor skills become more refined. Toddlers learn to use just a finger to point rather than involving the whole arm and hand. They can grasp a zipper tag between finger and thumb and pull it open and shut, and can twist knobs on the hi-fi. They learn to use a pencil more deliberately: by the end of the year they can make simple lines and semicircles as well as scribbles.

MENTAL LEAPS

These developing physical skills allow your child to explore the world and to get a better sense of how things work. They go hand in hand with brain development: burgeoning cognitive skills make themselves known in physical achievements, and exploration of the physical world stimulates the child's mind.

Toddlers naturally want to experiment with things, because this is how they learn about them. So they will press buttons on the washing machine, reach for door knobs, and post toast into the VCR. They will test everything – you can almost see them thinking, 'What happens if I press this?', or 'What does this do?'

INDIVIDUAL DEVELOPMENT
Children progress at different rates, but if you are worried at any time about any area of your child's growth and development, raise it with a health professional. You will be invited to a checkup to review your child's progress at around 18 months.

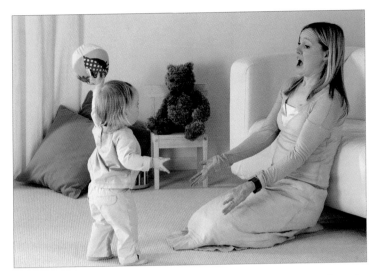

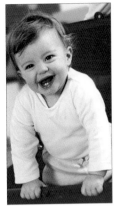

Once they've worked out how to do it, toddlers will love to make you laugh.

At some time in the second year children learn to throw overhand. Give your toddler a foam ball for safe throwing at home.

Memory steadily improves along with motor skills. Your child's new capacity to remember will show itself in play and the ability to anticipate events. If you are getting your coat to go out, your child may follow suit and go and stand by the door. If you were sweeping the floor this morning and have left the broom out, he or she may well grasp it and try to do the same in the afternoon or the next day. This is called deferred imitation.

Memory is, of course, essential for the development of language. There is a huge variation in the amount young toddlers speak, but most are able to name lots of familiar objects and to put two words together – 'Mummy phone', 'Louis ball', 'more milk' – by the end of the second year. You will notice that your toddler's ability to understand you is way ahead of his or her ability to talk – a child will fetch a teddy when you ask for it many months before he or she says the word.

EMOTIONAL DEVELOPMENT

Your baby gradually learns that he or she is an individual, separate from you. Sometimes this feels scary and may make a child anxious and clingy. But a toddler slowly gets more comfortable with the idea. After about 18 months, he or she will be happier to spend longer periods away from you.

A growing sense of self means that a child starts to assert his or her will by refusing to do things that don't appeal – expect to hear the word 'no' a lot. It can be quite sad to say goodbye to the compliant and unquestioning baby you have nurtured, but this new individualism is an essential part of growing up. Your child needs to be allowed to probe the limits of self-reliance, and will do so happily if you provide a loving, stable base to return to. Now, when you go to a parent-and-toddler group, your child will venture farther away from you, returning from time to time for reassurance that you are still there.

Although your toddler's behaviour is bound to test you at times, you'll notice a burgeoning awareness of other people that marks the start of socialization. This starts with you: your child will know when you are sad, for example, and will grasp which aspects of his or her behaviour please or displease you.

During his or her second year, a young child will find it easier to grasp a pencil and make marks.

Children are fascinated by zips, and work out how to manipulate them by about 18 months.

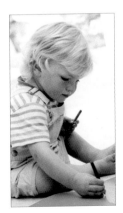

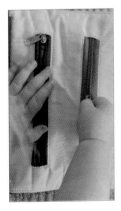

Your older toddler's development

Older toddlers are on the move all the time and they naturally have a lot more physical confidence than younger ones. Their improved sense of equilibrium means that by the age of two and a half they are proficient runners. By the end of the year they can jump off a step. They may also be able to stand on one leg for a few seconds, though they have to concentrate hard. They can kick and throw with much greater accuracy, throwing underarm as well as overarm, and they may be able to catch a ball (though they still miss more often than not).

CLIMBING CONFIDENCE

Older toddlers are much better at climbing, but how high your child climbs will depend on his or her individual sense of adventure. A child who is a natural risk taker may joyfully scramble up a climbing frame or on to a proper chair without considering how he or she is going to get down again. If this is the case, you will need to set limits. If your child is physically timid, he or she may be fearful of climbing. It may help your child to gain confidence if you encourage some practice on manageable pieces of play equipment, such as the first few rungs of the slide ladder, while you stand behind him or her.

If you have stairs in your home, your toddler will by now have had lots of practice at negotiating them. By the age of three, a child may walk up a flight of stairs as adults do, putting alternate feet on the steps. Coming down is trickier, and your child may continue to bring both feet on to each step until around four. If your home is on one level, then you might want to use a friend's home to get your child accustomed to negotiating stairs safely.

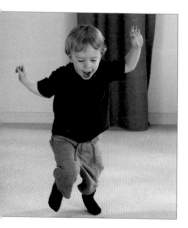

Jumping develops slowly. Most 18-month-olds can't manage to bend their knees and get themselves off the ground at the same time, but they may manage this feat by the age of two. Hopping comes much later.

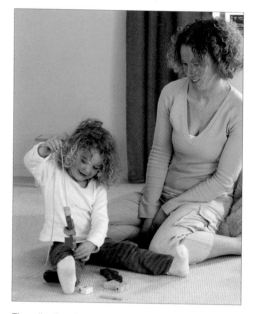

Threading beads on to a string requires a fair bit of manual dexterity. This toy is also great for counting games and learning the names of colours.

USING THE HANDS

At two, children can turn over one page of a book at a time, rather than two or three. They can also thread beads on to a string, provided the holes are large enough. And towers of bricks get higher: they can manage up to eight blocks by the age of two and a half. As children's hand movements continue to become more precise, they are able to tackle more everyday tasks: for example, doing up large buttons or toggles. Get your child to help you with jobs such as setting the table. Tackling everyday tasks will help his or her dexterity and build self-confidence.

Your child will have a lot more control when using a pencil or crayon: he or she won't be able to draw a

RIGHT- AND LEFT-HANDEDNESS

Lots of children are ambidextrous until the age of three. But you may notice that your child shows a definite preference for using the right or left hand when eating or playing.

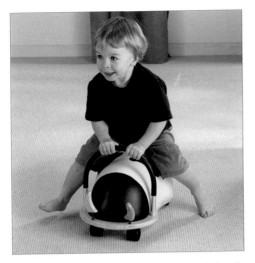

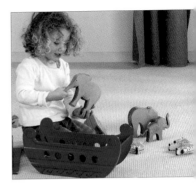

Left: A ride-on toy is good for balance and improves an older toddler's physical confidence.

Right: Your toddler will practise sorting in play: for example, he or she may group toys by colour or size, or put all the animals from a Noah's ark into their pairs.

picture yet, but will do lots of lines, dots and circles. By the end of the year, your child can probably manage a pair of children's safety scissors (supervised by you), though only to cut simple strips rather than complicated outlines at first. Using scissors is a complex manoeuvre, involving forethought, dexterity and concentration. Your toddler will have taken a big step forward when he or she can manipulate a pair of scissors.

MENTAL LEAPS

Your toddler has now garnered enough knowledge about how things work to be able to organize and sort things: he or she may place bricks in a line, say, or put toy animals in one box and toy cars in another. Older toddlers are able to 'think' about things that aren't right in front of them, which means they can be much more imaginative in play. Now your child doesn't necessarily need a toy as inspiration – he or she is able to pretend that a cardboard box, say, is a car or a house. In the toddler's make-believe world, ideas are drawn from everything – the daily routine, the people he or she knows, television shows and story

books. Your child's memory has improved to the extent that if you interrupt in the middle of a game, the child will be able to return to it and pick up where he or she left off. Language skills are developing rapidly and he or she will probably be talking in simple sentences by the age of three. You'll also see your toddler playing sorting games with toys, showing the natural urge to classify and categorize that is a very important skill for life: to function in the world, we need to be able to tell what's hot from what's cold, who is friendly and who is not, what is ours and what is someone else's.

EMOTIONAL DEVELOPMENT

During their third year, children develop a much better sense of the world and their place within it. Until now they have seen everything in relation to themselves. Now they start to realize that other people have needs, too. They also become more affectionate.

Toddlers develop a much stronger sense of self from about two years. This goes hand-in-hand with a new possessiveness. Another important part of the sense of self is an awareness of gender. This starts as early as 18 months, and children are sure in the knowledge that they are boys or girls by the age of three. They may start to behave in stereotypical ways at this point, particularly if they feel that this is what is expected of them.

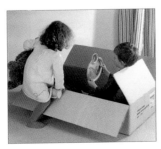

Who needs expensive toys when a large cardboard box can be a car...

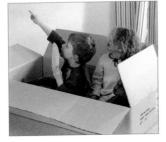

... a spaceship navigating the universe of the living room...

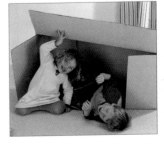

... or a special den in which to hide away from the grown-ups?

An expanding family

Young children love stability and routine, but they inevitably have to deal with change and new challenges from time to time. Probably the biggest upheaval of a child's early life is the arrival of a baby brother or sister, and sensitive handling is necessary to help a toddler accept a new baby.

PREPARING FOR A NEW BABY

Pack away any of your child's baby gear long before the arrival of the new baby. That way, your toddler is less likely to feel that the baby is taking things that belong to him or her when you get them out again. The toddler will also enjoy looking at them all again and helping you decide which toys to put out for the new baby.

Tell your child that you have a baby in your tummy once you start getting large – before other people let it slip. Older children may like to feel the baby kick or to listen to its heartbeat at your antenatal checkups. But ultrasound pictures can look bizarre, so don't show the scan unless you think your child is up to it.

Introducing a second child into your family can have its tricky moments, but your oldest will learn to accept his or her sibling in time.

WEANING A TODDLER

If you are still breastfeeding your toddler when you become pregnant, it is fine to continue. Some mothers decide to feed both their newborn and toddler at the same time (tandem feeding). However, if you decide to wean your toddler before the birth, it is best to start several months beforehand. The most natural way to wean is using the principle of 'never offer, never refuse': nurse your toddler if he or she asks, but don't offer a feed. This can work well for some children, but you may also need to do the following as well.

- Give your child a drink and a snack before your usual nursing times.
- Think about when your child likes to nurse. Change your routine so that he or she will naturally ask to nurse less often.
- If your child nurses irregularly, try postponing the feed and then provide a distraction by going out together or playing a game.
- If you usually feed on waking and at bedtime, get the child's dad or someone else to take over at these times.

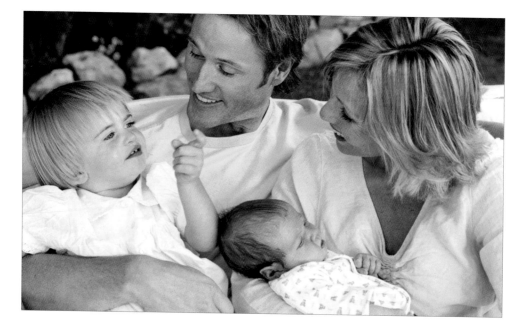

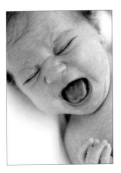

Left: Looking after a new baby and a toddler is hard work, so make sure you get enough rest.

Right: Encourage an older child to play nicely with a new baby and exclaim at how the baby seems to like him or her the most.

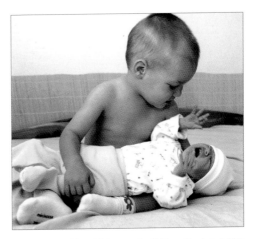

Don't make any major changes to your child's routine near the delivery date. Potty training, or moving a toddler to his or her own room or into a proper bed, should happen either a few months before the birth or once the child has got used to the new baby.

Talk to your child about what life will be like when the baby comes. It can help to reminisce about his or her own babyhood: tell stories about how your toddler kept you up all night. Give your child the opportunity to ask questions and voice any concerns, and be honest but reassuring in your answers – for example, agree that things will be different when the new baby comes, but talk about all the things that will stay the same too. If you have friends with small babies, it is a good idea to take your child with you to visit them. If possible, let him or her see other mothers breastfeeding and explain what is happening.

Let your toddler know who will care for him or her while you have the baby. It is much better to get a familiar person to come to your home rather than sending your child to stay with someone. However, if he or she has to go and stay elsewhere, be sure to arrange a couple of practice runs before the birth. If you plan to have the baby at home, you will still need a trusted person to care for your child. Childbirth is intense and messy, even when it is going well: you will need all your energy to focus on your contractions, and your child could be traumatized by witnessing his or her mummy in labour.

INTRODUCING A NEW SIBLING

After the birth, have your arms free for hugs when you see your child for the first time – put the baby in a cot or basket for a while. Tell your toddler how much you've missed him or her. If you are coming home from hospital, get someone else to carry the new baby into your home so that you can give your full attention to your older child. Look at the baby together. Children often find small babies fascinating, and your toddler may enjoy examining the funny squashed-up face or tiny wrinkly fingers with you. Let the toddler stroke the baby gently, and say how much the baby likes it; show your child how the baby will grip his or her finger to say hello.

Give your older child a small gift 'from the baby'. You can put this at the foot of the baby's cot for your child to discover. You may also like to give a gift from Mummy and Daddy at some point over the next few days – a present can be a tangible reminder of how much you love your child. For an older child, it can be helpful to choose a gift that subtly reaffirms his or her place in the home, such as a new duvet cover or a special cup. Remind grandparents and close friends to say hello to your older child before cooing over the newborn. If they are bringing a gift for the baby, suggest it would be good if they brought something small for the older child as well.

AS TIME GOES ON

Emphasize how lucky the baby is to have your older child as a sibling, rather than how nice it is for the toddler to have a playmate. Try not to go on too much about the 'big brother/sister' role – your child doesn't want to be seen as an adjunct to the new baby, and don't expect your child to feel instant love for your new baby. Help him or her enjoy the strangeness of the new baby instead – have a joke about the stinky nappies, the baby's funny little sneezes and yawns. Your child is bound to feel jealous of the new baby from time to time. Acknowledge this feeling and reaffirm how much you love him or her, but be firm that any rough behaviour around the baby is not to be tolerated.

Make the baby's feeding time a special time for your older child too – you can read stories, chat, do a jigsaw or listen to a story tape together while feeding. Let your older child help you care for the baby by fetching nappies or pushing the buggy, and praise him or her for helping.

Stick to your normal routines – bedtime, mealtimes and so on – as much as possible. Spend some time alone with your older child if you can: ideally, go on one outing a week while a grandparent or your partner babysits. Choose something you have always done together.

Helping toddlers play

It is during toddlerhood that children learn to learn: patterns acquired now will stay with them into their school years. But don't feel that you have to hothouse them with endless classes, planned activities and flash cards – too much structured time can be tiring for your child and doesn't leave enough time for imaginative play.

Your child will learn best in a stimulating and loving environment, with plenty of time for unhurried, self-directed play. Play will teach your toddler all he or she needs to know about problem solving, making judgments, being creative, gaining self-confidence, taking risks, developing empathy and – eventually – sharing. Here are some ways to help a toddler enjoy play.

Give your child your undivided attention when you play with him or her. Sit on the floor and do what the child wants. There's no substitute for one-on-one time, and play helps to build a good relationship.

Have fun together. Play is supposed to be enjoyable, and your child will love it if you introduce an element of humour into games.

Follow your child's lead. If your child is playing a game of make-believe, then do what he or she asks you – don't say how things ought to be. If your child needs your help to build a castle, let him or her be the architect and decide which brick goes where. Being in charge of the game helps to boost your child's self-confidence and encourages problem solving.

Don't interfere if your child is playing happily. Wait until he or she needs or asks for your input, and don't interfere or make suggestions.

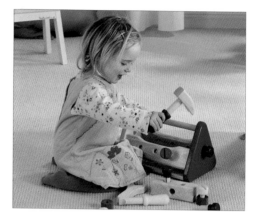

Construction toys are lots of fun, and a kit like this will cover several months of your toddler's development.

BALANCING A CHILD'S PERSONALITY TRAITS

By the time your child is two you may have a clear idea of his or her personality. Your child needs to be loved for who he or she is, but you can still use playtime constructively. If your child can't concentrate for long, for example, help by choosing an activity that he or she enjoys and then praising the child for sticking with it. Look out for the moment when the child gets bored and alter the activity slightly to reignite his or her interest.

Children are often interested in counting at an early age. They may be quick to recognize numbers long before they understand what they are for.

Rough and tumble is good for children, so long as they are enjoying it. It can help to make girls more physically confident and can help boys to manage aggression.

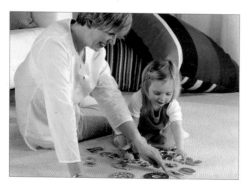

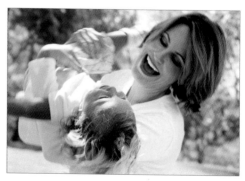

TODDLERS AND TELEVISION

Television has a mesmerizing effect, so it is tempting to allow your child to watch it when you need a break. But watching a lot of television on a regular basis can affect a toddler's ability to concentrate. A study by the American Academy of Pediatrics found that the likelihood of a child developing attention problems at school went up by 10 per cent for every hour of television watched each day – so a child watching three hours a day was 30 per cent more likely to have attention deficit disorder (ADD) by the age of seven. Excessive television at an early age has also been linked to obesity and aggression.

- Don't put a child under two in front of the television. Many children this age won't be interested in watching anyway.
- Limit older toddlers to 30 minutes at a time.
- Choose your child's viewing carefully. Children's programmes often have an educational theme and most children prefer them to adult programmes.
- Be wary of allowing your child to see advertisements. Watch videos instead of commercial programmes.
- Stay with your older toddler while he or she watches a programme and talk about it afterwards.
- Never have the television on in the background while your child is playing.

YOUR CHILD'S TOYS

Toys are more inviting if they are organized than if they are piled in a messy heap. Make tidying up part of play – your child can have just as much fun putting toys back in the box as emptying it. It's a good idea to rotate toys: if you put some away in a cupboard for a while your child will be much more interested in them when they reappear.

Provide some creative play materials, such as play dough or clay, paints, craft materials and dressing-up clothes. Let your child play with natural materials, such as snow, sand, water, mud and grass, as much as possible. Don't feel that you need to invest in electronic

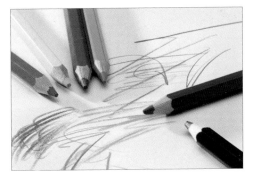

Making marks on paper is something that most children love to do, and it is an important precursor of writing, so keep chunky pencils, crayons and paper at hand.

'educational' toys. High-tech toys are very appealing to young children, but flashing lights and robotic sounds offer less potential for creative play than simple toys and play materials.

Encourage your child to play with a wide range of toys, including those aimed at the opposite gender. Different toys encourage different skills, so limiting your child early on could discourage some aspects of development: for example, playing with dolls can help with social skills, while using construction blocks helps with visual-spatial skills. Look for books that show, say, girls being brave and boys being sensitive to help your child get a broad understanding of how boys and girls behave.

It is important that your child's toys and books should accurately represent his or her world. For example, most dolls are based on Caucasian people, so if you are black or Asian, seek out toys that reflect your skin colour and make sure your child has books that feature people of your ethnic group. Studies show children can become aware of differences in skin colour by the age of two.

If you need to get on with other things, make sure your toddler has something fun to do. But don't expect your child to stay occupied for long periods.

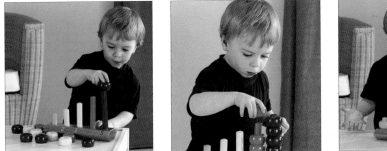
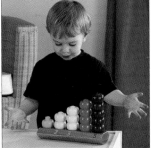

Ideas for play

Give your child a good balance of different forms of play. Toddlers need plenty of running around to let off steam, but they also need quiet activities such as looking at books or playing with bricks to help build concentration. Here are some ideas.

PHYSICAL PLAY

Toddlers have boundless energy, so give them lots of opportunity to expend it. You'll find a toddler easier to manage if he or she gets plenty of physical activity. Spend time outdoors every day if you can. Go to the park, where your child can run, jump and climb. Take your child to the local swimming pool or to a toddler gym (soft room) or go to a dancing class for older toddlers. Take short walks together and point out things that you see, hear or smell – the more children use their senses, the more they learn. On windy days, give an older toddler a length of ribbon and get the child to run so that it streams behind him or her. Some small children take a lively interest in the wildlife that can be found in a garden or park – the woodlice, worms, birds and spiders. You can foster this interest by feeding the ducks or visiting farms and zoos.

If you are stuck indoors with a fidgety toddler, push the furniture out of the way and have a mini-exercise class: touch toes, do star jumps (jumping with legs and arms wide open), run, hop, jump, spin around. Dance to some fast music: your two year old may well have a favourite tune you can dance to. Make a mini-obstacle course: create a tunnel out of a couple of chairs and a blanket, put down large open boxes for your child to crawl through and make a mountain of pillows to climb. For a calming down activity, try doing a few simple yoga poses.

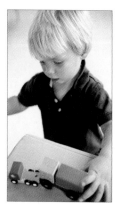

Once children develop the ability to play imaginatively, they can amuse themselves for much longer. A railway set or garage with toy cars will provide fun for many years to come as your child's play adapts to his or her growing abilities.

MAKE YOUR OWN PLAY DOUGH

Toddlers love playing with dough and it's easy to make your own. The dough will last a month or so if you store it in an airtight box in the refrigerator.

250g/8oz water
250g/8oz plain flour
30ml/2 tbsp cream of tartar
a few drops of food colouring
15ml/1 tbsp sunflower or other cooking oil
125g/4oz salt

Put all the ingredients in a small saucepan, place over a medium heat and stir until the mixture forms a smooth dough. Remove from the pan and leave to cool before using.

MESSY PLAY

Making a mess is tremendous fun, teaches your child about textures and encourages free expression. Make it a rule that your child covers up with an apron or similar (an older child's shirt, worn back-to-front, works well) and lay newspaper over the table or floor if you are using paints.

Water. Fill a washing-up bowl with water and let your child play with it, supervised, in the garden. Old yoghurt pots, bottles, straws, a funnel, spoons and a colander are all good to play with. If you have a patio, give your child a paintbrush for 'drawing' on the paving, or show him or her how to step in the water and make wet footprints.

Sand. Fill a washing-up bowl with clean sand. Show your child how to make patterns in it. Provide a small jug of water to wet the sand so that your child can build mountains, make 'cakes' and so on.

Painting. Younger toddlers can paint with their fingers, pieces of sponge, corks, cotton reels or potato printers. Give your child one colour to start with, and then another so that he or she can see what happens when the two are mixed. Your child may also like to do handprints (which make great cards for relatives). Use non-toxic finger paints or powder paints mixed with water and washing-up liquid (to make them thicker and easier to manage). Two year olds may be able to manage a chunky brush (or chunky non-toxic felt-tip pens).

DRESSING UP

Children enjoy dressing up from about 18 months. Make a collection of items from your own and your friends' or relatives' wardrobes and put them in a special dressing-up box, which you can bring out as a treat or on a rainy afternoon. Hats are good; other favoured items are sunglasses, short strings of beads, bracelets and other jewellery (check for safety), old handbags or briefcases, short nightdresses (for princess outfits), old jackets, gloves, boots, shawls and even odd lengths of glittering or shiny fabric.

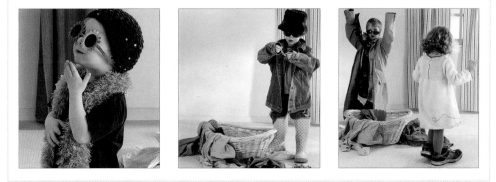

Sticking. You'll need a non-toxic glue pen, plus some small pieces of paper snipped from a magazine, bits of string, wool, ribbon and foil, dried leaves, crumpled tissues, scraps of fabric or cotton wool (cotton balls). Lentils, seeds, dried pasta shapes, loose tea leaves or desiccated coconut can all be shaken on to glued paper.

Model making. This is great fun for older toddlers. You can use all kinds of packaging: cardboard rolls, egg boxes, cereal boxes, corks, yoghurt pots and so on.

IMAGINATIVE PLAY

Toddlers have a natural instinct for copying and love pretend play. It helps them to understand their world and encourages them to use their imaginations.

Domestic play. Pretending to do chores will be a favourite game for several years. Include your child in everyday tasks when you can, such as dusting, watering plants or 'cooking'. Having a little helper may slow you down, but makes housework more fun. Most household items will be too heavy for your child to play with so you may want to invest in some toy domestic items.

Small world toys. Farmyards, dolls' houses, train sets, garages and so on will give your child hours of fun. Small toddlers will sort the items into groups; older ones may start to role-play with them.

Dolls and soft toys. These will be co-opted into pretend play – and may be assigned the role of a naughty toddler. Don't be surprised if they get shouted at and hit: this is how children act out aggression and difficult feelings.

Nearly fill small plastic bottles with sand and screw the lids on tight to make skittles; arrange them in a corridor and take turns to knock them over with a soft ball.

To make a potato printer, cut a potato in half and use a sharp knife to trace a shape into the cut face – simple shapes work best. Cut round the shape from the side and remove the unwanted pieces. Dip the shape into paint and use as a stamp.

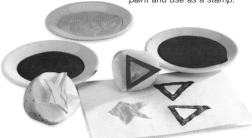

Learning to socialize

Your child's world expands gradually. As a baby, he or she was most interested in you and one or two other important people. Little by little, with your encouragement, your child has learned to interact with people such as relatives, friends, visitors and friendly passers-by. All children need to learn how to get on with other people. It's good to get your child used to being around different grown-ups and other children. This allows a toddler to get used to the idea that not everything revolves around him or her, and encourages the development of empathy, kindness and cooperation.

Most children become more sociable between the ages of 18 months and three years. But they vary greatly in how willing they are to engage with other people. Let your child develop at his or her own pace.

WHEN CHILDREN MAKE FRIENDS
Babies show interest in other children early on, but they don't know how to build relationships with each other. When your baby stretched out a hand to touch another baby's face, he or she was exploring it as much as trying to make friends.

Toddlers often respond to overtures from fun adults or older children. If your toddler has an older sibling or sees another older child regularly, the screams of delighted

Once children work out that it is more fun to play with a friend than alone, they naturally start to exhibit more cooperative and friendly behaviour.

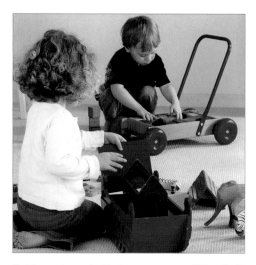

Toddlers enjoy each other's company, even if they don't play together. They may walk side by side, or sit next to each other playing with different toys. The natural instinct to be with people of the same age develops into more collaborative behaviour over time.

anticipation may show just how pleased he or she is to know them. But toddlers don't really engage with children of their own age until they are over two. They start to enjoy each other's company from about 18 months, but at

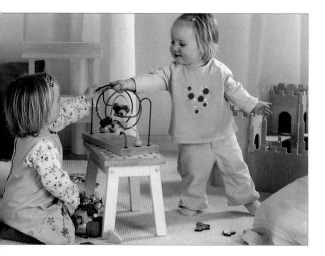

HELPING A SHY TODDLER
Some children are naturally shy and need gentle encouragement to socialize.
- Don't label your child 'shy' or talk about your child's shyness in his or her hearing.
- Keep social events manageable – tea at a friend's house, a small music group.
- Give your child lots of cuddles to help him or her feel secure. But don't withdraw from the group into a corner together.
- Hold your child when a visitor arrives. Ask the child to say 'hello' or wave and give lots of praise if he or she manages it.
- Look for ways to build your child's confidence: increase activities that he or she enjoys and give lots of attention and praise.

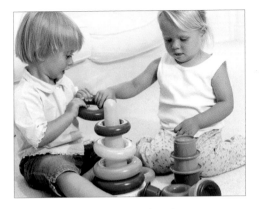

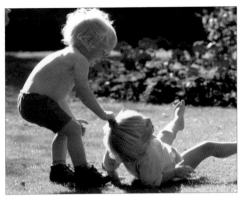

It's good to play games that involve rules or encompass turn-taking. Spell it out – say 'Now it's Joe's turn', 'Now it's Imogen's turn' – to drive home the message.

Violent outbursts are very common and need to be dealt with calmly and promptly. If your child is doing this often, you need to stick close by to pre-empt attacks.

this point they tend to play alongside each other rather than with each other (this is called parallel play). They are drawn more by the activity on offer than their liking for a particular child.

Young children are completely self-orientated. They are not aware that other people have feelings, so don't expect them to share their toys or to recognize another child's possessions: if your young toddler wants a toy, he or she will just snatch it from a companion.

BUILDING SOCIAL SKILLS

It is not until they are about three that toddlers will choose to play with a particular child, regardless of the activity. By this age, children have started to realize that other people have feelings and needs of their own. As a result, they may start to demonstrate some cooperative and considerate behaviour when playing. But playing nicely is a skill that takes time to acquire: a three year old is at the start of this process and won't be very good at it yet.

Adult supervision is still necessary to ensure that the play experience is a pleasant one for everyone. Don't leave toddlers to play on their own; you need to show them how to play together and be within earshot and visual contact to step in when conflict arises.

Encourage turn-taking. Tell one child that he or she can play with, say, the shape sorter for a little while and then it will be the other child's turn. To reinforce this (difficult) message, play games that involve taking turns or being 'out'.

Have clear rules. For example, say there must be no snatching or hitting. Be on the lookout for warning signs – if you can see that one child is about to take another's toy, intervene beforehand. Say, 'Joe, you seem to want Mike's car. He's playing with that one, but let's see if we can find you a car too.'

Avoid conflict. If other children are coming to your home, put away any toys that are particularly important to your child (older toddlers can choose which ones to put away). For older toddlers, it's helpful to introduce some activities that the children can do alongside one another, such as helping make biscuits or drawing with crayons.

Praise children for cooperative behaviour. Tell them how kind they are if they give another child a toy to play with or let another child have the first go on the slide.

Be a good role model. If you speak politely to other people, you are showing your toddler how to behave.

TRICKY BEHAVIOUR

Most toddlers lash out at other children from time to time – biting, hitting, kicking, pulling hair and so on. Like tantrums, this behaviour is mostly due to their inability to express their feelings, and it is a surefire way to get your attention. If your child hits out at another child:

- Remove your child swiftly from the situation.
- Make eye contact and tell your child in a firm voice that this behaviour is unacceptable – for example, 'No biting. Biting is wrong.'
- If possible, turn back to the injured party and give him or her lots of attention. But welcome your own child back with a hug quite soon.
- Never inflict the same behaviour on your child as a means of demonstrating why it is wrong. This merely sends the confusing message that biting, say, is in fact acceptable after all.
- Remember to give lots of praise when your child is playing nicely.
- Acknowledge the other parent/carer and say sorry. Even though most children hit out at some point, it is hard to see your own child hurt – a simple apology can smooth over any upset.

Talk time

Nothing is more natural than speaking. Children learn language simply by being around people who talk to them and to each other. The current thinking is that the ability to speak and understand speech is imprinted on the brain. In other words, all toddlers have an instinct for language. They recognize it for what it is and acquire it without the need to be taught. More than this, they begin to generate sentences and coin words of their own almost as soon as they learn to speak: a child may, entirely spontaneously, dub two grandmothers 'Nanny-one-cat' and 'Nanny-two-cats' to distinguish them. This is proof that children learn not merely by copying what they hear: they are born with an ability to make sense of the pops, hisses, grunts and whistles that make up human speech.

LANGUAGE MILESTONES

Your child is likely to say his or her first word at around one year old. The first words are usually naming words, but some children learn expressions such as 'Oops' or 'Oh dear' first. The words will be unclear, and may not be understood by anyone outside the family: children often

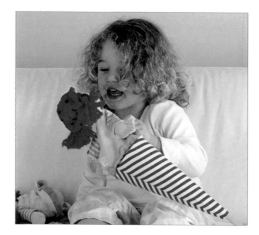

Children may start to use language in play from the age of about 18 months, and as they grow older will act out stories using conversation and dialogue.

BOOKS

Sharing books is a wonderful way of introducing new words and helping your child to understand more about the world. For younger toddlers, choose board books featuring children doing everyday things (going to bed, eating, playing) or animals. For older toddlers, choose books about counting, colours, shapes and sizes. Older toddlers will like books with simple stories or rhymes they can memorize.

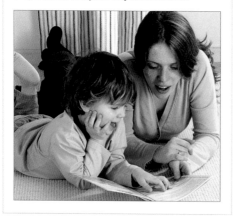

just say the first or last consonant of a word such as 'ca' for 'car' or 'guh' for 'dog'. New words are added very slowly, perhaps just one or two a month at first. But you may notice that your toddler uses the same word to mean different things and varies his or her intonation to communicate more effectively – for example, putting a rising inflection on 'do-og?' to indicate a question.

By about 18 months, toddlers can understand many words: they can point out a variety of things in books and in their surroundings, they know the names of key people and understand lots of what you say. But their active vocabulary – the words they say – is likely to be around ten words. Language learning often happens in fits and starts, and children may learn lots of new words in the second six months of the year. By the age of two, they can be using 30–50 words regularly: 'mine' and 'no' are two favourites. They also discover how to put words together to communicate better. Most children start to say two-word sentences by the age of two – this is called 'telegraphic speech'.

In the third year, the use of language becomes much more sophisticated: children can tell stories, chant nursery rhymes and little songs and hold a conversation. 'Why?' will soon become your child's favourite way of prolonging conversations. At three, children's vocabulary may consist of well over 300 words (some may know up to 1,000 different words by this age). They can string

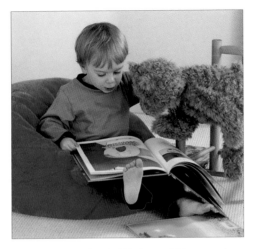

the age of two, and language development often occurs in spurts. But if you suspect that your child's language abilities aren't progressing as they should, then do talk to a health professional. Your child can be referred to a speech therapist if necessary.

ENCOURAGING LANGUAGE

You don't need to 'teach' your child to speak, but you can certainly encourage language development.

Talk lots. Studies show that children who are spoken to a lot when they are young have better vocabularies and higher IQs. Talk about what you or your child are doing. When you are out and about, point out things of interest: the red bus, the noisy pigeons and so on. If you have twins, be sure to address them individually.

Listen carefully. Toddlers' pronunciation is indistinct, so you have to concentrate to understand what they are saying. Repeating back what your child says or expanding on it shows that you are listening.

Don't answer for your child. If you ask your child a question, give him or her enough time to respond rather than jumping in. Don't finish your toddler's sentences.

Have fun with word play. Children love songs, nursery rhymes and finger games such as 'Round and round the garden' and 'This little piggy'.

Talk about feelings. Being able to name his or her feelings will help your child to cope with them. Say things like, 'Did you feel cross when I took your pencil away?' and 'You have a big smile, are you feeling happy?'

Leave books on a low shelf that your child can reach: you may be surprised at how often he or she chooses a book rather than a more active toy.

three, four or more words together in simple sentences: 'Mummy go work now.' They may start to use pronouns ('I', 'you') as well as connecting words such as 'and' and 'but'. Their pronunciation is clear enough to enable strangers as well as family members to understand them most of the time. They have become, in other words, social beings, able to express themselves and contribute their thoughts to society at large.

DELAYED SPEECH

The pace of language acquisition varies widely. Girls tend to speak earlier and use more words than boys, sociable toddlers talk more than shy ones and younger children in large families tend to acquire language more slowly than only or oldest children. Twins commonly experience delays in their language development: they may develop their own language, or one twin may talk for the other. It is quite possible for an intelligent child to say very little by

If you talk to your child a lot about what he or she is doing or can see, you will naturally introduce useful new words. Older toddlers love counting games: count their toy animals, cars, socks and so on.

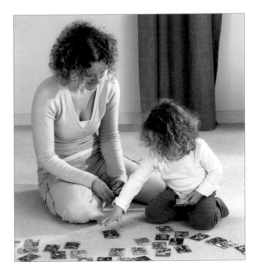

TWO LANGUAGES

Bilingual children learn as quickly as monolingual ones, but they may start by speaking a strange amalgam of both languages – picking and choosing words from each. It may seem that they are acquiring English more slowly than their contemporaries at first, but if this happens they will usually catch up by the age of two. Bilingualism never means that a child grows up less proficient in the language of his or her home country, and a native speaker's knowledge of more than one tongue will be a lifelong advantage.

The preschool years

❝ It is important to nurture your child's self-esteem, celebrate what is special and help him or her cope with things that they find difficult. **❞**

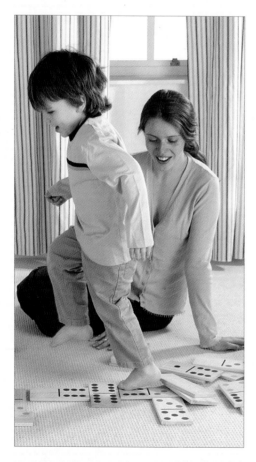

A toddler has very few social graces: when it comes to understanding the needs of other people, he or she is more like a baby than a mini-adult. But, very slowly, he or she starts to blossom into a more reasonable and social little being – someone who can think about other people. From the age of three, toddlers shows the first signs of empathy. He or she is open to persuasion, and any temper tantrums become less frequent.

A four year old realizes that people have feelings that must be respected, and is able to initiate friendships. He or she will share toys, invent games of their own, play for extended periods, and develop favourite pastimes. Preschool children become more aware of the differences between themselves and other people and will start to compare themselves to others. Succeeding or failing, and winning or losing all become more important issues at this stage, and it is important to nurture your child's self-esteem, celebrate what is special and help him or her to cope with things that they find difficult.

Preschool children will still have sudden mood swings, but generally will begin to become more rational and easier to negotiate with.

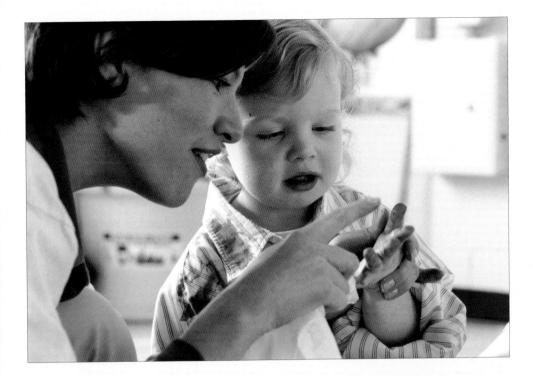

Young children love to learn, and now they have the language skills to help them. These years are a good preparation for the time when your child goes to school. Even the first term at school is a far more structured environment than your child has been accustomed to, so it is not surprising that many children get extremely tired in their first weeks and months in a school-day routine.

Good sleeping habits and a healthy diet, established over these early years, will help your child to cope. Your child will also get a new sense of himself or herself as a member of a group. Mixing with other children in the preschool years helps with this process, and all that play will have given him or her a love of learning that will help in the first steps of formal education.

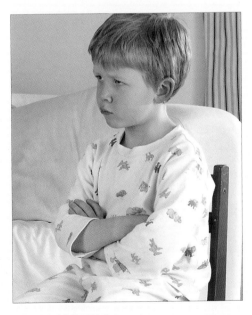

Top: As children's lives develop, people other than you will bring stimulus and interest. Your pre-school child will benefit from these expanding horizons.

A young child is still likely to be unreasonable and grumpy, but uncontrollable tantrums should lessen as he or she becomes more able to communicate.

Food and the preschooler

Young children can be surprisingly sensible eaters. If you offer them lots of healthy foods, they will generally take enough for their needs and select a reasonably balanced diet. So even if your child is one of the many who turns his or her nose up at vegetables, you will probably find that a reliable liking for several types of fruit compensates for this.

Helping your child to develop a positive relationship with food is part of good parenting, but it isn't always easy, especially as your child starts to socialize more. Relatives and friends are bound to offer sweets, crisps and so on from time to time. Three to five year olds will probably be exposed to advertising for junk foods that is deliberately targeted at them. And they are likely to see other children eating these foods, which will naturally make them want to have some too.

The best way to cultivate your child's interest in good food is to involve him or her in choosing or preparing it. Even a trip to a supermarket can be fun.

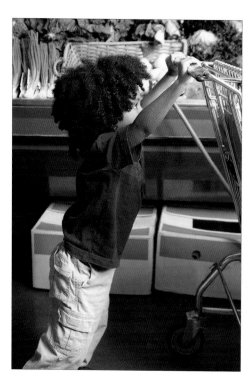

Children learn best by example, so to absorb the rudiments of table etiquette your child should share family mealtimes. Around the age of four, a child learns to handle a knife and fork well, but this is easier if they are special child-sized ones.

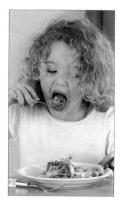

ESTABLISHING GOOD EATING HABITS

To help your child take a sensible and positive attitude to food, you need to set a good example yourself. If choosing and eating good nutritious food is the norm in your household, your children will naturally be inclined to adopt good eating habits. Explain that certain foods are good for you and others aren't, but don't give your child long lectures about healthy eating: he or she will switch off. Instead, get your child involved in choosing and preparing food to help develop an interest in it: let him or her pick out which fruit to buy when you are shopping and do some simple cooking together.

Avoid loading particular foods with emotional significance. People often give children sweets as rewards or bribes for good behaviour or to cheer them up when they are upset. It's better if your child views them just as another pleasant food. Equally, don't ban foods completely or you will make them seem even more desirable. An occasional trip to a fast-food restaurant won't ruin your child's palate.

Choose healthier snack foods: baked low-salt pretzels are better than flavoured crisps; chocolate, which quickly dissolves in the mouth, is better than boiled sweets, which linger. Have plenty of healthy snacks available:

IRON
Some preschool children don't get enough iron. The richest sources are red meat, but eggs, red kidney beans, canned fish, dried fruit and green leafy vegetables are also good. Serve foods rich in vitamin C at the same time to help the body absorb the iron.

BRAIN FOOD

Give your child two portions of fish a week, including one portion of oily fish such as salmon, mackerel, trout or tuna. Fish oils have been shown to help with concentration, social skills and behaviour.

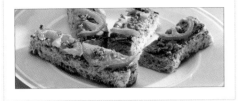

Milk and other dairy foods are still an important part of your child's diet: give three servings a day. A 200ml/¹/₃ pint glass of milk, a pot of yoghurt and a chunk of cheese provides your child with enough calcium.

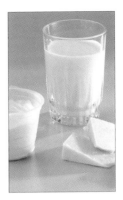

sticks of cheese, fresh fruit, mini-sandwiches, oatcakes, rice cakes and so on, and allow your child free access to these foods.

Give your child lots of water to drink as well as milk. If you want to give juice, dilute it well (one part juice to five parts water) and restrict it to mealtimes. Don't keep fizzy drinks (soda) or sweetened fruit drinks at home. If your child occasionally has these when out, try to make sure they are the ordinary versions rather than diet ones: the latter contain artificial sweeteners (such as aspartame), which are not recommended for young children.

Don't give your child ready-made convenience foods, which tend to be high in salt and made with inferior ingredients. You can make your own, much healthier versions of popular children's dishes: for example make chicken nuggets by dipping organic chicken pieces in whisked egg white then rolling them in breadcrumbs and baking in the oven; grill your own burgers, which are easily made from lean mince, wholemeal breadcrumbs, minced onions and herbs, bound together with egg. Roast thick-cut chips in the oven rather than fry them, and blot off the oil with kitchen paper, if you want to.

CHILDREN AND WEIGHT

Toddlers gradually slim down as they grow up, but you'll notice that your preschool child gets tubbier from time to time. This is because a child's body is designed to put on weight (puppy fat) just before a growth spurt. The energy stored in the fat will be burned off as it fuels the growing process. A small proportion of children put on weight without gaining height. This is the first step towards childhood obesity, an ever more acute problem in modern society. So if your child is overweight, you should address this, but follow these important guidelines.

Don't put a young child on a diet. It is better for a child to grow into the weight than to try to lose it.

Don't talk about losing weight. Don't comment on your child's body in a negative way.

Do increase physical activity. Do something active every day: get out to the park more often, play chasing games, go swimming, get your child a bike.

Do maintain healthy food habits, but still allow your child other treats from time to time.

Do give semi-skimmed milk rather than full-fat milk.

Do give small portions at mealtimes. Give your child another helping if he or she wants it, but never push extra food on your child or insist that everything is eaten.

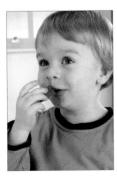
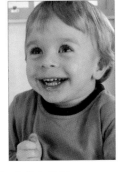

Banning sweet treats altogether is likely to be counterproductive – the occasional piece of chocolate will give huge enjoyment.

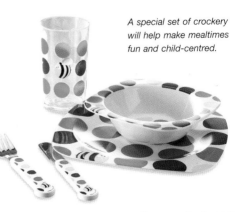

A special set of crockery will help make mealtimes fun and child-centred.

Sleep for preschool children

Many preschool children positively enjoy going to bed. Unlike toddlers, who don't like to be separated from their parents, older children can really appreciate the calm and routine of bedtime.

The need for sleep varies from child to child, but most preschool children need 11–13 hours' sleep a night. If your child doesn't get enough sleep, he or she is likely to be tired and irritable during the day. And your sleep will inevitably be affected, too. To encourage good sleeping habits, stick to a set bedtime and have a consistent bedtime routine. Help your child to wind down by avoiding rough play and noisy games and ruling out television, which can be physically and emotionally stimulating, for the hour before bedtime. Help your child to make a calm transition by giving a warning that bedtime is coming up. While young children probably need a five-minute warning followed by a one-minute

Reading a story together before bed is a wonderful way for your child to wind down and to enjoy being close to you at the end of the day.

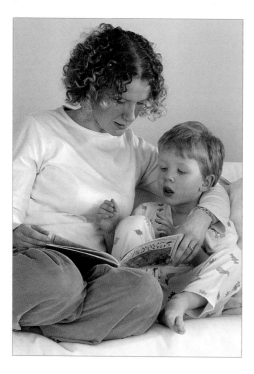

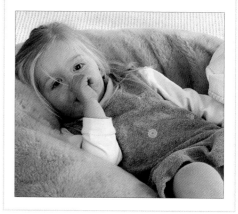

DAYTIME NAPS
Some children continue to have a daytime nap until they go to school, but most have stopped napping by the age of four. When your child first gives up a daytime nap, he or she is bound to get tired and irritable by the end of the day. You can help to manage this fatigue by ensuring that your child has regular meals and snacks and drinks lots of fluid. Balancing physical activities with quieter ones will also help. Some parents find that their preschool children are happy to go to bed for half an hour or so after lunch for some 'quiet time' instead of a nap: this is a great habit to instil.

warning, older children benefit from longer warnings (15–30 minutes), and may want to choose a final activity before the bedtime routine starts. Give your child your undivided attention as he or she prepares for bed. Most children love their bedtime story and goodnight kiss. Bedtime is also a valuable opportunity for your child to tell you about the day or confide something that is worrying him or her.

Be clear that lights-out means sleep time, and don't let your child string out bedtime by asking for 'one more story'. Leave your child to drop off alone, but for reassurance say that you'll be back in five minutes to check if he or she is asleep. If the child is still awake when you go back, say you'll be back in another five minutes. Have a firm rule that once in bed, your child stays there and should call you if he or she needs anything. The exception is needing to go to the bathroom.

SLEEP PROBLEMS

Some sleep disturbances are a fact of childhood: a nationwide survey of American children found that about 70 per cent experienced one or more of the following sleep problems most weeks.

Nightmares. Children between three and five have vivid imaginations but don't yet understand where the boundary lies between the physical world and their own inner universe, so nightmares are common. They need swift comfort and reassurance after a bad dream. It's important to tell your child that dreams aren't real and can't hurt, but you may need to switch on the light so that you can prove that there are, say, no monsters in the room. A small number of children have regular nightmares, which may be triggered by stress, changes in their routine or upsetting events. Helping children to talk about how they are feeling is helpful, and comforters and nightlights provide extra reassurance.

Night terrors. Unlike nightmares, which happen late at night, night terrors tend to occur an hour or two after the child has gone to sleep. They can be scary to witness because the child's eyes are open but he or she appears to be terrified. Don't try to wake your child, but stay with him or her. The child will settle when the dream ends, and won't remember it the next day. Night terrors can be connected with lack of sleep, so making bedtime earlier may help. Factors such as stress and sleeping in a strange environment can also trigger them.

Sleepwalking. Sleepwalking is very common in children. They usually do it an hour or two after going to bed. Don't wake a child who is sleepwalking, but make sure he or

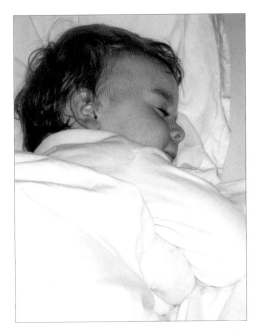

Sleep is essential for maintaining physical and mental health, so it is important to teach your child good sleeping habits from an early age.

she cannot come to any harm. Sleepwalking is associated with lack of sleep.

Snoring. Most children snore from time to time, and around 10 per cent snore often. If your child snores regularly and loudly, and also seems to have difficulty breathing, he or she could have sleep apnoea. In this condition, the child momentarily stops breathing and starts suddenly with a gasp or snort. This stop-start breathing affects sleep, so your child may be cranky or tired during the day. If you think your child may have sleep apnoea, see your doctor for a referral to a sleep specialist.

YOUR CHILD'S BEDROOM

It will help your child to sleep well if he or she sees their bedroom as a pleasant place to be, so don't use it as a place to send them as punishment. A nicely decorated room that is kept reasonably tidy and clean is naturally appealing, and you can choose an attractive bedcover that your child will like – or you can let him or her choose it. Keep a selection of toys and books within reach of the bed, so that he or she can amuse himself when he wakes up. A light that he or she can switch on from the security of the bed can help a feeling of security. If he or she is scared of the dark or has nightmares, then try leaving a dim nightlight on. He or she may have a special soft toy or comfort object that you can suggest they sleep with.

Make sure your child has calmed down before you begin the bedtime routine. If he or she is involved in a game, give a warning that bath time is in five minutes.

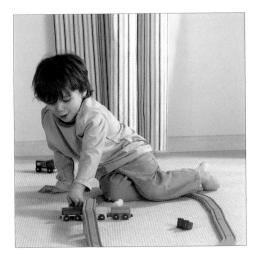

Physical and mental development

Three year olds have mastered the basic physical skills: they can walk, run, jump and climb easily. But can still be clumsy and uncoordinated. Over the next year or two, their balance will improve to the extent that they can walk along a low wall without falling off it. They'll also learn to hop (some time around their fourth birthday), but skipping – a complicated movement – will take longer to master. They may learn to ride a bike if given lots of help.

The upper body gets much stronger and children learn to pull themselves up by their hands. If they are confident in the water, they may learn to swim. It's a good idea to get your child into the habit of having lots of physical activity at an early age, so get out to the park and play plenty of games, chase and so on.

Hand and finger control become more precise: by the age of four, children tend to grasp a pen between thumb and finger as adults do. This allows them to draw with much greater accuracy: a four year old can usually copy simple geometric shapes and colour inside the lines. Everyday tasks such as getting dressed, putting on shoes and washing the face and hands will be achieved more easily, though adult help is often needed. Some children are able to clean their own teeth at four or five, but still need supervision.

Developmental reviews (well-child visits) will check hearing, eyesight and progress, and give you an opportunity to discuss your child's daily life.

Many children learn to recognize numbers from quite a young age and may like to play simple number-recognition games such as dominoes.

WATCHING TELEVISION
Children over the age of three can benefit from watching some television: research by the American Academy of Pediatrics found that children who watched educational television actually did better in some maths and language tests. But too much television will stop them learning through more active play, so limit your child to an hour's viewing a day, of children's videos or educational programmes.

MENTAL PROGRESS
Preschool children gradually gain much better recall of recent events. Their sense of time is also developing, and their new ability to think about future events means that they can start to plan ahead.

Language develops rapidly now and most young children enjoy learning new words. Your conversations will get more interesting and you'll notice that your child starts to use adjectives and adverbs as well as nouns and verbs. He or she will enjoy all sorts of language play: made-up words, silly songs, jokes, rhymes and stories.

Your child can now express curiosity about the world in language, so prepare to be bombarded with questions. 'Why?' is the familiar cry of the preschool child. Answer these questions as simply as you can. Sometimes children ask why? to continue the conversation rather than because they want a specific answer. Encourage your child to frame a genuine query in a whole sentence.

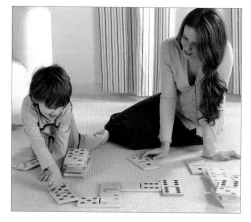

TEACHING NUMBERS AND LETTERS
You don't need to teach your preschool child to read or do sums, but it is helpful to get him or her familiar with letters and numbers. Show your child the letters that make up his or her name: stick magnetic letters or numbers on the fridge. Help your child learn about numbers by pointing out that he or she is playing with two teddies, but only one doll, for example; look at house and bus numbers when you are out and about.

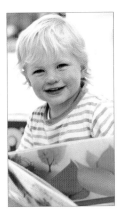

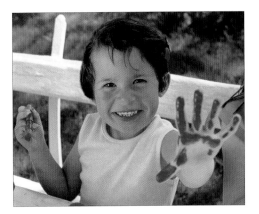

Left: If books are a part of a baby's life right from the early months, it is likely that your developing toddler will entertain himself or herself by looking at the pictures in books, as well as asking you to read the story.

Right: At first, children paint for the fun of it, then they give their art a label. Finally they draw something specific.

TOYS AND GAMES

Choose toys with long-lasting appeal, which can be used in different ways as your child gets older. Good toys for this age group include dolls, extendable railway sets, small construction blocks, balls, musical instruments and non-toxic felt-tip pens. Avoid buying toy guns: a young boy will almost certainly make his own make-believe weapons using his fingers or sticks, but research shows that having toy guns encourages aggressive play. Preschool children enjoy make-believe. They want to play at being other people, rather than just imitating their parents' actions, as toddlers do. Expect to see your mannerisms exaggerated in games of mummies and daddies and to see some rather sexist divisions of labour.

Three and four year olds can get a lot out of playing board games or simple card games, such as 'pairs', in which they have to turn over matching picture cards. These games naturally involve turn-taking, and they also are a good way to introduce the concept of winning and losing. But losing is hard for most children, so it is good to let them win most of the time.

ENJOYING BOOKS AND MUSIC

Your child will get a lot out of story books: look out for books with detailed illustrations that offer more scope for discussion. It's also worth getting a couple of illustrated children's reference books: you are unlikely to be able to answer all the questions that your child has about the world, and it is good for children to see that books offer exciting information they want to know about.

Have fun with music: there's evidence to suggest that active music-making can help with language and mathematical ability, concentration and memory. Sing together (songs that involve movement are particularly good), get your child a musical instrument such as a keyboard, toy piano or xylophone, dance together (a child will love to stand on your feet and hold your hands while you dance), and look for a dance or creative movement class for under-fives in your area. Play recordings at home and seek out live music you can enjoy for short periods.

Your child is now old enough to do some simple cooking, which offers real-life practice in weighing, measuring and pouring.

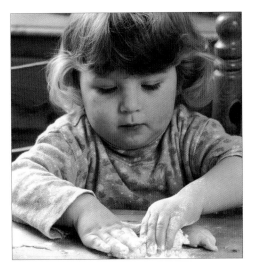

HOW CHILDREN DRAW PEOPLE
Children's representations of the human figure all follow the same progressive pattern. At first, children will draw a circle for the head with two vertical lines representing legs. They may add dots for eyes and marks for the mouth and nose. By four, a torso is usually present and the figure may have arms. By five, the figure has a trunk, arms have hands, legs have feet, and there may be clothing on the body.

Yoga for children

Yoga is a beautiful discipline that involves using the body in a completely different way to other forms of exercise. Children don't have the focus to practise it as adults do: you can't expect a preschooler to sit quietly for long. But they will get a lot out of a short yoga session that focuses on having fun.

BENEFITS OF YOGA

Children are naturally supple, but they start to stiffen up once they go to school and spend most of the day sitting, then spend lots of time watching television or playing computer games. Yoga helps them to stretch their bodies and maintain flexibility, good posture and muscle strength. It teaches good balance, coordination and natural awareness of the body, which can reduce clumsiness. It is non-competitive but can be challenging, so it can increase children's physical confidence.

Lots of the poses are based on animal movements or other elements of nature. Imagining themselves as different creatures, trees or mountains can help children to become more aware of their environment and more sensitive to it.

Yoga works on the mind as well as the body. It induces a feeling of natural calm and relaxation, and may help your child to sleep better. It also builds the mental focus of children, including those who are hyperactive. It teaches that being quiet can be enjoyable. There are lots

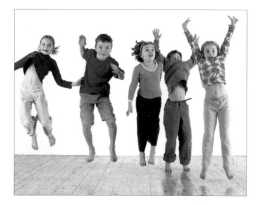

A good yoga class will offer an outlet for youthful exuberance and help children to channel their natural energy in a positive way.

of health benefits, too: yoga encourages good breathing (it may be helpful for those children who have asthma or get chesty), it also helps the digestion and boosts the immune system.

YOGA AT HOME

You don't have to be an expert to teach your child simple yoga poses. Find a quiet area of the home (or go outside), clear away clutter, which can be distracting, and make sure you are both able to stretch out safely. Wear comfortable clothing that doesn't restrict your movements, and have bare feet.

Do a quick warm-up by running on the spot or doing some star jumps to help your child release excess energy. Then try some of these poses: keep the atmosphere playful and move quite quickly from one posture to the next to keep your child interested. Getting your child to make noises (such as barking like a dog) or to imagine what each pose is based on will help him or her to maintain the poses for longer. Try to end the session with a few moments' rest.

CHILDREN'S YOGA CLASSES

A good yoga teacher for children will use the classic postures as the basis for games or to create a magical story: children may swim like fishes or roar like lions. Look for an atmosphere that is creative and dynamic. Some classes take children from the age of two, but most are for the over-threes.

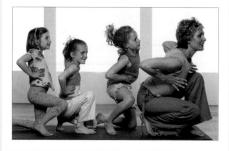

CAUTION

Don't get children doing headstands or shoulderstands – their neck muscles are not strong enough. Never push a child into a posture, or you could cause damage.

Cat stretch

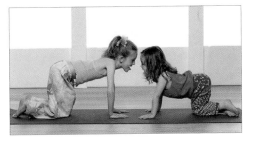

Go on to all fours, on your hands and knees; you are going to be cat who has just woken up. Stretch like a cat – let your head drop down and arch your back and stre-e-e-tch. Now bring your head up, let your back drop down and miaow, miaow, miaow. Do both again. Walk around the room being cats.

Dog pose

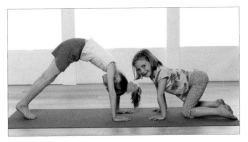

Get on to your hands and knees. Then go on to your toes and straighten your legs: you are a dog stretching after a sleep. Push your hands and your toes into the floor and stre-e-e-tch. Now imagine you see a tiny mouse under your nose: bark to shoo it away. Thank goodness, you can stretch again. Oh-oh, here comes the mouse again...

Roar like a lion

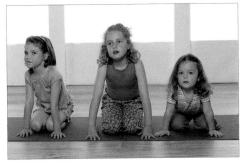

1 Kneel on the floor with your legs together, then sit back, with your hands on the floor in front of you.

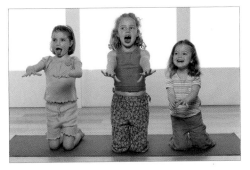

2 Get ready to be a scary lion. Kneel up, stick your tongue out and roar... 'Raaaah!' Hold out those sharp claws.

Bridge

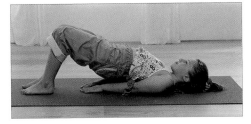

Lie on your back with your arms by your sides. Now bend your knees and bring your heels up to your bottom. Keep your feet and knees apart. Lift up your bottom and turn your body into a bridge: you've got to be really strong so that all the people can walk over you. Keep your bottom up: let the ships sail underneath you. Lower your bridge and repeat a couple more times.

Give yourself a cuddle

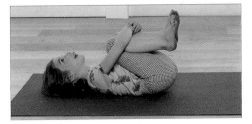

Lie on your back, bend your knees so that you can put your feet flat on the floor. Now bring up your knees so you can hug them. Give them a squeeze – bring them right to your chest: give yourself a lovely cuddle, mmmmmmm. Now try rocking from side to side, like you are a little turtle on its back: ooh this is comfy. Now stretch out your legs again and sl-ee-eeee-p.

Encouraging good behaviour

Small children don't have any real sense of what is right and what is wrong. But they do have a desire to please their parents or carers and they understand that older people have authority over them. You can channel your child's instinct to please you into good behaviour in the following ways.

Set a good example. Children love to imitate, and they naturally think that what you do is right. So you must set an example of good behaviour yourself: if you want your child to speak politely to others, you must do so too; if you don't want your child to shout or hit out at others, don't shout at or hit your child.

Encourage a level of responsibility. Give your child opportunities to help you: wiping up the drink he or she has spilled, fetching your bag when you are going out.

Acknowledge good behaviour. Show that you are pleased when your child is doing things that you approve of, such as giving another child some of his or her apple slices, or playing nicely with toys.

Disapprove of bad behaviour. When your child does something you dislike, say so. Keep it simple: 'You kicked Ellie. Kicking is wrong because it hurts people.' Talk about the behaviour itself as being wrong, rather than the child being 'naughty' or 'bad'. Don't unintentionally 'reward' bad behaviour by giving your child extra attention because of it.

BEHAVIOUR AND DIET
Lots of parents see a link between certain foods and their child's behaviour. Fizzy drinks (soda), processed foods and lots of sugar can all have a negative impact, while regular meals and healthy snacks help to regulate a child's blood sugar levels and moods. Fish oils have also been shown to have a beneficial effect on behaviour: a children's fish-oil supplement may be worth considering.

Be fair. Give your child the opportunity to learn what is unacceptable. A small child may be confused if you tell him or her off for, say, drawing on the walls when in the child's eyes it is no different from the perfectly permissible business of scribbling on an old newspaper. What is more, small children naturally believe that the naughtiness of a given action is related to the enormity of the consequences, rather than to the intention to do harm. So you need to make a distinction between deliberate acts (such as hitting others) and accidental ones (such as knocking over a vase). It will take time for this to sink in, so be patient, forgiving, consistent and persistent.

Stay in control. If you get angry, or shout at or smack your child, you have lost control. Your child may do what

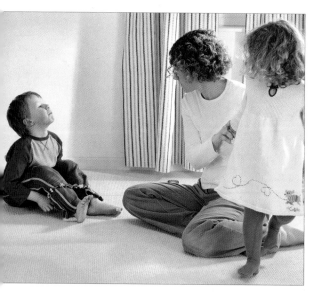

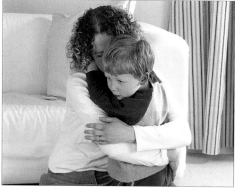

If there has been a dispute between two children, make sure that after you have mediated and reprimanded there is forgiveness. Make space and time for apologies and making up. Don't stay angry for too long on principle. Once you have made your point let everyone recover from it and move on.

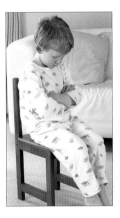

Time out is a great technique to help your child learn that their negative behaviour will have negative consequences. It isn't a punishment so much as a chance for your child to calm down and reflect on his or her actions.

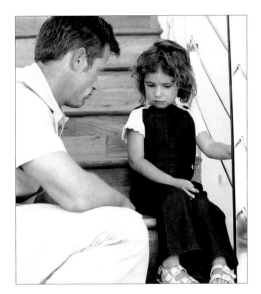

If you need to reprimand your child, squat down so that you are at the child's level. Say the behaviour is wrong in a calm but firm voice. Don't shout from on high.

you say from fear but this won't help him or her to learn how to behave well. If you think you are going to lose your temper, tell your child that you are getting angry and are leaving the room to calm down. And if you do lose it (as almost all parents do at some time), it's best to acknowledge the fact and apologize.

FEELING THE CONSEQUENCES

A good way to help preschool children develop better behaviour is to let them feel the consequences of their actions. If your child refuses to eat dinner, for example, you could try going out and not taking snacks with you. Once a child experiences the consequence of refusing food – being hungry – he or she may be more inclined to eat dinner next time.

The consequence has to be linked to the behaviour, and must be proportionate to it. So, you might let your child go out without food, but you won't keep him or her

out for hours. Keep your attitude calm and sympathetic – 'What a shame you are hungry, that's probably because you didn't eat your dinner' will drive the message home.

THE TIME-OUT METHOD

If your child is doing something that he or she knows is wrong, then the time-out method can be very helpful. It involves putting the child in a safe place until he or she is ready to behave reasonably. To make it work, you have to observe all the steps, in the order given here. In particular, don't miss out the warning stage.

1 Tell your child not to do something: 'Peter, stop kicking the table.' If the behaviour continues, say, 'Peter, I told you to stop kicking the table. You either stop now or go for some time out.'

2 If the child does it again, remove him or her to your safe place: this could be a room with a door you can shut, the bottom stair or a quiet corner of the house. Tell the child he or she is to sit there until ready to behave nicely. Alternatively, tell your child to sit there for a set period – one minute for each year of age is a good formula: a four-year-old should stay for four minutes, and so on.

3 When your child comes out or time is up, ask him or her to say sorry. If the child does this, have a hug and make up. If the child refuses, put him or her back into the time-out spot and repeat until you get an apology.

5 Some children run out of the safe place immediately. Simply lead your child back again quietly and calmly, as often as it takes. Don't lose your cool.

LYING AND STEALING

Telling lies is very common in the over-threes: it is a sign of their growing imaginations and a normal developmental stage. Young children make up lots of fantastic stories because they have difficulty distinguishing between fact and fiction. They may also lie to get themselves out of trouble. It will help your child to be honest if you are understanding about naughtiness and don't overreact to misdemeanours or accidents.

Similarly, you may find that your child squirrels away things that don't belong to him or her. Young children have only a vague idea about possessions, so your child doesn't understand why this is wrong. Calmly explaining that we don't take things from other people because it makes them sad will help. In older children, stealing can sometimes be a sign that the child feels he or she is lacking attention or love.

Sociability in the wider world

Children gradually develop empathy from the age of about three: they realize that other people not only have feelings but may react or feel differently than they would do themselves in the same situations. Once they have made this intellectual leap, they are able to make proper friendships and their social skills improve. With your help, your child will start to show behaviour that is more cooperative and thoughtful.

ENCOURAGING FRIENDSHIPS

Friends will become increasingly important to your child from now on. Going to nursery or playgroup, or having regular playtimes with other children, will give your child lots of opportunities to interact with other children.

Teach your child to take turns and not to snatch things from another child. If small children are playing a game that involves turn-taking, an adult should supervise.

Your child needs to be able to voice his or her needs honestly. Children with good language skills naturally find it easier to manage in group situations, so set aside time each day to talk to your child without interruptions. Encourage a shy child to speak loudly and clearly. When with other children, try to get him or her to come up with solutions for conflict. Say something like, 'You and Mike both want the toy and you are getting cross. How can we make both you and Mike happy?' Suggest taking turns, playing together, and other possible solutions if your child isn't able to come up with any.

Teach your child to stand up for himself or herself when necessary. Young children need to know that they can say 'No' to another child or refuse to give up a toy if someone else tries to grab it. Practise ways of doing this in a reasonable way. But don't let your child think he or she has to do this all alone: children need to know that they can ask an adult for help. Help your child feel secure in a new situation, such as preschool nursery, by introducing him or her to it gradually and make sure he or she knows which adult is in charge in group situations.

Encourage empathy – helping children to recognize other people's feelings spurs them to be kind and cooperative. So say, 'If you take Joey's tractor, he'll be sad. But alongside this encouragement to behave well, let your child know that you understand that doing things for other people can be difficult.

BOOSTING SELF-ESTEEM

Children who feel good about themselves naturally do well in group situations and will also cope better with the challenges of school. Here are some ways to boost self-esteem in your child.

- Talk to your child about what is special about him or her.
- Point out things that your child is good at.
- Don't tease your child about things he or she finds difficult; be sympathetic.
- Encourage your child to talk about his or her emotions.
- Make sure your child knows that he or she is loved even when behaving badly: it is the behaviour that you don't like, not the child.
- Show your child that his or her opinions are important by listening and acknowledging what he or she says (even if you don't do what the child wants).
- Give your child some sense of mastery over a situation by letting him or her make simple choices between two or three equally satisfactory options.

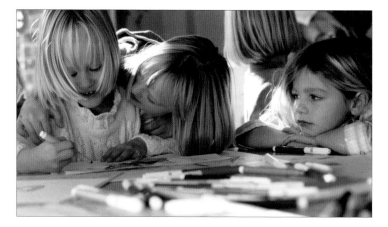

If you feel your child is struggling to integrate at nursery, talk to him or her about ways to start an interaction with someone else: try telling a story about another child who wants to join in a game, and get your child to suggest some strategies.

CHOOSING A NURSERY

Some group care can be beneficial for children over the age of three because it gives them the opportunity to develop good social skills before they go to school. It also sets up a positive pattern for learning. An American study that followed children through their early school years found that those who received high-quality nursery care did better in language and maths. They also tended to have better concentration, were more sociable and demonstrated less problem behaviour. If you are choosing a nursery for your child, look for one where:

- the atmosphere is friendly and happy
- the nursery is clean and well-organized
- the children seem to be enjoying their activities
- the children seem happy to make requests from staff
- the staff speak warmly about and to their charges
- the majority of staff are trained
- the facilities and activities on offer suit your child's personality – for example, for a very active child, look for a nursery with a soft room and outdoor play area.

STARTING NURSERY

If your child has never been to nursery before, it is bound to feel strange at first. It will help your child to cope if he or she is already used to being in groups of children (such as parent-and-toddler groups).

Attend a trial session so that your child can meet the staff and learn where everything is while you are there. Stay in the background as much as possible. If your child seems to be settling happily, then tell him or her you are going out (to visit the shops) and will be back soon. Say goodbye calmly and confidently – it won't help your child cope if he or she can see that you are worried about leaving, and sneaking off without saying you are going will

Learning to manage in a group situation is an essential life skill. Going to preschool can give your child valuable experience of this before he or she goes to school.

MALE ROLE MODELS

Most children are cared for by their mothers, and nursery workers and preschool teachers are also predominantly female. It's important that children spend time playing with their fathers, and that those whose fathers are absent most or all of the time develop strong relationships with other trustworthy male relatives or family friends. This is particularly important for boys. It's also very good for young boys if their fathers read to them and, later on, take an interest in their schoolwork.

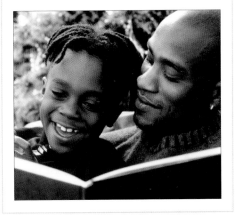

shake your child's confidence. Make a judgment on how long to stay away: err on the side of caution the first time.

Some children need a few trial sessions: gradually increase the length of time you leave the nursery. If your child cries when you leave, call to check whether he or she has settled soon afterwards (most children do). It can be helpful to follow the same 'goodbye' and 'hello' ritual each day to ease the stress of the transition, and many children like to keep a favourite toy with them.

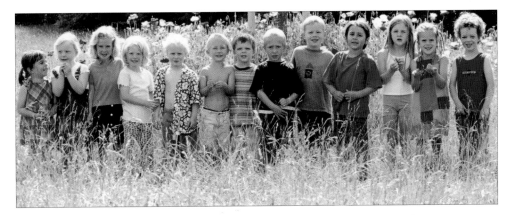

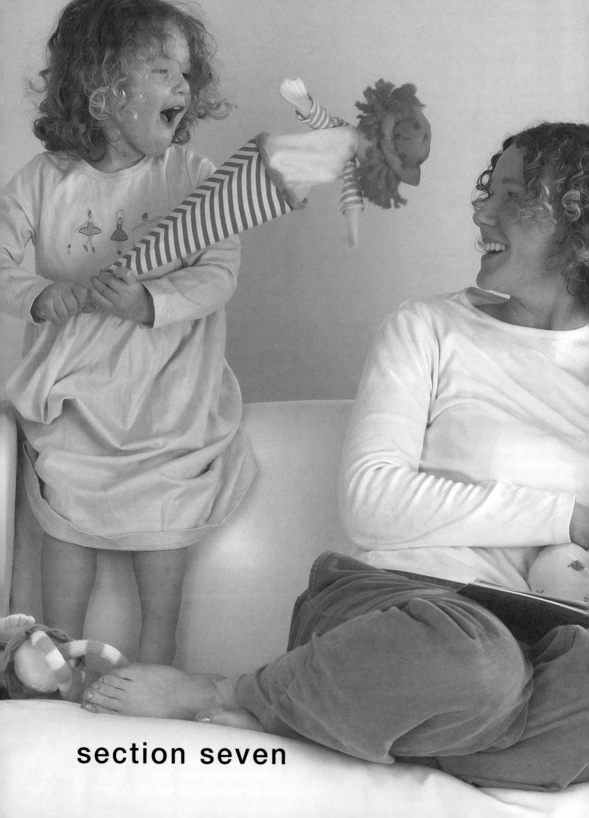

section seven

health, safety and good food

Good diet will help to protect your child from disease, but when he or she does fall ill, as children are bound to do from time to time, there are plenty of natural treatments that do not involve using chemically refined medicines. With health, as with food; what you put into your child's body matters.

Health and safety

“ Children need to feel loved and secure in order to develop good mental health, which also contributes to physical well-being. ”

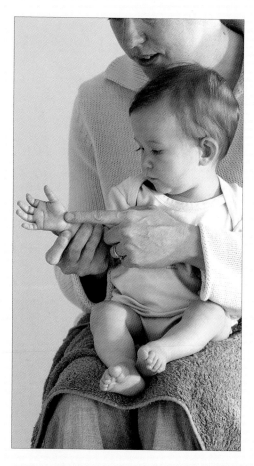

A healthy lifestyle will go a long way towards making your child's immune system strong, so that he or she can fight off bugs and recover from minor ailments quickly.

Give your child a healthy balanced diet of home-cooked food. Using fresh, locally produced, organic produce will minimize the amount of pesticides your child is exposed to and will help to ensure he or she gets as many nutrients as possible. Fresh garlic in the diet is helpful: it has natural antibiotic properties. Encourage your child to drink lots of water. Proper hydration is essential for general well-being, and may help reduce the risk of disease. Filter tap water before giving it to your child if you can.

It's important to facilitate good sleeping habits. Children need a lot more sleep than adults: up to 16 hours for newborns, and around 12 hours for three year olds. And make exercise part of your child's daily life. Most children spend about 90 per cent of their time indoors, so some physical activity outdoors will build muscle strength and get them

Natural remedies such as aromatherapy oils can relieve common symptoms, but check that your child won't react to them by doing a patch test before use.

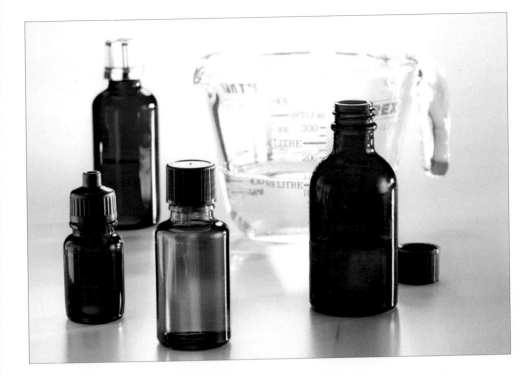

breathing fresh air. Babies benefit from being taken out every day and from spending time on the floor, where they can move their arms and legs freely.

Make your home as healthy an environment as possible, by reducing your use of chemical-laden household products and taking basic safety precautions. Avoid unnecessary risks. Observe basic hygiene when preparing your child's food to prevent stomach upsets, and keep your child away from people with infectious diseases.

Finally, give your child lots of unreserved love and affection. It's known that babies need plenty of physical contact in order to thrive; children, too, need to feel loved, valued and secure in order to develop good mental health, which also contributes to physical well-being.

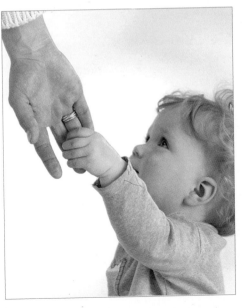

Top: Reducing the amount of noxious chemicals you use in the home is an important aspect of healthy living. For a natural air freshener, try aromatherapy oils.

All parents want to do the best for their children, and an abundance of love and affection lays the foundation for good mental health.

Immunization and supplements

The subject of immunization causes parents a lot of anxiety, but in a sense there is nothing unnatural about it: what you are doing is introducing a small dose of a disease into the body so that the immune system can develop antibodies to it. This is exactly what the body does when it encounters a disease 'accidentally', except that with vaccination the body does not go through the dangers and unpleasantness of illness.

There is no doubt that we all have benefited from a widespread vaccination programme: smallpox has been eradicated worldwide, and diseases such as polio and diphtheria are now largely unknown in developed countries. However, there is much debate about the wisdom of vaccinating very young children. Some natural practitioners say that the standard practice of immunizing babies against several diseases at once overloads their immature immune systems and can lead to an increased risk of problems such as asthma, eczema and allergy later on. And parents worry about the possibility of side effects. Controversy over the MMR jab, which was linked to autism in one British study, caused many parents to decide not to give it to their children. This study has been widely discredited and intensive research has not found a link. Generally speaking, the risk of serious side effects from a vaccine is much smaller than the risk from diseases such as measles.

Every parent has to make an individual decision about what is right for a child. There are four options:

Following the standard vaccination programme. This is what the vast majority of doctors recommend.

Delaying vaccinations. Some people prefer to give vaccinations when the child is older, to give the immune system a chance to strengthen. This may make you feel more comfortable, especially if there is a family history

WHEN NOT TO VACCINATE
If your child is ill, you should delay vaccination. Always tell the person giving the vaccination if your child is unwell or is taking medication. Vaccination is not appropriate in the following cases.
• Children who have a high temperature.
• Children who have a weakened immune system.
• Children who have had an allergic reaction to a previous immunization or who are allergic to ingredients used in the vaccine.
• Children who have had fits.

of allergy or allergy-related illnesses. However, your child will obviously not be protected in the meantime.

Having selected vaccinations. Some parents prefer to avoid giving children all-in-one shots, and choose not to vaccinate against certain diseases. It is worth bearing in mind that single-vaccine injections may not have been tested as rigorously as the standard injections.

Not vaccinating. If you feel strongly that vaccination is not right for your child, then you may decide not to do it

VACCINATION AFTER-EFFECTS
Your child may experience some minor side effects after a vaccination: fever, feeling irritable, and redness and soreness in the injection site are common. Call your doctor if his or her temperature goes above 39°C/102°F. Some children have an allergic reaction after the immunization; for this reason, you will asked to wait in the doctor's surgery for a short period after the injection has been given.

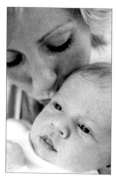

Vaccination jabs are usually given in the thigh. Some children barely notice them; others get upset but can usually be quickly soothed.

Giving children a specially developed multi-vitamin supplement will ensure that they receive the right amount of vitamins and minerals in their diet.

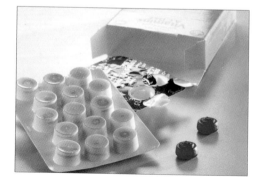

at all. Ensuring your child is as healthy as possible is vital: a child with a robust immune system is likely to react to infection less severely. Seek advice from a naturopath, nutritional therapist or homeopath on ways to help support your child's immune system.

NUTRITIONAL SUPPLEMENTS FOR CHILDREN
Many nutritionists maintain that you can get all the nutrients you need from a good mixed diet. However, the mineral and vitamin content of fresh produce has dropped in recent years as the soil in which food is grown has become depleted. Giving children a daily multimineral, multivitamin supplement helps to ensure that they get enough health-giving trace elements, such as zinc.

Minerals work in combination inside the body, so it is not a good idea to give single-mineral supplements without professional advice: giving a dose of one mineral could lead to a deficiency in another. Giving high doses of certain vitamins can also be dangerous. If you think that your child needs a particular nutrient, it is best to seek advice from a qualified nutritional therapist or your doctor.

Probiotics work to replenish levels of good bacteria in the gut, which help with digestion. They can be very useful if your child has had a stomach upset or been on antibiotics. Fish oils (omega-3), or a vegetarian equivalent such as flaxseed, can be beneficial if your child will not eat oily fish. A deficiency in omega-3 oils may contribute to behavioural problems (including hyperactivity) and conditions such as eczema and asthma.

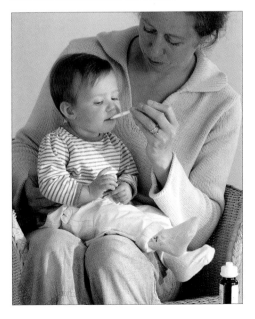

A liquid vitamin formulation, which is gentle on the stomach and suitable for children, can be bought from health food stores; babies can be given vitamin drops.

Natural medication

There's no doubt that modern medicine can be useful when your child is very ill. But it is wise to refrain from giving medication when it is not strictly necessary. Some medicines – such as cough mixtures – interrupt the workings of the immune system. Others, such as antibiotics, tend to be overused to the extent that they can be rendered impotent.

Natural remedies and common-sense measures can be just as good as conventional medicines in soothing certain symptoms and encouraging healing. And complementary therapies can encourage the body's natural ability to mend itself. Parents often feel more comfortable using natural methods to treat their children because they tend to have a gentler action than conventional medicines. But it is essential to take a balanced view. For example, not all natural remedies are gentle: some are toxic if taken in large quantities or are not advisable for babies or young children. And if your child is seriously ill, natural remedies are unlikely to help and urgent medical attention should always be sought.

GIVING MEDICATION

Doctors have different attitudes towards natural remedies and complementary therapies. If possible, find a doctor who is open-minded and try to build a good and respectful relationship so that you can discuss alternative methods. If you know that your doctor generally agrees with a cautious approach to medication, you will also feel more confident about taking advice if he or she urges conventional treatment.

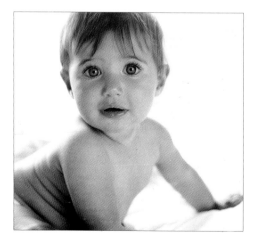

Always ask how a medicine works if you are going to give it to your baby. You should know why you are giving it. Ask whether there are any side effects, so you can be on the lookout for them. If your baby is already on medication – or is taking natural remedies – always mention it to the doctor. Check that the medicine is really necessary in your baby's case. Sometimes a doctor may prescribe medication because that is what most parents expect, not because he or she feels it is essential treatment. Ask whether alternative medicines or approaches could work. Your doctor may be happy for you to delay giving antibiotics, say, for 24 hours to see if your child's condition improves on its own.

When you do give medication, don't forget to give every dose on time. Set an alarm to remind you, and keep a record of every dose you give. Don't stop the medication if your baby starts to feel better. Antibiotics, for example, need to be taken for a set number of days in order to kill the bacteria and prevent infection recurring. On the other hand, sometimes the recommended course is longer than strictly necessary, to allow for a margin of error: check with your doctor whether you could stop a course a day or two earlier.

HIGH TEMPERATURE

The conventional response to a temperature is to give paracetamol (acetaminophen) in order to bring it down again. It is worth considering whether this is necessary, and whether simple natural measures may be sufficient. Fever is part of the body's natural response to infection. It helps to increase the number of disease-fighting white blood cells in the bloodstream, and boosts the level of the antiviral substance interferon. Once the immune system has beaten the infection, the body's thermostat will reset itself and your baby's temperature will return to normal.

A child may have a raised temperature simply because he or she has too many clothes on. Taking off a layer or two and opening a window may be all you need to do to combat a slightly raised temperature. Teething and vaccination may also cause a rise in body temperature.

> **CAUTION**
> A very high temperature in a child can cause a fit (febrile convulsion). In the event of a seizure, lay your child on one side and remove anything in his or her mouth. Call an ambulance.

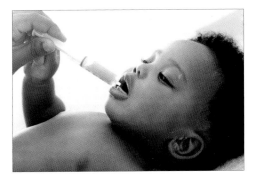

If you need to give a young baby medicine, use a sterilized syringe. Hold it against your baby's bottom lip and depress the plunger slowly so that the medicine doesn't hit the back of the throat hard.

Your child needs a strong immune system in order to cope with all the bugs he or she comes across in daily life. One study found that the more fevers children had in the first year of life, the less likely they were to develop allergies later on. So it may be unwise to give medicines that, in the long term, may interfere with this natural mechanism for dealing with disease.

WHEN TO CALL A DOCTOR
Seek medical advice if a baby under three months has a fever, or if a child has a fever that is over 39°C/102°F, lasts

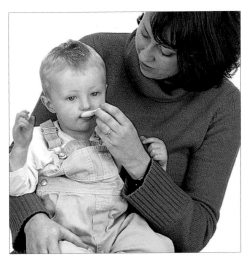

Older babies and children may prefer to take medicine from a spoon rather than syringe; use a proper measuring spoon to be sure of giving the correct dose.

for longer than 24 hours or seems to be steadily increasing. If you do decide to give medication, children's paracetamol (acetaminophen), suitable for babies over two months, is milder than chidren's ibuprofen. Never give a child aspirin, which is linked with the rare and potentially fatal disease Reye's syndrome.

MANAGING FEVER NATURALLY
A fever can be dangerous if it gets very high and a raised temperature can also be uncomfortable. Follow these steps to help to lower a fever naturally.

1 Remove your child's clothing. Turn down any heating and ventilate the room to cool it.

2 Sponge your child down using tepid water; don't use cold water, as this will cause the blood vessels to contract, and so raise the core temperature of the body. Leave the water to evaporate rather than drying with a towel.

3 Dress your child in minimum clothing and, if he or she is in bed, cover with a sheet or light blanket. Give lots of fluid: frequent breastfeeds or extra drinks of cooled, boiled water for a baby; lots of cool drinks for older children. Encourage your child to sip drinks, as gulping could induce vomiting.

4 Check your child's temperature in half an hour, and then every hour or two.

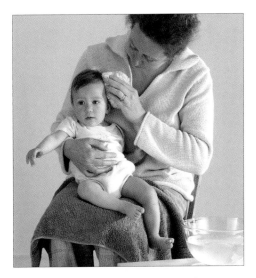

If you are sponging a child down to reduce fever, try adding 2 drops of lavender or chamomile essential oil dissolved in 20ml/4 tsp full-fat milk to the water: these oils reduce fever and encourage sleep.

Complementary therapies for children

Two types of treatment constitute complementary medicine. On the one hand, there are natural remedies that can be used to target particular ailments or symptoms, such as herbal teas and tinctures, essential oils, certain homeopathic pills and herbal creams. On the other hand, there are therapies such as acupuncture, osteopathy and homeopathy.

Natural therapies are holistic – they treat the body as a whole rather than targeting specific parts or symptoms. The body is seen as an organic and complex system in which an ailment may be caused by an imbalance in many parts; conversely many of the body's systems may need to be brought to bear to cure a specific hurt or sickness. For this reason, two children who seem to have the same symptoms may be given different treatments or remedies by the same complementary health practitioner.

There is often an assumption that natural remedies and therapies are always gentle and safe. But any treatment that is effective can be harmful if used incorrectly. Children can be more vulnerable to any side effects than adults, because their bodies are small and still developing. So it is essential to use complementary therapies and natural remedies wisely. Always check unusual symptoms with a doctor first.

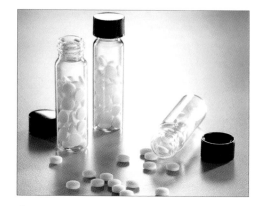

Always check that any natural remedy you buy over the counter is safe for children. If in doubt, or if your child has a chronic condition or severe symptoms, consult the relevant therapist. Check that the dosage is correct for your child.

USING COMPLEMENTARY THERAPIES SAFELY

When seeking treatment for your child, choose a complementary therapist who is qualified and trained. If possible, find one who specializes in treating children. Ask your doctor or other parents for a recommendation (but don't rely solely on someone else's opinion).

Where possible, pick a practitioner with several years' experience and make sure the therapist you choose is registered with the relevant professional association and that he or she is insured. Follow your instincts. If you do not feel comfortable with a particular therapist, don't let him or her treat your child. Beware of anyone promising miraculous results.

Tell your doctor about any natural therapies your child is having: some remedies can interfere with conventional medication. Likewise, always tell a complementary therapist about any medication your child is taking. Do not stop your child's medication because he or she is having complementary treatment.

HOMEOPATHY

Homeopathic medicine uses very gentle remedies derived from natural ingredients (plants, minerals and animal substances such as bee venom). The remedies have been

AROMATHERAPY FOR CHILDREN

Age	Suitable oils	Recommended dosage
0–3 months	Do not use essential oils	
3–6 months	Lavender and Roman chamomile	1 drop per 10ml/2 tsp carrier oil or full-fat milk, or use in a vaporizer
6–12 months	Lavender, Roman chamomile, mandarin, neroli, rose	1 drop per 10ml/2 tsp carrier oil or full-fat milk, or use in a vaporizer
12 months–3 years	Lavender, chamomile, tea tree, mandarin, neroli, orange, rose, rosewood	2 drops per 10ml/2 tsp carrier oil or full-fat milk, or use in a vaporizer

diluted many times over, so that only a minuscule part of the active ingredient remains. However, homeopaths say this is enough to stimulate the immune system and encourage the body's natural ability to heal itself. Homeopathy can be used for a wide range of childhood complaints, including teething, sleeplessness, digestive complaints, coughs and colds. Many doctors refer patients to homeopaths, and some are trained in homeopathy in addition to conventional medicine.

Homeopathic remedies are available from health food stores and pharmacists, so home treatment is possible, but homeopathic remedies are prescribed not just on the basis of the symptoms but also according to personality, habits, build and so on. For this reason, it is usually better to consult a qualified homeopath, who can prescribe the correct constitutional remedy for your child.

A homeopath can also advise you on dosage. The paradox at the heart of homeopathy is that the more diluted the remedy the more powerful its effects: a remedy marked 200c is more dilute than one marked 6c. As a general rule, you should stick to remedies of 6c and 30c when treating at home. These are usually given three to six times a day, depending on the severity of the symptoms. Give 30c for no more than three days, 6c for up to a week, but stop when symptoms improve. Give one remedy at a time.

AROMATHERAPY

Essential oils, distilled or pressed from the flowers, leaves, bark or other parts of plants, have therapeutic properties, and can be helpful for skin problems, anxiety and sleeplessness. But they are highly concentrated so only a few are suitable for children. The best ways to use

Natural and conventional approaches to health are not mutually exclusive and are often used side by side.

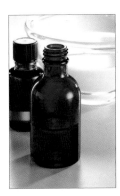
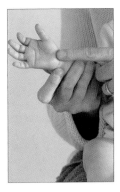

Essential oils should never be applied neat to a child's delicate skin. Always dilute them in either full-fat milk or in a suitable carrier oil before using.

Do a patch test before using an aromatherapy oil in a massage oil: add a drop of the diluted oil to your child's wrist and wait 24 hours to see if any reaction occurs.

them is to dilute them well in a carrier (such as olive oil, sunflower oil or full-fat milk) and then apply the aromatic oil to the skin or mix into the bathwater. Another very gentle way of using them is in a vaporizer.

Always use pure essential oils, preferably those that are made from organically grown plants. Do a patch test on your child before using aromatherapy oils in massage oil: if there is a reaction, it is best to avoid using that essential oil on your child for now. If the skin is fine, that particular oil is safe to use but you will have to test any others in the same way.

Lavender and chamomile are very gentle essential oils and can be used on children over three months.

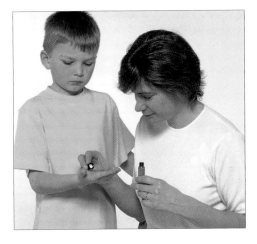

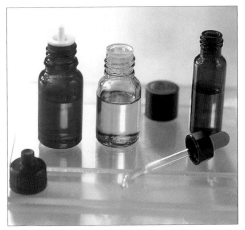

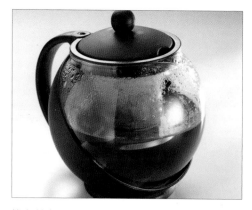

Herbal infusions are a gentle way of giving herbs to a child. The tea should be weak enough to be palatable, you can sweeten it with honey for an older child.

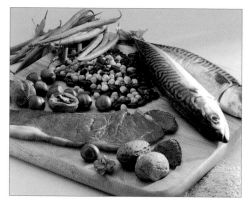

A nutritional therapist can help you to ensure that seemingly healthy food in your child's diet is not the root cause of a lingering health problem.

MEDICAL HERBALISM

Herbal medicine is the oldest form of medicine. Many conventional medicines are based on isolated plant ingredients, but herbalists believe that it is better to use whole parts of the plant – roots, leaves, berries, seeds and so on. The idea is that the many active ingredients in plants work together to promote healing in a gentle and holistic way.

Childhood complaints such as skin problems, asthma, coughs and colds can all be helped with herbal medicine. As with homeopathy, a herbalist will take into account your child's personality and behaviour traits as well as the symptoms when prescribing a remedy.

Herbal remedies come in the form of creams, tinctures, syrups and capsules. Some have well-known effects and can be used in home treatment. But many herbal remedies can be toxic so it is essential that you do not give one to your child unless you know it to be safe. If your child suffers any ill effects when taking a herbal remedy, stop giving it immediately and contact your herbalist and your doctor.

ACUPUNCTURE OR ACUPRESSURE

These Chinese therapies are based on the idea that well-being depends on the free flow of life energy (chi) through the body. In acupuncture, fine needles are inserted – usually painlessly – into specific points on the body in order to release blockages or quicken a sluggish flow. However, the points can also be stimulated by finger pressure (acupressure), and most acupuncturists would treat children in this way rather than with needles.

The principles that underlie acupuncture are very different to those that inform western medicine, but scientific research has shown it to be highly effective in easing pain and reducing the symptoms of common problems such as constipation, sleeplessness or anxiety. Many doctors are now happy to refer patients to acupuncturists for treatment.

NUTRITIONAL THERAPY

Good diet is fundamental to a healthy life, but particular foods can sometimes be the underlying cause of many childhood complaints: for example, a series of ear infections may be linked to an intolerance of dairy foods. A nutritional therapist will help you to ascertain whether your child is intolerant of particular foods, or deficient in certain nutrients.

You will usually be asked to complete a diet and lifestyle questionnaire before the first appointment. A nutritional therapist may carry out tests, and will come up with an eating plan tailored to your child's particular

---

MAKING A HERBAL INFUSION

To make a herbal tea for a child over one year, put ¼ tsp dried leaves or ⅛ tsp fresh leaves in a cup or small teapot. Pour over 200ml/⅓ pint boiling water and cover. Leave to steep for 10 minutes, then strain. Give a small cupful (about 50ml/2fl oz) to your child.

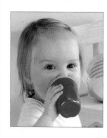

Store the rest in a sterilized screwtop jar in the refrigerator and use within 24 hours. Give no more than three cups a day.

If you want to add the infusion to your child's bath, make ten times the quantity.

NATUROPATHY

Naturopaths use a wide range of natural treatments, including nutritional therapy, herbal remedies and water treatments (hydrotherapy). Some naturopaths may also be trained in homeopathy or osteopathy.

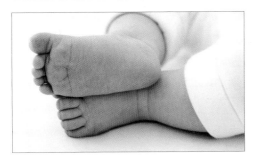

Children can respond well to reflexology, and it is helpful to start when they are young and to have the therapist come to your home so that your child is in a familiar environment.

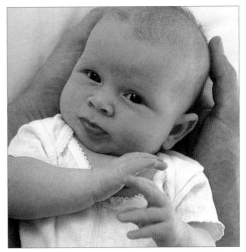

A cranial osteopath lays his or her hands on a baby's skull and uses featherlight touch to manipulate it. If you have this treatment yourself, you will find that you are barely aware of what the practitioner is doing.

needs. He or she may recommend eliminating certain foods for a while and then re-introducing them to check for intolerances. You will usually have to return for several appointments during this process. You may also be given natural supplements such as grapefruit-seed extract for your child to take.

CRANIAL OSTEOPATHY

Cranial osteopaths believe that many physical health problems can result from tiny misalignments in the bones of the skull. They use very gentle touch to manipulate the bones and surrounding tissues into their correct place. Some also practise cranial-sacral therapy, which involves working on the spine and sacrum as well as the head.

SEEING A PRACTITIONER

A complementary health practitioner should take a full medical history of your baby or child from you before starting any treatment. He or she will also ask about various aspects of your child's daily lifestyle and habits: such as bowel movements, sleep patterns, diet, likes and dislikes, and general behaviour. The treatment should always be gentle, and you should be able to stay with your child throughout. After the treatment, symptoms may occasionally get worse for a day or two before they start to improve. Call the therapist or your doctor if anything unusual occurs that worries you. Most therapists recommend several follow-up treatments.

Cranial osteopathy and cranial-sacral therapy are particularly good for babies, especially those who have had difficult births. A baby's head is naturally compressed as it travels down the birth canal, and then gradually regains its normal shape over the next few days. Cranial osteopaths say that sometimes this process leaves slight distortions in the skull that cause tension in the body and may be a root cause of sleeplessness, colic, wind and other digestive problems in babies. They believe that it can also be the cause of problems such as recurrent ear infections, frequent blocked-up noses and headaches in young children.

Cranial osteopathy and cranial-sacral therapy are widely used on babies and young children. These treatments are very safe in the hands of a qualified practitioner. However, always go to a qualified osteopath for treatment; not all cranial-sacral therapists have had the rigorous training that osteopaths have.

REFLEXOLOGY

Like acupuncture, reflexology works on energy points. It is based on the idea that the body is divided into ten energy zones, which run from head to feet, and that all the parts of the body can be influenced by working on the feet. Practitioners use a variety of gentle massage techniques to stimulate energy points here, and the effect is generally very soothing.

Reflexology can be good for colic, bowel problems and digestive complaints, skin problems, breathing disorders, sleeplessness and hyperactivity.

Natural first aid

All children have tumbles and minor accidents, and you are bound to have to deal with grazed knees, burns and cuts. Natural remedies help speed healing and can also soothe an unhappy child. But don't hesitate to get medical attention if your child has had a bad fall or if you cannot easily treat the injury yourself.

A NATURAL FIRST-AID BOX

These are some of the most useful natural remedies to have to hand.

Aloe vera gel. A herbal remedy for burns and rashes. Aloe vera has natural antiseptic, antibiotic and anti-inflammatory properties. You can also use the fresh sap of an aloe vera leaf.

Arnica. This homeopathic remedy

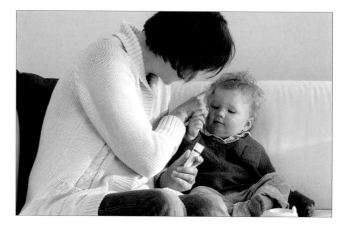

STANDARD FIRST-AID ITEMS

You can buy a first-aid kit from pharmacists, but it is easy to make your own. Get a rigid, closable box and fill it with the following basic items: scissors, safety pins, tweezers, cotton wool, bandages, absorbent dressings, gauze dressings and assorted plasters.

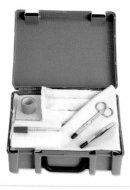

comes in cream and tablet form, and it is worth getting both. The cream is good for bruises; the tablets are also helpful for bruises as well as sprains, shock after an injury, and nosebleeds.

Calendula cream. A natural antifungal and antiseptic cream that fights infection. Calendula is good for minor skin complaints such as burns, blisters and insect bites and stings.

Chamomilla. A homeopathic remedy for teething pain and sleeplessness. Diluted chamomile tea can also be useful, both to sip and for compresses.

Distilled witch hazel. A widely available liquid herbal remedy that is good for bites, stings, bruises and sprains.

Lavender oil. A multipurpose essential oil that has antibacterial and anti-inflammatory qualities; it is good for sleeplessness, minor skin problems and headaches.

Rescue Remedy. This gentle blend of flower essences is great for calming upset children after an accident. Put four drops in water and give to your child to sip.

Most children enjoy having a 'magic' cream smoothed over their hurts. Arnica will help to speed healing from bruising.

Roman chamomile oil. A soothing essential oil that helps with sleeplessness, muscle strain and skin problems.

Tea tree oil. An antibacterial and antifungal essential oil that helps to prevent infection.

Honey has been used for centuries as a natural antiseptic, it also has anti-inflammatory qualities, and is a natural antihistamine.

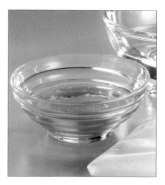

MAKING A LAVENDER COMPRESS

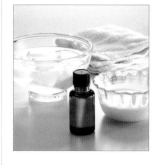

1 Fill a bowl with very cold water and add a handful of ice cubes.
2 Add a few drops of lavender oil diluted in 15ml/1 tbsp full-fat milk.
3 Dip a clean facecloth into the scented water.
4 Squeeze out excess water and apply to the bruised area. Dip the cloth frequently to keep it cold. Apply for a maximum of 10 minutes in total. Reapply every few hours as necessary.

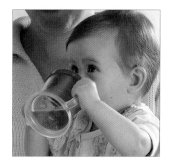

A few drops of Rescue Remedy added to a cup of water can help soothe minor shocks and upsets.

CUTS AND GRAZES

Most cuts are minor wounds that heal quickly but you should always clean the damaged skin to prevent infection. Grazes often occur when the child has slid along the ground after a fall, so they may contain bits of dirt or grit, which will all need to be removed.

What to do. Fill a small bowl with warm water, add a couple of drops of tea tree oil and use to bathe the wound, or simply wash under running water. Press a folded pad of gauze or similar over the area to stop bleeding (don't use cotton wool (cotton balls) as the fibres may stick). Smooth a little Calendula cream over the cleaned area before covering with a plaster. You can also apply honey: ideally use manuka honey, which has a marked antibacterial and anti-inflammatory action.

When to seek help. Seek medical attention if the cut is very deep, there are objects embedded in it that you cannot easily remove, it doesn't stop bleeding when a dressing is applied or if it covers a large area.

BRUISES

When the blood vessels under the skin are damaged, blood seeps out into the surrounding tissues, causing bruising. Some children bruise more easily than others. Including more fruits and vegetables in the diet can help, since these foods are known to contain vitamin C and bioflavonoids, which help to strengthen the walls of blood vessels.

What to do. Apply a cold lavender compress to the skin for a few minutes to reduce swelling. A packet of frozen peas wrapped in a towel will also work well. Don't hold a compress against your child's skin for longer than 10 minutes. To encourage healing, smooth Arnica cream on the bruise three times a day. You can also give an Arnica tablet immediately after the injury to help with the shock, and every two hours during daytime for the next 48 hours.

When to seek help. See a doctor if you suspect a broken bone, or if the pain is worse 24 hours later. Frequent bruising is occasionally due to a problem with blood clotting: see your doctor if your child bruises very easily and unusually.

NOSEBLEEDS

A nosebleed happens when the delicate blood vessels that line the nose are damaged by a blow, frequent nose-blowing or picking, or inflammation caused by a cold. If your child has nosebleeds often, try giving more fruits and vegetables to increase his or her intake of vitamin C and bioflavonoids.

What to do. Get your child to lean forwards (not backwards), and gently pinch the fleshy part just under the bridge of the nose for 10–15 minutes. Release, repeat if bleeding continues. Arnica tablets can be given after a nosebleed, or daily for frequent bleeds. Rescue Remedy helps soothe any shock.

When to seek help. Take your child to hospital if a nosebleed occurs after a blow to the head, or if the bleeding doesn't stop within half an hour. See a doctor if your child has frequent nosebleeds.

A pack of frozen peas wrapped in a muslin makes a makeshift icepack.

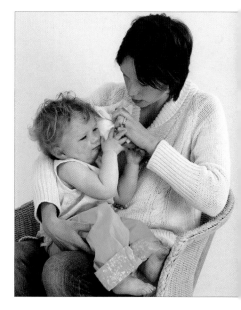

CHOKING

A sudden fit of coughing may mean your child is choking on a piece of food or other small item. The natural instinct to give someone who is choking a slap on the back is a good one, but encourage a child to cough first – this is often enough to remove an obstruction. Check the mouth and remove the obstruction if you can see it: don't feel for it with your fingers – you may damage the throat or push the obstruction in further.

If you do need to slap the child on the back, get him to bend over (or bend him over your knee) and slap between the shoulderblades. If a baby is choking, hold him face-down along your forearm so that the head is facing downwards and use two fingers to tap sharply between the shoulder blades.

All parents worry about choking and it is worth learning how to do chest compressions and life-saving procedures in the very unlikely event that back slaps don't clear the obstruction. You can do a simple first-aid course specifically for babies and children; this usually involves practising the techniques on a life-sized model. Courses are run by voluntary organizations such as St John Ambulance (Red Cross) and are aimed at parents and carers. Often there are child care facilities.

SPRAINS AND STRAINS

A sprain is an injury to the ligaments of a joint, while a strain is an injury to a muscle. It's quite difficult to tell the difference between a strain or sprain and a fracture, especially in young children, whose bones may bend rather than break. If in doubt, seek medical advice.

What to do. Get your child to sit or lie down. Apply a cold lavender or chamomile compress or ice pack for up to 10 minutes. Place a thick wad of cotton wool or other soft pad against the injury and bandage firmly, or put on an elastic bandage to compress. Then elevate the

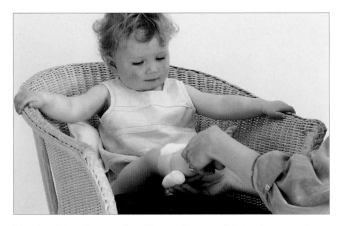

injured part to reduce swelling. Give Arnica for shock and to encourage healing; Rhus tox is another good homeopathic remedy for sprains and strains. Apply Arnica cream or comfrey ointment over the area (only if the skin is unbroken). Rescue Remedy will help soothe any upset.

Caution. Be sure that you do not bandage so tightly that you cut off the circulation. To check, press on an uninjured area of skin below the bandaged area. If it takes more than three seconds for colour to return, your bandage is probably too tight.

When to seek help. Get medical advice if you suspect a fracture or if the pain doesn't subside at all after the treatment.

WASP AND BEE STINGS

These stings can be very painful.
What to do. If you can see a sting in

Arnica cream and tablets help to speed healing for a strain or sprain.

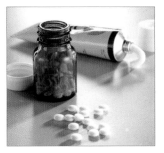

If you need to bandage a sprain, use a thick wad of gauze or cotton wool to cushion the wound first.

your child's skin, remove it carefully. Put a little iced water in a bowl and add a few drops of lavender or tea tree oil diluted in 15ml/1 tbsp full-fat milk. Dip cotton wool in the water and apply to the area every 10 minutes or so until the pain subsides. Other easily available natural remedies for bee stings include witch hazel, bicarbonate of soda or crushed garlic; wasp stings can be helped by applying witch hazel, cider vinegar or lemon juice. The homeopathic remedy Apis can be given to help with the after-effects of a sting.

When to seek help. If your child is allergic to wasp or bee stings, he or she may go into anaphylactic shock, needing urgent medical attention.

INSECT BITES

Gnat, ant or mosquito bites can be very itchy.
What to do. Witch hazel is a good treatment for insect bites. Rescue Remedy can be applied to the bite. Mosquito bites can be soothed with cider vinegar or lemon juice.
Prevention. Before dusk, when mosquitoes are most active, cover up your child in clothes of closely woven, lightly coloured fabric. You can get eucalyptus-based repellents

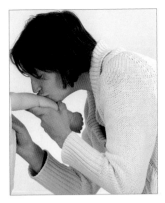

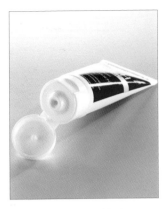

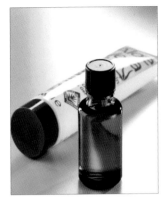

Remove a bee sting by scraping it off with a credit card or by pressing your thumb into the neighbouring skin and pushing it sideways. Don't try to pull it out with tweezers: this can squeeze any poison left in the sting into your child's skin. Suck out any poison before treating.

suitable for children from health food stores. Burning citronella oil in a vaporizer or using citronella candles is also helpful.

BURNS
Minor (first-degree) burns affect only the top layer of skin, which reddens but does not blister or swell. They can be treated at home.

What to do. Place the burned area under cold, running water for 10 minutes. Apply aloe vera gel, Calendula cream, or lavender oil

Acidic lemon juice or cider vinegar can take the sting out of a mosquito bite.

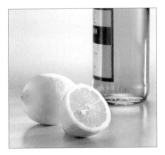

You can get witchhazel in the traditional tincture form or in handy tubes of gel.

diluted in full-fat milk to ease pain and speed healing. Give Rescue Remedy or Arnica for the shock.

When to seek help. If the burn is larger than the child's palm or if the pain gets worse after treatment, seek immediate medical advice. If the skin is moist, swollen or blistered, the burn may have reached underlying areas of skin (second-degree burn); if the child feels no pain after a burn but the area is red, white, yellow or darkened, the nerves may be damaged (third-degree burn). Seek urgent medical advice.

SUNBURN
It's important to protect your child's delicate skin from the sun. If it gets too much sunlight, the skin will be red, hot and sore.

What to do. Bathe the skin in cool water to which you have added a couple of drops of lavender oil diluted in full-fat milk. Add a few drops of lavender oil to aloe vera gel and smooth over the affected area. The homeopathic remedy Sol is good for mild sunburn.

When to seek help. Seek immediate medical advice if the skin has blistered, or if your child develops a high temperature (39°C/102°F or above).

Aloe vera gel and lavender essential oil are two natural remedies for minor burns.

SUNSTROKE
A sunburned child may also develop heatstroke, with a raised temperature, headache, nausea, dizziness and general aches.

What to do. Cool your child down by sponging with tepid water. Give plenty of cool drinks to sip: water, diluted fruit juice or a rehydration drink (available from pharmacists). The homeopathic remedies Sol or Belladonna may be given.

When to seek help. Act quickly to get immediate medical help if your child's temperature is very high (39°C/102°F).

FOREIGN OBJECTS IN THE EYE
Children can easily rub grit or other irritants into their eyes.

What to do. If you can see a piece of grit in your child's eye, get the child to put his or her head on one side with the affected side uppermost. Holding the eyelids open with your fingers, very slowly pour tepid water into the upper corner of the eye so that water covers the whole eye. If the grit doesn't move, try lifting it off with the corner of a damp handkerchief.

When to seek help. Seek immediate medical attention if something is stuck to the surface of the eye or embedded in it.

When your baby is sick

Babies can't tell you when they are sick, but as a parent you quickly become adept at reading the early signs. The first hint of illness is usually clinginess: your baby may want to be held all the time. This is a very natural response: the baby knows that something is wrong and wants you to take care of him or her. Babies are usually listless when they are ill: yours may be content to lie quietly in your arms and may be needing to sleep more than usual.

Other signs of illness include:

Looking unwell. A sick baby usually looks poorly, with a pathetic expression and dull eyes.

Reduced appetite. Sick babies tend to feed a lot less than normal: this won't harm your baby so long as he or she is taking enough fluid to prevent dehydration.

Irritability. Your baby may cry more than usual or in an unusual way. This can be a sign of pain.

Fever. Illness usually (but not always) goes hand-in-hand with a raised temperature, which causes babies to breathe more quickly than usual.

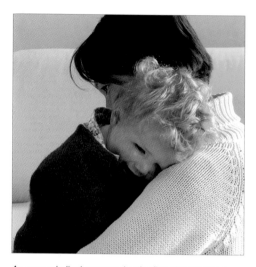

An unusual clinginess may be the first sign that your baby is ill. He or she instinctively knows that he needs to stay close to you.

WHEN TO SEEK HELP

It can be difficult to assess a baby's condition. Similar symptoms occur in serious and non-serious illnesses, and although symptoms are often more severe in a very sick baby, this is not always the case. It is best always to seek medical advice if you think your baby is ill, is refusing feeds or has unusual symptoms. Always see a doctor if a baby under three months has a fever.

Seek immediate medical help if your baby:

- has a seizure (fit)
- is limp and seems unaware of your presence
- is unusually drowsy and hard to wake up
- seems to be getting weaker or sicker by the hour
- is breathing very fast or noisily, or with difficulty, or if the skin between the ribs is sucked in as he or she breathes
- has a temperature over 39°C/102°F, especially if there is also a rash
- turns blue or becomes very pale, blotchy or ashen (if your baby is dark-skinned, check the palms)
- has a bulging or sunken fontanelle (the soft spot on the top of the head)
- has a purplish-red rash that doesn't disappear when you press a glass to it.

Rash. Skin rashes are a symptom of many illnesses and other conditions such as food sensitivity. Occasionally, they may have a serious cause, so it is essential to have an unexplained rash checked by a medical practitioner.

Diarrhoea and vomiting. Babies can be sick when they have an ear, chest or throat infection, and they may pass loose, smelly stools when they have a viral infection. Vomiting and diarrhoea occurring together usually indicate food poisoning or gastroenteritis.

TAKING YOUR BABY'S TEMPERATURE

A normal body temperature is 37°C/98.6°F, when taken by mouth. But it varies slightly depending on the time of day: a temperature taken in the morning will usually be slightly lower than one taken in the afternoon.

Poorly children need lots of fluids to prevent dehydration. A refreshing squeeze of lemon adds a little natural antiseptic to the drink.

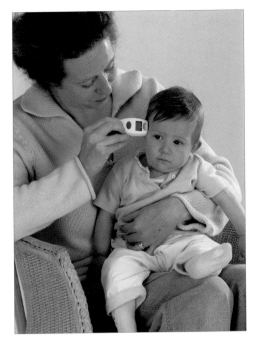

A digital thermometer gives you an accurate reading of your child's temperature in an instant without your having to disturb him or her.

You can often tell that your child has a temperature simply by feeling the forehead. But it is best to get an accurate reading using a thermometer. Get a digital one that bleeps when an accurate reading has been taken: glass thermometers contain mercury, which is highly toxic if released into the atmosphere.

Under the arm. This is an easy way to take a baby's temperature. A normal temperature here is 36.4°C/97.4°F; anything over 37°C/98.6°F is a fever. Put your baby on your lap, place the thermometer under his or her arm and hold the arm against the baby's body to keep it in place.

Ear sensor. A digital ear thermometer takes a reading by measuring heat in the ear canal. It only takes a second and is not intrusive, but it is expensive.

Indicator strips. An indicator strip gives you the temperature of your baby's skin – not the body – so it is not an accurate measure.

CARING FOR A POORLY BABY

Sleep is a wonderful cure-all, and babies are naturally inclined to sleep more when poorly. But your baby

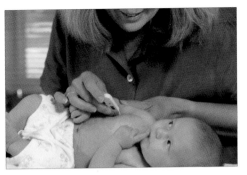

Using a digital thermometer under the arm is a safe and accurate method of reading your child's temperature.

probably won't want to be far from you. Be patient and keep the baby in your arms as much as possible: let the baby doze on you if that is what he or she needs. If your baby normally sleeps in a different room to you, then it is often a good idea to move the cot back in to your room so that you can monitor his or her condition more easily. Alternatively, sleep in the baby's room for a night or two.

Take steps to manage any fever and give frequent fluids to prevent dehydration: fever, diarrhoea, vomiting, coughing, crying or loss of appetite can all make your baby dehydrated. It's best to give fluids in small amounts to prevent your baby from vomiting it back up again. If you are breastfeeding, nurse often. Otherwise, give cooled, boiled water in addition to feeds (unless otherwise advised). If your baby is over six months, you can add a squeeze of lemon juice to the water – it has naturally antiseptic properties.

Don't feel that you have to keep your baby indoors: fresh air can be beneficial even if with a fever. Wrap the baby up well and go out for short periods.

Let a poorly child sleep as much as he or she needs: rest is one of the best natural medicines we have.

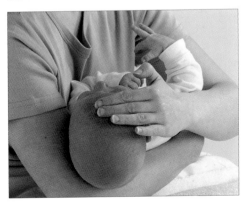

When your child is sick

As your child gets older, it becomes easier to assess what is wrong: now he or she can point to a sore throat, or tell you exactly where it hurts or how they feel. You will still have to rely on the outward signs of illness, too, however. If your child is unusually irritable, not interested in eating or suddenly drinking more than usual, something may be wrong.

You will probably have a good sense of how poorly your child is. Don't hesitate to contact your doctor if you think the child may be seriously ill or if you are not sure what is wrong. If you think the illness may be infectious, tell the reception staff who can arrange for you to sit away from other patients.

CARING FOR A POORLY CHILD

Rest is the best way of managing most illness. If your child doesn't want to stay in bed, then let him or her sit with you: read stories, do jigsaws or simply let the child nap on the sofa. Put light, comfortable clothing on your child: pyjamas and a light cardigan or dressing gown. If the child is in bed, change the sheets regularly. Open the window from time to time to air the room. Disinfect the room using a natural spray (see box).

Be prepared for your child to revert to babyish behaviour traits: a young child who is just potty-trained, for example, may revert to nappies. Be patient if he or she is fractious and irritable.

SYMPTOM SORTER

Symptoms with or without fever	Could be
Runny nose, cough or sneezing	Cold
All the above plus aches and pains	Flu
Sore throat and pain on swallowing	Throat infection
Runny or blocked nose, pain in ear or (in young child) crying and pulling on ear	Ear infection
Cough, phlegm	Bronchitis
Cough, phlegm and or rapid or difficult breathing	Bronchiolitis
Itchy red spots that blister	Chickenpox
Frequent urination and pain or burning when passing water	Infection in urinary tract
Diarrhoea and/or vomiting	Food poisoning or gastroenteritis

If your child has a fever, take steps to reduce it. Give lots of fluids, preferably water with a little added fresh lemon juice. Failing this, try diluted fruit juice even if you don't usually give it: juice is a good way to get vitamins into your child and encourage him or her to drink.

Children who are poorly often don't want to eat. This won't harm your child, and it's best not to encourage

---

WHEN TO SEEK HELP
Contact a doctor if your child:
- has an unexplained rash
- has a high or persistent fever
- is breathing very fast or noisily
- is unusually sleepy and cannot be roused
- is making you feel concerned.

Go to hospital or call an ambulance if your child:
- cannot breathe properly
- has a fit or is unconscious
- has severe leg pain, cold hands or feet with a high body temperature, very pale skin or blue-tinged skin around the lips (early signs of bacterial meningitis)
- has a headache, stiff neck, aversion to bright light or a purplish-red rash that does not disappear when pressed with a glass (later signs of bacterial meningitis)

AIR FRESHENER
For a natural room spray to refresh the air in your child's room, use 5 drops each of lavender, thyme linalol and eucalyptus smithi essential oils to 150ml/$\frac{1}{4}$ pint water. Pour into a plant spray bottle, shake well, and spray into the air.

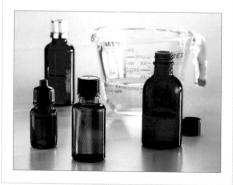

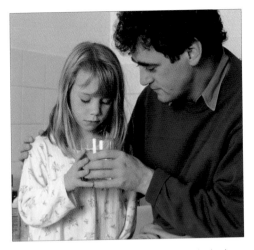

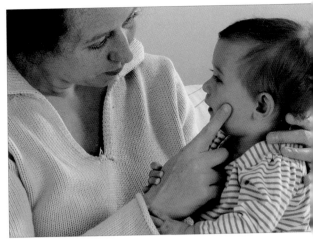

Being sick and having diarrhoea dehydrates the body, so make sure your child drinks enough water after vomitting. Encourage them to take small sips of cooled, boiled water and repeat at intervals.

Trust your own instincts: if something tells you that your child is seriously ill, act on your intuition. You know your child better than anyone else, so you may pick up on clues that may not be obvious to other people.

eating: his or her body may need to put all its energy into fighting off an infection. Once your child starts to feel better, the appetite may return. Give foods that are easy to eat and gentle on the stomach: a thick, smooth home-made vegetable or chicken soup, mashed potato, natural yoghurt with mashed-up banana, or a smoothie made with fruit juice, yoghurt and honey.

A HOSPITAL STAY

A stay in hospital is bound to be disorientating and intimidating for a young child. Prepare your child as much as you can by talking about what will happen. Sharing a book about a child who has to go to hospital could help. If possible, go on a visit to the ward where your child will be staying – see if he or she can meet some of the nurses and other staff who work there and see some of the fun things – such as the television above each bed. Be as

matter-of-fact as you can: it is important that your child doesn't pick up on your anxiety. But do acknowledge any feelings of fear or worry your child may have.

Take familiar items with you: your child's favourite toy or comforter, pyjamas, bowl and spoon, as well as the essentials. Take snacks, water, a book and comfortable clothing for yourself as well. Stay with your child in hospital: even if you have to sleep in an armchair, it will make your child feel much better if you are there. If you cannot be there all the time, ask another trusted relative or friend that the child knows well to fill in for you. Make sure that you are present when your child is examined by a doctor. Even if your child seems to cope well with being in hospital, don't be surprised if he or she displays some signs of disturbance once you get home. It is common for children to be clingy or naughty, even aggressive, after an unsettling experience. Be patient and this will pass.

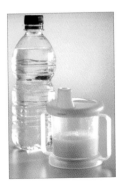

Left: Diluted juice is a good way of boosting a poorly child's energy levels. Use freshly squeezed juice if you can; it has more nutrients.

Right: During illness or convalesence, tempt a poor appetite with food that is easy to eat – a banana and yoghurt smoothie is ideal.

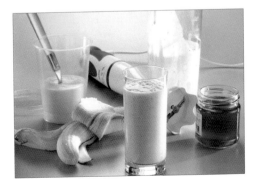

Common problems: colds, coughs and breathing disorders

Children get more coughs and colds than adults. Most children catch between six and eight colds a year until they build up immunity. And as the airways of a child are much smaller than those of adults, they are more vulnerable to infection.

COLDS

It is viruses that cause colds, so antibiotics do not help. A cold usually lasts a week or two, but can go on for longer in young children. Symptoms include a blocked-up or runny nose, sticky eyes, sore throat, a tickly cough (especially at night) and slight fever.

What to do. You can't hasten a cold's progress, but you can make your child more comfortable. Keep him or her warm, but open windows regularly to get fresh air circulating. Take your child out (well wrapped up) on short trips. Increase the humidity in the child's room to help with breathing: put a damp towel on the radiator, place a bowl of water near the radiator or other heat source or use a vaporizer.

Give lots of fluids. Children over a year old can have hot honey and lemon, which is soothing for the throat and a good source of vitamin C. Weak elderflower tea acts as a decongestant. Dilute fruit juices can also be a good way of encouraging a child to drink. Unsweetened blackcurrant diluted with warm water is good if your child has a cold: it is packed with vitamin C.

- If your child is eating, cut out dairy products (which are mucus-forming) while symptoms remain, but give alternative sources of calcium such as tofu, ground nuts and seeds, and leafy green vegetables. Babies will still need their usual milk.
- Get older children to blow their nose regularly, to stop mucus dripping down the back of the throat.
- Consider giving a homeopathic remedy to soothe symptoms. The following are common cold remedies: Aconite, given in the first 24 hours; Allium cepa, when there is lots of watery discharge from the nose and eyes; Pulsatilla, when there is thick, greenish mucus.

When to seek help. Seek medical advice if you spot other unusual signs, such as wheezing or earache, if the symptoms are very severe or if your child gets more poorly after a few days.

COUGHS

Coughing is how the body removes irritants or mucus from the breathing apparatus, so it is best to avoid over-the-counter medications that are designed to suppress this natural mechanism. If your child suddenly starts coughing violently, consider whether he or she may have inhaled a foreign object. Take steps to remove it from the airway (see first aid for choking).

What to do. If your child is coughing, the suggestions given for colds above are helpful, together with the following:

- Humidify all rooms by placing a bowl of water under the radiator or heat source.
- Avoid taking your child outdoors if the weather is cold and damp.
- For babies over three months, put a drop of essential oil of

For colds, give drinks of diluted blackcurrant, orange or lemon juice sweetened with a little honey.

There are many homeopathic remedies for different types of cough and cold symptoms.

Eucalyptus oil is a good natural decongestant, but you need only a drop on a tissue.

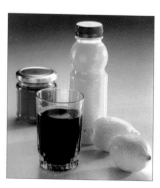

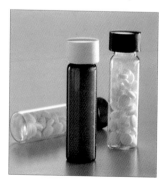

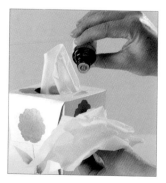

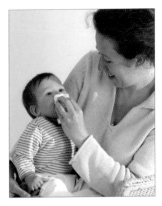

Use soft cotton wool (cotton balls) rather than tissues to wipe a child's nose to stop it getting sore.

eucalyptus smithi (not eucalyptus globulus, which is stronger) on a handkerchief and leave it in your child's room, out of reach.

- For children over one year, give diluted warm blackcurrant juice to soothe a sore throat, or thyme tea remedy (see box). If children are eating, include mild spices such as cinnamon or ginger in their food to help loosen mucus. Pineapple is also good because it contains bromeline, which is a natural anti-inflammatory.
- Consider giving one of the many homeopathic remedies used to relieve symptoms. A homeopath will help you pinpoint the right one for your child. Common remedies include: Aconite, for a dry cough that comes on at night; Bryonia, for a dry, painful cough (worse on inhalation) that follows a cold; Ipepac, for a cough that is accompanied by vomiting up phlegm; Phosphorus, for a dry, tickly cough that is worse at night; Pulsatilla, for a cough that produces yellow or green phlegm

When to seek help. Coughing can be a minor ailment or a symptom of some much more serious illnesses such as bronchiolitis and bronchitis. Always see a doctor if a cough occurs in a young baby, or if it is

severe, prolonged or accompanied by wheezing, noisy breathing or fast breathing.

CROUP

A barking cough and noisy breathing on inhalation are the key signs of croup, which is most common among children aged between six months and three years.

What to do. There are two ways to improve the breathing: take your child into a steamy room (run the hot shower and taps in the bathroom to create steam) or wrap the child up well and go outside into the cold air. Different approaches work for different children, so do which works best for your child.

THYME TEA REMEDY

This traditional remedy can help to ease a dry cough and loosen mucus. If possible, use New Zealand manuka honey, which has particular therapeutic properties.

Add a small handful of finely chopped thyme leaves to a cup of boiling water, steep until cool, then strain. Add honey to sweeten, then pour into a sterilized jar. Give 1 tsp three or four times a day. Keep in the refrigerator for up to 3 days.

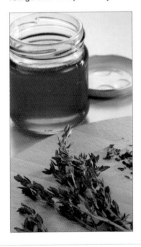

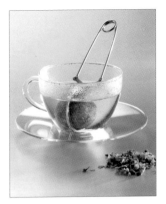

For flu, try giving your child weak lime flower tea, which helps to treat fever and reduce nasal catarrh.

BRONCHIOLITIS

This viral infection is most common in babies under twelve months, and affects the smallest airways in the lungs (the bronchioles). It starts as a cold and fever and develops into coughing, fast breathing (more than 50 breaths a minute) and wheezing.

What to do. See your doctor quickly: sometimes hospital treatment is needed.

BRONCHITIS

This infection of the large airways (bronchi) is common in toddlers and children. The symptoms are similar to those of bronchiolitis. Deficiencies in vitamin C and zinc can be an underlying cause for recurrent lung problems such as bronchitis.

What to do. Medical advice should be sought. Giving a multivitamin multimineral supplement in addition may help.

FLU

The symptoms of flu include a high temperature, aches and pains, cold symptoms, vomiting and/or diarrhoea and general malaise.

What to do. See your doctor for a diagnosis. Lime flower and elderflower tea – or a combination of both – are good for flu. They should be drunk warm, well diluted.

Common problems: asthma and eczema

Asthma and eczema are now very common in young children. Both are the result of oversensitivity of the immune system, which cause it to react to substances that have no effect on other people. They often occur together, and affected children are also more likely to suffer from food allergies.

Nobody quite knows why asthma and eczema have become so prevalent, but it may be because improved living standards have reduced the amount of germs children come into contact with, with the result that their immune systems are less robust. The increase in pollution, both outdoors and indoors, is also a likely factor. One Australian study found that exposure to the volatile organic chemicals (VOCs) found in paint and other

CHECKLIST OF ASTHMA TRIGGERS
- Dust mites
- Pollen
- Pet dander (animal hair and skin scales)
- Certain foods, especially eggs, dairy products, chocolate, wheat, citrus fruits and corn
- Mould spores
- Colds and other respiratory infections
- Cigarette smoke or exhaust fumes
- Fumes from air fresheners, household cleaners, perfumes, dry-cleaning solvents, paints, glues and pesticides
- Cold air
- Exercise
- Stress and anxiety.

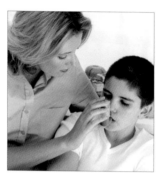

Asthma medicine is given via an inhaler and can quickly reduce symptoms of an attack. Children using inhalers need supervising by a responsible adult.

products increased the risk of childhood asthma. Exclusive breastfeeding in the first months of life can reduce the likelihood of both asthma and eczema developing.

ASTHMA

Growing numbers of children suffer from the recurrent attacks of breathlessness and wheezing that characterize asthma. In asthmatic children, the small airways in the lungs are hypersensitive: they narrow when they come into contact with, say, small amounts of smoke or pollutants. Asthma usually gets better as the child gets older. A child who is diagnosed with asthma will be given inhalers to prevent attacks and relieve symptoms. Natural therapies can help to support conventional medical treatment.

What to do. Try to identify possible triggers for your child's asthma and take steps to avoid them. Your doctor can arrange tests to check for allergy to substances such as dust mites. Improve the air quality in your home and keep it free of dust (but

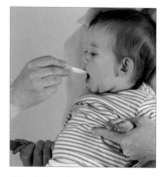

Fish oils have been shown to ease symptoms of both asthma and eczema. In one study, three out of four children given fish oil found that their symptoms improved.

vacuum when your child is out of the way). Choose a synthetic pillow and duvet with allergen-proof covers for your child's bed, and wash the bedding often in hot water. Limit toys in the cot to one or two, and wash them each week at 60°C/140°F or put in a plastic bag in the freezer overnight to kill dust mites.

Make sure that your child has a healthy diet including lots of fresh fruits and vegetables: this has been shown to be good for lung function. Choose organic produce wherever possible to reduce your child's exposure to pesticides. Do not put salt in your child's food, and avoid processed foods that contain added salt and additives such as tartrazine, which may exacerbate asthma. Consider consulting a nutritional therapist to help you uncover any possible food intolerances, and give a multivitamin, multimineral supplement: low levels of vitamin C, vitamin B6, vitamin B12, magnesium and zinc can exacerbate the symptoms. Homeopathy may help. Arsenicum, Ipecac, Nat sulph and

Pulsatilla are all prescribed to relieve mild asthma attacks, but you should see a homeopath for a specific remedy for your child. Herbal medicine has several remedies for asthma. A medical herbalist can advise you on the best herbs to use (alongside conventional treatment). Acupuncture may be helpful for some asthma sufferers, and yoga or breathing exercises may help.

ECZEMA

There are different types of eczema: those that usually affect children are seborrhoeic eczema (cradle cap) and the itchy atopic eczema, which one child in five develops. Atopic eczema can affect any part of the body, but is most common on the face, armpits, elbows, hands and knees. During an acute attack, the skin reddens, becomes extremely itchy and can blister and weep. It may be thick, dry and flaky at other times.

What to do. See your doctor, as it's essential to manage your child's eczema to prevent infection. Eczema reduces the skin's ability to act as a barrier, and bacteria are more likely to stick to dry, flaky skin.

Avoid irritating the skin. For example, choose clothing or bedding made from cotton, launder

Keep your child's fingernails short to stop him or her scratching areas of skin affected by eczema and causing infection.

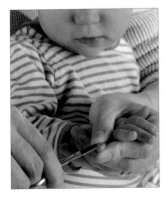

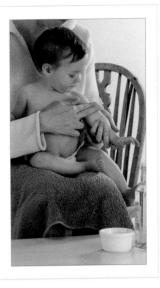

OILS FOR ECZEMA

Aromatherapy oils may help with mild eczema symptoms. Try this simple recipe. You can also make a cool compress using the same oils to soothe itching.

2 drops chamomile essential oil
2 drops lavender essential oil
45ml/3 tbsp hypoallergenic lotion

Mix together all the ingredients and then apply to the affected skin in a thin layer. Be sure to do a patch test 24 hours before you first use the lotion.
You can also make a cool compress using the same oils diluted in a simple carrier oil such as olive oil to soothe itching.

with non-biological washing powders and use an extra rinse cycle on your washing machine. Avoid soap and bath products. Keep your child as cool as possible, as heat and sweating exacerbate eczema. Cut his or her fingernails short to help prevent scratching (put cotton mittens on babies and young children at night).

Keep your child's skin clean and moisturized. Give lukewarm (not hot) daily baths to remove dry skin scales and cleanse the skin. Use an emollient such as a handful of oatmeal tied in a muslin square (you can add a drop of lavender or chamomile essential oil). Different creams work for different children. Hemp seed oil cream is one good natural alternative to try, as is olive oil. Apply a thin layer and let it soak in rather than rubbing it in (which can increase itching).

Increase oils in your child's diet. Add a spoonful of hemp seed oil to your child's food each day and give oily fish or a supplement. Give lots of water to keep your child well hydrated. Consider food sensitivity as an underlying factor, and see a qualified nutritional therapist to help

you pinpoint any problem foods. Milk, wheat, nuts, citrus fruits, fish and eggs are the most likely culprits, and sugar can exacerbate eczema. As with asthma, a multivitamin, multimineral supplement may be helpful, and a child-friendly probiotic will help to improve the balance of good bacteria in the gut, which can also be beneficial.

A probiotic drink that is suitable for children may help with eczema.

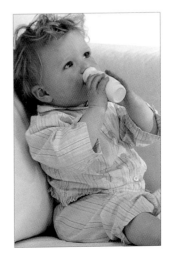

Common problems: digestive disorders

Children have sensitive digestive systems that react quickly to get rid of unwanted substances: they are much more prone to diarrhoea and vomiting than adults. These unpleasant symptoms are basically the body's way of cleansing itself, so medications to stop them are generally unhelpful. Your main aim should be to reduce discomfort and prevent dehydration.

Tummy ache is unusual in very young children, so it is best to report it to a doctor to rule out the possibility of appendicitis. In older

Most children become distressed after vomiting. Give your child a glass of cool water to sip: add a few drops of Rescue Remedy to calm and reassure.

children, it can have a physical or emotional cause: gastroenteritis, overeating or anxiety can all be responsible. Sometimes it can be triggered by other infections, such as tonsillitis. Call a doctor if your child is in severe pain, there is blood in his or her stools or if tummy ache and fever occur together.

DIARRHOEA

Your child may get a short bout of diarrhoea (frequent, loose, unpleasant-smelling stools) after having a lot of fruit or fruit juice, after eating a food he or she is intolerant to, when teething or with a cold. A course of antibiotics can also be a trigger. Diarrhoea can be a sign of food poisoning or gastroenteritis, especially if accompanied by

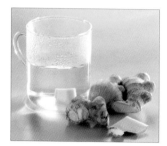

Fresh ginger is a natural remedy for nausea. All you need do is steep a piece of the fresh root in a cup of hot water for a few minutes.

vomiting. In most cases, it lasts 24 hours or less and clears up by itself. **What to do.** Give frequent drinks for sipping. Let a nursing baby breastfeed on demand and give a bottle-fed baby extra drinks of cooled, boiled water. Plain water should be sufficient in mild cases, but you can also give a rehydration drink (available from pharmacists) if necessary. Antispasmodic herbal teas, such as chamomile or fennel, can ease abdominal pains. Diluted unsweetened blackcurrant juice helps to fight infection in the gut.

For a soothing tummy massage, add one drop chamomile essential oil to 15ml/1 tbsp olive or sunflower oil. Gently massage the tummy, with clockwise circular strokes.

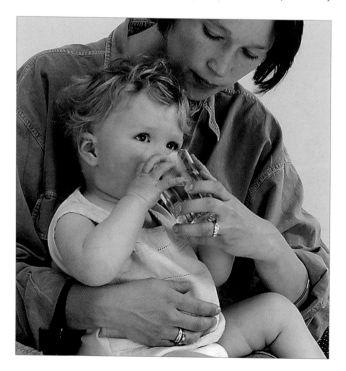

DEHYDRATION
Seek immediate help if your child shows signs of dehydration: dry mouth, sunken eyes, loose skin and dry nappies. The soft spot on the top of a baby's head (the fontanelle) may become depressed.

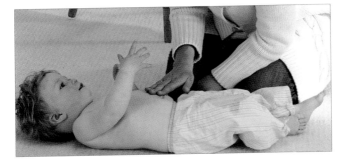

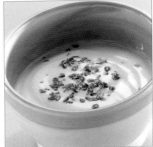

A gentle tummy massage, following the path of the intestines, can help to get the bowels moving.

Fibre-rich ground flaxseed can help with constipation. Add a little to natural yoghurt or in a smoothie.

Consider giving a suitable probiotic to help balance the bacteria in the gut. This can help reduce the duration of a bout of diarrhoea. If the diarrhoea occurred after you introduced a new food into your child's diet, make a note of it. If the symptoms re-occur the next time you give the food, then your child is almost certainly sensitive to it and it is best avoided.

When to seek help. Contact a doctor if a baby has diarrhoea for more than a few hours or if it lasts longer than 24 hours in an older child. Also, seek medical help if the diarrhoea is very severe, if there is blood in the stools, if your child seems dehydrated or has persistent stomach ache or if you think he or she has taken something toxic.

VOMITING

Like diarrhoea, vomiting can have many causes. If your child is doing both, the most likely cause is gastroenteritis or food poisoning. Vomiting on its own can be the result of the child having eaten too much (or a baby having taken too much milk) or can be part of a feverish illness. A baby with a cold may be sick, to expel phlegm from the body. **What to do**. Treat as for diarrhoea (but avoid giving a tummy massage). Encourage your child to sip rather than to gulp liquid to help it stay down. Ginger is particularly good for

nausea and vomiting: you can make a simple ginger tea by steeping a block of peeled, bruised garlic in a cup of hot water.

When to seek help. Contact your doctor if a baby vomits repeatedly or violently, or if vomiting and diarrhoea occur together. Seek medical advice for an older child if vomiting is very frequent, lasts longer than 24 hours, or if there is blood in the vomit.

CONSTIPATION

If your child suddenly goes for longer than normal between bowel movements, and then produces hard, dry, pebble-like stools, he or she is constipated.

What to do. Increase the vegetables and fruits in your child's diet (but cut out bananas): broccoli, leafy green vegetables and dried apricots are particularly helpful. Give older children whole grains: porridge oats and rye bread are better than wholewheat bread, which can irritate the lining of the gut. Most important

If your child is hungry after vomiting or diarrhoea, plain boiled rice is very gentle on the stomach.

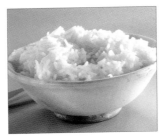

of all, make sure your child is well hydrated: give extra cups of water and remind the child to drink them.

Consider sprinkling a little ground flaxseed (available from health food stores) on your child's cereal, or put 5ml/1 tsp flaxseed oil into your child's food or in a fruit smoothie. Flaxseeds are rich in fibre and are a natural lubricant. Give live yoghurt if the balance of the intestinal flora has been upset by a bout of gastroenteritis or a course of antibiotics. Or consider giving a child-friendly probiotic supplement.

Massage can soothe cramping and encourage the bowels to move: stroke your hand over the abdomen, making an arch shape in a clockwise direction so that you are following the line of the intestines. For children over one year, you can use a massage oil of orange essential oil diluted in a carrier oil. Reflexology treatment can be helpful: one Scottish study found that regular treatment helped to relieve chronic constipation in children.

If constipation is a recurring problem, consider whether food sensitivity could be a root cause. An Italian study found that sensitivity to cow's milk caused chronic constipation in some children.

When to seek help. Seek medical advice if your child does not have a bowel movement for several days, or if the problem is recurrent.

Common problems: skin rashes and ear infections

Rashes are a feature of many childhood infections, both non-serious and serious. It's quite hard to distinguish between different rashes, so it is best to check them out with your doctor.

CHICKENPOX

The first symptoms of chickenpox are usually tiredness, fever and loss of appetite. Within a day or two, small, flat red spots appear, usually on the back, stomach and chest. They can spread to the face and head in a day or two. The red spots join up and blister, becoming intensely itchy. They scab over within 24 hours, as more spots appear.

Chickenpox is infectious from two days before the spots appear until scabs have formed on all the spots. It takes 10–21 days for the symptoms to appear after infection. One attack usually confers lifelong immunity. Chickenpox can be very dangerous for unborn children if the mother is not immune, so if your child has been in contact with a pregnant woman, let her know, so that she can contact her doctor.

Chickenpox spots blister and then scab. They are itchy, but discourage your child from scratching in case of infection and scarring.

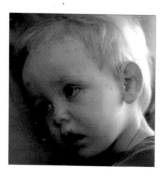

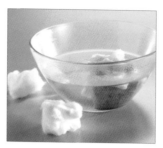

Make an elderflower infusion, dip cotton wool in the bowl and dab on the spots for relief from itching.

What to do. Encourage your child to rest as much as possible and take steps to manage any fever. Use calendula cream or calomine lotion on the spots to relieve itching, or dab them with elderflower tea or a solution of 5ml/1 tsp distilled witch hazel in a cup of warm water. Give lots of fruits and vegetables to boost your child's immune system, and add raw garlic to food if your child will eat it. Consider giving the following homeopathic remedies:
- Aconite, for the initial symptoms of tiredness and fever
- Belladonna, for the early stages if temperature is high and the child is flushed and very thirsty
- Rhus tox, for itching and any restlessness

> **RELIEVING ITCHING CHICKENPOX SPOTS**
> A lukewarm oatmeal bath can be soothing. Place a handful of oatmeal in a muslin square or the foot of a nylon stocking, add 2 drops each of chamomile and lavender essential oils, tie up and place in the water. Give several baths a day.

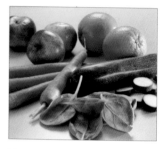

Encourage your child to eat lots of healthy fruits and vegetables to promote healing.

Protect your child's skin from direct sunlight for a couple of weeks after the scabs fall off, to avoid any danger of scarring.

When to seek help. See your doctor if a baby is affected, if the attack is severe, if the spots become inflamed or if you are pregnant and are not sure that you are immune.

HEAT RASH

Young children have immature sweat glands, which are easily blocked. Heat rash usually appears as small red bumps, sometimes with a blister in the centre, that appear on areas exposed to sunlight or areas that sweat a lot.

What to do. Cool your child down: remove clothing, sponge down or give the child a tepid bath. Good topical treatments include aloe vera gel, distilled witch hazel, Calendula cream or a lavender or chamomile compress. The homeopathic remedy Sol can also be helpful.

IMPETIGO

This infectious skin condition usually starts off around the mouth or nose. It takes the form of red blisters, which soon burst and form a golden crust on reddened, weeping skin.

GLUE EAR

This is a condition in which thick, sticky fluid accumulates in the middle ear, leading to hearing problems. It can be linked to repeated ear or throat infections, which block the Eustachian tube. If it is persistent, the conventional treatment is the insertion of a plastic grommet to allow fluid to drain. But the procedure involves a general anaesthetic and has itself been linked to hearing problems. Repeated ear infections are often a cause, so take steps to avoid them (see above). Many complementary health practitioners believe that glue ear is linked to food sensitivity, particularly an intolerance of dairy foods, or to passive smoking.

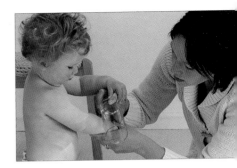

What to do. Bathing the skin with warm salt water can help to reduce itching; tea tree oil added neat to water can also help with itching and can limit the infection. Give garlic perles every two hours for a day or two, then reduce to three times a day, to help resolve the infection. The homeopathic remedies Ant crud or Arsenicum can be useful.

Be scrupulous about hygiene: do not share face towels or pillows and keep your child away from other children while infectious.

EAR INFECTIONS

Children are prone to ear infections, particularly after a cold or throat infection. The Eustachian tube, the drainage canal that links the nose, ear and throat, is very narrow. If it becomes blocked, fluid accumulates and viruses and bacteria multiply. The main symptoms are pain, hearing loss and fever. A small child

Warmth can soothe the pain of an earache; use a covered hot water bottle or a lavender compress.

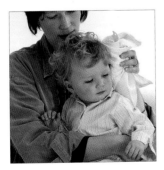

may tug on the ear, but most simply cry and seem unwell.

Seek medical advice straight away if you suspect your child has an ear infection. It needs prompt treatment – usually antibiotics – to prevent the infection spreading. Take steps to prevent recurrence, so your child does not have to take repeated courses of antibiotics.

What you can do. Warm the affected ear by holding a warm lavender compress or a covered hot-water bottle against it. Dilute lavender essential oil in olive or sunflower oil and smooth into the skin around the ear and neck.

For children over one year, give plenty of warm drinks such as honey and lemon and fresh blackcurrant juice; you can give a herbal tea combining chamomile (antiseptic and relaxing), elderflower or lemon balm (to reduce mucus) and lime flowers (to bring down fever) three times a day. Garlic can help relieve infection: add fresh garlic to your child's food if possible, or give garlic perles. If your child has taken antibiotics, give live yoghurt every day for a month to help rebalance the bacteria in the gut.

Raise the head of the cot or bed to help fluid drain from the Eustachian tube. Avoid washing your child's hair or going swimming while symptoms persist. Consider giving a homeopathic remedy, such as:

- Aconite, at the onset of symptoms, especially if the child has a blocked nose, fever and is thirsty
- Belladonna, for earache that is

To test for a meningitis rash, press a clear glass against it, if the spots do not disappear seek immediate medical aid.

worse at night and better when the child sits upright

- Chamomilia, for earache that accompanies teething, is causing extreme pain and irritability
- Pulsatilla, for earache with a cold that is worse at night.

If your child gets repeated ear infections, keep his or her ears, throat and neck warm at all times: wrap the child up well in cold weather. Give the remedies mentioned above at the first signs of a cold, to try to head off infections, but seek advice from a homeopath for a remedy specifically tailored to your child. Consider food sensitivity as a possible cause. Dairy products are the most common culprits, but wheat, eggs and chocolate could also be triggers in some children.

Make sure your child is eating a healthy, balanced diet, with plenty of fresh fruits and vegetables, zinc-rich foods such as meat and poultry, and lots of garlic. Do not give sugar, which depresses the immune system. Warm drinks of honey and lemon or diluted fresh blackcurrant juice support the immune system and encourage mucus to clear. Consider giving a multivitamin, multimineral supplement.

When to seek help. See a doctor if you suspect an ear infection, or if blood or clear liquid is discharged from the ear.

Food allergy and intolerance

Though often confused, food allergy and food intolerance are two different things. In food allergy, the immune system mistakenly identifies the food as a foreign invader. This can cause an extreme and sometimes life-threatening reaction. Food allergy may affect up to 8 per cent of children, but most grow out of it: just 2 per cent of adults are affected. Children with a food allergy are more likely to suffer from other allergy-related problems such as eczema or asthma, which also tend to diminish with age.

Food intolerances are harder to pin down. Symptoms vary widely, even in the same individual. They are usually milder and can occur hours or days after the food is eaten. Some may be delayed reactions by the immune system, others are caused by the body's inability to digest the food properly. For these reasons, many doctors are sceptical even about the existence of many food intolerances, while many nutritional therapists believe them to be a factor in a wide range of common childhood ailments.

WARNING

Children with severe allergies can go into anaphylactic shock, in which their blood pressure drops and they become unconscious. Anaphylaxis can be fatal unless the victim is treated with a shot of adrenaline (epinephrine): call an ambulance immediately. Parents and teachers of children with a severe allergy need to carry an adrenaline shot with them so it can be administered at any time.

COMMON FOOD ALLERGENS

Any food can trigger a reaction, but about 90 per cent of food allergies are caused by one of the following eight foods:

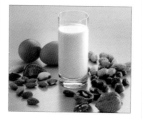

Cow's milk; eggs; peanuts; wheat; soya; tree nuts (such as walnuts, brazil nuts, hazelnuts, almonds and pecans);

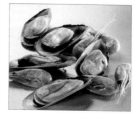

Fish and shellfish.

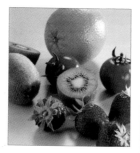

Other common allergenic foods include strawberries, kiwi fruit, tomatoes, oranges, chocolate and soya.

SYMPTOMS

Common symptoms of food allergy include:

- swelling of the lips and throat
- skin rash, eczema or itching
- swelling of the eyelids
- vomiting or diarrhoea
- wheezing or breathing difficulties.

If a child is intolerant – as opposed to allergic – to a food, the symptoms are usually more general, though some are similar to those of an allergic reaction. They include:

- fatigue
- vomiting and diarrhoea
- bloating and wind
- eczema or skin rashes (especially around the mouth)
- wheezing
- muscular aches and pains
- frequent colds or ear infections
- temper tantrums or behaviour problems
- sleeplessness
- cravings (perhaps for the very food the child is intolerant of).

WHAT TO DO

If you suspect that your child may be allergic to a food, the first step is to visit your doctor to arrange for a test. Tests usually take the form of a blood test or a prick test (in which the skin is scratched and a tiny amount of the allergen introduced to see if a reaction occurs). If your child tests positive for an allergy, the only option is to cut the food out of the diet and replace it with healthy alternatives. If there is any doubt, an elimination diet can determine the suspect food. Cutting a food out of the diet is not as easy as it sounds. Someone with an allergy to soya, for example, will also need to avoid foods labelled tempeh, tamori, textured vegetable protein, and so

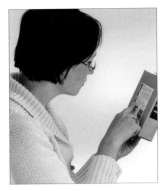

If your child has a food allergy, you will get used to reading the lists of ingredients on food labels: many problem foods crop up in a surprising variety of forms and names. You can find information on food labelling on food allergy websites.

on. A dietician can tell you what you need to look for on food labels.

It is more difficult to test for food intolerances than allergies As a starting point, try keeping a food diary for two weeks, listing everything your child eats and any symptoms. This can sometimes help you to get a better idea of whether

Sweets are full of colourings, preservatives, sugars and artificial sweeteners, all of which can cause behavioural reactions, and certainly have no nutritional value.

your child does indeed have a food intolerance.

If you think this is the case, see your doctor and asked to be referred to an allergy specialist or a dietician. An allergy specialist can help you to check for intolerance by removing the suspect foods from your child's diet for five to ten days, and then re-introducing them. The short period of abstinence should be scrupulously observed in order to be sure that all traces of the food have passed through the digestive system. This has the effect of making any reaction when the food is re-introduced stronger and more immediate, making diagnosis easier.

Although the process sounds simple, it is best to have professional advice when you undertake it: it is very easy to make the mistake of assuming a child has a food intolerance when this is not the case, which could lead you to restrict his or her diet unnecessarily. A specialist will also help ensure that your child is getting essential nutrients while following an exclusion diet.

Where an intolerance is diagnosed, eliminating the problem food is the usual remedy, as with allergies. However, in the case of intolerance, when a food is excluded from the diet, the body tends to build up tolerance to it. This means that the child may be able to eat it again in small quantities not too frequently.

ELIMINATING FOODS
Don't be tempted to exclude important foods such as milk from your child's diet without professional advice. It can be difficult to provide alternative sources of, say calcium. Children can become malnourished while following a severely restricted diet.

If your child does have a food sensitivity, make sure he or she has a good balanced diet, and takes regular meals and snacks to keep blood-sugar levels steady. Consider giving a multivitamin, multimineral supplement and a suitable probiotic drink to encourage good digestion. It's important to get your child to chew food properly (this makes it easier to digest).

You can help to build your child's tolerance to a problem food such as wheat by eliminating it from the diet for a couple of months. After this, the child may have no trouble eating occasional pieces of bread.

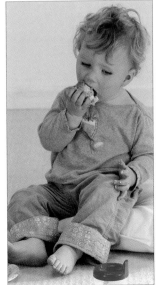

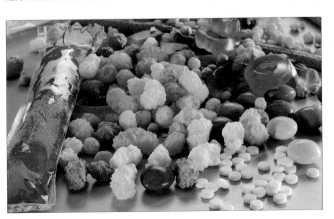

A healthy home

We are all exposed to toxic chemicals every day: they are in the air we breathe, our food and drink and the toiletries and household products we use. Because our homes are enclosed spaces, toxin levels can build up and the air can actually be more polluted than it is outdoors. Ordinary household dust can contain a mixture of solvents, hormone-disrupting chemicals, heavy metals, solvents, pesticides and flame retardants. Children spend a lot of their time indoors and they are more likely to be affected by pollution than adults. So it is important to ensure that your home is a healthy environment for your child to grow up in.

Here are some basic steps for a healthy home.
• Ban smoking at home.
• Open your windows regularly.
• Keep pets out of sleeping areas. If your child is allergic to your pet, you may have to keep it out of all living areas or find it a new home.
• Wipe your feet when you come in, and leave your shoes by the door to avoid bringing dirt, heavy metals and toxic chemicals indoors.
• Choose furniture made from untreated natural materials.
• Wash curtains, other soft furnishings and bedclothes regularly.

Keeping your home dust-free will help to protect your child from inhaling pollutants. But use natural products rather than spray polishes and carpet cleaners.

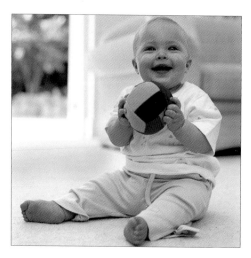

NATURAL CLEANING PRODUCTS

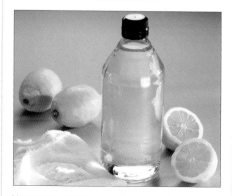

You can use ordinary ingredients to tackle many cleaning jobs around the home.
Bicarbonate of soda (baking soda). Sprinkle this on a damp sponge and use to clean surfaces. For stubborn stains, mix it with a little water and leave for 20 minutes before wiping off. Add 30ml/2 tbsp bicarbonate of soda to a cup of vinegar and add to the toilet bowl. Leave for at least 15 minutes, then clean with a brush. To clean a drain, add half a cup of bicarbonate then half a cup of vinegar. Leave for 15 minutes, then pour down a kettle of boiling water.
White vinegar. This is great for cleaning windows. Add half a cup of vinegar to 1 litre/2 pints warm water and apply with a soft cloth, then buff with crumpled newspaper. Vinegar can also be used for descaling appliances: add equal parts of vinegar and water to a kettle and leave overnight. Throw out the vinegar, boil the kettle and discard the water before using again.
Lemon juice. Lemon is an excellent natural brightening agent and cleanser. Add half a cup of lemon juice to a bucket of water and soak white or coloured clothes overnight before washing as usual.

• Keep your home as dust-free as possible. Consider buying a vacuum cleaner with a high-efficiency particulate air (HEPA) filter. Keep children out of the way while you dust and vacuum.
• Dry clothes outside or in a properly ventilated space. Avoid putting them around the house (on radiators and so on); the moisture will be released into the air and may cause the growth of mould spores in your walls.

DECORATING

If you are planning a nursery for your baby or revamping a child's bedroom, seek out non-toxic decorating products and furnishings. Babies and children spend a lot of time on or near the floor, so choose a natural covering such as wood or cork rather than laminate or vinyl, which may contain harmful chemicals. Hard flooring is the best option because carpet traps dust, which can lead to a build-up of airborne toxins and dust mites. But if you want to use carpet for warmth, choose wool, sisal or coir with a natural backing, and vacuum regularly.

Regular paints contain volatile organic compounds (VOCs), which give off noxious vapours after being applied. Choose water-based low-VOC paints, keep the room well ventilated during and after decorating and don't let your child sleep in the room for a few days after painting it. Better still, use organic paints made from natural materials such as linseed, casein and mineral pigments. These take longer to dry and can be harder to use, but they are safe for allergy- and asthma-sufferers.

If you are picking furniture for a child's room, avoid items made from MDF, laminated wood or chipboard, which contain formaldehyde. Choose furniture made from untreated hardwood from sustainable sources instead. Use natural materials for your child's bedding. For example, get a mattress made from organic latex, wool and cotton, and sheets of unbleached organic cotton.

CUT THE CHEMICALS

Reducing the amount of chemicals you use in the home will lower the risk of your child coming into contact with something harmful.

- If your kitchen cupboard is a jumble of different products, go through it and get rid of any products you don't use. General cleaners may leave a residue on your surfaces, which your child may then touch: so avoid those labelled 'irritant' and choose gentle eco-friendly products or natural cleaning alternatives instead.

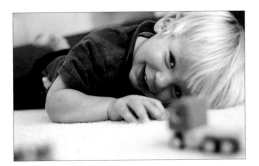

Young children inevitably spend a lot of time on the floor, so it is worth investing in natural coverings that are free from unnecessary chemicals.

- In the same way, go through your bathroom cupboards and throw out any products that you do not need. Avoid wearing perfume, hairspray and a plethora of other products to reduce the amount of chemicals your child breathes in. He or she will prefer your natural smell in any case. Put only natural substances on your baby or toddler – he or she can do without bubble baths, wipes, talc and harsh soaps.
- Get rid of garden pesticides, weed killers and so on. Many common garden products – including creosote – have now been banned, so it is best to dispose of any products you have had for several years. Consider gardening organically to help protect your child from hazardous chemicals. For example, use saucers of beer sunk into the soil to trap slugs rather than poisonous pellets (which a young child could eat).

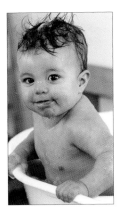

Left: Avoid using unnecessary toiletries. Many bubble baths contain detergent, which irritates the skin, while the ingredients for baby wipes may include propylene glycol – a chemical that is also present in anti-freeze.

Right: Make sure your child spends some time outside every day, whatever the weather.

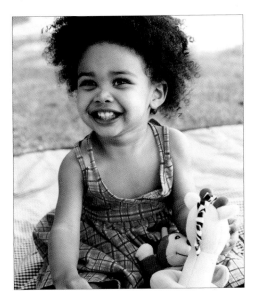

Safety in the home

Young children are naturally curious and have little sense of danger, so it is up to you to make their environment safe. To make your home child-friendly, you need to develop an eye for potential disaster. The best way to do this is to crawl around so that you see each room from a child's perspective. Notice what dangles down, what can be pulled or poked, opened or climbed, and then take steps to make it safe. Be prepared to refine your childproofing at the major stages of your child's development – crawling, walking and so on.

Young children need constant adult supervision: they shouldn't be left in a room alone even for a few minutes. Take extra care when you are under pressure, entertaining guests or trying to get ready to go out: accidents are more likely to happen when you are distracted. It's a good idea to get your child used to a playpen from an early age, so that you have somewhere to put him or her when you need to concentrate on something else.

Babies have a knack of exploring that little bit further when you least expect it, so you need to keep a watchful eye on them at all times.

FIRE!
Smoke inhalation, burns and scalds are all common injuries in childhood. Contact your local fire service for individual advice on protecting your home from fire (fire officers may be willing to fit smoke alarms free of charge).
• Don't overload sockets.
• Don't use an extension lead that isn't powerful enough for the appliance; large appliances should not be plugged into extension leads. Put extension leads away after use.
• Don't leave candles or aromatherapy vaporizers that use a naked flame burning: it's safest not to use them at all. Get in the habit of putting matches and lighters well out of reach.
• Do put smoke alarms on every floor; install a carbon monoxide alarm too.
• Do cover all open fires with a fixed fireguard. Use radiator covers too.
• Do switch off appliances at the socket when they are not in use.

Babies and young children love to rummage through handbags. Be on the safe side and don't ever keep sharp items such as nail clippers or scissors in yours, and make sure any medications you use are in child-safety containers.

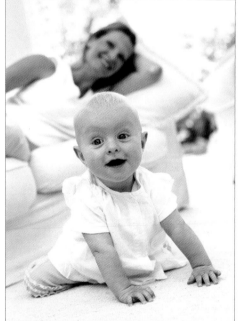

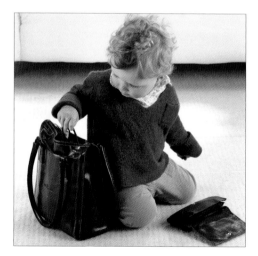

KEEPING ACTIVE CHILDREN SAFE

- Fit stairgates at the top and bottom of stairs once your child is ready to crawl.
- Check your banisters are safe: you need vertical spindles (horizontal ones can serve as a ladder), no more than 10cm/4in apart.
- Put locks on any windows that your child could open.
- Make sure that the locks on the doors to your home are set higher than your child can reach. If not, fit a high bolt and use it.
- Put plug covers on all unused electrical sockets. Turn off the switch at the socket when you are not using it, and replace any worn flexes.
- Cover any child-level glass with safety film.
- Put corner covers on any tables. Consider getting rid of low coffee tables altogether.
- Don't have any flimsy furniture that your child could pull over on top of him or her. Attach freestanding bookshelves to the wall.
- Constantly check floors and other areas for small items that your child could choke on: coins, marbles, pen tops, buttons, rubber tyres from toy cars, small squidgy balls and burst or uninflated balloons are all potential hazards to your child.

IN THE BEDROOM

Children's bedrooms are generally safer than other parts of the home, because they are usually decorated and furnished with the child in mind. But there are some basic things to bear in mind:

The best time to iron is when your child is in bed. If you do need to iron at other times, keep your child well away (in a playpen or behind a safety gate) and put the iron out of reach as soon as you have finished. Put it away when it has cooled down.

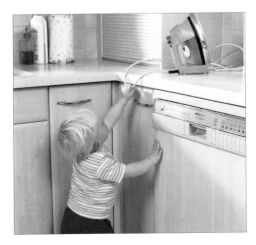

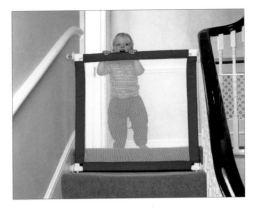

Fit a stairgate at the top and bottom of stairs until your child can safely navigate them independently. Let children practise going up and coming down from time to time: teach your child to come down bottom first.

- Make sure your child's cot is a safe place. The bars should be no more than 7cm/2¾in apart, and the mattress should fit snugly. Don't give a child under one year a duvet or pillows.
- Position the cot or bed away from windows and radiators.
- Don't put anything under the window (such as low cupboards, bookshelves or toy boxes) that your child could use as a step. Don't forget to fit window locks in your child's room.
- Use a radiator cover to protect your child from burns. Alternatively, turn the thermostat down and cover the radiator with a large towel.

SAFETY WITH TOYS

- Don't let your child play with a toy intended for an older child; age ranges are recommended for safety reasons.
- Don't give toys with long strings to a baby: they are a strangling hazard. Musical cot toys with strings should be removed before the child can get on hands and knees.
- Remove all packaging and labels before giving a toy to your child.
- Check second-hand toys carefully. Old toys may have been made to less stringent safety standards or contain chemicals that are no longer allowed.
- Get rid of broken toys that cannot be repaired.
- If you need to change the batteries in a toy, change all of them: old batteries can get overheated if they are next to new ones.
- Don't get a toy chest that can be locked or one with a hinged lid – it could slam on your child's head.

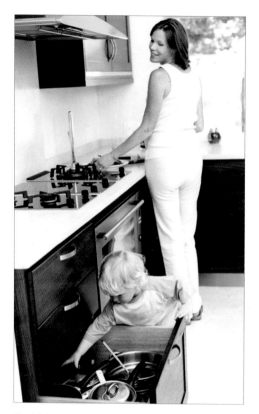

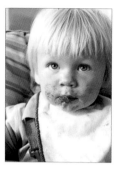

Make sure that your child is sitting in a highchair or booster seat that is appropriate for his or her age, and that they are safely strapped in at mealtimes.

Fit childproof locks to kitchen cupboards and drawers within your child's reach, especially if you store breakable, heavy or harmful items there. But consider letting a child use one cupboard or drawer for play.

IN THE KITCHEN

The kitchen is full of items that are potential hazards for inquisitive children. You need to get into the habit of tidying up after yourself and closing cupboard doors and drawers once you have got what you need. If you can, keep your child out of the kitchen when you are cooking: you may be able to use a stair gate to fence off the cooking area or fit in a playpen to keep your child safe.

Store plastic bags and clingfilm out of reach: young children instinctively want to wear a bag like a hat. Keep knives somewhere safe. Fit locks to low-level cupboards and drawers. Store dishwasher tablets (which are particularly noxious) and other cleaning products in a locked cupboard, and make sure that your child knows this is the 'nasty cupboard'. If a child does swallow something toxic, get medical advice urgently. If you need to go to hospital, take the packaging with you.

When you are cooking, turn saucepan handles to the back of the hob, and use the rear burners when possible.

Hob guards can make cooking and lifting pans awkward, so are not advisable. Give up deep-fat frying, which is very dangerous, or invest in an electric fryer. Have a small fire extinguisher and a fire blanket to hand.

Put the kitchen bin somewhere your child cannot access. Clean up spills quickly, to avoid slipping, and watch for toys, particularly wheeled ones, left in the kitchen. Ban tablecloths for now, and push chairs in under the table so that your child doesn't use them as a step.

EATING SAFELY

Always get your child to sit down when eating, as he or she is more likely to choke if running around and eating at the same time. Encourage your child to chew well and to eat slowly.

Chop foods that are firm and round. Sausages and hot dogs can block the windpipe, so cut them lengthways and then into small pieces. Cut fruit and raw vegetables into small pieces, not rounds, and quarter grapes before giving them to your toddler. Never give whole nuts to a child under five; popcorn, boiled or sticky sweets and peanut butter eaten from the spoon (rather than spread thinly on toast) are also choking hazards.

Always strap your child into a highchair or booster seat: a five-point harness is safest. Don't use a chair that can be attached directly on to the kitchen table; it may work its way loose unnoticed.

IN THE BATHROOM

Most young children love water, but it is important that you supervise them at all times when they are in the bath and that you don't leave a filled bath unattended: a child can drown in even shallow water and your toddler may be better at climbing than you think. If you need to do something, such as answer the door or attend to another child's needs, get your child out of the bath and take him or her with you.

Keep the toilet seat cover down. A toilet seat lock is useful if your child develops a desire to throw toys and other items down the toilet. Keep mouthwashes, cleaners, razors and medicines in a locked cabinet. Get

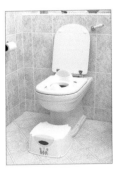

Left: Once your child is toilet trained, you will need to get a step so that he or she can reach the toilet safely and independently.

Right: A garden is a wonderful place for a child to play, so long as it has been made safe.

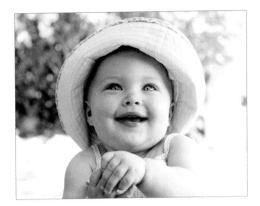

rid of glass thermometers that contain mercury; take them to a pharmacist for safe disposal. Consider turning the hot water temperature down to less than 55°C/130°F.

IN THE GARDEN

A garden allows children to play chasing and ball games much more safely than indoors. And it introduces them to some of the simple wonders of nature: flowers, trees, insects and birds. But you need to plan your garden carefully to ensure that it is safe. Make sure that your child cannot get out of the garden into neighbouring gardens or the street. Maintain fences or walls, make sure there are no gaps that your child can squeeze through, and lock gates after use.

Don't leave your child unattended near any water, even in a bucket. Drain paddling pools and turn them upside-down after use to prevent rainwater from collecting here. Turn any containers kept in the garden, such as dustbins or wheelbarrows, upside-down too.

If you have a slide or climbing frame in the garden, place it on grass rather than a hard surface and check it regularly for safety. Lock away any garden chemicals in a safe place. Always keep garden products in the original bottle so that you know what they are; never decant them into, say, a lemonade bottle. Better still, get rid of them. Keep garden tools and lawnmowers locked away.

If you have a dog, don't allow it to urinate or defecate in the garden. Teach your child not to eat soil, which may be contaminated by cat faeces. Wash your child's hands after playing in the garden.

Discourage your child from picking flowers or from putting plant material into his or her mouth. Many plants are poisonous and may irritate the skin if they are touched and cause illness or even death if eaten. If you think a child has eaten a poisonous plant, take him or her to hospital (or call an ambulance), and take a sample of the plant with you.

POISONOUS PLANTS

Common garden plants that are toxic include yew, laburnum, lily of the valley, delphinium, deadly nightshade, foxgloves, ivy, hyacinth, mistletoe, daffodil, azalea, privet, rhododendron, toadstools and some mushrooms.

Don't have a pond: it is too easy for a young child to fall in and drown. If you already have one, the safest option is to fill it in; you could turn it into a sandpit.

Don't assume a gate will keep your child in a garden – this one has horizontal bars and an adventurous toddler could easily climb up it.

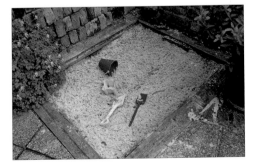

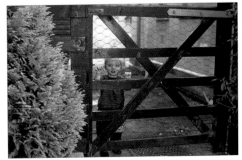

Safety when you are out

However safe you make your own home, you are bound to take your children to other people's homes that are less child-friendly. Get in the habit of scanning any room your child enters for possible hazards. Most people won't mind if you ask them to move something breakable from your child's reach or to move their coffee cup from the corner of a table. Be careful around animals that are unused to children: err on the side of caution and keep your child well away. If you plan to leave your child in another person's care, make sure that you are happy the environment is safe enough.

Be extra vigilant if there is a pond: about 80 per cent of drownings in garden ponds happen when children are visiting friends or relatives. If you go to a park where there is a pond or lake, keep very close to your child.

CAR JOURNEYS

All children should be fastened into properly fitted car seats for car journeys, however short. Never be tempted to take a trip holding your child in your lap; you will not be able to hold on to the child if your car is hit, and you could injure him or her with your body on impact.

Choose a car seat that meets recognized safety standards, and check with the manufacturer that it is suitable for your particular car. Check online to ensure that your car seat meets the regulations in your country. Don't buy a second-hand car seat: you won't know if it has been weakened in a previous accident, and it may have been made to less rigorous safety standards than a new seat.

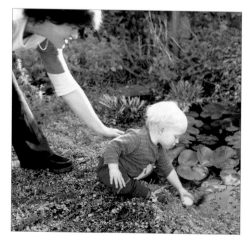

WHICH CAR SEAT?

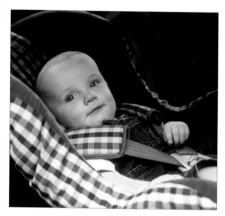

Babies (Group 0): Rear-facing seats are needed for babies from birth to 10–13kg/22–29lb. But it is best to avoid taking a very young baby on a long car journey if you can. Keep your baby in this first car seat until he or she outgrows it. You can get Group 0+ and 1 seats that are rearward-facing and suitable for a child up to the age of four. These are more protective in the event of a crash but take up more space.

Older babies and toddlers (Group 1): Forward-facing seats are suitable for children from about nine months (so long as they can sit up well unsupported and weigh at least 9kg/20lb). They last until the child is about four and weighs 18kg/40lb.

Young children (Group 2): Booster seats with a back and wings are suitable for children weighing 15–25kg/33–55lb, usually between the ages of four and six. They are best fitted in the back of the car rather than the front, and this is essential if there is an airbag in the front of the car. They don't have a separate harness as car seats do; instead the seatbelt goes around both the seat and the child.

Older children (Group 3): Children should use some sort of booster seat until they reach the age of 11. Booster cushions are used for children weighing 22–36kg/48–79lb.

Children are instinctively drawn by water. Never leave your child unattended in a garden with a pond; keep him or her in sight at all times.

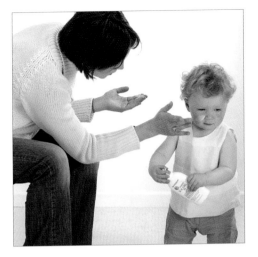

Around 10 minutes of sun early or late in the day helps your child to make essential vitamin D. But he or she needs a high-factor suncream at other times.

Many car seats are fitted incorrectly, so go to a specialist if you need help. If your car is new, go for an ISOFIX car seat, which is much easier to fit.

- Never fit a car seat in the front seat of a car if there is an airbag in front of it – the airbag could seriously harm (and possibly kill) your child if it inflates. It is safer to fit the seat in the back even if there is no airbag.
- Make sure that the seat belt goes through all guides on the seat.
- Check the seat belt is pulled tight before every journey: the seat shouldn't rock sideways or forwards when you try to move it.
- Don't have the buckle of the seatbelt resting on the frame of the car seat; it could snap open in an accident.
- Adjust the harness so it fits snugly. Check it at the start of every journey, as the fit will depend on what your child is wearing. Don't have the buckle resting on your child's tummy.
- If you are using a booster seat, make sure the seatbelt rests against your child's shoulder, not his neck, and from hip bone to hip bone.

OUT IN THE SUN

Children's skin is thinner than adults', so you need to be vigilant about protecting it from sunburn: damage to the skin now could have long-term effects. Babies under six months should be kept out of direct sunlight entirely. If your baby is in a buggy or pram, use a UV sunshade. If you are carrying a baby in a sling, cover his or her arms and legs with a light but closely woven fabric such as cotton and get a wide-brimmed hat.

SUN FOODS

Foods containing the antioxidant beta-carotene may help protect the skin from the harmful effects of the sun. Carrots, melons, mango, apricots and spinach are all good sources that are worth including in your child's summer diet.

Put sunscreen on the baby's hands and feet if they are exposed. Older babies and young children should be kept out of direct sunlight as much as possible during the hottest part of the day (10am–4pm on very hot days). Apply a high-factor sunscreen at least half an hour before you go outside. Use a sunscreen made from natural ingredients with an SPF of at least 20. This will be gentler on your child's skin than very high factor sunscreens that last three or four hours (but which may get rubbed off beforehand in any case). Apply a thick layer and let it sink into the skin rather than rubbing in. Reapply frequently. However, if you know that your child is going to be out in the sun for some time, especially in someone else's care, use a higher factor to be on the safe side. Remember that skin can still burn on warm cloudy days, or in the shade next to water or sand, which reflects sunlight.

Your child will need more fluids when it is hot. If you are breastfeeding, nurse frequently: your milk has a higher water content on hot days so your baby shouldn't need extra drinks.

Some children refuse to hold hands when they are out and about – in which case you will need reins or a wrist strap to keep them safe.

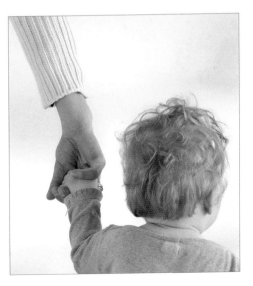

Meal planners
and recipes

❝ It is always good to include your young child in family meal times and it is easy to adapt your cooking for adults and young children. **❞**

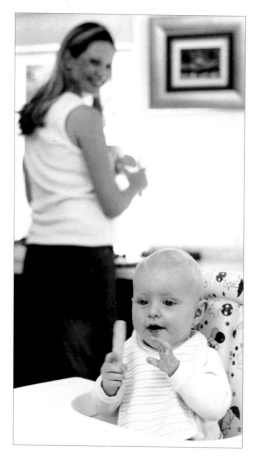

Cooking for children – like most other aspects of childcare – can be very pleasurable but also intensely frustrating. All parents have had the experience of seeing a lovingly prepared meal rejected entirely, flung on the floor or spat out in disgust. Children don't appreciate the effort that you put into making their meals. It's not a criticism of your cooking or your care.

It will take some of the tension out of meal times if you cook batches of food in advance and put them in the freezer. If there is a gap between the time when you cook the food and the time when you serve it, then you will take it less personally if your child merely toys with a couple of spoonfuls. This chapter includes some tried-and-tested recipes that can be spooned into small pots and frozen. Even if you have no home-cooked meals in the freezer, you don't have to resort to processed food. There are plenty of quick meals you can make without much effort: boiled rice with tiny chunks of cheese and peas, pasta with grated fresh tomato, scrambled eggs, and sardines

While your baby still instinctively tests things with his or her mouth, take advantage of this inquisitiveness and offer as many different textures and flavours as you can.

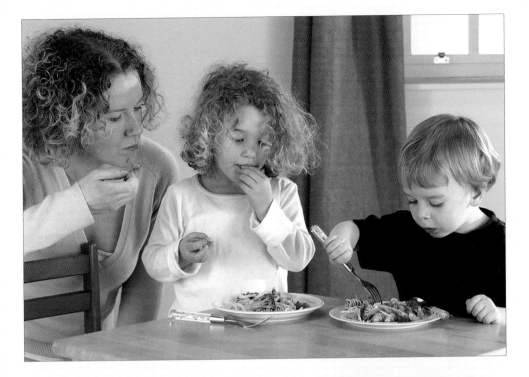

on toast. All these take a few minutes to prepare, and are often a child's favourite meals.

Of course, it is always good to include your young child in family meal times and it is easy to adapt your cooking to suit adults and young children. When you make soup or casseroles, for example, get into the habit of using homemade stock or a low-salt bouillon, and then add salt at the table to your own portion if you need it.

Children are amenable to a little spice in their food, but are unlikely to take to an intensely flavoured, fiery curry. If you are making a curry, stir in the hotter spices once you have taken out your child's portion. Always offer new foods or unusual tastes as something interesting to try rather than something they have to like and eat.

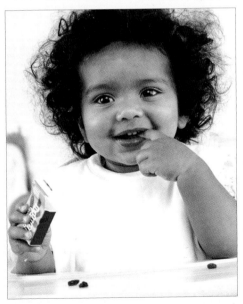

Top: As children get older they enjoy eating in company and start to appreciate the social side of meal times. Encourage this by eating with them whenever you can.

Children love sweet things, but keep their sugary snacks to a minimum and offer dried or fresh fruit rather than biscuits and cakes.

meal planners and recipes **459**

Meal planning for babies

First foods should be easy for babies to eat and digest, so baby rice, puréed root vegetables and pears and apples are ideal, but there is no strict rule about exactly which foods to give first, so it is fine if you want to chop and change. However, do make sure you don't introduce any foods that may cause an allergic reaction until the ages recommended in Chapter 5. The menu planner on the opposite page starts at six months: if you are starting solids earlier, you will have to adapt it slightly so that you don't introduce foods such as chicken, fish or wheat too early.

INTRODUCING SOLIDS

It helps your baby to adjust to new flavours if you mix each food with his or her usual milk or with milky baby rice for the first few times you give it.

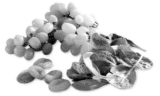

Giving fruits and vegetables of different colours will help your child to get a good range of vitamins.

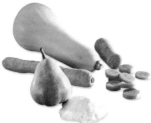

Meat, eggs, tomatoes and citrus fruits can be introduced once the baby is well established on solids.

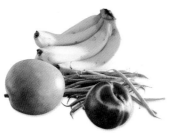

You can gradually introduce a wider variety of fruits and vegetables to your child.

Babies like sweet tastes, so root vegetables, pears and apples mixed with baby rice are good first foods.

Alternate the new food with foods you have already introduced, so that your baby gets used to having different tastes at every meal. You can combine purées, too, mixing squash and carrot, carrot and parsnip, parsnip and apple and so on. Be sure to leave three days before introducing each new food, to allow time for any reaction to show itself. However, once your baby is eating lots of different foods, you can introduce a flavouring such as garlic at the same time as, say, lentils. Remember that you shouldn't cut down on milk feeds until the end of the first year.

PLANNING YOUR MENUS

Once you have a few meals prepared and stored in the freezer, it's easy to give your baby a good and varied diet. Pasta or rice with butter, cheese and a few chopped

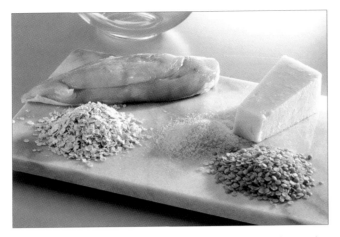

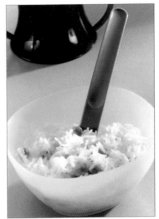

Grains are an important source of energy, while chicken, pulses and dairy foods are good protein foods.

vegetables mixed in, or mashed avocado, make a good quick meal if you run out. Your baby may need a few snacks as well as the usual milk in between meals. Use the menu planner as a guide, and remember that so long as you vary foods throughout a week, your baby will be getting a good mix of nutrients, even if on one day they refuse to eat anything other than grapes.

Breastfed babies will usually have more milk feeds, but a routine might look like this:

A good quick meal is rice with a spoonful of cooked vegetables and some grated cheese.

On waking Milk, then breakfast
11.30 am Lunch with water
2.30 pm Milk and afternoon snack
5.00 pm Supper with water
7.00 pm Milk

MENU PLANNER FOR A BABY FROM NINE TO TWELVE MONTHS

Adapt this to your needs and routine and vary it if you need to.

Day 1
Breakfast Oat porridge with banana
Lunch Tarragon chicken with potatoes
  Plain yoghurt
Snack Pear slices and toast fingers
Supper Vegetable soup with rice

Day 2
Breakfast Oat/millet porridge with pear purée
  Toast fingers
Lunch Lentil dhal with rice or quinoa and spinach
Snack Rice cakes and apple slices
Supper Pasta with peas, olive oil and cheese
  Mango purée

Day 3
Breakfast Wheat biscuit cereal with banana
Lunch Cauliflower and broccoli cheese
  Raspberry and apple purée
Snack Polenta fingers and pear slices
Supper Fish pilau

Day 4
Breakfast Oat porridge with mango and cinnamon
  Toast fingers
Lunch Beany bake
Snack Rice cakes, grapes
Supper Buttery rice with swede (rutabaga) purée and broccoli
  Natural yoghurt with fruit purée

Day 5
Breakfast Millet porridge with pear and banana
Lunch Ratatouille with pitta fingers
  Strawberries or raspberries with

Greek yoghurt
Snack Oatcakes and melon chunks
Supper Lamb casserole with rice

Day 6
Breakfast Wheat biscuit cereal with pear
Lunch Poached salmon with rice, sugar snap peas and cooked tomato
Snack Banana
Supper Vegetable soup and mini cream cheese sandwiches (add pineapple to the cheese and blend to a purée)

Day 7
Breakfast Oat porridge with banana
Lunch Couscous salad
  Apricot compote
Snack Polenta fingers and grapes
Supper Lightly fried chicken fillet, rice and steamed carrot sticks

Recipes for babies: six to nine months

Once your baby is eating a range of foods, you can start combining ingredients to make more interesting meals. Here are some suggestions for easy-to-cook, baby-friendly dishes.

BABY RICE

It's worth making your own baby rice once your baby is eating more than a couple of teaspoonfuls at a time. You won't get it as smooth as the commercial variety, but this is a good way to start introducing texture. Use white rice not brown.

50g/2oz white rice
breast or formula milk

Bring a small pan of water to the boil, add the rice and stir once. Leave to simmer for about 10 minutes, until the rice grains are tender. Drain the rice, then purée with your baby's usual milk.

COURGETTE PURÉE

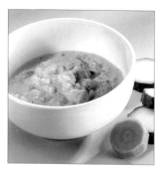

Steamed courgettes (zucchini) go well with sweet carrots. Leave the skin on the carrot if it is organic. This is a good purée to freeze in single-portion quantities.

1 courgette (zucchini)
1 carrot

Chop the courgette and peel and chop the carrot. Put the carrot in a steamer and cook for 5 minutes. Add the courgette and steam for another 10 minutes, until both vegetables are very soft. Purée with your baby's usual milk or use a little of the water used to steam the vegetables.

POTATO, SWEET POTATO AND SWEDE MASH

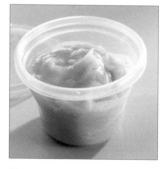

Most root vegetables purée well and have an easy texture and a nice sweet taste. You can try adding a pinch of garam masala to the combination to liven it up once your baby is well established on solid foods and is ready to experience new tastes.

2 large potatoes
quarter of a small swede
  (rutabaga)
1 small sweet potato

Peel and dice all the vegetables and steam them for 15–20 minutes, until soft. Blend or mash with your baby's usual milk until smooth.

VEGETABLE SOUP

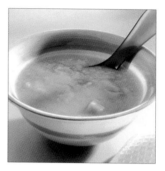

Soup slips down easily, so it is great for times when your baby is tired and doesn't want to eat much. This is a simple recipe that you can also use as a pasta sauce. Substitute celery for the leeks if you like, but in this case add half a chopped onion to the pan and fry for 2–3 minutes before adding the other vegetables.

2 medium leeks, cleaned
4 large potatoes
2 carrots
a little olive oil, for frying
1.2 litres/2 pints/5 cups vegetable
  stock
handful of parsley, finely chopped

Slice the leeks. Cut the potatoes into large chunks, and peel (unless organic) and slice the carrots.

Put a little olive oil in a pan over a low heat and add the vegetables. Cook for 5 minutes, stirring all the time. Add the stock, bring to a simmer, cover and cook for 25 minutes. Add the parsley and cook for 5 minutes, then blend.

FREEZING PURÉES

Most vegetable and fruit purées can be frozen, but you should add any milk after defrosting. It is also better not to use chicken stock for frozen meals, as it needs to be boiled when reheating.

STOCK

Most commercial stocks are too salty for babies. Good supermarkets and health food stores stock low-salt, good-quality bouillon, but, better still, make your own – it's pretty easy and once you get into the habit of doing it you won't want to go back to cubes. Store stock in the refrigerator for up to 4 days or freeze for up to 3 months.

For vegetable stock

Chop 1 celery stick, 1 large carrot, 1 large leek, 1 onion and 1 garlic clove. Put in a pan with 5 peppercorns, 2 sprigs of parsley (or parsley stalks), 2 sprigs of thyme and a bay leaf. Cover with 1.2 litres/2 pints/5 cups water, and bring to the boil. Skim off any froth, cover the pan, reduce the heat and simmer for 45 minutes. Leave to cool. Pour through a sieve lined with muslin (a baby muslin is ideal).

For chicken stock

Break up the carcass of a cooked chicken. Chop 1 onion, 1 carrot and 1 celery stick and place in a pan with the chicken bones, 5 peppercorns, 2 cloves, a small handful of parsley (or parsley stalks) and a bay leaf. Cover with 1.2 litres/2 pints/5 cups water, and bring to the boil. Skim off any froth, cover the pan, reduce the heat and simmer for 1 hour. Fish out the big bones, then strain through a muslin-lined sieve.

MEDITERRANEAN VEGETABLES

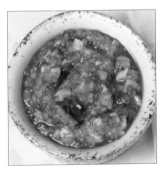

Red pepper has quite a strong flavour for babies, so you might want to try this recipe without it or with half the quantity the first time. Add some garlic with the vegetables for another flavour variation.

3 tomatoes
175g/6oz courgettes (zucchini)
75g/3oz button (white)
* mushrooms*
115g/4oz red (bell) pepper
20ml/4 tsp tomato ketchup
250ml/8fl oz/1 cup water
pinch of dried mixed herbs
40g/1½oz dried pasta shapes

Make a cross cut in each tomato, put in a small bowl and cover with boiling water. Leave for 1 minute, then drain and peel off the skins. Cut into quarters and scoop out the seeds from the tomatoes. Rinse and slice the courgette and mushrooms. Chop the pepper. Put the vegetables in a pan with the ketchup, water and herbs. Cover and simmer for 10 minutes, or until tender. Meanwhile cook the pasta in boiling water for 8–10 minutes, until tender. Drain. Mix the vegetables and pasta together and process or mash with a fork until the right consistency.

LENTIL DHAL

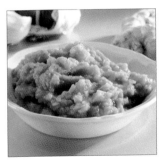

Babies love dhal. You can purée this one with a serving of baby rice and some sliced cooked spinach to make a balanced meal in one – it's good with a spoonful of bio-active yoghurt. You can also add a spoonful of dhal to vegetable soup to make it a more substantial meal.

50g/2oz red lentils, washed
small slice of ginger
half a clove of garlic (sliced
* lengthways)*
1 bay leaf
1 tomato (optional)

Place the lentils in a small pan. Pour in water up to a level about one and a half times the depth of the lentils. Add the ginger, garlic and bay leaf.

Bring to the boil, skim off any froth, reduce the heat, cover the pan and simmer for about 25 minutes or until the lentils are very tender.

Meanwhile, pour boiling water over the tomato, if using. Leave for a minute or two, remove the skin, cut in half, deseed and chop finely.

When the lentils are soft, discard the ginger and bay leaf, but mash the garlic into the dhal. Add the chopped tomato, if using, and cook for another 5 minutes. Blend if your baby is still eating smooth purées. **Variation**: For a spicier dhal, fry half an onion in vegetable oil until golden brown. Add 1.5ml/¼ tsp each of ground coriander and ground cumin and fry for a further minute or two. Add this to the dhal.

FISH CREOLE

White fish is a good first protein for your baby, it is easy to digest and the texture doesn't pose as much of a challenge as chicken. If you use fresh fish you can freeze the purée.

50g/2oz celery
50g/2oz red (bell) pepper
300ml/½ pint/1¼ cups water
50g/2oz/¼ cup long grain rice
10ml/2 tsp tomato ketchup
90g/3½oz frozen cod

Trim the celery and discard the core and seeds from the pepper. Rinse and chop the vegetables. Bring the water to the boil in a pan and add the vegetables, rice, ketchup and cod. Bring back to the boil, then reduce heat, cover and simmer for 15 minutes, until the rice is tender and the fish is cooked. Lift the fish out of the pan with a slotted spoon. Use a knife and fork to check for bones. Stir the fish back into the pan and then chop or process. Spoon a little fish mixture into a small bowl, test the temperature and cool if necessary, before giving to the baby. Cover the leftover fish creole and transfer to the refrigerator as soon as possible. Use within 24 hours.

CHICKEN, PARSNIP AND GREEN BEAN PURÉE

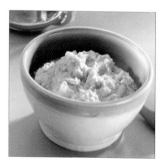

Any vegetable purée will go well with chicken, but parsnip has a wonderfully sweet taste that babies love. Use broccoli or leeks in place of the beans if you like.

1 parsnip
50g/2oz fine green beans
1 small chicken breast
a little olive oil, for frying

Cut the parsnip into quarters lengthways. Cut out the woody core from each piece then chop into small chunks. Top and tail the beans. Steam the parsnip for 5 minutes then add the green beans to the steamer and continue cooking for another 10 minutes, until soft.

Meanwhile, cut the chicken breast into small pieces. Heat a little olive oil in a frying pan, and fry the chicken for 6–7 minutes until cooked through. Combine the cooked chicken with the vegetables and blend or mash until smooth.

TURKEY STEW WITH CARROTS AND CORN

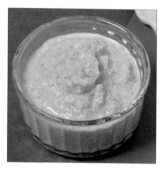

Using formula milk gives this purée a creamy texture that your baby will enjoy, while the carrot and corn will add sweetness.

175g/6oz potato
175g/6oz carrot
115g/4oz turkey breast, skinned
*   and boned*
50g/2oz/⅓ cup frozen corn
300ml/½ pint/1¼ cups formula
*   milk*

Trim and peel the potato and carrots, rinse under cold water and then chop into small cubes. Rinse the turkey breast and cut into thin strips. Place in a small pan with the potato and carrot, add the corn and milk. Cover and simmer for 20 minutes, until the turkey is cooked. Purée, mash or sieve (strain) the mixture until smooth.

Variation: Try using the same amount of sweet potato in place of the carrot. Sweet potato is really very sweet, so don't mix it with carrot. You can use chicken breast instead of turkey in this recipe.

PORK AND RUNNER BEANS

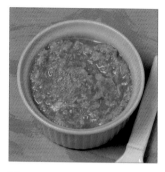

When you are reheating frozen dishes that contain meat, especially pork or chicken, you must ensure that the food is heated through. If fresh beans are not in season use broccoli instead.

115g/4oz lean pork
115g/4oz potato
115g/4oz carrot
75g/3oz runner (green) beans
pinch of dried sage
350ml/12fl oz/1½ cups water

Rinse the pork under cold water, trim away any fat and gristle and chop into small cubes. Peel the potato and carrot, trim the beans, rinse and chop. Put the pork, potato and carrot in a pan with the sage and water. Bring to the boil, cover and simmer for 30 minutes. Process or mash to the desired consistency.

LAMB HOTPOT

This is a tasty purée suitable for an older baby who is ready for some new tastes and textures. You can add a pinch of cumin and coriander if you wish.

115g/4oz potato
115g/4oz carrot
115g/4oz swede (rutabaga)
50g/2oz leek
115g/4oz lamb fillet
300ml/½ pint/1¼ cup water
pinch of dried rosemary

Peel the potato, carrot and swede, then rinse and chop into small cubes. Halve the leek lengthways, rinse well and slice. Place all the vegetables in a pan. Rinse the lamb under cold water and chop into small pieces, discarding any fat. Add the meat to the pan together with the water and rosemary. Bring to the boil, cover and simmer for 30 minutes or until the lamb is thoroughly cooked. Process or mash the ingredients to the desired consistency.

RASPBERRY AND APPLE PURÉE

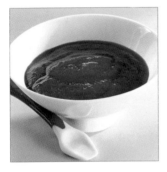

Simple fruit purées are a great way of getting vitamins into your baby.

1 eating apple, peeled and diced
115g/4oz raspberries

Place the fruit in a small pan with a tablespoon of water. Cook over a low heat for 5 minutes, or until soft. Purée the fruit, then pass through a sieve (strainer) to remove the seeds.

APRICOT COMPOTE

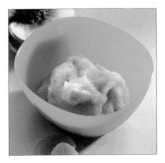

3 ready-to-eat dried apricots
1 eating apple, peeled and diced
1 large nectarine, stoned (pitted)

Chop the apricots and nectarine. Place all the fruits in a small pan with a little water. Simmer for about 10 minutes, until very soft, then purée.

APPLE AND ORANGE FOOL

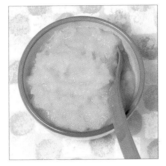

The custard made with formula milk gives a lovely creamy texture and flavour to this dessert. Use a good quality custard powder that doesn't contain excess colourings and additives.

2 eating apples
5ml/1 tsp grated orange rind and
*   15ml/1 tbsp orange juice*
15ml/1 tbsp custard powder
5ml/1 tsp caster (superfine) sugar
150ml/¼ pint/⅔ cup formula milk

Quarter, core and peel the apples. Slice and place the apples in a pan with the orange rind and juice. Cover and cook gently for 10 minutes, stirring occasionally until the apples are soft. Blend the custard powder and sugar with a little of the milk to make a smooth paste. Bring the remaining milk to the boil and stir into the custard mixture. Return the custard to the pan and slowly bring to the boil, stirring until thickened and smooth. Process or mash the apple to the desired consistency. Add the custard and stir to mix. Spoon a little into a bowl, test the temperature and cool if necessary,

before giving to the baby. Cover the remaining fool and transfer to the refrigerator as soon as possible. Use within 24 hours.

MARMITE BREAD STICKS

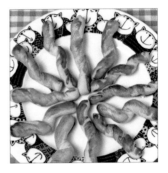

By the time your baby is 9 months old he or she will be ready for finger foods. Try these marmite bread sticks together with crudites of fresh vegetables such as celery, carrot and red pepper. This recipe makes around 36 sticks, you can freeze half and simply defrost as needed.

little oil, for greasing
150g/5oz packet pizza base mix
flour, for dusting
5ml/1 tsp Marmite (yeast extract
*   spread)*
1 egg yolk

Brush two baking sheets with a little oil. Put the pizza mix in a bowl and mix to a smooth dough as directed on the packet. Knead on a lightly floured surface for 5 minutes, then roll out to a 23cm/9in square. Cut into strips 7.5cm x 1cm/3 x ½in, twisting each to give a corkscrew effect. Arrange on the baking sheets, slightly spaced apart.

Mix the Marmite and egg yolk together and brush over the bread sticks. Loosely cover with oiled clear film (plastic wrap) and leave in a warm place for 30 minutes to rise. Preheat the oven to 220°C/425°F/Gas 7. Bake for 10 minutes, until risen. Leave to cool. Store for up to three days.

Recipes for babies: nine to twelve months

Once you have introduced a reasonable number of different foods, cooking for your baby becomes a lot more fun. Here are some baby-friendly meals that older children (and adults) will love too.

SIMPLE FISH PILAU

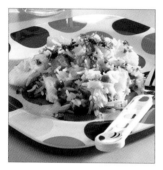

This is a simple fish dish that you can make just as easily with salmon.

200g/7oz cod or haddock fillet
milk to cover
1 onion, finely chopped
2 garlic cloves, crushed
a little olive oil, for frying
knob (pat) of butter
200g/7oz basmati rice
600ml/1 pint/2½ cups vegetable
  or fish stock
225g/8oz tomatoes
50g/2oz frozen peas
small handful of parsley, chopped
freshly ground black pepper

Place the fish in a small pan and cover with milk. Cook on a low heat until the fish is just opaque – about 5–7 minutes.

Heat a little olive oil in a frying pan. Add the onion and garlic and sweat for 6–7 minutes, until softened but not browned. Add the butter to the pan and let it melt, then add the rice, and stir until coated. Pour in half the stock and stir until it is absorbed into the rice, then add the rest a little at a time until the rice is cooked (about 25 minutes). Skin and deseed the tomatoes and chop, add with the peas to the rice mixture, and cook for a further 5 minutes.

Flake the cooked fish, removing any bones, and add to the rice with the herbs. Season with a twist of black pepper, and cook the pilau for a further 2–3 minutes, stirring.

FISH AND CHEESE PIE

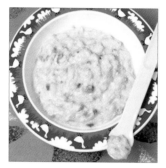

This is a great classic family recipe that has endless variations. This creamy version includes leeks and mushrooms, but you could use carrots and broccoli instead, according to taste.

225g/8oz potato
50g/2oz leek
50g/2oz button (white)
  mushrooms
90g/3½oz frozen skinless cod
250ml/8fl oz/1 cup formula milk
50g/2oz grated Cheddar,
  or mild cheese

Peel the potato, halve the leek and trim the mushrooms. Place all the vegetables in a colander and rinse well with cold water, drain, then chop the vegetables. Place the vegetables in a pan with the frozen cod and milk. Bring to the boil, cover and simmer for 15 minutes, until the fish is cooked and the potatoes are tender when pierced with a knife. Lift the fish out of the pan with a slotted spoon and break into pieces with a knife and fork, checking carefully for bones. Return the fish to the pan and stir in the grated cheese. Chop or process the mixture to give the desired consistency. Spoon a little into a bowl, test the temperature and cool if necessary, before serving to the baby. Cover the remaining fish pie and transfer to the refrigerator as soon as possible. Use within 24 hours.

TARRAGON CHICKEN

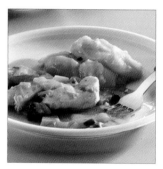

If you are bringing your child up to eat meat, chicken is likely to figure often on the menu. This easy stew contains leeks and mushrooms, but you can add other vegetables as well. Choose organic chicken.

2 large chicken breast fillets
2 medium leeks, washed
a little vegetable oil, for frying
knob (pat) of butter
450ml/¾ pint/scant 2 cups stock,
  or to cover
handful of parsley, chopped
1 sprig fresh tarragon (or a large

pinch of dried tarragon)
450g/1lb large flat mushrooms
5ml/1 tsp cornflour (cornstarch)
freshly ground black pepper

Cut the chicken into small chunks. Finely chop the leeks.

Heat the vegetable oil in a flameproof casserole or a deep heavy-bottomed frying pan. Fry the chicken in two or three batches over a medium heat for 6–7 minutes, until cooked through. Set aside.

Add the butter to the same pan and cook the leeks for 6–7 minutes until softened but not browned. Return the chicken to the pan. Add the stock and season with a couple of twists of black pepper. Add the herbs and leave to simmer for 10 minutes, uncovered, stirring from time to time, until slightly reduced. Chop the mushrooms very small and add to the pan. Cook for a further 6–7 minutes until cooked down.

When the stew is cooked, put about 50ml/2 fl oz/¼ cup water in a cup. Sprinkle in the cornflour and stir until dissolved. Add the mixture to the stew and cook for a further 2–3 minutes to thicken the sauce.

Variation: You can add 450g/1lb new potatoes, chopped into small pieces or grated, to the stew to make a complete meal. If you want to try new tastes and textures on your baby add other vegetables, try

half a green (bell) pepper or an aubergine (eggplant), diced or a little finely shredded cabbage or spinach. Cook the potatoes and any other vegetables with the leeks.

CHICKEN AND CELERY SUPPER

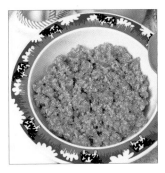

The celery adds a nice flavour to this chicken dish. For a slightly stronger flavour use the same amount of homemade chicken or vegetable stock instead of water, and substitute the same amount of tomato purée for the vegetable purée.

175g/6oz chicken thighs, skinned
    and boned
¼ onion
225g/8oz carrots
75g/3oz celery
5ml/1 tsp oil
10ml/2 tsp vegetable purée (paste)
250ml/8fl oz/1 cup water

Rinse the chicken under cold water, pat dry, trim off any fat and cut into chunks. Trim and rinse the vegetables and cut into small pieces. Heat the oil in a pan, add the chicken and onion, and fry for a few minutes, stirring until browned. Add the carrots, celery, vegetable purée and water. Bring to the boil, cover and simmer for 20 minutes, until tender. Chop or process the mixture to the desired consistency. If using a food processor, process the solids first and then add the liquid a little at a time.

LAMB COUSCOUS

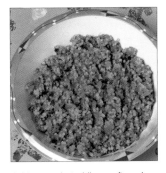

Babies and toddlers often love couscous, although some may take a while to get used to the texture. This is a good way of introducing it, mixed with more familiar ingredients. Use tomato purée if you can't find vegetable purée.

115g/4oz carrot
115g/4oz swede (rutabaga)
¼ onion
175g/6oz lamb fillet
5ml/1 tsp oil
10ml/2 tsp vegetable purée
    (paste)
30ml/2 tbsp currants or raisins
300ml/½ pint/1¼ cups water
50g/2oz couscous

Peel the carrot, swede and onion, rinse and chop. Rinse the lamb, trim off any fat, and chop. Heat the oil in a pan, and fry the lamb until browned. Add the vegetables, cook

---

FOOD ON THE GO
Sticks of cheese, mini sandwiches, easy-to-eat fruit or small pots of natural yoghurt are all ideal foods to take out with you. For a more substantial lunch, you could make an easy couscous or pasta salad.

Couscous salad
Pour a serving of couscous into a teacup and cover with boiling water. Add 5ml/1 tsp olive oil, cover and leave for 3–4 minutes for the grains to swell. Cook a few peas, and a chopped tomato in a pan with a tiny amount of water. Add to the couscous with some Cheddar cheese cut into tiny dice.

Pasta salad
Combine some cooked pasta shapes with some finely diced, cooked carrots and peas, flaked canned tuna, chopped parsley and a little olive oil.

for 2 minutes, then stir in the vegetable purée, currants and water. Cover and simmer for 25 minutes. Put the couscous in a sieve (strainer) and rinse under cold running water. Cover and steam the couscous over the lamb pan, for 5 minutes. Chop or process the lamb mixture to the desired consistency. Fluff the couscous up with a fork and add to the lamb mixture stirring well.

LAMB CASSEROLE

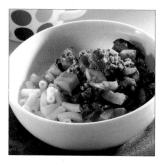

Red meat is the best source of iron, so it is good to include it in your child's diet. Lamb is easy to digest and most babies love it. Make sure you choose lean minced (ground) lamb, as lamb can be fatty. Choose organic meat if you can.

a little vegetable oil, for frying
450g/1lb minced (ground) lamb
1 large onion, finely chopped
2 large carrots, diced
2 courgettes (zucchini), diced
225g/8oz mushrooms, diced
300ml/½ pint/1¼ cups vegetable
*   stock*
400g/14oz can chopped tomatoes
5ml/1 tsp tomato purée (paste)
pinch of mixed herbs
5ml/1 tsp cornflour (cornstarch)

Heat a little vegetable oil in a flameproof casserole or a deep, heavy-bottomed frying pan. Brown the minced lamb in two or three batches for about 5 minutes over a high heat, stiring continuously. Remove the meat from the pan.

Lower the heat under the pan and add the chopped onion and carrot. Cook for 5–6 minutes, until softened. Add the courgettes and mushrooms and cook until soft. Return the meat to the pan, pour in the stock, canned tomatoes, tomato purée and herbs. Cover and simmer for 40 minutes. Stir from time to time.

Put about 50ml/2fl oz/¼ cup water in a cup. Sprinkle in the cornflour and stir until dissolved. Add the cornflour mixture to the stew and cook for a further 2–3 minutes to thicken the sauce.

PAPRIKA PORK

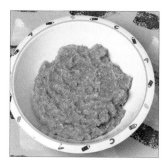

Commercially produced baked beans can be high in salt and sugar but if mixed with other ingredients are a good occasional food for your baby. Paprika gives a warm spicy note to this dish.

175g/6oz lean pork
75g/3oz carrot
175g/6oz potato
¼ onion
¼ red (bell) pepper
5ml/1tsp oil
2.5ml/½ tsp paprika
150g/5oz/⅔ cup baked beans
150ml/¼ pint/⅔ cup water

Preheat the oven to 180ºC/350ºF/ Gas 4. Rinse the pork under cold water, pat dry and trim away any fat or gristle. Cut the pork into small cubes. Peel the carrot, potato and onion. Cut, core and seed the pepper. Rinse, then chop into small

pieces. Heat the oil in a flameproof casserole, add the pork and fry, stirring, until browned. Add the vegetables, cook for 2 minutes, then add the paprika, baked beans and water. Bring back to the boil, cover and cook in the oven for 1¼ hours. Chop or process the casserole to the desired consistency, then spoon a little into a bowl.

TAGLIATELLE AND CHEESE WITH BROCCOLI AND HAM

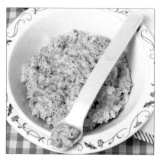

Babies and children love pasta, and of course it is one of the quickest and easiest of meals to prepare. This recipe can be prepared in 10 minutes, so is a great standby for busy days.

115g/4oz broccoli
50g/2oz thinly sliced ham
50g/2oz Cheddar or mild cheese
300ml/½ pint/1¼ cups formula
*   milk*
50g/2oz tagliatelle

Rinse the broccoli and cut into small florets, chopping the stalks. Chop the ham and grate the cheese. Pour the formula milk into a pan, bring to the boil and add the tagliatelle. Simmer uncovered for 10 minutes. Add the broccoli and cook for 5 minutes, until tender. Add the sliced ham and grated cheese to the broccoli and pasta, stirring until the cheese has melted. Chop or process the mixture to the desired consistency and then spoon a little into a bowl.

CAULIFLOWER AND BROCCOLI CHEESE

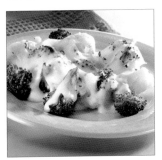

You can add this cheese sauce to any cooked vegetables, or pasta. Use formula or full-fat cow's milk, and choose a cheese with a good flavour – babies like stronger tastes than you might think.

1 small cauliflower, in florets
1 head of broccoli, in florets

For the cheese sauce
50g/2oz butter
20ml/4 tsp flour
300ml/½ pint/1¼ cups whole milk
115g/4oz Cheddar cheese,
  grated
dab of English (hot) mustard
  (enough to cover the tip of
  a teaspoon)
pinch of cayenne pepper

Steam the vegetables for about 10–12 minutes until soft.
    Meanwhile, to make the sauce, melt the butter in a small pan. Stir in the flour for 1 minute, until the flour is completely cooked. Very slowly pour in the milk, stirring all the time. It will go into a lump at first, but keep stirring and adding the milk slowly. Bring the mixture slowly to the boil, then take the pan off the heat. Add the cheese, mustard and cayenne pepper. Keep stirring.
    Add the sauce to the vegetables. Purée in a blender or mash well with a fork, depending on the age of your baby. If you are cooking for an older child, leave the florets whole.

RATATOUILLE

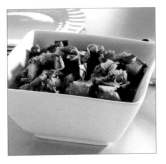

This is great with mashed potato, rice or buttery pasta.

½ small onion, chopped
a little olive oil, for frying
1 clove garlic, chopped
1 red (bell) pepper, diced
2 courgettes (zucchini), diced
1 aubergine (eggplant), diced
2 large mushrooms, diced
4 tomatoes, peeled and chopped
5ml/1 tsp tomato purée (paste)
small handful of basil, chopped

Fry the onion in a little olive oil for 6–7 minutes. Add the garlic, diced red pepper, courgette, aubergine and mushrooms and cook for 8 minutes. Add the tomatoes, tomato purée and basil, and cook for a further 15 minutes, stirring from time to time.

VANILLA CUSTARDS

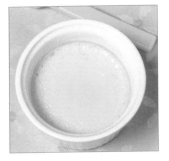

Only give your baby dishes with sugar as an occasional treat. This custard is a good way to introduce egg to your baby's diet.

1 egg
5ml/1 tsp caster (superfine) sugar
few drops vanilla essence
  (extract)
150ml/¼ pint/⅔ cup formula or
  cow's milk

Preheat the oven to 180°C/350°F/ Gas 4. Using a fork, beat the egg, sugar and vanilla essence together in a bowl. Pour the milk into a small pan and heat until it is just on the point of boiling. Gradually stir the milk into the egg mixture, whisking or beating until smooth. Strain into two ramekin dishesand place in a roasting pan. Add enough boiling water to come halfway up the sides of the dishes. Bake for 15–20 minutes, or until the custard has set. Cool to room temperature before serving, or refrigerate as soon as possible. Serve within 24 hours.

BREAD FINGERS WITH EGG

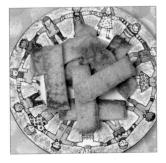

These bread fingers are delicious, and your baby will enjoy them as finger food or part of a meal.

2 slices bread, crusts removed
1 egg
30ml/2 tbsp formula or cow's milk
little butter and oil, for frying

Beat the egg and milk in a dish and dip the bread into it. Heat a little butter and oil in a frying pan. Add the bread and fry until browned on both sides. Cool, and cut into fingers.

Meal planning for toddlers and older children

This two-week plan gives a good, mixed diet with plenty of variety: it uses some simple meals together with recipes from the preceding and following pages. It's a good idea to keep introducing new recipes and ingredients from time to time. But don't worry if your child rejects the unfamiliar at first – children often need to see a new food a few times before they decide to try it.

Day 1
Breakfast Oat porridge with pear
  Plain yoghurt
Morning snack Toast with yeast extract, cheese chunks and apple
Lunch Lightly fried chicken, quinoa or rice and peas
Afternoon snack Oatcakes spread with butter and a few raisins
Supper Hummus, vegetable dippers and pitta fingers

Day 2
Breakfast Oat or millet porridge with banana and cinnamon
Morning snack Polenta fingers, cheese slices and apple
Lunch Pasta with pepper sauce
Afternoon snack Pancakes (older children can help to make them)
Supper Fishcakes and green beans
  Mango and yoghurt

Tuna pizza

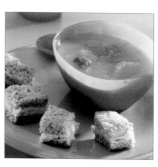

Vegetable soup with sandwiches.

Day 3
Breakfast Wheat biscuit cereal with apple slices
Morning snack Polenta fingers and grapes
Lunch Sardines on toast
Afternoon snack Rice cakes and grapes
Supper Vegetable soup and mini sandwiches

Day 4
Breakfast Oat porridge and mango
Morning snack Mashed banana on toast
Lunch Fish pilau
  Raspberry and apple purée with yoghurt or fromage frais
Afternoon snack Oatcakes and melon chunks
Supper Pasta with basic tomato sauce

Day 5
Breakfast Millet porridge with raisins and cinnamon
Morning snack Mini nut butter sandwiches
Lunch Homemade pizza with vegetable topping
  Natural yoghurt and/or fruit
Afternoon snack Carrot and cucumber sticks and cheese sticks
Supper Tarragon chicken with steamed potatoes

Day 6
Breakfast Wheat biscuit cereal with pear
Morning snack Toast with yeast extract, grapes
Lunch Spanish omelette with vegetable sticks
Afternoon snack Mini pitta with hummus, grated carrot, shredded lettuce and diced tomatoes
Supper Lamb casserole

Day 7
Breakfast Oat porridge with banana
Morning snack Rice cakes and apple slices
Lunch Borscht served with herby garlic bread or pitta fingers
Afternoon snack Spanish omelette (leftover)

Hummus with vegetables and pitta.

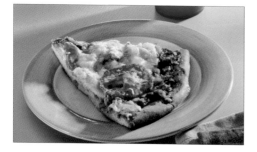

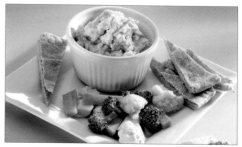

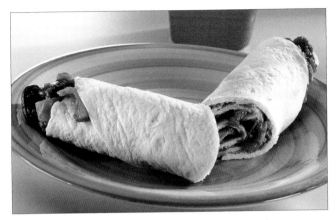

Flatbreads filled with beany bake.

Supper Beany bake in flatbreads with grated cheese

Day 8
Breakfast Wheat biscuit cereal and a plum
Morning snack Polenta fingers with apple slices
Lunch Poached salmon with mashed potatoes, steamed green beans and carrots
Afternoon snack Oatcake and pear
Supper Scrambled eggs on toast

Day 9
Breakfast Yoghurt, pear and toast with yeast extract
Morning snack Rice cakes and apricot or plum
Lunch Butter bean purée on toast
  Grapes and cheese slices

Fish cakes and peas.

Afternoon snack Carrot sticks and hummus
Supper Vegetable soup with a few added haricot (navy) beans

Day 10
Breakfast Millet and oat porridge with apricot compote
Morning snack Oatcakes spread with cream cheese
Lunch Ratatouille with rice or rolled up in flatbreads
Afternoon snack Banana and rice cakes
Supper Dhal with shredded spinach, rice and green beans

Day 11
Breakfast Wheat biscuit cereal with banana
Morning snack Mini sandwiches with peanut butter and grated apple
Lunch Fried chicken fillet, couscous salad and broccoli
  Papaya slices
Afternoon snack Rice cakes and

nectarine slices
Supper Macaroni cheese with peas and carrots

Day 12
Breakfast Oat porridge with apple purée and cinnamon
Morning snack Yoghurt and banana
Lunch Easy fishcakes made with haddock
  Fruit salad of mixed soft fruits sweetened with a little orange juice
Afternoon snack Rice cakes and pear slices
Supper Pasta with pesto

Day 13
Breakfast Scrambled egg on toast, pear slices
Morning snack Rice cakes, raisins and plain yoghurt
Lunch Cauliflower and broccoli cheese
Afternoon snack Polenta slices and an apricot, or apricot purée
Supper Shepherd's pie (Lamb casserole topped with mash)

Day 14
Breakfast Oat porridge with pear and raisins
Morning snack Banana and breadsticks
Lunch Fish pilau made with salmon
  Plain yoghurt
Afternoon snack Apple and cheese sticks
Supper Vegetable soup with pitta fingers

Pasta and pesto with cheese.

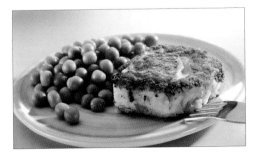

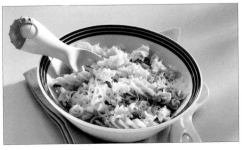

Recipes for toddlers and older children

In theory, older children can eat pretty much what adults do. But you may find that your meals are a bit too spicy or salty for your toddler. The following recipes are good for all the family, but they can also be frozen in small portions for the occasions when you want to eat different things or at different times from your child. When eating the same food as your toddler, add salt and pepper to your plate after serving it, don't be tempted to add salt during cooking, children's salt intake should be very low.

BUTTER BEAN PURÉE

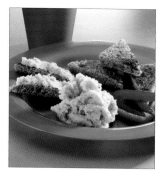

This purée goes wonderfully on toast, or with vegetable dippers You can add a pinch of paprika or garam masala to spice up the purée.

small can of butter (lima) beans
50g/2oz Cheddar cheese
30ml/2 tbsp olive oil
½ garlic clove, crushed
10ml/2 tsp very finely chopped
  parsley

Mash the butter beans and grate the cheese. Stir the olive oil into the beans with the crushed garlic clove, parsley and cheese. Blend to a thick purée.

SPANISH OMELETTE

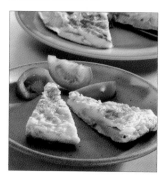

This is an almost universally popular dish. Serve it with sliced tomatoes and carrot sticks. You'll need a small, deep frying pan (about 20cm/8in), and a larger one to fry the onions and potatoes. The omelette is best eaten at room temperature.

1 medium onion
450g/1lb potatoes
30ml2 tbsp olive oil
4 large eggs
splash of milk
pinch of sea salt
good twist of black pepper
small pinch of cayenne pepper

Halve the onion then slice it thinly into half moons. Peel and slice the potatoes. Heat the oil in a large frying pan and cook the potatoes and onions over a medium heat for 8–10 minutes. Keep stirring so they soften without browning. Turn the heat as low as possible, cover the pan and leave to cook for 20 minutes, stirring occasionally, until soft. Meanwhile, beat the eggs lightly with the milk and seasoning and set aside.

Transfer the cooked potatoes and onions to a small, deep frying pan and place on the same low heat.

Give the pan 1–2 minutes to heat up, then pour in the omelette mixture. It should run into all the gaps between the potatoes and onions. Cook gently, uncovered, for 20 minutes, or until the mixture is cooked through.

When the omelette is done brown the top under the grill for 2–3 minutes. Place a plate over the pan and turn out the omelette. Leave it to cool for 10 minutes or so – it may fall apart if you try to cut it straight away.

QUICK HUMMUS

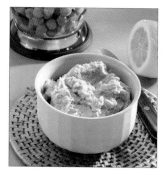

Toddlers love dips, and they are a good way to get them eating raw vegetables. Try thin sticks of carrot, red (bell) pepper, celery or lightly cooked green beans, broccoli and cauliflower florets. Hummus won't freeze but it will keep for a couple of days in the refrigerator.

400g/14oz can chickpeas
½ clove garlic
squeeze of lemon juice
30–45ml/2–3 tbsp Greek (US
  strained plain) yoghurt

Blend the chickpeas with the garlic and lemon juice until smooth. Add enough Greek yoghurt to make a good consistency, transfer to an air tight container and refrigerate.

EASY FISHCAKES

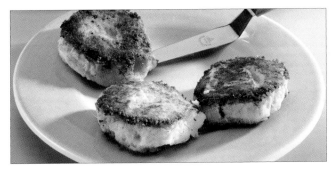

You can make these with any fish – fresh salmon, cod or haddock, or canned salmon or tuna. If you are using canned fish, halve the quantity specified here, as it has a much stronger flavour. The mashed potato should be cold, so this is a good way of using up leftovers.

450g/1lb potatoes
knob (pat) of butter
milk (see recipe)
200g/7oz salmon fillets, skinned
15ml/1 tbsp capers (optional)
handful of parsley or dill, finely
  chopped
flour
vegetable oil, for frying

Peel the potatoes and cut into even-sized chunks. Place them in a large pan of water and bring to the boil. Simmer for about 20 minutes or until cooked. Drain, mash with butter and a little milk, then leave to cool.

Place the salmon in a small pan and cover with milk. Bring to a simmer and poach gently for about 6–7 minutes, or until the salmon flesh is opaque all the way through. Drain the fish and flake it very carefully, removing any bones.

Mix the mashed potato and fish together well, adding the capers, if using, and the parsley or dill. Shape the mixture into about six small balls.

Sprinkle the flour on to a plate. Heat some vegetable oil in a large frying pan. Roll each fish ball in flour then place in the hot oil. Cook for about 5 minutes on each side, until golden, pressing the balls down as they cook to make nicely shaped cakes. Drain on kitchen paper, to remove any excess oil.

If you freeze some fishcakes do so before frying, then fry as required when thoroughly defrosted.

PEPPERED BEEF CASSEROLE

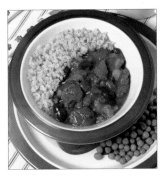

This is a tasty main course meal that could feed the whole famiily. Adding beans to the meat gives added vegetable protein and is a good texture to introduce your toddler to.

115g/4oz lean braising steak
¼ small onion
¼ small red (bell) pepper
¼ small yellow (bell) pepper
5ml/1 tsp oil
30ml/2 tbsp canned red kidney
  beans, drained and rinsed
5ml/1 tsp plain (all-purpose) flour
150ml/¼ pint/⅔ cup lamb stock
15ml/1 tbsp tomato ketchup

HERBY GARLIC BREAD

Any idea that children don't like garlic is quickly dispelled when garlic bread is on offer. If you don't need a whole loaf, cut the prepared bread into portions, wrap each in foil and freeze. This is good with pretty much any soup or vegetable stew.

French loaf
2 cloves garlic, crushed
Handful of parsley and
oregano, finely chopped
250g/9oz unsalted butter,
softened

Preheat the oven to 180°C/350°F/Gas 4. Cut the bread into 1cm/½in slices, but don't cut right the way through, so that the base of the loaf stays in once piece. Stir the garlic and herbs into the butter, combining well. Spread the garlic butter on both sides of each slice, and spread any leftover butter over the top of the loaf. Wrap the bread tightly in foil and bake for 20 minutes.

5ml/1 tsp Worcestershire sauce
a few drops of oil
couscous and peas, to serve

Preheat the oven to 180°C/350°F/Gas 4. Rinse the meat under cold water and pat dry. Trim away any fat and cut into small cubes.

Chop the onion, remove the seeds and core from the peppers and cut into small cubes.

Fry the meat in a little olive oil until browned. Add the onions, peppers and kidney beans, then stir in the flour, lamb stock, tomato ketchup, Worcestershire sauce. Bring to the boil, stirring, then reduce the heat, cover and simmer for about 1½ hours, or until the meat is tender.

Spoon the casserole on to two plates or dishes and serve with couscous and peas.

STICKY CHICKEN

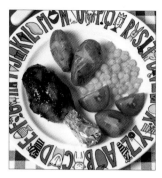

Now that your toddler is eating by themselves, give them fun lunches like these tasty chicken drumsticks and mini jacket potatoes. to use their newly developed skills on. This would make a good picnic or lunch on the go too.

4 chicken drumsticks
10ml/2 tsp oil
5ml/1 tsp soy sauce
15ml/1 tbsp smooth peanut
   butter
15ml/1 tbsp tomato ketchup
small baked potatoes, corn and
   tomato wedges, to serve

Preheat the oven to 200°C/ 400°F/Gas 6 and line a small shallow baking tin (pan) with foil. Rinse the drumsticks under cold water, pat dry and peel off the skin. Cut three or four slashes in the meat and place in the tin.

Blend the remaining ingredients and spread thickly over the top of the chicken drumsticks. Cook in the oven for 15 minutes.

Turn the drumsticks over and baste with the peanut butter mixture and meat juices.

Cook for a further 20 minutes or until the juices run clear when the chicken is pierced with a knife.

Cool slightly, then wrap a small piece of foil around the base of each drumstick. Arrange on plates and serve with small baked potatoes, hot corn, and tomato wedges.

BASIC TOMATO SAUCE

This sauce is good for pasta and pizza topping. The sugar balances the acidity of the tomatoes, but you can leave it out. For a more substantial pasta sauce, add flaked canned tuna. Any vegetable can be added to this sauce.

15ml/1 tbsp olive oil
½ onion, chopped
1 clove garlic, finely chopped
400g/14oz can plum tomatoes
5ml/1 tsp tomato purée (paste)
   or sun-dried tomato paste
Pinch of dried oregano
1 bay leaf
2.5ml/½ tsp sugar

Heat the oil in a pan and soften the onion and garlic in it. Cook over a low heat and do not let them brown.

Pour in the tomatoes, breaking them up, and add the rest of the ingredients. Cook, covered, over a low heat for 30–40 minutes, until thick, stirring from time to time. Blend the sauce until smooth, or use it as it is served with pasta or rice.

SHEPHERD'S PIE

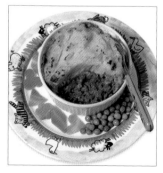

A classic meal that all children, and adults too, enjoy eating. Use carrots instead of parsnips in the mash if you want, you could also use celeriac or butternut squash.

½ small onion
175g/6oz lean minced (ground)
   beef
10ml/2 tsp plain (all-purpose)
   flour
30ml/2 tbsp tomato ketchup
150ml/¼ pint/⅔ cup beef stock
pinch of mixed herbs
50g/2oz swede (rutabaga)
½ small parsnip, about 50g/2oz
1 medium potato, about 115g/4oz
10ml/2 tsp milk
15g/½oz/1 tbsp butter or
   margarine
½ carrot
40g/1½oz/3 tbsp frozen peas
salt and pepper (optional)

Preheat oven to 190°C/375°F/ Gas 5. Finely chop the onion, and place in a small pan with the mince and dry fry over a low heat, stirring, until the mince is evenly browned.

Add the flour, stirring, then add the ketchup, stock, mixed herbs and seasoning, if using. Bring to the boil, cover and simmer gently for 30 minutes, stirring occasionally.

Meanwhile, chop the swede, parsnip and potato, and cook for 20 minutes, until tender. Drain. Mash with the milk and half of the butter or margarine.

Spoon the meat mixture into two 250ml/8fl oz/1 cup ovenproof dishes. Place the mashed vegetables on top, fluffing them up with a fork. Dot with butter or margarine.

Place both the pies on a baking sheet and cook for 25–30 minutes, until browned on top and bubbly.

Peel and thinly slice the carrot lengthways. Stamp out shapes with petits fours cutters. Cook in a pan of boiling water with the peas for 5 minutes. Drain and serve with the shepherd's pies. Remember that baked pies are very hot when they come out of the oven. Alllow to cool properly before you serve.

FISH AND CHEESE PIES

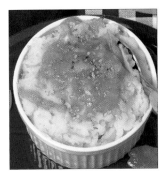

These little individual pies are easy to reheat in the oven, but if you are going to freeze them use fresh, not frozen, fish to make them with.

1 medium potato, about 150g/5oz
25g/1oz green cabbage
115g/4oz cod or hoki fillets
25g/1oz/2 tbsp frozen corn
150ml/¼ pint/⅔ cup milk
15ml/1 tbsp butter or margarine
15ml/1 tbsp plain (all-purpose)
  flour
25g/1oz/¼ cup grated Red
  Leicester or mild cheese
5ml/1 tsp sesame seeds

carrots and mangetouts
  (snowpeas), to serve

Peel and cut the potato into chunks and shred the cabbage. Cut any skin away from the fish fillets and rinse under cold water.

Bring a pan of water to the boil, add the potato and cook for 10 minutes. Add the cabbage and cook for a further 5 minutes until tender. Drain.

Meanwhile, place the fish fillets, the corn and all but 10ml/2 tsp of the milk in a second pan. Bring to the boil, then cover the pan and simmer very gently for 8–10 minutes, until the fish flakes easily when pressed with a knife.

Strain the fish and corn, reserving the cooking liquid. Wash the pan, then melt the butter or margarine in the pan.

Stir in the flour, then gradually add the reserved cooking liquid and bring to the boil, stirring until thickened and smooth.

Encourage your child to see eating meals as a social activity, something to be enjoyed.

Add the fish and corn with half of the grated cheese. Spoon into two small ovenproof dishes.

Mash the potato and cabbage with the remaining 10ml/2 tsp milk. Stir in half of the remaining cheese and spoon the mixture over the fish.

Sprinkle with the sesame seeds and the remaining cheese.

Cook under a preheated grill until the topping is browned. Cool slightly before serving with fresh vegetables.

BASIC PIZZA DOUGH

Making your own pizzas is easy, and older children will enjoy putting on their own toppings. This recipe makes enough dough for two pizzas, or four mini ones. Freeze the spare bases – you can add the toppings and cook them from frozen later on.

350g/12oz strong (hard wheat)
  plain white flour
1 sachet easy-blend yeast
5ml/1 tsp salt
30ml/2 tbsp olive oil
200ml/7 fl oz lukewarm water

Place the flour in a bowl and add the yeast and salt. Make a well in the middle and pour in the oil and water. Mix using a wooden spoon, then your hands, to make a smooth ball.

Sprinkle a little flour on the work surface and knead the dough for 5 minutes. Cover with a damp, clean cloth and leave to rest for 5 minutes, then knead for another 5 minutes, until the dough has a slight sheen and is smooth.

Place it in an oiled bowl and cover with a warm, damp cloth. Leave in a warm place for an hour or so, until the dough has doubled in size. Knead and shape into the required number of bases.

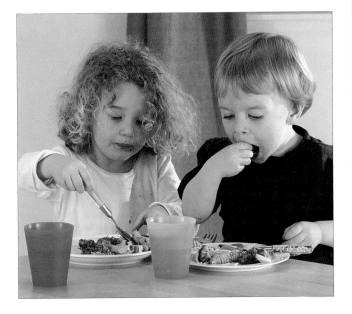

SURPRISE FISH PARCELS

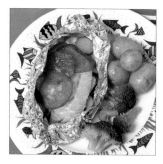

This is a lovely, simple recipe that retains all the goodness and flavour of the fish and vegetables in a foil parcel. You can cook any firm-fleshed fish fillets in this way, try salmon or unsmoked haddock.

½ small courgette (zucchini)
175g/6oz smoked haddock or cod
1 small tomato
knob (pat) of butter or margarine
pinch of dried mixed herbs
new potatoes and broccoli,
  to serve

Preheat the oven to 200°C/ 400°F/Gas 6. Tear off two pieces of foil, then trim and thinly slice the courgette and divide equally between the two pieces of foil.

Cut the skin away from the fish, remove any bones, cut into two equal pieces and rinse under cold water. Pat the fish dry and place on top of the courgettes.

Slice the tomato and arrange slices on top of each piece of haddock. Add a little butter or margarine to each and sprinkle with mixed herbs.

Wrap the foil around the fish and tightly seal the edges of each piece to make two parcels, then place the parcels on a baking sheet and cook them in the oven for around 15–20 minutes, depending on the thickness of the fish. To test if they are cooked, open up one of the parcels and insert a knife into the centre. If the fish flakes pull easily,

away from each other then the fish is ready. Cool slightly, then arrange the parcels on plates and serve with new potatoes and broccoli.

PORK AND LENTIL CASSEROLE

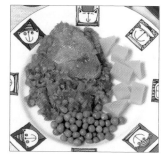

Adding lentils to a meat dish in this way is a great way to introduce vegetable proteins. Young children really enjoy red lentils, and they are easy to cook, very nutritious, and need no pre-soaking.

175g/6oz boneless spare-rib
  pork chop
¼ small onion
1 small carrot, about 50g/2oz
5ml/1 tsp oil
1 small garlic clove, crushed
25g/1oz red lentils
90ml/6 tbsp canned chopped
  tomatoes
90ml/6 tbsp chicken stock
salt and pepper (optional)
swede (rutabaga) and peas,
  to serve

Preheat the oven to 180°C/350°F/ Gas 4. Trim off any excess fat from the pork and cut in half. Finely chop the onion and dice the carrot.

Heat the oil in a frying pan, add the pork and onion and fry until the pork is browned on both sides.

Add the garlic, lentils and carrot and stir gently to mix.

Pour in the chopped tomatoes, stock and seasoning, if using, and cook briefly to bring to the boil. Transfer to a casserole, cover and cook in the oven for 1¼ hours.

Spoon portions on to serving plates or shallow dishes and cool slightly. Serve with diced buttered swede and peas.

BEANY BAKE

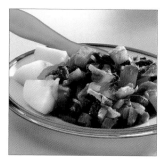

This is a good recipe for the whole family. Older children may like to eat it in flatbreads (Mexican tortillas) with cheese sprinkled on top.

1 onion, chopped
1 green (bell) pepper, chopped
1 garlic clove, crushed

a little vegetable oil, for frying
10ml/2 tsp ground cumin
400g/14oz can chopped tomatoes
5ml/1 tsp tomato purée (paste)
½ small swede (rutabaga), diced
3 carrots, diced
150g/5oz mushrooms, chopped
2 sticks celery, chopped
120ml/4fl oz/½ cup vegetable
    stock
400g/14oz can red kidney beans
handful of coriander (cilantro) or
    parsley, finely chopped

Preheat the oven to 180°C/350°F/ Gas 4. Heat a little vegetable oil in a flameproof casserole. Add the onion, pepper and garlic and cook for 6–7 minutes, until softened. Add the cumin and cook for another 1 minute.

Add the canned tomatoes, tomato purée, swede, carrots, mushrooms and celery, together with the stock, and season with a couple of twists of black pepper. Cover and cook in the oven for 30 minutes, stirring halfway through the cooking.

Add the kidney beans and cook for another 15 minutes, until the beans are heated through and the vegetables are tender. Stir in the coriander or parsley before serving.

PEPPER PASTA SAUCE

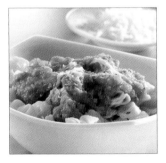

Sweet (bell) peppers are rich in vitamin C, and make a fabulous, quick, healthy sauce for pasta. Grate a little Cheddar cheese over the pasta too, if you like.

1 onion
1 garlic clove
1 red pepper
1 yellow pepper
15ml/1 tbsp olive oil
2 large tomatoes
small handful fresh basil

Chop the onion and garlic and deseed and slice the peppers. Heat the olive oil in a frying pan and cook the onion, garlic and peppers for 15 minutes over a low heat, until soft.

Meanwhile, skin, deseed and chop the tomatoes. Add them to the sauce and increase the heat. When it is bubbling, tear the basil leaves and stir them in, and cook for another minute or two, stirring. Add a dash of water if necessary. Blend to a purée.

PIZZA

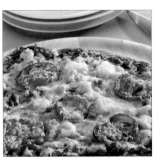

Pizza is popular with all ages, and if you make it yourself rather than rely on storebought or takeaway pizzas, you can make it into a nutritious as well as enjoyable meal. This is a great meal to cook with your children, as they will love flattening out the dough, and adding their choice of topping.

1 quantity of basic pizza dough
1 quantity of basic tomato sauce
toppings of your choice

Preheat the oven to 230°C/450°F/ Gas 8. Divide the dough into two or four balls and roll each one out to a circle about 1cm/½in thick. Put the pizza on an oiled baking sheet and push the edges up a little to keep the topping in place. Spread a little basic tomato sauce over the base then add the toppings (see below).

Cook for about 12 minutes, until the base is cooked and the topping is bubbling hot.

Pizza toppings: sliced mushrooms, drained, tinned corn, sliced pitted olives, sliced (bell) peppers, sliced tomatoes, cooked peas, steamed, sliced broccoli florets, blobs of pesto, thinly sliced cooked potatoes, flaked canned tuna, small prawns (shrimp), sliced ham, cooked chicken. Top with sliced mozzarella or grated Cheddar or parmesan or cheese, or a mixture of these.

SARDINES ON TOAST

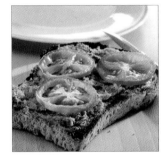

This is a tasty quick meal, and a great way to get your child to eat oily fish. Sardines contain bones that are edible and a good source of calcium, but mash the fish well before using.

small can of sardines
1 large tomato
2 slices wholemeal (whole-
    wheat) bread

Preheat the grill. Halve the fish, remove the backbones if you wish. Mash well. Slice the tomato thinly.

Brown one side of the bread slices under the grill then spread the mashed fish over the uncooked side. Top with slices of tomato. Grill (broil) until the fish is heated through. Cut off any charred bits of toast.

Family meals

Eating together as a family takes on a new dimension as your family grows and there's a baby, a fussy toddler, and parents to feed at the same time. Eat together as much as you can, it will help your children develop positive and healthy eating habits, as well as improving their sociability and eating skills. Rather than preparing different dishes opt instead to cook three versions of the same basic set of ingredients. The following recipes are for a baby aged nine months and over, a toddler or small child aged up to four years, and two adults eating together.

SPANISH PAELLA

400g/14oz cod fillet
115g/4oz fish cocktail or a
    mixture of prawns (shrimp),
    mussels and squid
15ml/1 tbsp olive oil
1 onion, chopped
1 garlic clove, crushed
150g/5oz/⅔ cup long grain
    white rice
pinch of saffron or turmeric
few sprigs of fresh thyme or
    a pinch of dried thyme
225g/8oz can tomatoes
½ red (bell) pepper, cored,
    seeded and chopped
½ green (bell) pepper, cored,
    seeded and chopped
50g/2oz frozen peas
30ml/2 tbsp fresh chopped
    parsley
salt and ground black pepper

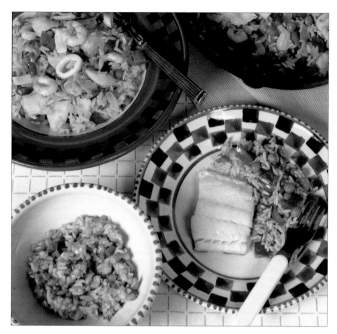

1 Remove any skin from the cod fillet. Place the fish cocktail in a sieve (strainer), and rinse well with cold water.

2 Heat the oil in a frying pan, add the onion and fry until lightly browned, stirring occasionally. Add the garlic and 115g/4oz/½ cup of the rice and cook for 1 minute.

3 Add the saffron or turmeric, thyme, two of the canned tomatoes, 350ml/12fl oz/1½ cups water, and salt and pepper. Bring to the boil and cook for 5 minutes.

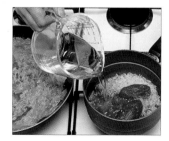

4 Put the remaining rice and canned tomatoes in a small pan with 90ml/ 6 tbsp water. Cover the pan and cook for about 5 minutes.

5 Add 15ml/1 tbsp of the peppers and 15ml/1 tbsp of the peas to the small pan. Add all the remaining chopped vegetables to the large pan.

6 Place 115g/4oz of the fish in a metal sieve (strainer), cutting in half if necessary. Place above a small pan of boiling water, cover and steam for 5 minutes. Add the remaining fish to the paella, cover, and cook for 5 minutes.

7 Add the fish cocktail to the paella, cover the pan and cook for a further 3 minutes.

8 Stir the chopped parsley into the paella and spoon on to two warmed serving plates for the adults.

9 Spoon half of the tomato rice mixture and half the fish on to a plate for the child and process the remaining fish and rice to the desired consistency for the baby.

10 Spoon into a dish and check both children's meals for bones. Test the temperature of the children's food before serving.

SALMON AND COD KEBABS

200g/7oz salmon steak
275g/10oz cod fillet
15ml/1 tbsp lemon juice
10ml/2 tsp olive oil
2.5ml/½ tsp Dijon mustard
350g/12oz new potatoes
200g/7oz frozen peas
50g/2oz/4 tbsp butter
15–30ml/1–2 tbsp milk
3 tomatoes, chopped, seeds
    discarded
¼ round (butterhead) lettuce,
    finely shredded
salt and ground black pepper

For the mustard sauce
1 sprig fresh dill
20ml/4 tsp mayonnaise
5ml/1 tsp Dijon mustard
5ml/1 tsp lemon juice
2.5ml/½ tsp soft dark brown
    sugar

1 Rinse the salmon steak and cod fillet under cold water and pat dry with kitchen paper.

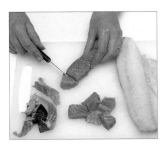

2 Cut the salmon steak in half, cutting around the central bone. Cut away the skin and then cut into chunky cubes, making sure you remove any bones. Remove the skin from the cod and cut into similar sized pieces.

3 Cut a few pieces of fish into smaller pieces and thread on to five cocktail sticks (toothpicks). Thread the remaining fish pieces on to long wooden skewers.

4 Mix together the lemon juice, oil, Dijon mustard and a little salt and pepper to taste in a small bowl and set aside.

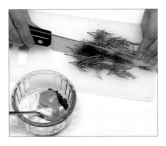

5 Finely chop the dill and place in a bowl with the other ingredients for the sauce, and mix. Set aside.

6 Scrub the potatoes, halve any large ones and then cook in lightly salted water for 15 minutes, or until they are tender.

7 Place the peas and half of the butter in a frying pan, cover and cook very gently for 5 minutes.

8 Preheat the grill (broiler), place the kebabs on a baking sheet and brush the larger kebabs with the lemon, oil and mustard mixture. Grill (broil) for 5 minutes, until the fish is cooked, turning once.

9 Remove the fish from two cocktail sticks and mix in a small bowl with a few new potatoes and 15ml/1 tbsp of the peas. Chop or process with a little milk to the desired consistency, then transfer to a baby bowl.

10 Arrange the toddler's kebabs on a small serving plate with a few potatoes, 30ml/2 tbsp peas and a small amount of chopped tomato. Remove the cocktail sticks from the kebabs before serving.

11 Add the tomatoes to the remaining peas and cook for 2 minutes, stir in the lettuce and cook for 1 minute. Spoon on to serving plates for the adults, add the kebabs and potatoes, and serve.

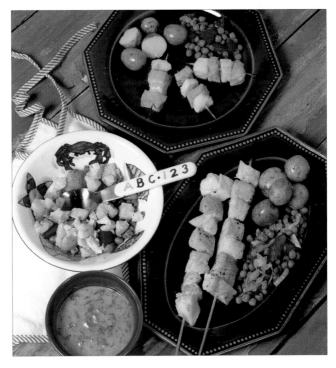

FISH CAKES

450g/1lb potatoes, cut into pieces
450g/1lb cod fillet
75g/3oz prepared spinach leaves
75ml/2fl oz/¼ cup full-fat
  (whole) milk
25g/1oz/2 tbsp butter
1 egg
50g/2oz/1 cup fresh breadcrumbs
25g/1oz drained sun-dried
  tomatoes
25g/1oz drained stuffed olives
115g/4oz Greek (US strained
  plain) yogurt
3 tomatoes, cut into wedges
½ small onion, thinly sliced
15ml/1 tbsp frozen peas, cooked
vegetable oil, for frying
salt and pepper
lemon and tomato wedges, sliced
  onion and green salad, to serve

1 Half fill a large pan or steamer base with water, add the potatoes and bring to the boil. Place the cod in a steamer top or in a colander above the pan. Cover and cook for 8–10 minutes, or until the fish flakes easily when pressed.

2 Take the fish out of the steamer and place on a plate. Add the spinach to the steamer, cook for 3 minutes, until just wilted, and transfer to a dish. Test the potatoes, cook them for 1–2 minutes more if necessary, then drain and mash them with 30ml/2 tbsp of the milk and the butter.

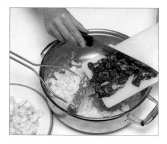

3 Peel away the skin from the fish, and break into small flakes, carefully removing any bones. Chop the spinach and add to the potato with the fish.

4 For the baby, spoon 45ml/3 tbsp of the mixture into a bowl and mash with another 30ml/2 tbsp of milk. Add a little salt and pepper, if liked, to the remaining fish mixture.

5 For the older child, shape three tablespoons of mixture into three small rounds with floured hands. For the adults, shape the remaining mixture into four cakes.

6 Beat the egg and the remaining milk on a plate. Place the breadcrumbs on a second plate and dip both the toddler and the adult fish cakes first into the egg and then into the crumb mixture.

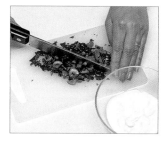

7 Chop the sun-dried tomatoes and stuffed olives and stir into the yogurt with a little salt and pepper. Spoon into a small dish.

8 Heat some oil in a frying pan and fry the small cakes for 2–3 minutes on each side until browned. Drain well and arrange on a child's plate. Add tomato wedges for tails and peas for eyes.

9 Fry the adult fish cakes, in more oil if necessary, for 3–4 minutes on each side, until browned and heated through. Drain and serve with the dip, lemon and tomato wedges, thinly sliced onion and a green salad. Reheat the baby portion if necessary, but test the temperature of the children's food before serving.

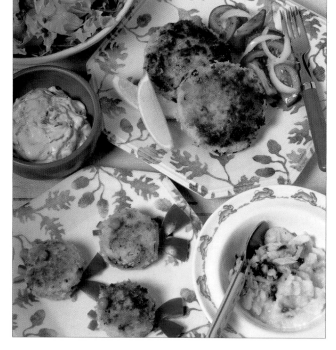

TUNA FLORENTINE

50g/2oz pasta shapes
175g/6oz fresh spinach leaves
50g/2oz frozen mixed vegetables
200g/7oz can tuna in brine
2 eggs
buttered toast and grilled (broiled)
  tomatoes, to serve

For the sauce

25g/1oz/2 tbsp butter
45ml/3 tbsp plain (all-purpose)
  flour
300ml/½ pint/1¼ cups milk
50g/2oz/½ cup grated Cheddar or
  mild cheese

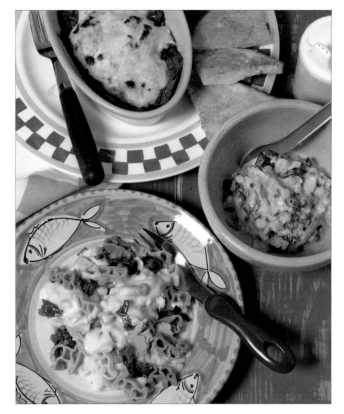

1 Cook the pasta in boiling water for 10 minutes. Meanwhile, tear off any spinach stalks, wash the leaves in plenty of cold water and place in a steamer or colander.

2 Stir the frozen vegetables into the pasta as it is cooking, and then place the spinach in the steamer over the top. Cover and cook for the last 3 minutes, or until the spinach has just wilted.

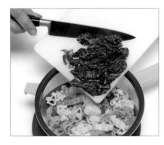

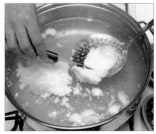

3 Drain the pasta and vegetables through a sieve (strainer). Chop one quarter of the spinach and add to the pasta and vegetables, dividing the remainder between two shallow 300ml/½ pint/1¼ cup ovenproof dishes for the adults.

4 Drain the tuna and divide among the dishes and sieve (strain).

5 Refill the pasta pan with water, bring to the boil.

6 When the water is simmering, break the eggs one at a time into the water and cook gently until the egg whites are set. Remove the eggs with a slotted spoon, and shake off all the water. Arrange the eggs on top of the tuna for the adults.

7 To make the sauce, melt the butter in a small pan, stir in the flour, then gradually add the milk and bring to the boil, stirring until thick and smooth.

8 Stir the cheese into the sauce, reserving a little for the topping. Spoon the sauce over the adults' portions until the eggs are covered. Stir the children's pasta, vegetables and tuna into the remaining sauce and mix together.

9 Spoon the pasta on to a plate for the toddler and chop or process the remainder for the baby, adding a little extra milk, if necessary, to make the desired consistency. Spoon into a dish. Test the temperature of the children's food before serving.

10 Preheat the grill (broiler), sprinkle the adults' portions with the reserved cheese and grill for 4–5 minutes, until browned.

11 Serve with buttered toast and grilled (broiled) tomatoes.

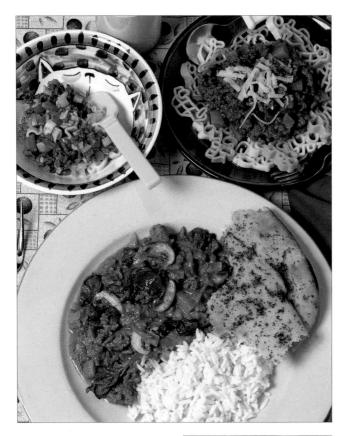

4 Meanwhile place the coconut or coconut milk in a small bowl, add 120ml/4fl oz/½ cup of boiling water and stir until dissolved. Wipe and slice the mushrooms, and wash and drain the spinach, discarding any large stalks.

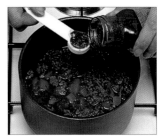

5 Transfer one-third of the meat mixture to another pan. Stir the coconut mixture, curry paste and salt and pepper into the remaining meat mixture and cook for about 5 minutes, stirring.

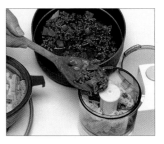

6 Mash or process one-third of the pasta and reserved meat mixture to the desired consistency for the baby and spoon into a small dish.

7 Spoon the remaining pasta and reserved meat mixture into a small bowl for the older child.

8 Stir the mushrooms and spinach into the curried beef and cook for 3–4 minutes, until the spinach has just wilted. Spoon on to warmed serving plates for the adults and serve with boiled rice and warmed naan bread. Sprinkle the toddler's portion with a little grated cheese. Test the temperature of the children's food before serving.

BEEF KORMA

350g/12oz lean minced (ground)
    beef
1 onion, chopped
1 carrot, chopped
1 garlic clove, crushed
400g/14oz can tomatoes
pinch of dried mixed herbs
25g/1oz pasta shapes
50g/2oz creamed coconut or
    120ml/4fl oz/½ cup coconut
    milk
50g/2oz button (white)
    mushrooms
50g/2oz fresh spinach leaves
15ml/1 tbsp hot curry paste
salt and freshly ground black
    pepper
boiled rice, warm naan bread and
    a little grated Cheddar cheese,
    to serve

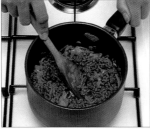

1 Dry fry the meat and onion in a medium-size pan, stirring until the beef has browned.

2 Add the carrot, garlic, tomatoes and herbs, bring to the boil, stirring, and then cover and simmer for about 30 minutes, stirring occasionally.

3 Cook the pasta in a small pan of boiling water for 10 minutes, until tender. Drain.

MOUSSAKA

1 onion, chopped
350g/12oz minced (ground) lamb
400g/14oz can tomatoes
1 bay leaf
1 medium aubergine (eggplant),
* sliced*
2 medium potatoes
1 medium courgette (zucchini),
* sliced*
30ml/2 tbsp olive oil
2.5ml/½ tsp grated nutmeg
2.5ml/½ tsp ground cinnamon
2 garlic cloves, crushed
salt and freshly ground black
* pepper*

For the sauce
30ml/2 tbsp butter
30ml/2 tbsp plain (all-purpose)
* flour*
200ml/7fl oz/scant 1 cup milk
pinch of grated nutmeg
15ml/1 tbsp freshly grated
* Parmesan cheese*
20ml/4 tsp fresh breadcrumbs

1 Dry fry the onion and lamb in a pan, stirring, until browned. Add the tomatoes and bay leaf, bring to the boil, stirring, then cover and simmer for 30 minutes.

2 Place the aubergine slices in a single layer on a baking sheet, sprinkle with a little salt and set aside for 20 minutes. Preheat oven to 200°C/400°F/Gas 6.

3 Slice the potatoes thinly and cook them in boiling water for 3 minutes. Add the courgette and cook for 2 minutes, until tender.

4 Remove most of the slices with a slotted spoon and place in a colander, leaving just enough for the baby portion. Cook these for 2–3 minutes more until soft, then drain.

5 Rinse the salt off the aubergine and dry. Heat the oil in a frying pan and fry until browned on both sides.

6 Spoon 45ml/3 tbsp of the meat mixture into a bowl with the baby vegetables and chop or purée to the desired consistency.

7 Spoon 60ml/4 tbsp of the meat mixture into an ovenproof dish for the older child. Arrange four slices of potato, a slice of aubergine and three slices of courgette on top.

8 Stir the spices, garlic and seasoning into the remaining lamb mixture, and cook for 1 minute and then spoon the mixture into a 1.2 litre/2 pint/5 cup shallow ovenproof dish discarding the bay leaf.

9 Arrange the remaining potatoes overlapping on top of the lamb, then add the aubergine slices, tucking the courgette slices in between the aubergines in a random pattern.

10 To make the sauce, melt the butter in a pan, stir in the flour, then gradually add the milk and bring to the boil, stirring until thickened and smooth. Add a pinch of nutmeg and a little salt and pepper.

11 Pour a little sauce over the toddler's portion, then pour the rest over the adult portions. Sprinkle the larger dish with Parmesan cheese and 15ml/1 tbsp breadcrumbs, sprinkle the remaining breadcrumbs over the toddler's portion.

12 Cook the moussakas in the oven. The larger dish will take 45 minutes, while the toddler's portion will take about 25 minutes.

13 Reheat the baby portion, and test the temperature of the children's food before serving.

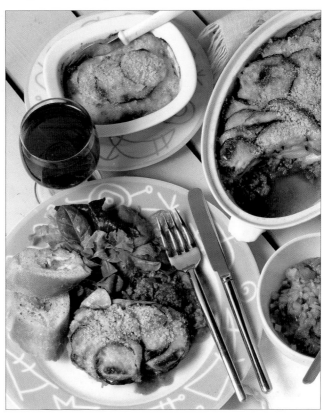

BOBOTIE WITH BAKED POTATOES AND BROCCOLI

3 medium baking potatoes
1 onion, chopped
350g/12oz lean minced (ground)
  beef
1 garlic clove, crushed
10ml/2 tsp mild curry paste
10ml/2 tsp wine vinegar
90ml/6 tbsp fresh breadcrumbs
15ml/1 tbsp tomato purée (paste)
25g/1oz sultanas (golden raisins)
15ml/1 tbsp mango chutney
1 medium banana, sliced
2 eggs
20ml/4 tsp turmeric
120ml/4fl oz/½ cup skimmed milk
4 small bay leaves
225g/8oz broccoli, cut into florets
30ml/2 tbsp fromage frais or
  Greek (US strained plain) yogurt
200g/7oz can baked beans
salt and freshly ground black
  pepper

1 Preheat the oven to 180°C/350°F/ Gas 4. Scrub the potatoes, insert a skewer into each and bake for 1½ hours, until tender.

2 Place the chopped onion and 225g/ 8oz of the beef in a pan and stir fry, until browned all over.

3 Add the garlic and curry paste, stir well and cook for 1 minute, then remove from the heat and stir in the vinegar, 60ml/4 tbsp of the breadcrumbs, the tomato purée, sultanas and a little salt and pepper.

4 Chop up any large pieces of mango chutney and stir into the meat mixture with the banana slices. Spoon into a 900ml/1½ pint/3¾ cup ovenproof dish and press into an even layer with the back of a spoon. Place the dish on a baking sheet, cover loosely with foil and cook in the oven for 20 minutes.

5 Meanwhile, mix the remaining beef with the remaining breadcrumbs, then beat the eggs together and stir 15ml/1 tbsp into the meat. Make eight small meatballs about the size of a grape for the baby. Form the remaining beef into a 7.5cm/3in burger, using an upturned cookie cutter as a mould.

6 Blend the turmeric, milk and a little salt and pepper with the remaining eggs. Remove the cover from the bobotie, and lay the bay leaves over the meat.

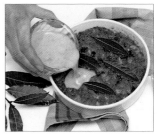

7 Pour the egg mixture over. Return to the oven for a further 30 minutes, until well risen and set.

8 When the adults' portion is ready, heat the grill (broiler) and cook the burger and meatballs until browned, turning once. The burger will take 8–10 minutes, while the meatballs will take about 5 minutes.

9 Cook the broccoli in boiling water until tender and drain.

10 Cut the bobotie for the adults into wedges and serve with baked potatoes topped with fromage frais or Greek yogurt and broccoli.

11 Serve the toddler's burger with half a potato, warmed baked beans and a few broccoli florets. Serve the baby's meatballs with chunky pieces of peeled potato and broccoli. Spoon a few baked beans into a small dish for the baby. Test the temperature of the food before serving to the children.

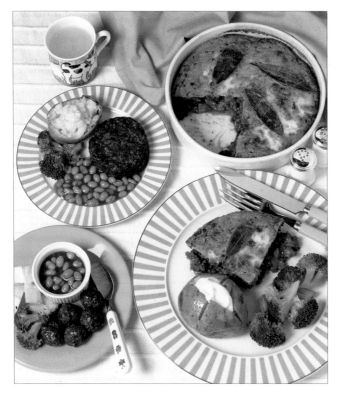

CHILLI CON CARNE

3 medium baking potatoes
1 onion, chopped
450g/1lb lean minced (ground)
   beef
1 carrot, chopped
½ red (bell) pepper, cored,
   seeded and diced
400g/14oz can tomatoes
10ml/2 tsp tomato purée (paste)
150ml/¼ pint/⅔ cup beef stock
3 small bay leaves
30ml/2 tbsp olive oil
115g/4oz button (white)
   mushrooms, sliced
2 garlic cloves, crushed
10ml/2 tsp mild chilli powder
2.5ml/½ tsp ground cumin
5ml/1 tsp ground coriander
200g/7oz can red kidney beans,
   drained
40g/1½oz frozen mixed
   vegetables
15ml/1 tbsp milk
generous knob (pat) of butter
60ml/4 tbsp fromage frais or
   Greek (US strained plain) yogurt
15ml/1 tbsp chopped fresh
   coriander (cilantro) leaves
salt and freshly ground black
   pepper
green salad, to serve

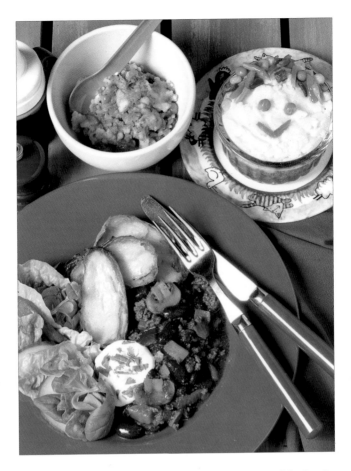

1 Preheat the oven to 180°C/350°F/Gas 4. Scrub and prick the potatoes and cook in the oven for 1½ hours. Dry fry the onion and beef in a pan until browned. Add the chopped carrot and red pepper and cook for 2 minutes.

2 Add the tomatoes, tomato purée and stock and bring to the boil. Transfer one quarter of the mixture to a 600ml/1 pint/2½ cup casserole dish, add 1 of the bay leaves, cover with a lid and set aside.

3 Spoon the remaining meat mixture into a 1.2 litre/2 pint/ 5 cup casserole. Heat 15ml/1 tbsp of the oil in the same pan and fry the mushrooms and garlic for 3 minutes.

4 Stir in the spices and seasoning, cook for 1 minute, then add the drained red kidney beans and the remaining bay leaves and stir into the meat mixture. Cover and cook both dishes in the oven for 1 hour.

5 When the potatoes are cooked, cut into halves or quarters and scoop out the potato, leaving a thin layer of potato on the skin.

6 Brush the potato skins with the remaining oil and grill (broil) for 10 minutes, until browned. Boil the frozen vegetables for 3 minutes.

7 Mash the potato with the milk and a knob of butter. Spoon the meat from the smaller casserole into an

ovenproof ramekin dish for the toddler and the rest into a bowl for the baby. Top both with some of the mashed potato.

8 Drain the vegetables, arrange pea eyes, a carrot mouth and mixed vegetable hair on the toddler's dish.

9 Spoon the remaining vegetables into a baby bowl and chop or process to the desired consistency. Test the temperature of the children's food before serving.

10 Spoon the adults' chilli on to warmed serving plates, add the potato skins and top with fromage frais or Greek yogurt and chopped coriander. Serve with a green salad.

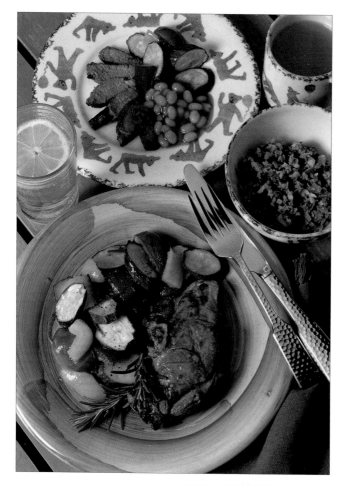

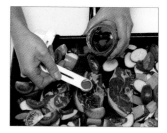

2 Arrange the vegetables around the lamb. Season two of the chops for the adults with garlic, honey, rosemary and salt and pepper, and drizzle oil over the vegetables.

3 Cook under a hot grill for 12–14 minutes, turning once, until the lamb is well browned and cooked through and the vegetables are browned.

4 Warm the baked beans in a small pan. Transfer the unseasoned chop to a chopping board and cut away the bone. Thinly slice half the meat for the toddler and arrange on a plate with some vegetables and 30–45ml/ 2–3 tbsp baked beans.

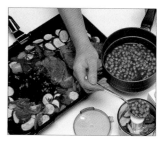

5 Chop or process the remaining lamb with four slices of courgette, two small pieces of pepper, two peeled tomato quarters and 15–30ml/1–2 tbsp of baked beans, adding a little boiled water if too dry. Spoon into a dish for the baby and test the temperature of the children's food before serving.

6 For the adult's portions, discard the cooked rosemary. Spoon the pan juices over the chops and garnish with fresh rosemary. Serve with crusty bread.

MEDITERRANEAN LAMB

3 lamb chump chops
350g/12oz courgettes (zucchini)
½ yellow (bell) pepper
½ red (bell) pepper
3 tomatoes
1 garlic clove, crushed
15ml/1 tbsp clear honey
few sprigs of fresh rosemary, plus
*   extra to garnish*
15ml/1 tbsp olive oil
200g/7oz can baked beans
salt and freshly ground black
*   pepper*
crusty bread, to serve

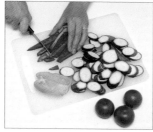

1 Rinse the chops under cold water, pat dry, trim off fat and place in the base of a grill (broiler) pan. Trim and slice the courgettes, cut away the core and seeds from the peppers and then rinse and cut into chunky pieces. Rinse and cut the tomatoes into quarters.

LAMB HOTPOT

350g/12oz lamb fillet
1 onion
1 carrot
175g/6oz swede (rutabaga)
15ml/1 tbsp sunflower oil
30ml/2 tbsp plain (all-purpose)
    flour
450ml/¾ pint/scant 2 cups lamb
    stock
15ml/1 tbsp fresh sage or 1.5ml/
    ¼ tsp dried
½ dessert apple
275g/10oz potatoes
15g/½oz/1 tbsp butter
225g/8oz Brussels sprouts
salt and ground black pepper

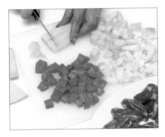

1 Preheat the oven to 180°C/350°F/ Gas 4. Rinse the lamb under cold water, pat dry, trim away any fat and then slice thinly. Peel and chop the onion, carrot and swede.

2 Heat the oil in a large frying pan and fry the lamb, turning until browned on both sides. Lift the lamb out of the pan, draining off any excess oil, and transfer one-third to a small 600ml/1 pint/2½ cup casserole dish for the children and the rest to a 1.2 litre/2 pint/5 cup casserole dish for the adults.

3 Add the vegetables to the pan and fry for 5 minutes, stirring until lightly browned.

4 Stir in the flour, then add the stock and sage. Bring to the boil, stirring, then divide between the two casserole dishes.

5 Core, peel and chop the apple and add both to the larger casserole dish with a little seasoning.

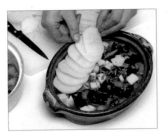

6 Thinly slice the potatoes and arrange overlapping slices over both casserole dishes. Dot with butter and season the larger dish.

7 Cover and cook in the oven for 1¼ hours. For a brown topping, remove the lid and grill (broil) for a few minutes at the end of cooking, until browned. Cook the Brussels sprouts in boiling water for 8–10 minutes, until tender, and drain.

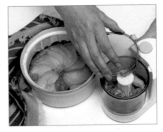

8 Chop or process half the hotpot from the small casserole, with a few sprouts for the baby, adding extra gravy if needed, until the desired consistency is reached. Spoon into a baby dish.

9 Spoon the remaining child's hotpot on to a plate, add a few sprouts and cut up any large pieces. Test the temperature of the children's food before serving.

10 Spoon the hotpot for the adults on to serving plates and serve with Brussels sprouts.

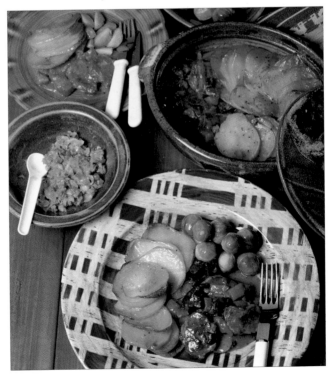

OSSO BUCCO PORK WITH RICE

3 pork spare rib chops, about
   500g/1¼lb
15ml/1 tbsp olive oil
1 onion, chopped
1 large carrot, chopped
2 celery sticks, thinly sliced
2 garlic cloves, crushed
400g/14oz can tomatoes
few sprigs fresh thyme or 1.5ml/
   ¼ tsp dried
grated rind and juice of ½ lemon
150g/5oz/⅔ cup long grain rice
pinch of turmeric
115g/4oz green beans
knob (pat) of butter
20ml/4 tbsp freshly grated
   Parmesan cheese
salt and freshly ground black
   pepper
1 or 2 sprigs parsley

1 Preheat the oven to 180°C/
350°F/Gas 4. Rinse the chops under
cold water and pat dry.

2 Heat the oil in a large frying pan,
add the pork, brown on both sides
and transfer to a casserole dish.

3 Add the onion, carrot and celery
to the frying pan and fry for
3 minutes, until lightly browned.

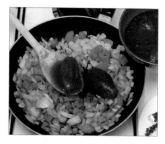

4 Add half the garlic, the tomatoes,
thyme and lemon juice and bring to
the boil, stirring. Pour the mixture
over the pork, cover and cook in the
oven for 1½ hours, or until tender.

5 Half fill two small pans with water
and bring to the boil. Add 115g/4oz/

½ cup rice to one with a pinch of
turmeric and salt, add the remaining
rice to the second pan. Return to the
boil, and simmer.

6 Trim the beans and steam above
the larger pan of rice for 8 minutes,
or until the rice is tender.

7 Drain both the pans of rice, return
the yellow rice to the pan and add
the butter, Parmesan cheese and a
little pepper. Mix together well and
keep warm.

8 Dice one chop, discarding any
bone if necessary. Spoon a little of
the white rice on to a plate for the
toddler and add half of the diced
chop. Add a few vegetables and a
spoonful of the sauce.

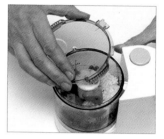

9 Process the other half of chop,
some vegetables, rice and sauce to
the desired consistency and turn into
a small bowl for the baby.

10 Spoon the yellow rice on to the
adults' plates and add a pork chop
to each. Season the sauce to taste
and then spoon the sauce and
vegetables over the meat, discarding
the thyme sprigs if used.

11 Finely chop the parsley and
sprinkle it over the pork with the
lemon rind and the remaining
crushed garlic.

12 Serve the adults' and toddler's
portions with green beans. Test the
temperature of the children's food
before serving.

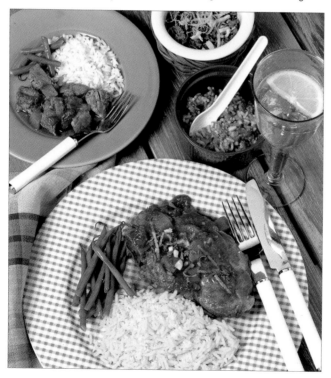

SAUSAGE CASSEROLE

450g/1lb large sausages
15ml/1 tbsp vegetable oil
1 onion, chopped
225g/8oz carrots, chopped
400g/14oz can mixed beans in
    water, drained
15ml/1 tbsp plain (all-purpose)
    flour
450ml/¾ pint/scant 2 cups beef
    stock
15ml/1 tbsp Worcestershire sauce
15ml/1 tbsp tomato purée (paste)
15ml/1 tbsp soft brown sugar
10ml/2 tsp Dijon mustard
1 bay leaf
1 dried chilli, chopped
3 medium baking potatoes
salt and ground black pepper
butter and sprigs of fresh parsley,
    to serve

1 Preheat the oven to 180°C/350°F/Gas 4. Prick and separate the sausages.

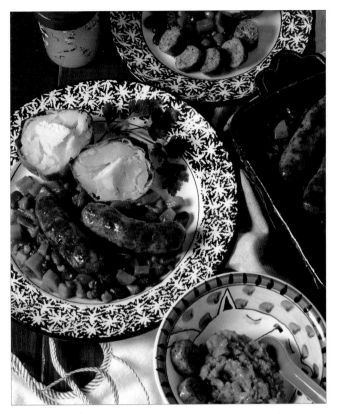

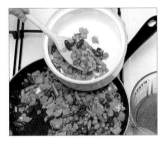

2 Heat the oil in a frying pan, add the sausages and cook over a high heat until evenly browned but not cooked through. Drain and transfer to a plate.

3 Add the chopped onion and carrots to the pan and fry until lightly browned. Add the drained beans and flour, stir well and then spoon one-third of the mixture into a small casserole. Stir in 150ml/ ¼ pint/⅔ cup stock, 5ml/1 tsp tomato purée and 5ml/1 tsp sugar.

4 Add the Worcestershire sauce, remaining beef stock, tomato purée

and sugar to the pan, together with the mustard, bay leaf and chopped chilli. Season and bring to the boil, then pour into a large casserole.

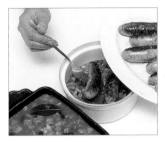

5 Add two sausages to the small casserole and the rest to the larger dish. Cover both and cook in the oven for 1½ hours.

6 Scrub and prick the potatoes and cook on a shelf above the casserole for 1½ hours, until tender.

7 Spoon two-thirds of the child's casserole on to a plate for the toddler. Slice the sausages and give him or her two-thirds. Halve one of the baked potatoes, add a knob (pat) of butter and place it on the toddler's plate.

8 Scoop the potato from the other half and mash or process with the remaining child's beans to the desired consistency for the baby.

9 Spoon into a dish and serve the remaining sausage slices alongside as finger food. Test the temperature of the children's food before serving.

10 Spoon the adults' casserole on to warmed plates. Halve the other potatoes and add to the plates. To serve top with a knob of butter and garnish with parsley.

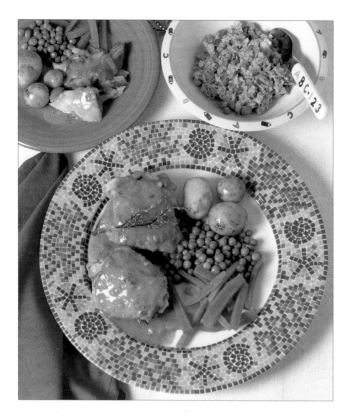

4 Pour over the chicken, cover and cook in the oven for 1 hour, or until tender.

5 Meanwhile, scrub the potatoes and cut any large ones in half. Cut the carrot into matchsticks.

6 Cook the potatoes in boiling water 15 minutes before the chicken is ready and cook the carrot and peas in a separate pan of boiling water for 5 minutes. Drain.

7 Take one chicken thigh out of the casserole, remove the skin and cut the meat away from the bone. Place in a food processor or blender with some of the vegetables and gravy and chop or process to the desired consistency. Turn into a baby bowl.

8 Take a second chicken thigh out of the casserole for the toddler, remove the skin and bone and slice if necessary.

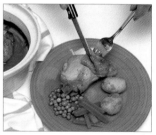

9 Arrange on a plate with some of the vegetables and gravy. Test the temperature of the children's food before serving.

10 Arrange two chicken thighs on warmed serving plates for the adults. Stir the mustard, orange rind and juice, fromage frais or yogurt, and seasoning into the hot sauce and then spoon over the chicken.

11 Serve immediately, with the vegetables, garnished with a sprig of thyme or parsley.

CHICKEN AND THYME CASSEROLE

6 chicken thighs
15ml/1 tbsp olive oil
1 onion, chopped
30ml/2 tbsp plain (all-purpose) flour
300ml/½ pint/1¼ cups chicken stock
few sprigs fresh thyme or 1.5ml/ ¼ tsp dried

To serve
350g/12oz new potatoes
1 large carrot
115g/4oz/¾ cup frozen peas
5ml/1 tsp Dijon mustard
grated rind and juice of ½ orange
60ml/4 tbsp fromage frais or natural (plain) yogurt
salt and freshly ground black pepper
fresh thyme or parsley, to garnish

1 Preheat the oven to 180°C/ 350°F/Gas 4. Rinse the chicken under cold water and pat dry.

2 Heat the oil in a large frying pan, add the chicken and brown on both sides, then transfer to a casserole.

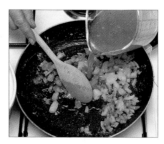

3 Add the onion and fry, stirring until lightly browned. Stir in the flour, then add the stock and thyme and bring to the boil, stirring.

TANDOORI-STYLE CHICKEN

6 chicken thighs
150g/5oz natural (plain) yogurt
6.5ml/1¼ tsp paprika
5ml/1 tsp hot curry paste
5ml/1 tsp coriander seeds,
　roughly crushed
2.5ml/½ tsp cumin seeds, roughly
　crushed
2.5ml/½ tsp turmeric
pinch of dried mixed herbs
5ml/2 tsp vegetable oil

To serve
350g/12oz new potatoes
3 celery sticks
10cm/4in piece cucumber
15ml/1 tbsp olive oil
5ml/1 tsp white wine vinegar
5ml/1 tsp mint
salt and freshly ground black
　pepper
few sprigs of watercress, knob
　(pat) of butter and cherry
　tomatoes, to serve

1 Cut away the skin from the chicken thighs and slash the meat two or three times with a small knife. Rinse under cold water and pat dry.

2 Place four thighs in a shallow dish, the other two on a plate. Place the yogurt, 5ml/1 tsp of the paprika, the curry paste, both seeds and almost all the turmeric into a small bowl and mix together. Spoon over the four chicken thighs.

3 Sprinkle the remaining paprika and the mixed herbs over the other chicken thighs and sprinkle the remaining pinch of turmeric over one thigh. Cover both dishes loosely with clear film (plastic wrap) and chill in the refrigerator for 2–3 hours.

4 Preheat the oven to 200°C/400°F/Gas 6. Arrange the chicken thighs on a roasting rack set over a small roasting pan and drizzle oil over the herbed chicken. Pour a little boiling water into the base of the pan

and cook for 45–50 minutes, until the juices run clear when the chicken is pierced with a skewer.

5 Meanwhile, scrub the potatoes and halve any large ones. Cook in a pan of boiling water for 15 minutes, until tender.

6 Cut one celery stick and a small piece of cucumber into matchsticks. Chop or shred the remaining celery and cucumber.

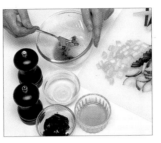

7 Blend together the oil, vinegar, mint and seasoning in a bowl and add the chopped or shredded celery,

cucumber and watercress, tossing well to coat.

8 Drain the potatoes and toss in a little butter. Divide the potatoes among the adults' plates, toddler's dish and the baby bowl.

9 Cut the chicken off the bone of one thigh for the toddler and arrange the pieces on a plate with half of the celery and cucumber sticks.

10 Cut the second chicken thigh into tiny pieces for the baby, and allow to cool. Add to the bowl with the cooled potatoes and vegetable sticks and allow the baby to feed him or herself. Add a few halved tomatoes to each child's portion. Test the temperature of the children's food before serving.

11 For the adults, arrange the remaining chicken thighs on warmed serving plates with the potatoes. Serve with the piquant salad.

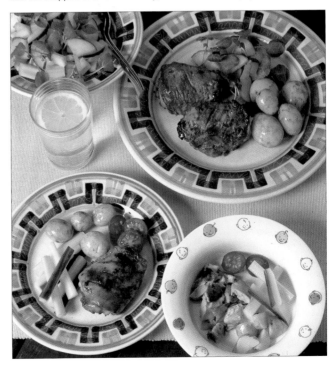

CHICKEN WRAPPERS

3 boneless, skinless chicken
  breasts
5ml/1 tsp pesto
40g/1½oz thinly sliced ham
50g/2oz Cheddar or mild cheese
350g/12oz new potatoes
175g/6oz green beans
15g/½oz/1 tbsp butter
10ml/2 tsp olive oil
1 tomato, cut into wedges
6 stoned (pitted) black olives,
  sliced
10ml/2 tsp plain (all-purpose)
  flour
150ml/¼ pint/⅔ cup chicken stock
15ml/1 tbsp crème fraîche

1 Rinse the chicken under cold water and pat dry. Put the chicken breasts between two pieces of clear film (plastic wrap) and bat them out with a rolling pin.

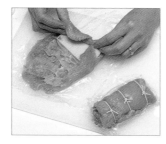

2 Spread pesto over two of the chicken breasts and divide the ham among all three. Cut the cheese into three thick slices, then add one to each piece of chicken. Roll up so that the cheese is completely enclosed, then secure with string.

3 Scrub the potatoes, halve any large ones and cook in a pan of boiling water for 15 minutes, until tender. Trim the beans and cook in a pan of boiling water for 10 minutes.

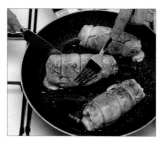

4 Meanwhile, heat the butter and oil in a large frying pan, add the chicken and cook for about 10 minutes, turning several times, until well browned and cooked through.

5 Lift the chicken out of the pan, keeping the pieces with pesto warm, and leaving the other to cool slightly.

6 Stir the flour in to the pan and cook for 1 minute. Gradually stir in the stock and bring to the boil, stirring until thickened. Add the tomato and olives.

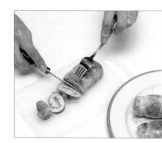

7 Snip the string off the chicken and slice the children's breast thinly. Arrange four slices on a child's plate with a couple of spoonfuls of sauce a few potatoes and green beans.

8 Chop or process the remaining cut chicken with 30ml/2 tbsp of the sauce, a potato and three green beans to the desired consistency. Test the temperature of the children's food before serving.

9 Arrange the remaining chicken on plates. Add the crème fraîche or sour cream to the pan, and heat gently. Spoon over the chicken and serve.

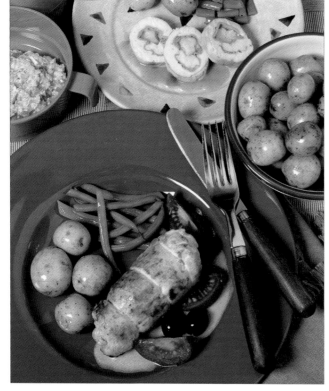

PAN-FRIED TURKEY WITH CORIANDER

3 turkey breast steaks
1 onion
1 red (bell) pepper, cored and
  seeded
15ml/1 tbsp vegetable oil
5ml/1 tsp plain (all-purpose) flour
150ml/¼ pint/⅔ cup chicken stock
30ml/2 tbsp frozen corn
150g/5oz/⅔ cup long grain white
  rice
1 garlic clove
1 dried chilli
50g/2oz creamed coconut or
  200ml/7fl oz/1 cup coconut
  cream
30ml/2 tbsp chopped fresh
  coriander (cilantro)
fresh coriander sprigs, to garnish
fresh lime wedges, to serve

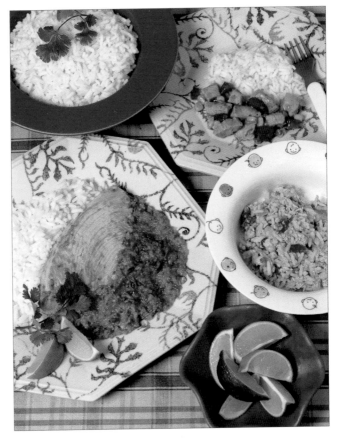

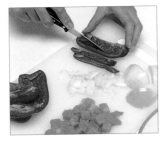

1 Rinse the turkey steaks under cold water, and pat dry. Chop one of the steaks, finely chop one quarter of the onion and dice one quarter of the red pepper. Heat 5ml/1 tsp of the oil in a frying pan and fry the chopped turkey and onion until browned.

2 Stir in the flour, add the stock, corn and chopped pepper, bring to the boil, and simmer for 10 minutes.

3 Cook the long grain rice in boiling water for 8–10 minutes, or until just tender. Drain.

4 Meanwhile, finely chop the remaining onion and red pepper with the garlic and chilli, including the seeds if you like hot food.

5 Put the coconut cream into a bowl, pour on 200ml/7fl oz/1 cup boiling water and stir until dissolved.

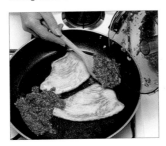

6 Heat the remaining oil in a large frying pan. Brown the turkey breasts on one side, turn over and add the pepper paste. Fry for 5 minutes, until the second side of the turkey has also browned.

7 Pour the coconut milk or diluted cream over the turkey and cook for 2–3 minutes, stirring until the sauce has thickened slightly. Sprinkle with the chopped fresh coriander.

8 Chop or process one-third of the children's portion with 30ml/2 tbsp rice until the desired consistency is reached. Spoon into a baby bowl.

9 Spoon the child's portion on to a child's plate and serve with a little rice. Test the temperature of the children's food before serving.

10 Spoon the rest of the rice on to warmed serving plates for the adults, and add the turkey and sauce. Garnish with coriander sprigs and serve with lime wedges.

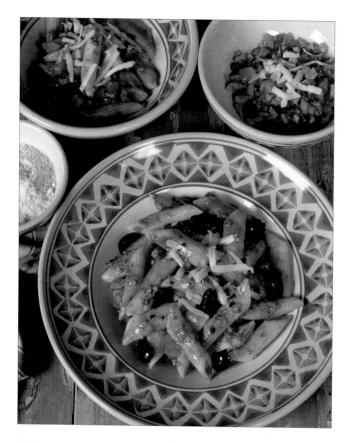

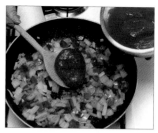

4 Add the tomatoes and sugar and cook for 5 minutes, stirring occasionally, until the tomatoes are broken up and pulpy. Drain the pasta, return to the pan and stir in the tomato sauce.

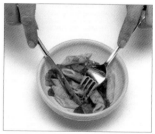

5 Spoon 45–60ml/3–4 tbsp of the mixture into a bowl or processor and chop or process to the desired consistency for the baby. Spoon 75–90ml/5–6 tbsp of the mixture into a bowl for the toddler.

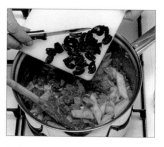

6 Quarter the olives and stir into the remaining pasta with the pesto, chilli seeds if using, and a little salt and pepper. Spoon into dishes.

7 Sprinkle the grated parmesan cheese over all the dishes, and serve the adults' portions with a green salad. Test the temperature of the children's food before serving.

PENNE WITH TOMATO SAUCE

150g/5oz penne or pasta quills
1 onion
2 celery sticks
1 red (bell) pepper
15ml/1 tbsp olive oil
1 garlic clove, crushed
400g/14oz can tomatoes
2.5ml/½ tsp caster (superfine)
  sugar
8 stoned (pitted) black olives
10ml/2 tsp pesto
1.5ml/¼ tsp dried chilli seeds
  (optional)
50g/2oz/½ cup grated Cheddar or
  mild cheese
salt and freshly ground black
  pepper
10ml/2 tsp freshly grated
  Parmesan cheese, to serve
green salad, to serve (optional)

1 Cook the pasta in salted boiling water for about 10–12 minutes, until just tender.

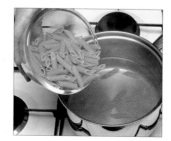

2 Meanwhile, chop the onion and the celery. Cut the pepper in half, then scoop out the core and seeds and dice the pepper finely.

3 Heat the oil in a second pan, add the vegetables and garlic and stir-fry for 5 minutes, until lightly browned.

CHEESE VEGETABLE CRUMBLE

1 onion
225g/8oz carrot
175g/6oz swede (rutabaga)
175g/6oz parsnip
15ml/1 tbsp olive oil
220g/7½oz can red kidney beans
10ml/2 tsp paprika
5ml/1 tsp ground cumin
15ml/1 tbsp plain (all-purpose)
   flour
300ml/½ pint/1¼ cups vegetable
   stock
225g/8oz broccoli, to serve

For the topping
115g/4oz Cheddar or mild cheese
50g/2oz wholemeal (whole-wheat)
   flour
50g/2oz plain (all-purpose) flour
50g/2oz margarine
30ml/2 tbsp sesame seeds
25g/1oz blanched almonds
salt and freshly ground black
   pepper

1 Preheat the oven to 190°C/ 375°F/Gas 5. Peel and roughly chop the onion. Then peel and cut the carrot, swede and parsnip into small cubes. Heat the oil in a large pan and fry the vegetables for 5 minutes, stirring until lightly browned.

2 Drain the kidney beans and add to the pan with the spices and flour. Stir well, add the stock, then cover and simmer for 10 minutes.

3 Meanwhile, make the topping. Cut a few squares of cheese for the baby and grate the rest. Put the two flours in a bowl, add the margarine and rub in with your fingertips until the mixture resembles fine breadcrumbs. Stir in the grated cheese and sesame seeds.

4 Spoon a little of the vegetable mixture into a 300ml/½ pint/ 1¼ cup ovenproof dish for the toddler. Spoon the remaining mixture into a 900ml/1½ pint/ 3¾ cup ovenproof pie dish for the adults, leaving a little

vegetable mixture in the pan for the baby. Season the adults' portion with a little salt and pepper.

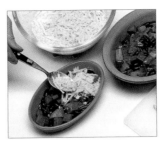

5 Spoon 45ml/3 tbsp of crumble over the older child's portion. Roughly chop the almonds, add to the remaining crumble with a little salt and pepper and spoon over the large dish. Bake in the oven for 20 minutes for the small dish, and 30 minutes for the large dish.

6 Add 90ml/3fl oz water to the baby's portion, cover and cook for 10 minutes, stirring occasionally, until the vegetables are very tender. Mash or process to the desired consistency and spoon into a bowl.

7 Cut the broccoli into florets and cook in a little water for 5 minutes, or until just tender; drain. Spoon the toddler's portion on to a small plate.

8 Serve the broccoli to all members of the family, allowing the baby to pick up and eat the broccoli and cubed cheese as finger food. Check the temperature before serving to the children.

Note: Never give whole nuts to children under five, as they are a choking hazard.

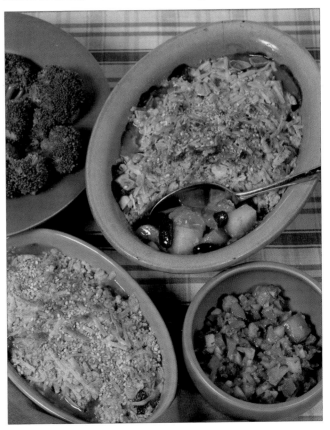

VEGETABLE TAGINE

1 onion
225g/8oz carrots
225g/8oz swede (rutabaga)
75g/3oz prunes
20ml/4 tsp olive oil
425g/15oz can chickpeas
2.5ml/½ tsp turmeric
10ml/2 tsp plain (all-purpose)
    flour, plus extra for dusting
2 garlic cloves, finely chopped
450ml/¾ pint/2 scant cups
    chicken stock
15ml/1 tbsp tomato purée (paste)
2cm/¾in piece fresh root ginger
2.5ml/½ tsp ground cinnamon
3 cloves
115g/4oz couscous
8 green beans
2 frozen peas
piece of tomato
knob (pat) of butter
salt and freshly ground black
    pepper
fresh coriander (cilantro),
    to garnish

1 Peel and chop the onion, and peel and dice the carrots and swede. Cut the prunes into chunky pieces, discarding the stones (pits).

2 Heat 15ml/3 tsp of the olive oil in a large pan, add the onion and fry until lightly browned. Stir in the carrot and swede and fry for 3 minutes, stirring.

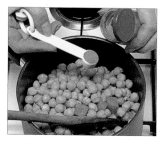

3 Drain the chickpeas and stir into the pan with the turmeric, flour and garlic. Add 300ml/½ pint/ 1¼ cup of the stock, tomato purée, and prunes. Bring to the boil, cover and simmer for 20 minutes, stirring occasionally.

4 Place three heaped spoonfuls of mixture in a bowl or food processor, draining off most of the liquid. Mash or process and then form the mixture into a burger with floured hands.

5 Chop or process two heaped spoonfuls of mixture and sauce to the desired consistency for the baby and spoon into a bowl.

6 Finely chop the root ginger and stir into the remaining vegetable mixture with the cinnamon, cloves, remaining stock and seasoning.

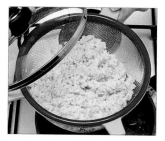

7 Place the couscous in a sieve (strainer), rinse with boiling water and fluff up the grains with a fork. Place the sieve above the vegetables, cover and steam for 5 minutes.

8 Fry the veggie burger in the remaining oil until browned on both sides.

9 Trim and cook the beans and peas for 5 minutes. Drain and arrange on a plate like an octopus, with a piece of tomato for a mouth and peas for eyes.

10 Stir the butter into the couscous and fluff up the grains with a fork.

11 Spoon the couscous on to warmed serving plates for adults, add the chick pea and vegetable mixture and garnish with a sprig of coriander. Check the temperature of the children's food before serving.

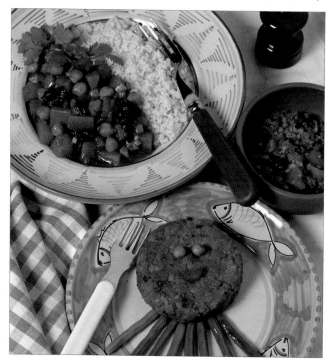

STILTON AND LEEK TART

175g/6oz/1½ cups plain (all-
    purpose) flour
75g/3oz/6 tbsp butter
1 carrot
2 slices ham
10cm/4in piece of cucumber
mixed green salad leaves, to
    serve

For the filling

25g/1oz/2 tbsp butter
115g/4oz trimmed leek, thinly
    sliced
75g/3oz Stilton (blue) cheese,
    diced
3 eggs
175ml/6fl oz/¾ cup milk
40g/1½oz Cheddar or mild
    cheese, grated
pinch of paprika
salt and pepper

1 Put the flour in a bowl with a pinch of salt. Cut the butter into pieces and rub into the flour with your fingertips until the mixture resembles fine breadcrumbs.

2 Mix to a smooth dough with 30–35ml/6–7 tsp water, knead lightly and roll out thinly on a floured surface. Use to line an 18cm/7in flan dish, trimming round the edge and reserving the trimmings.

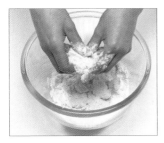

3 Re-roll the trimmings and then cut out six 7.5cm/3in circles, using a fluted cookie cutter. Press the pastry circles into sections of a patty tin (muffin pan) and chill all of the tarts. Preheat the oven to 190°C/ 375°F/Gas 5.

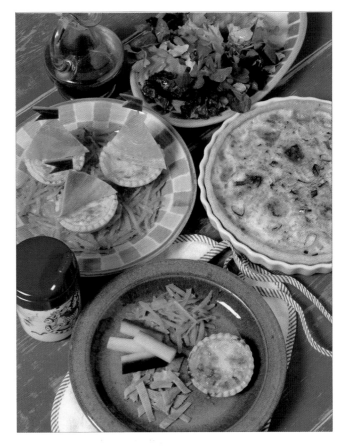

4 For the filling, melt the butter in a small frying pan and fry the leek for 4–5 minutes, until soft, stirring frequently. Stir in the diced Stilton, then spread over the base of the large tart.

5 Beat the eggs and milk together in a small bowl and season with salt and pepper.

6 Divide the Cheddar among the small tartlet shells and pour egg mixture over. Pour the remaining egg over the leek and Stilton tart and sprinkle with paprika.

7 Cook the small tartlets for 15 minutes and the large tart for 30–35 minutes, until well risen and browned. Leave to cool.

8 Peel and coarsely grate the carrot. Cut the ham into triangles for "sails". Cut the ham trimmings into small strips for the baby. Cut the cucumber into matchsticks.

9 Place a spoonful of carrot, some cucumber, a small tart and some ham trimmings in the baby dish.

10 Spread the remaining carrot on to a plate for the older child, place the tarts on top and secure the ham "sails" with cocktail sticks (toothpicks) Serve any remaining tarts the next day.

11 Cut the large tart into wedges and serve with a mixed leaf salad.

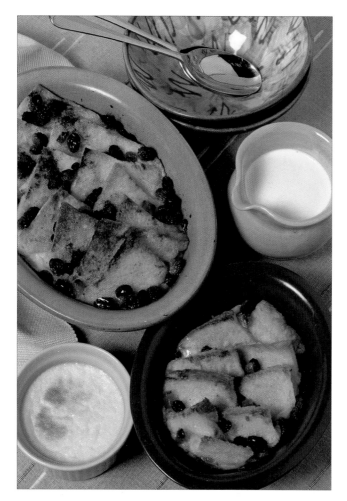

2 Spread the bread with butter and cut one slice into mini triangles. Layer in a 150ml/¼ pint/⅔ cup pie dish with plain apricots and sultanas and 5ml/1 tsp of the sugar.

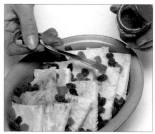

3 Cut the remaining bread into larger triangles and layer in a 900ml/1½ pint/3¾ cup pie dish with the sherried fruits and all but 5ml/1 tsp of the remaining sugar. Sprinkle with cinnamon. Put the last 5ml/1 tsp sugar in a ramekin dish.

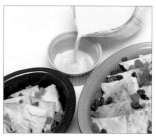

4 Beat the eggs, milk and vanilla together and pour into the ramekin and two pie dishes.

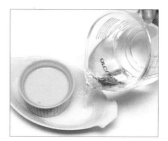

5 Stand the ramekin dish in an ovenproof dish and half fill with hot water. Cook the small pudding and the ramekin for 25–30 minutes, and the larger pudding for 35 minutes. Serve the adult portions with cream.

BREAD AND BUTTER PUDDING

3 dried apricots
45ml/3 tbsp sultanas (golden raisins)
30ml/2 tbsp sherry
7 slices white bread, crusts removed
25g/1oz/½ tbsp butter, softened
30ml/2 tbsp caster (superfine) sugar
pinch of ground cinnamon
4 eggs
300ml/½ pint/1¼ cups milk
few drops of vanilla extract
pouring cream, to serve

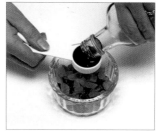

1 Chop two dried apricots and place in a small bowl with 30ml/2 tbsp of the sultanas and the sherry. Set aside for about 2 hours. Chop the remaining apricot and mix with the remaining sultanas. Preheat the oven to 190°C/375°F/Gas 5.

EVE'S PUDDING

500g/1¼lb cooking apples
50g/2oz/¼ cup caster (superfine)
  sugar
50g/2oz frozen or canned
  blackberries

For the topping
50g/2oz/4 tbsp butter or
  margarine
50g/2oz/¼ cup caster (superfine)
  sugar
50g/2oz/⅓ cup self-raising (self-
  rising) flour
1 egg
½ lemon, rind only
15ml/1 tbsp lemon juice
icing (confectioners') sugar, for
  dusting
custard, to serve

1 Preheat the oven to 180°C/350°F/
Gas 4. Peel and slice the cooking
apples, discarding the core, and
then place in a pan with the caster
sugar and 15ml/1 tbsp water. Cover
and cook gently for 5 minutes, until
the apple slices are almost tender
but still whole.

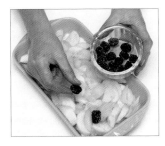

2 Half fill a 150ml/¼ pint/⅔ cup
ovenproof ramekin with cooked
apple for the toddler and mash
30ml/2 tbsp of apple for the baby
in a small bowl.

3 Put the remaining apple slices
into a 600ml/1 pint/2½ cup ovenproof
dish, and scatter the blackberries
over the apple slices.

4 To make the topping, place the
butter or margarine, sugar, flour and

egg in a bowl and beat until smooth.
Spoon a little of the pudding mixture
over the toddler's ramekin so that
the mixture is almost to the top.

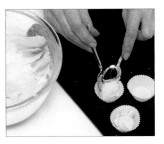

6 Half fill three petits fours cases
with the pudding mixture. Grate the
lemon rind and stir with the juice into
the remaining mixture.

7 Spoon the pudding mixture over
the large dish, levelling the surface.

8 Put the small cakes, toddler and
adult dishes on a baking sheet and
bake in the oven for 8–10 minutes for
the small cakes, 20 minutes for the
ramekin and 30 minutes for the
larger dish, until they are well risen
and golden brown.

9 Dust the toddler's and adults'
portions with icing sugar and leave
to cool slightly before serving with
the custard. Warm the baby's portion
if liked, and test the temperature
before serving. Take the cakes out of
their paper cases before you give
them to a child.

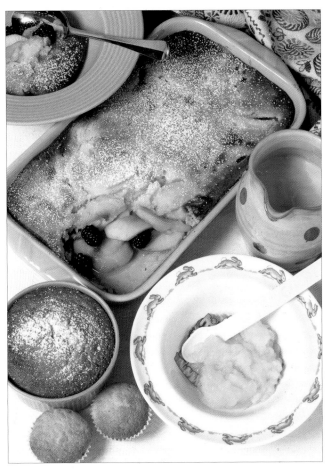

PLUM CRUMBLE

450g/1lb ripe red plums
25g/1oz/2 tbsp caster (superfine)
sugar

For the topping

115g/4oz/1 cup plain (all-purpose)
flour
50g/2oz/4 tbsp butter, diced
25g/1oz/2 tbsp caster (superfine)
sugar
10ml/2 tsp chocolate dots
75g/3oz marzipan
30ml/2 tbsp rolled oats
30ml/2 tbsp flaked (sliced)
almonds
custard, to serve

1 Preheat the oven to 190°C/375°F/Gas 5. Wash the plums, cut into quarters and remove the stones (pits). Place in a pan with the sugar and 30ml/2 tbsp water, cover and simmer for 10 minutes.

2 Drain and spoon six plum quarters on to a chopping board and chop finely. Spoon the plums into a small baby dish with a little juice from the pan.

3 Drain and roughly chop six more of the plum quarters and place in a 150ml/¼ pint/⅔ cup ovenproof ramekin dish with a little of the juice from the pan.

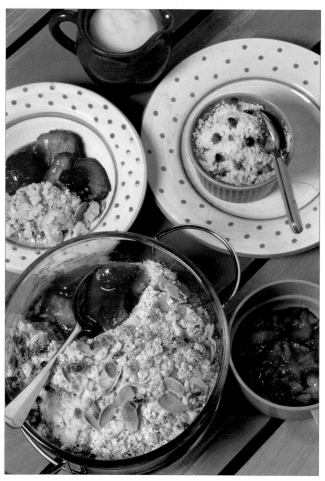

4 Spoon the remaining plums into a 750ml/1¼ pint/3⅔ cup ovenproof dish for the adults.

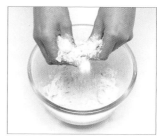

5 Make the topping. Place the flour in a bowl, rub in the butter and then stir in the sugar.

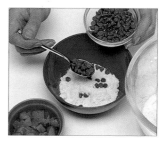

6 Mix 45ml/3 tbsp of the crumble mixture with the chocolate dots, then spoon over the ramekin.

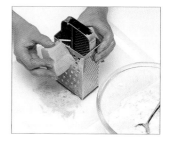

7 Coarsely grate the marzipan and stir into the remaining crumble with the oats and almonds. Spoon over the adults' portion.

8 Place the toddler and adult portions on a baking sheet and cook for 20–25 minutes, until golden. Cool slightly before serving. Warm the baby's portion if liked. Check the temperature of the children's food before serving. Serve with custard.

HONEY AND SUMMER FRUIT MOUSSE

10ml/2 tsp powdered gelatine
500g/1¼lb bag frozen summer
    fruits, defrosted
20ml/4 tsp caster (superfine)
    sugar
500g/1¼lb tub fromage frais or
    Greek (US strained plain) yogurt
150ml/¼ pint/⅔ cup whipping
    cream
25ml/1½ tbsp clear honey

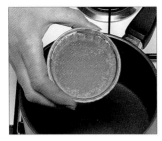

1 Put 30ml/2 tbsp cold water in a cup and sprinkle the gelatine over, making sure that all grains of gelatine have been absorbed. Soak for 5 minutes, then heat in a pan of simmering water until the gelatine dissolves and the liquid is clear. Cool slightly.

2 For the baby, process or liquidize 50g/2oz of fruit to a purée and stir in 5ml/1 tsp sugar. Mix 45ml/3 tbsp fromage frais or yogurt with 5ml/1 tsp sugar in a separate bowl.

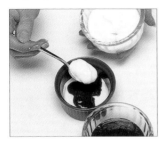

3 Put alternate spoonfuls of fromage frais or yogurt and purée into a small dish for the baby. Swirl the mixtures together with a teaspoon. Chill until required.

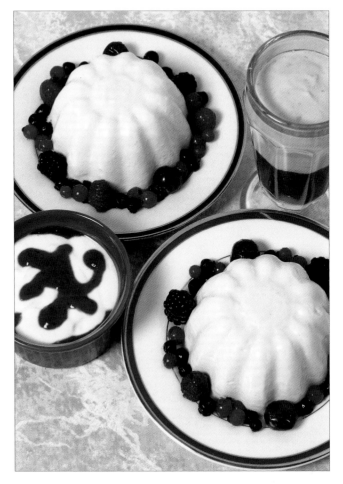

4 For the toddler, process 50g/2oz fruit with 5ml/1 tsp sugar. Mix 60ml/4 tbsp fromage frais or yogurt with 5ml/1 tsp sugar, then stir in 10ml/2 tsp fruit purée.

5 Stir 5ml/1 tsp gelatine into the fruit purée and 5ml/1 tsp into the fromage frais or yogurt mixture. Spoon the fruit into the base of a and chill until set.

6 For the adults, whip the cream until softly peaking. Fold in the remaining fromage frais or yogurt and honey and add the remaining gelatine. Pour into two 250ml/8fl oz/1 cup moulds. Chill until set.

7 Spoon the remaining fromage frais or yogurt mixture over the set fruit layer in the serving glass for the toddler and chill until set.

8 To serve, dip one of the dishes for the adults in hot water, count to 15, then loosen the edges with your fingertips, invert on to a large plate and, holding mould and plate together, jerk to release the mousse and remove the mould. Repeat with the other mould.

9 Spoon the remaining fruits and some of the juice around the desserts and serve.

Useful contacts

UK

Allergy UK
Allergy UK
Planwell House
LEFA Business Park
Edgington Way
Sidcup, Kent
DA14 5BH
tel: 01322 619898
www.allergyuk.org

Association of Breastfeeding Mothers
PO Box 207
Bridgewater TA6 7YT
0870 401 7711
tel: 0300 330 5453

Association of Reflexologists
5 Fore Street
Taunton, Somerset
TA1 1HX
tel: 01823 351010
www.aor.org.uk

Asthma UK
18 Mansell Street
London
E1 8AA
tel: 020 7786 4900
www.asthma.org.uk

Bach Centre
Mount Vernon
Baker's Lane
Brightwell-cum-Sotwell
Oxon OX10 0PZ
tel: 01491 834678
www.bachcentre.com

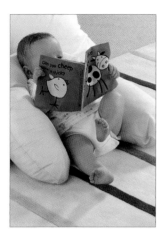

Bliss
2nd Floor, Chapter House
18-20 Crucifix Lane
London SE1 3JW
tel: 020 7378 1122
www.bliss.org.uk
support for parents of premature babies

Breastfeeding Network
tel: 0300 100 0212
www.breastfeedingnetwork.org.uk
Information on breastfeeding

The British Acupuncture Council
63 Jeddo Road
London W12 9HQ
tel: 020 8735 0400
www.acupuncture.org.uk

The British Homeopathic Association
Hahnemann House
29 Park Street West
Luton LU1 3BE
tel: 01582 408675
www.britishhomeopathy.org

The British Hypnotherapy Association
30 Cotsford Avenue
New Maldon, Surrey, KT3 5EU
tel: 020 8942 3988
www.hypnotherapy-association.org

The British Register of Complementary Practitioners (BRCP)
ICNM, Can Mezzanine
32-36 Loman Street
London SE1 0EH
tel: 020 7922 7980
www.icnm.org.uk

Child Accident Prevention Trust
Canterbury Court
1-3 Brixton Riad
London SW9 6DE
tel: 020 7608 3828
www.capt.org.uk

Cry-sis
BM Cry-sis
London WC1N 3XX
tel: 08451 228 669
www.cry-sis.org.uk
Helpline for parents with crying babies and toddlers

Eneuresis Resource and Information Centre (ERIC)
tel: 0117 960 3060
www.eric.org.uk
Advice on bedwetting and soiling

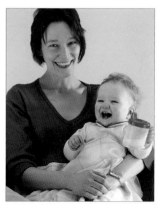

Foresight
The Association for the Promotion of Preconceptual Care
3 Lower Queens Road
Clevedon, BS21 6LX
tel: 01275 878953
www.foresight-preconception.org.uk

General Chiropractic Council
44 Wicklow Street
London WC1X 9HL
tel: 020 7713 5155
www.gcc-uk.org

The General Osteopathic Council
Osteopathy House
176 Tower Bridge Road
London SE1 3LU
tel: 020 7357 6655
www.osteopathy.org.uk

Gingerbread
520 Highgate Studios
53-79 Highgate Road
London NW5 1TL
tel: 0808 802 0925
www.gingerbread.org.uk
Local support groups for single-parent families

The Human Fertilisation and Embryology Authority
103-105 Bunhill Road
London EC1Y 8HF
tel: 020 7291 8200
www.hfea.gov.uk/ForPatients

Infertility Network UK
Charter House
43 St Leonard's Road
Bexhill-on-Sea, TN40 1JA
tel: 0800 008 7464
www.infertilitynetworkuk.com

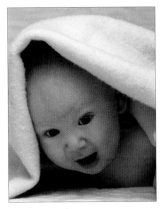

The International Federation of Aromatherapists
20A The Mall
London W5 2PJ
tel: 020 8567 2243
www.ifaroma.org

Iyengar Yoga Institute
223a Randolph Avenue
London W9 1NL
tel: 020 7624 3080
www.iyi.org.uk

JABS
1 Gawsworth Road
Golborne
Warrington WA3 3RF
tel: 01942 713565
www.jabs.org.uk
Alternative advice on vaccination

La Leche League
129a Middleton Boulevard
Wollaton Park
Nottingham NBG8 1FW
tel 0845 120 2918
www.laleche.org.uk
Breastfeeding support

Miscarriage Association
17 Wentworth Terrace
Wakefield WF1 3QW
tel: 01924 200799
www.miscarriageassociation.org.uk

The Multiple Births Foundation
Queen Charlotte's & Chelsea Hospital
Du Cane Road
London W12 0HS
tel: 020 3313 3519
www.multiplebirths.org.uk

National Childbirth Trust
Alexandra House
Oldham Terrace
Acton, London W3 6NH
tel: 0300 330 0700
www.nct.org.uk
Breastfeeding and postnatal problems

National Childminding Association
www.childcare.co.uk
Advice on finding a registered
childminder

National Eczema Society
Hill House
Highgate Hill
London N19 5NA
tel: 0800 089 1122
www.eczema.org

The National Institute of Medical Herbalists
Clover House
James Court, South Street
Exeter EX1 1EE
tel: 01392 426022
www.nimh.org.uk

Relate
tel: 0845 1304010
www.relate.org.uk
Relationship counselling

Royal College of Obstetricians and Gynaecologists
27 Sussex Place
London NW1 4RG
tel: 020 7772 6200
www.rcog.org.uk

St John Ambulance
27 St Johns Lane
London EC1M 4BU
08700 10 49 50
www.sja.org.uk
Information on first aid courses,
including baby and child resuscitation

The School of Meditation
158 Holland Park Avenue
London W11 4UH
tel: 020 7603 6116
www.schoolofmeditation.org

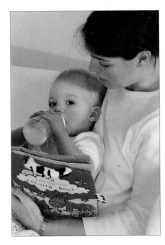

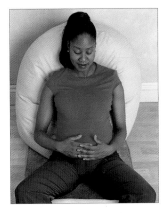

Single Parents Action Network
The Silai Centre
176-178 Easton Road
Bristol BS5 0ES
tel: 0117 9514231
www.spanuk.org.uk

The Society of Teachers of the Alexander Technique
Grove Business Centre, Unit W48
560-568 High Road
London N17 9TA
tel: 020 8885 6524
www.stat.org.uk
Help with posture and back pain

Twins and Multiple Birth Association (TAMBA)
Manor House, Church Hill
Aldershot GU12 4JU
tel 01252 332344
www.tamba.org.uk

Women's Environmental Network
20 Club Row
London E2 7EY
tel: 020 7481 9004
www.wen.org.uk
For information on using environmentally
friendly real nappies

USA

American Association of Oriental Medicine
PO Box 96503 #44114
Washington, DC 200900-6503
tel: 866 455 7999
www.aaaomonline.org

American Chiropractic Association
1701 Clarendon Boulevard
Arlington VA 22209
tel: 703 276 8800
www.acatoday.org

The American College of
Obstetricians and Gynecologists
409 12th Street NW
Washington DC 200024-2188
tel: 202 638 5577
www.acog.org

American Herbalists Guild
125 South Lexington Avenue
Suite 101
Asheville, NC28801
tel: 617 520 4375
www.americanherbalistsguild.com

American Holistic Medical
Association
5313 Colorado Street
Duluth, NMN 55804
tel: 218 525 5651
www.aihm.org

American Institute of
Hypnotherapy
1805 E Garry Avenue
Suite 100, Santa Ana CA 92705
tel: 714 261 6400
www.aih.cc

American Massage Therapy
Association
500 Davis Street, Suite 900
Evanston, IL 60201-4695
tel: 847 864 0123
www.amtamassage.org

American Osteopathic
Association
142 East Ontario Street
Chicago IL 60611
tel: 312 202 8000
www.osteopathic.org

American Red Cross
2025 E Street, NW
Washington DC 20006
tel: 202 303 4498
www.redcross.org

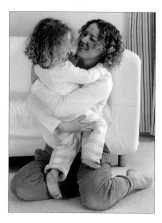

Food Allergy Initiative
7925 Jones Branch Drive
Suite 1100
McLean, VA22102
tel: 703 691 3179
www.foodallergy.org

International Association of
Yoga Therapists
PO Box 426
Manton CA 96059
tel: 530 474 5700
www.iayt.org

International Institute of Reflexology
PO Box 12642
St Petersburg FL 33733
tel: 813 343 4811
www.reflexology-usa.net

La Leche League
PO Box 4079, Schaumburg
Ilinois 60168-4079
tel: 1 877 452 5324
www.lllusa.org
Promotes breastfeeding

National Association of
Childbearing Centers
3123 Gottschall Road
Perkiomenville PA 18074
tel: 215 234 8068
www.birthcenters.org

National Center for Homeopathy
7918 Jones Branch Drive
Suite 33
McLean VA 22102
tel: 703 506 7667
www.nationalcenterforhomeopathy.org

National Organization of Mothers
of Twins
PO Box 700860
Plymouth
Michigan 48170-0955
www.nomotc.org

Safe Kids Worldwide
1301 Pennsylvania Avenue NW
Suite 1000
Washington DC 20004
tel: 202 662 0600
www.safekids.org
Advice on keeping children safe in the
home and outside

National Women's Health Network
1413 K Street NW, 4th Floor
Washington DC 20005
tel: 202 682 2640
www.nwhn.org

Resolve (fertility problems)
The National Infertility Association
7918 Jones Branch Road, Suite 300
McLean VA 22102
tel: 703 556 7172
www.resolve.org

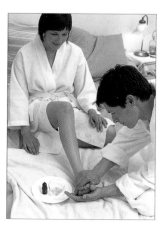

CANADA

Canadian Examining Board of
Health Care Practitioners Inc
658 Danforth Avenue
Suite 204, Toronto
Ontario M4J 5B9
tel: 416 466 9755
www.canadianexaminingboard.com

Canadian Women's Health
Network
Suite 203, 419 Graham Avenue
Winnipeg, Manitoba R3C 0M3
tel: 204 942 5500
www.cwhn.ca

Anaphylaxis Canada
2005 Sheppard Avenue East
Suite 800
Toronto, Ontario M2J 5BA
tel: 866 785 5660
www.anaphylaxis.org

Infertility Network
160 Pickering Street
Toronto, Ontario M4E 3J7
tel: 416 691 3611
www.infertilitynetwork.org

La Leche League Canada
12050 Main Street W
PO Box 700, Winchester
Ontario K0C 2K0
tel: 613 774 4900
www.lllc.ca

Multiple Births Canada
tel: 612 834 8946
www.multiplebirthscanada.org

Safe Kids Canada
2110 Kipling Avenue, North
PO Box 551
Etobicoke Ontario M9W 4KO
tel: 888 499 4444
www.safekidscanada.com

St John Ambulance Canada
1900 City Park Drive, Suite 400
Ottawa, Ontario K1J 1A3
tel: 613 236 7461
www.sja.ca

AUSTRALIA

Allergy & Anaphylaxis Australia
Suite 204, Level 2
16 Hunter Street Mall
Hornsby NSW 2077
tel: 1300 728 000
www.allergyfacts.org.au

Austprem
www.austprem.org.au
Internet-based support for parents of
preterm babies

Australian Breastfeeding Association
1818 Malvern Road
East Malvern
Victoria 3145
tel: 03 9885 0855
www.breastfeeding.asn.au
Telephone numbers of breastfeeding
counsellors are posted on the website.

Complementary Medicine Association
Suite 14b
5 Michigan Drive
Oxenford QLD 4210
tel: 07 5580 5990
www.cma.asn.au

**The Australian Multiple Births
Association (AMBA)**
Po Box 105
Coogee, NSW 2034
tel: 1300 886 499
www.amba.org.au

Australian Women's Health Network
PO Box 188
Drysdale Vic 3222
www.awhn.org.au

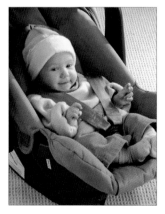

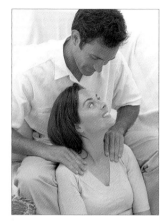

Fertility Society of Australia
119 Buckhurst Street
South Melbourne, VIC 3205
tel: 3 9645 6359
www.fertilitysociety.com.au

Kidsafe Australia
50 Bramston Terrace
Herston, QLD 4006
tel: 7 3854 1829
www.kidsafe.com.au

La Leche League
www.lalecheleague.org/australia

St John Ambulance
10-12 Campion Street
Deakin ACT 2600
tel: 1300 360 455
www.stjohn.org.au

NEW ZEALAND

Allergy New Zealand
441a Mount Eden Road
Mount Eden 1024
tel: 9 623 3912
www.allergy.org.nz

La Leche League
PO Box 50780
Porirua 5240
tel: 4 471 0690
www.lalecheleague.org.nz

St John Ambulance
PO Box 10 043, Wellington
tel: 0800 785 646
www.stjohn.org.nz
First aid courses

**The New Zealand Health
Information Network**
PO Box 337
Christchurch 8015
tel: 03 980 4646
www.nzhealth.net.nz

Fertility New Zealand
PO Box 28262
Remuera, Auckland 1541
tel: 0800 333 306
www.fertilitynz.ord.nz

**New Zealand Multiple Birth
Association**
PO Box 1258
Wellington
New Zealand
tel: 0800 489 467
www.multiples.org.nz

Early Buds
Early Buds
1/B Waiwhero Street
Mangakakahi, Rotorua 3015
tel: 027 348 8433
www.earlybuds.org.nz
Support for parents of premature and
poorly babies

Safekids Aotearoa
PO Box 26488
Epsom, Auckland 1344
tel: 9 630 9955
www.safekids.org.nz

SOUTH AFRICA

www.activebirth.co.za

African Health Anthology
www.nisc.co.za

WEBSITES
www.bygpub.com
www.babyfriendly.org.uk
www.talk-about-twins.com
www.tripletconnection.org
www.mumsnet.com
www.unicef.org
www.familylives.org.uk
www.netmums.com
www.parents.com
www.newdadssurvivalguide.com

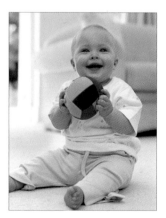

Further reading

Hilary Boyd *Working Woman's Pregnancy* (Mitchell Beazley, 2001)

Nikki Bradford *The Miraculous World of Your Unborn Baby* (Salamander, London, 1998 and by Contemporary Books, USA, 1998)

Miranda Castro *Homeopathy for Pregnancy, Birth and Your Baby's First Year* (St Martin's Press, New York, 1992)

Penelope Leach, *Your Baby and Child* (Penguin, 1977)

Jan Parker and Jan Stimpson, *Raising Happy Children* (Hodder and Stoughton, 1999)

William Sears, Martha Sears, *The Baby Book* (Little, Brown and Company, 2003)

Dr Benjamen Spock and Dr Robert Needham, *Dr Spock's Baby and Child Care* (Simon and Schuster, 2005)

BREASTFEEDING

La Leche League, *The Womanly Art of Breastfeeding* (Plume Books, 2004)

Norma Jane Bumgarner, *Mothering Your Nursing Toddler* (La Leche League, 1980)

Clare Byam-Cook, *What to Expect if You Are Breastfeeding and What If You Can't* (Vermillion, 2001)

P Stanway, *Breast is Best* (Pan, 2005)

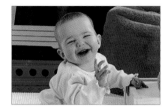

FEEDING YOUR BABY AND TODDLER

Rachael Anne Hill, *Real Food for Kids* (Ryland, Peters and Small, 2005)

Annabel Karmel, *Feeding your Baby and Toddler* (Dorling Kindersley, 1999)

Sara Lewis, *Veggie Food for Kids* (Hamlyn, 2003)

SLEEP, CRYING AND BEHAVIOUR

Jo Frost, *Supernanny: How to Get the Best from Your Children* (Hodder and Stoughton, 2005)

Penny Hames, *Help Your Baby to Sleep* (Harper Collins, 2002)

Penny Hames, *Toddler Tantrums* (Harper Collins, 2002)

Deborah Jackson, *When Your Baby Cries* (Hodder and Stoughton, 2004)

Elizabeth Pantley *The No-Cry Sleep Solution* (McGraw Hill, 2002)

DEVELOPMENT AND ACTIVITIES

Lynne Murray and Liz Andrews, *The Social Baby: Understanding Babies' Communication from Birth* (CP Publishing, 2005)

Françoise Barbira Freedman, *Water Babies* (Lorenz Books, 2001)

Peter Walker, *Baby Massage* (Carroll and Brown, 2005)

Stella Wellar, *Yoga for Children* (Harper Collins, 1996)

HEALTH CARE

Dr John Briffa, *Natural Health for Kids* (Michael Joseph, 2004)

Susan Clark, *What Really Works for Kids: The Insider Guide for Mums and Dads* (Bantam Press, 2002)

Françoise Barbira Freedman, *Postnatal Yoga* (Lorenz Books, 2000)

Joseph Garcia-Prats and Sharon Simmons Hornfischer, *What To Do When Your Baby Is Premature* (Three Rivers Press, 2000)

BEING A PARENT

Kate Figes, *Life After Birth: What Even Your Friends Won't Tell You About Motherhood* (Viking, 1998)

Sean French, *Fatherhood: Men Writing About Fatherhood* (Virago, 1992)

Acknowledgements

Thanks to the following agencies for supplying additional images (all those not listed below are © Anness Publishing Ltd): t=top; b=bottom; c=centre; l=left; r=right

Photographs in the book were taken by Scott Morrison, and are the property of Anness Publishing Ltd. Photographs also taken by: Jo Harrison: 273tl, 287tm, 288b, 291t, 315b, 333t, 335t, 338b, 341tr, 341tl, 355b, 382b, 385b. Christine Hanscombe: 350bl, 350br, 351 both. John Freeman: 414–15 all. Alamy: 236rm, 258t & bl, 261tr, 272t, 281tl, 284t, 285t (both), 288t, 289tr, 304b, 324t, 331 both, 334t, 336, 337 both, 340 both, 242, 347tr, 364b, 369b, 371tl, 372b, 373br, 374, 375tl, 381b, 383b, 386, 387 both, 397tr, 403tr, 408b, 413tr & b, 417tr, 431tr, 437tr, 439tl, 442tl, 446b, 456t. *Science Photo Library:* p47tl /BSIP, Chassenet; p62 /BSIP, HARDAS; p69bl & br /James King-Holmes; p72br /Alexander Tsiaras; p73tl /James King-Holmes; p87tr P. Saada/Eurelios; p106b /Ruth Jenkinson/MIDIRS; p119tl /Neil Bromhall; p137tr /Faye Norman; p142b /Hank Morgan; p153t /GE Medical Systems; p169bl /Ian Hooton; p170b /Ruth Jenkinson/MIDIRS; p181tl /Mark Clarke; p183t /Petit Format; p195tr /Ruth Jenkinson/MIDIRS; p200 /Tracy Dominey; p201br /Hank Morgan; p202tr /Mark de Fraeye; p210 /Simon Fraser; p216br /Mark Thomas; p269bl. *Corbis:* p45bl /Larry Williams; p49 /Norbert Schaefer; p51cr /Royalty-free; p55tr /Royalty-free; p71t Corbis only; p109t /Tom and Dee Ann McCarthy; p115tr /Angela Wood; p115br /Larry Williams and Associates; p151tr /Larry Williams; p179br /Douglas Kirkland; p186b /Mug Shots; p199br /Larry Williams; pp208, 235tr, 245tr, 263tr, 287br, 314bl, 407t, 418, 419 both.

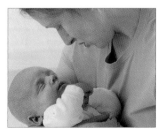

Index

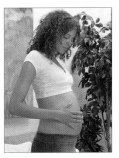
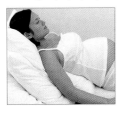

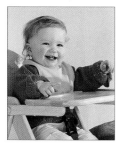

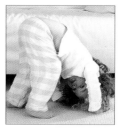

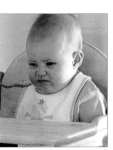

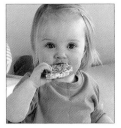

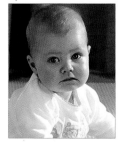
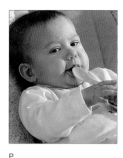

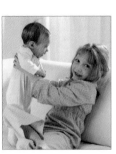

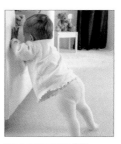

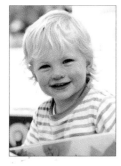

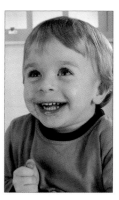